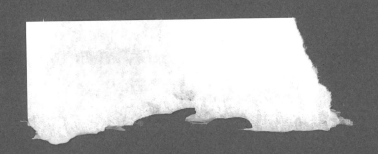

The Founders of Operative Surgery

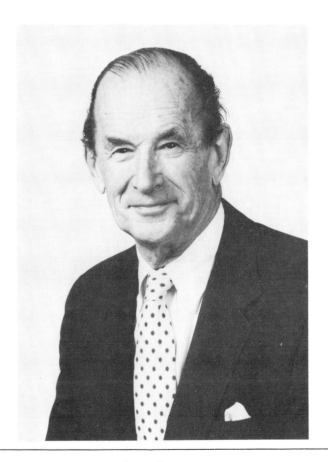

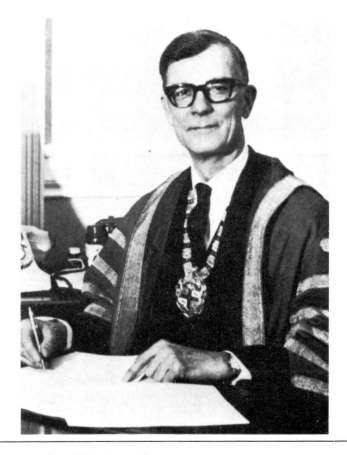

Charles Granville Rob MC, MChir, FRCS, FACS
Professor of Surgery, Uniformed Services University of the
Health Sciences, E Edward Hébert School of Medicine,
Bethesda, Maryland
Quondam: Professor of Surgery, St Mary's Hospital Medical
School, London 1950–1960
Professor and Chairman, Department of Surgery, University of
Rochester, New York, 1960–1978
Professor of Surgery, East Carolina University, 1978–1983

Lord Smith of Marlow KBE, MS, FRCS, Hon DSc
(Exeter and Leeds), Hon MD (Zurich), Hon FRACS,
Hon FRCS(Ed), Hon FRCS (Glas), Hon FACS, Hon FRCS(Can),
Hon FRCSI, Hon FRCS(SA), Hon FDS, Past President, RSM
Honorary Consulting Surgeon, St George's Hospital, London
Quondam: Surgeon, St George's Hospital, London,
1946–1978
President of the Royal College of Surgeons of England,
1973–1977

Rob & Smith's

Operative Surgery

Orthopaedics   Part 2

Fourth Edition

Rob & Smith's
Operative Surgery

General Editors

Hugh Dudley ChM, FRCS(Ed), FRACS, FRCS
Emeritus Professor, St Mary's Hospital, London, UK

David C. Carter MD, FRCS(Ed), FRCS(Glas)
Regius Professor of Clinical Surgery, Royal Infirmary, Edinburgh, UK

R. C. G. Russell MS, FRCS
Consultant Surgeon, Middlesex Hospital, St John's Hospital for Diseases of the Skin; Royal National Nose, Throat and Ear Hospital, London, UK

Rob & Smith's
Operative Surgery

Orthopaedics   Part 2

Fourth Edition

Edited by

George Bentley ChM, FRCS
Professor of Orthopaedic Surgery, The Institute of Orthopaedics, University of London; Honorary Consultant Orthopaedic Surgeon, The Royal National Orthopaedic Hospital, Stanmore, Middlesex and the Middlesex Hospital, London, UK

Robert B. Greer III MD, FACS
Professor and Chairman of Orthopaedic Surgery, Pennsylvania State University College of Medicine, Hershey, Pennsylvania 17033, USA

Butterworth–Heinemann
London   Boston   Sydney   Wellington   Singapore

Butterworth–Heinemann Ltd
PO Box 63, Westbury House, Bury Street, Guildford, Surrey GU2 5BH, UK

 PART OF REED INTERNATIONAL BOOKS

OXFORD   LONDON   GUILDFORD   BOSTON
MUNICH   NEW DELHI   SINGAPORE   SYDNEY
TOKYO   TORONTO   WELLINGTON

First published 1991

British Library Cataloguing in Publication Data

Rob & Smith's operative surgery. – 4th ed: Orthopaedics
    1. Medicine. Surgery. Operations
    I. Bentley, George   II. Greer, Robert B. III.
    III. Rob, Charles *1913-*
    IV. Smith, Rodney Smith *Baron 1914-*
    Operative Surgery
    617.91

    ISBN 0-7506-1029-8 (Set)
    ISBN 0-7506-1480-3 (Part 1)
    ISBN 0-7506-1490-0 (Part 2)

Library of Congress Cataloging-in-Publication Data

(Revised for vol. 13)

Rob & Smith's operative surgery.

    Rev. ed. of: Operative surgery. 3rd ed. 1976–
    Includes bibliographies and index.
    Contents: [1] Alimentary tract and abdominal wall.
1. General principles, oesophagus, stomach, duodenum,
small intestine, abdominal wall, hernia/edited by
Hugh Dudley — [13] Orthopaedics/[edited by] George
Bentley, Robert B. Greer III.
    1. Surgery, Operative. I. Rob, Charles.
II. Dudley, Hugh A. F. (Hugh Arnold Freeman).
III. Pories, Walter J. IV. Carter, David C. (David
Craig). V. Operative surgery. [DNLM: 1. Surgery,
Operative. I. Smith of Marlow, Rodney Smith, Baron,
1914--   . WO 500 061 1982]
RD32.06   1983   617'.91   83-14465
ISBN 0-7506-1029-8 (Set)
        0-7506-1480-3 (Part 1)
        0-7506-1490-0 (Part 2)

Composition by Genesis Typesetting, Laser Quay, Rochester, Kent
Printed and bound by Hartnoll Ltd, Bodmin, Cornwall

Volumes and Editors

Alimentary Tract and Abdominal Wall

1 General Principles · Oesophagus · Stomach · Duodenum · Small Intestine · Abdominal Wall · Hernia

Hugh Dudley ChM, FRCS(Ed), FRACS, FRCS
Emeritus Professor, St Mary's Hospital, London, UK

2 Liver · Portal Hypertension · Spleen · Biliary Tract · Pancreas

Hugh Dudley ChM, FRCS(Ed), FRACS, FRCS
Emeritus Professor, St Mary's Hospital, London, UK

3 Colon, Rectum and Anus

Ian P. Todd MS, MD(Tor), FRCS, DCH
Consulting Surgeon, St Bartholomew's Hospital, London;
Consultant Surgeon, St Mark's Hospital and
King Edward VII Hospital for Officers, London, UK

L. P. Fielding FRCS
Chief of Surgery, St Mary's Hospital, Waterbury, Connecticut, USA;
Associate Professor of Surgery, Yale University, Connecticut, USA

Cardiac Surgery

Stuart W. Jamieson FRCS, FACS
Professor and Head, Cardiothoracic Surgery,
University of Minnesota, Minneapolis, Minnesota, USA

Norman E. Shumway MD, PhD, FRCS
Professor and Chairman, Department of Cardiovascular Surgery,
Stanford University School of Medicine, California, USA

The Ear

John C. Ballantyne FRCS, HonFRCSI, DLO
Consultant Ear, Nose and Throat Surgeon,
Royal Free and King Edward VII Hospital for Officers, London, UK;
Honorary Consultant in Otolaryngology to the Army

Andrew Morrison FRCS, DLO
Senior Consultant Otolaryngologist, The London Hospital, UK

General Principles, Breast and Extracranial Endocrines

Hugh Dudley ChM, FRCS(Ed), FRACS, FRCS
Emeritus Professor, St Mary's Hospital, London, UK

Walter J. Pories MD, FACS
Professor and Chairman, Department of Surgery, School of Medicine,
East Carolina University, Greenville, North Carolina, USA

Gynaecology and Obstetrics

J. M. Monaghan FRCS(Ed), FRCOG
Consultant Gynaecological Surgeon, Head of the Regional
Department of Gynaecological Oncology, Queen Elizabeth Hospital,
Gateshead, Tyne and Wear, UK

The Hand

Rolfe Birch FRCS
Consultant Orthopaedic Surgeon, PNI Unit and Hand Clinic,
Royal National Orthopaedic Hospital, Stanmore, Middlesex, and
St Mary's Hospital, London, UK

Donal Brooks MA, FRCS, FRSCI
Consulting Orthopaedic Surgeon, University College Hospital,
London and Royal National Orthopaedic Hospital, Stanmore,
Middlesex, UK; Civilian Consultant in Hand Surgery to the Royal Navy
and Royal Air Force, UK

Neurosurgery

Lindsay Symon TD, FRCS
Professor of Neurosurgery, Gough-Cooper Department of
Neurological Surgery, Institute of Neurology, National Hospitals for
Nervous Diseases, London, UK

David G. T. Thomas MRCP, FRCSE
Senior Lecturer and Consultant Neurosurgeon,
Institute of Neurology, National Hospitals for Nervous Diseases,
London, UK

Kemp Clark MD, FACS
Professor of Neurosurgery, Division of Neurological Surgery,
Southwestern Medical School, Dallas, Texas, USA

Nose and Throat

John C. Ballantyne FRCS, HonFRCSI, DLO
Consultant Ear, Nose and Throat Surgeon,
Royal Free and King Edward VII Hospital for Officers, London, UK;
Honorary Consultant in Otolaryngology to the Army

D. F. N. Harrison MD, MS, FRCS, FRACS
Professor of Laryngology and Otology,
Royal National Throat, Nose and Ear Hospital, London, UK

Ophthalmic Surgery

Thomas A. Rice MD
Assistant Clinical Professor of Ophthalmology,
Case Western Reserve University School of Medicine,
Cleveland, Ohio, USA; formerly of the Wilmer Ophthalmological
Institute, The Johns Hopkins School of Medicine, Maryland, USA

Ronald G. Michels MD
Professor of Ophthalmology, The Wilmer Ophthalmological Institute,
The Johns Hopkins University School of Medicine,
Maryland, USA

Walter W. J. Stark MD
Professor of Ophthalmology, The Wilmer Ophthalmological Institute,
The Johns Hopkins University School of Medicine,
Maryland, USA

Orthopaedics

George Bentley ChM, FRCS
Professor of Orthopaedic Surgery, The Institute of Orthopaedics,
University of London; Honorary Consultant Orhtopaedic Surgeon,
The Royal National Orthopaedic Hospital, Stanmore, Middlesex, and
The Middlesex Hospital, London, UK

Robert B. Greer III MD, FACS
Professor and Chairman of Orthopaedic Surgery, Pennsylvania State
University College of Medicine, Hershey, Pennsylvania, USA

Paediatric Surgery

L. Spitz PhD, FRCS(Ed), FRCS(Eng), FAAP(Hon)
Nuffield Professor of Paediatric Surgery, Institute of Child Health,
University of London; Consultant Paediatric Surgeon, London, UK

H. Homewood Nixon MA, FRCS(Eng), FRCSI(Hon), FACS(Hon), FAAP(Hon)
Consultant Paediatric Surgeon, The Hospital for Sick Children,
Great Ormond Street, London and St Mary's Hospital, Paddington,
London, UK

Plastic Surgery

T. L. Barclay ChM, FRCS
Consultant Plastic Surgeon, St Luke's Hospital,
Bradford, West Yorkshire, UK

Desmond A. Kernahan MD
Chief, Division of Plastic Surgery,
The Children's Memorial Hospital, Chicago, Illinois, USA

Thoracic Surgery

The late J. W. Jackson MCh, FRCS
Formerly Consultant Thoracic Surgeon, Harefield Hospital,
Middlesex, UK

D. K. C. Cooper MD, PhD, FRCS
Department of Cardiac Surgery, University of Cape Town
Medical School, Cape Town, South Africa

Trauma Surgery

Howard R. Champion FRCS(Ed), FACS
Chief, Trauma Service; Director, Surgery Critical Care Services, The
Washington Hospital Center, Washington DC; Professor of Surgery,
Chief of Division of Surgery for Trauma, Department of Surgery,
Uniformed Services University of the Health Sciences, Bethesda,
Maryland, USA

John V. Robbs ChM, FRCS(Ed)
Professor of Surgery; Head, Metropolitan Vascular Services;
Head, Division of Surgery, University of Natal, Durban, Natal, South
Africa

Donald D. Trunkey MD, FACS
Chairman, Department of Surgery, University of Portland, Portland,
Oregon, USA

Urology

W. Scott McDougal MD
Professor and Chairman, Department of Urology,
Vanderbilt University Medical Center, Nashville, Tennessee, USA

Vascular Surgery

James A. DeWeese MD
Professor and Chairman, Division of Cardiothoracic Surgery,
University of Rochester Medical Center, Rochester, New York, USA

Head and Neck

Ian McGregor ChM, FRCS
Formerly Director, Plastic and Oral Surgery Unit, Canniesburn
Hospital, Glasgow, UK

David J. Howard FRCS, FRCS(Ed)
Deputy Director, Professorial Unit, Institute of Laryngology and
Otology, London and the Royal National Throat, Nose and Ear
Hospital, London, UK

Contributors

C. E. Ackroyd MA, FRCS
Consultant Orthopaedic Surgeon, Southmead Hospital, Bristol, UK

J. Crawford Adams MD, MS, FRCS
Consulting Orthopaedic Surgeon, St Mary's Hospital, London, UK

Paul Aichroth MS, FRCS
Consultant Orthopaedic Surgeon, Westminster Hospital and
Westminster Children's Hospital, London and Queen Mary's Hospital,
Roehampton, UK

Peter C. Amadio MD
Assistant Professor of Clinical Orthopaedics, SUNY, Stony Brook, and
Active Staff, St. John's Episcopal Hospital, Smithtown, New York, USA

J. C. Angel FRCS
Consultant Orthopaedic Surgeon, Royal National Orthopaedic and
Edgware General Hospitals, Middlesex, UK

G. C. Bannister MChOrth, FRCS
Consultant Senior Lecturer, Southmead Hospital, Bristol, UK

N. J. Barton FRCS
Consultant Hand Surgeon, Nottingham University Hospital and
Harlow Wood Orthopaedic Hospital, Mansfield, Nottinghamshire,
UK

E. H. Bates FRCS, FRACS
Chairman, Section of Orthopaedics, Prince of Wales Children's
Hospital, Sydney, Australia

J. I. L. Bayley FRCS
Consultant Orthopaedic Surgeon, Royal National Orthopaedic
Hospital, Stanmore, Middlesex, UK

Sir George Bedbrook OBE, OStJ, MS(Melb), HonMD(WA),
HonFRCS(Ed), HonDTech(Wait), FRCS, FRACS, DPRM(Syd),
FCRM(Hon)
Emeritus Consultant Orthopaedic Surgeon and Spinal Surgeon, Royal
Perth Hospital and Spinal Unit, Royal Perth Rehabilitation Hospital,
Western Australia

George Bentley ChM, FRCS
Professor of Orthopaedic Surgery, The Institute of Orthopaedics,
University of London; Honorary Consultant Orthopaedic Surgeon, The
Royal National Orthopaedic Hospital, Stanmore, Middlesex, and the
Middlesex Hospital, London, UK

Rolfe Birch MChir, FRCS
Consultant Orthopaedic Surgeon, St. Mary's Hospital, London and
The Royal National Orthopaedic Hospital, Stanmore, Middlesex, UK

M. D. Brough MA, FRCS
Consultant Plastic Surgeon, University College Hospital, Royal Free
Hospital, Whittington Hospital and Royal Northern Hospital, London,
UK

Paul T. Calvert MA, FRCS
Consultant Orthopaedic Surgeon, St George's Hospital, Blackshaw
Road, London, UK

A. Catterall MChir, FRCS
Consultant Orthopaedic Surgeon, Charing Cross Hospital, London,
and Royal National Orthopaedic Hospital, Stanmore, Middlesex, UK

The late Sir John Charnley CBE, FRS, FRCS, FACS
Formerly Emeritus Professor of Orthopaedic Surgery, University of
Manchester; Honorary Orthopaedic Surgeon, Centre for Hip Surgery,
Wrightington Hospital, Wigan; Consultant Orthopaedic Surgeon, King
Edward VII Hospital, Midhurst, Sussex, UK

S. C. Chen FRCS
Consultant Orthopaedic Surgeon, Enfield Group of Hospitals,
Middlesex, UK

Neil Citron MChir, FRCS
Consultant Orthopaedic Surgeon, St Helier's Hospital, Carshalton,
Surrey, UK

C. L. Colton FRCS, FRCS(Ed)
Consultant Orthopaedic Surgeon, University Hospital, Queen's
Medical Centre, Nottingham, UK

H. V. Crock AO, MD, MS, FRCS, FRACS
Honorary Consultant, Royal Postgraduate Medical School,
Hammersmith Hospital, London, UK

H. Alan Crockard FRCS, FRCS(Ed)
Consultant Neurosurgeon, The National Hospitals for Nervous
Diseases, Maida Vale, London, UK

James E. Culver MD
Head, Section of Hand Surgery, Department of Orthopaedic Surgery,
Cleveland Clinic Foundation, Cleveland, Ohio, USA

J. C. Dorgan MCh Orth, FRCS
Consultant Orthopaedic Surgeon, Royal Liverpool Childrens Hospital
and Royal Liverpool Hospital, Liverpool, UK

G. S. E. Dowd MD, MChOrth, FRCS
Consultant Orthopaedic Surgeon, St Bartholomew's and Homerton
Hospitals, London, UK

R. B. Duthie CBE, MA, ChM, FRCS
Nuffield Professor of Orthopaedic Surgery, Nuffield Department of
Orthopaedic Surgery, University of Oxford, UK

Michael Edgar MChir, FRCS
Consultant Orthopaedic Surgeon, The Middlesex Hospital, London,
and The Royal National Orthopaedic Hospital, Stanmore, Middlesex,
UK

Philip M. Faris MD
Clinical Associate Professor, Department of Orthopaedic Surgery, Louisiana State University Medical Center, USA

Malcolm W. Fidler MS, FRCS
Consultant Orthopaedic Surgeon, Onze Lieve Vrouwe Gasthuis and Netherlands Cancer Institute, Amsterdam, The Netherlands

J. A. Fixsen MChir, FRCS
Consultant Orthopaedic Surgeon, The Hospital for Sick Children, Great Ormond Street and St Bartholomew's Hospital, London, UK

Anthony J. B. Fogg FRCS
Consultant Orthopaedic Surgeon, Princess Margaret Hospital, Swindon, UK

Mark C. Gebhardt MD
Assistant Professor of Orthopaedic Surgery, Harvard Medical School, Massachusetts General Hospital and the Children's Hospital, Boston, Massachusetts, USA

William N. Gilmour FRCS, FRACS
Emeritus Consultant Surgeon, Royal Perth Hospital and Princess Margaret Hospital for Children, Perth, Australia

M. J. Griffith MChOrth, FRCS, FRCS(Ed)
Consultant Orthopaedic Surgeon, West Wales General Hospital, Carmarthen, UK

David L. Hamblen PhD, FRCS
Professor of Orthopaedic Surgery, Western Infirmary, Glasgow, UK

Philip H. Hardcastle FRCS(Ed), FRACS
Consultant Surgeon, Spinal Unit, Royal Perth Rehabilitation Hospital, Perth, Western Australia

Kevin Hardinge MChOrth, FRCS
Hunterian Professor, Royal College of Surgeons of England; Honorary Lecturer, Victoria University of Manchester; Consultant Orthopaedic Surgeon, Centre for Hip Surgery, Wrightington Hospital, Wigan, UK

Michael H. Heckman MD
Consultant Surgeon, South Texas Sports Medicine and Orthopaedics, Corpus Christi, Texas; and Department of Orthopaedic Surgery, University of Texas Health Science Center, San Antonio, Texas, USA

B. Helal MChOrth, FRCS
Honorary Consultant Orthopaedic Surgeon, The Royal London Hospital and the Royal National Orthopaedic Hospital, London, and Enfield Group of Hospitals, Middlesex, UK

Adrian N. Henry MCh, FRCS, FRCSI
Formerly Senior Consultant Orthopaedic Surgeon, Guy's Hospital, London, UK

Sean P. F. Hughes MS, FRCS
Professor of Orthopaedic Surgery, University of Edinburgh; Clinical Research Unit, Princess Margaret Rose Orthopaedic Hospital, Edinburgh, UK

James M. Hunter MD
Clinical Professor of Orthopaedic Surgery, Thomas Jefferson University and Chief, Hand Surgery Service, Department of Orthopaedics, Thomas Jefferson Hospital, Philadelphia, Pennsylvania, USA

John N. Insall MD
Professor of Orthopaedic Surgery, Cornell University Medical College and Director, The Knee Service, The Hospital for Special Surgery, New York, USA

Andrew M. Jackson FRCS
Consultant Orthopaedic Surgeon, University College Hospital and The Hospital for Sick Children, Great Ormond Street, London, UK

J. P. Jackson FRCS
Emeritus Orthopaedic Surgeon, University Hospital, Nottingham and Harlow Wood Orthopaedic Hospital, Mansfield, Nottinghamshire, UK

Robert W. Jackson MD, MS(Tor), FRCS(C)
Chief of Staff/Surgery, Orthopaedic and Arthritic Hospital, 43 Wellesley Street East, Toronto and Professor of Surgery, University of Toronto, Toronto, Canada

Julian Jessop FRCS
Lecturer, University Department of Orthopaedic Surgery, The Institute of Orthopaedics, Royal National Orthopaedic Hospital, Stanmore, Middlesex, UK

H. B. S. Kemp MS, FRCS
Consultant Orthopaedic Surgeon, The Middlesex Hospital, London and The Royal National Orthopaedic Hospital, Stanmore, Middlesex, UK

J. Kenwright FRCS
Consultant Orthopaedic Surgeon, The Nuffield Orthopaedic Centre, Oxford, UK

Kevin King FRCS, FRACS
Director, Department of Orthopaedic Surgery, The Royal Melbourne Hospital, Victoria, Australia

E. O'Gorman Kirwan FRCS, FRCS(Ed)
Consultant Orthopaedic Surgeon, University College Hospital, and Royal National Orthopaedic Hospital, London, UK

Leslie Klenerman ChM, FRCS
Professor and Head of University Department of Orthopaedic and Accident Surgery, Royal Liverpool Hospital, Liverpool, UK

Sanford S. Kunkel MD
Orthopaedic Surgeon, Methodist Hospital, Indiana, USA

V. G. Langkamer FRCS
Orthopaedic Registrar, Southmead Hospital, Bristol, UK

R. J. Langstaff
Honorary Senior Registrar, University Hospital, Queen's Medical Centre, Nottingham, UK; Senior Specialist (Orthopaedics), Royal Air Force Medical Services

Robert D. Leffert MD
Associate Professor of Orthopaedic Surgery, Harvard Medical School; Chief of Surgical Upper Extremity Rehabilitation Unit and Department of Rehabilitation Medicine, White 10, Massachusetts General Hospital, Boston, Massachusetts 02114, USA

John C. Y. Leong FRCS, FRCS(Ed), FRACS
Professor of Orthopaedic Surgery, University of Hong Kong

I. J. Leslie MChOrth, FRCS
Department of Orthopaedic and Traumatic Surgery, Bristol Royal Infirmary, Bristol, UK

E. Letournel MD
Professor of Orthopaedic Surgery and Traumatology, Centre Medico-Chirurgical de la Porte de Choisy, Paris, France

Alan Lettin MS, FRCS
Consultant Orthopaedic Surgeon, St Bartholomew's Hospital, London and Royal National Orthopaedic Hospital, Stanmore, Middlesex, UK

P. S. London *MBE*, FRCS, MFOM, FACEM(Hon)
Formerly Surgeon, Birmingham Accident Hospital, Birmingham, UK

J. S. P. Lumley MS, FRCS, FMAA(Hon), FGA
Professor of Vascular Surgery, St Bartholomew's Hospital, London, UK

M. F. Macnicol FRCS, MCh, FRCS Ed(Orth)
Consultant Orthopaedic Surgeon, Princess Margaret Rose
Orthopaedic Hospital, Edinburgh, UK

Henry J. Mankin MD
Edith M. Ashley Professor of Orthopaedic Surgery, Harvard Medical
School; Chief, Orthopaedic Service, Massachusetts General Hospital,
Boston, Massachusetts, USA

R. A. B. Mollan MD, FRCS(Ed), FRCSI
Professor of Orthopaedic Surgery, Queen's University of Belfast, UK

T. R. Morley FRCS
Consultant Orthopaedic Surgeon, The Hospital for Sick Children,
Great Ormond Street, London, and The Royal National Orthopaedic
Hospital, Stanmore, Middlesex, UK

I. W. Nelson MA, FRCS
Clinical Lecturer, Nuffield Department of Orthopaedic Surgery,
University of Oxford, UK

J. P. O'Brien PhD, FRCS(Ed), FACS, FRACS
Consultant Surgeon in Spinal Disorders, 149 Harley Street, London,
UK

The late Sir Henry Osmond-Clarke *KCVO*, *CBE*, FRCS(I),
FRCS
Former Orthopaedic Surgeon to Her Majesty Queen Elizabeth II;
Consulting Orthopaedic Surgeon, The Royal London Hospital, London
and Robert Jones and Agnes Hunt Orthopaedic Hospital, Oswestry,
UK

H. Piggott FRCS
Consultant Orthopaedic Surgeon, United Birmingham Hospitals,
Royal Orthopaedic Hospital, Birmingham, and Warwickshire
Orthopaedic Hospital, Coleshill, Warwickshire, UK

Andrew O. Ransford FRCS
Consultant Orthopaedic Surgeon, Royal National Orthopaedic
Hospital, London, UK

Harold J. Richards FRCS
Formerly Consultant in the Surgery of Orthopaedics and Trauma,
University Hospital of Wales and Prince of Wales Orthopaedic
Hospital, Cardiff, UK

John T. Scales *OBE*, FRCS, CIMechE
Emeritus Professor of Biomedical Engineering, The Royal National
Orthopaedic Hospital, Stanmore, Middlesex, UK

Thomas P. Sculco MD
The Hospital for Special Surgery, 535 East 70th Street, New York, NY
10021, USA

Campbell Semple FRCS
Consultant Hand Surgeon, Western Infirmary, Glasgow, UK

W. J. W. Sharrard MD, ChM, FRCS
Emeritus Consultant Orthopaedic Surgeon, Royal Hallamshire
Hospital and Children's Hospital, Sheffield; Professor of Orthopaedic
Surgery, University of Sheffield, UK

E. W. Somerville FRCS(Ed), FRCS
Emeritus Consultant Orthopaedic Surgeon, Nuffield Orthopaedic
Centre, Oxford, UK

W. M. Steel FRCS(Ed)
Consultant Orthopaedic Surgeon, Department of Postgraduate
Medicine, University of Keele, Hartshill, Stoke-on-Trent, UK

John D. M. Stewart MA, FRCS
Consultant Orthopaedic Surgeon, Chichester District Health
Authority, West Sussex, UK

Ian Stother FRCS(Ed), FRCS(Glas)
Consultant Orthopaedic Surgeon, Glasgow Royal Infirmary and The
Glasgow Nuffield Hospital, Glasgow, UK

Michael Sullivan FRCS
Consultant Orthopaedic Surgeon, Royal National Orthopaedic
Hospital, London, UK

John P. W. Varian FRCS, FRACS(Orth)
Consultant Hand Surgeon, Blackrock Clinic, Dublin, Ireland

William Angus Wallace FRCS(Ed), FRCS(Ed)Orth
Professor of Orthopaedic and Accident Surgery, University of
Nottingham, Queen's Medical Centre, Nottingham, UK

W. Waugh MChir, FRCS
Emeritus Professor of Orthopaedic and Accident Surgery, University of
Nottingham; Honorary Consultant Orthopaedic Surgeon, Harlow
Wood Orthopaedic Hospital, Mansfield, Nottinghamshire, UK

Paul C. Weaver MD, FRCS, FRCS(Ed)
Consultant Surgeon (Surgical Oncology), Portsmouth and South East
Hampshire Group of Hospitals, Portsmouth; Clinical Teacher,
University of Southampton, UK

J. K. Webb FRCS
Consultant Orthopaedic Surgeon, University Hospital, Queen's
Medical Centre, Nottingham, UK

P. J. Webb FRCS
Consultant Orthopaedic Surgeon, The Hospital For Sick Children,
Great Ormond Street, London, and The Royal National Orthopaedic
Hospital, Stanmore, Middlesex, UK

Thomas E. Whitesides Jr MD
Professor of Orthopaedics, Department of Orthopaedic Surgery,
Emory University School of Medicine, Atlanta, Georgia, USA

Alan H. Wilde MD
Chairman, Department of Orthopaedic Surgery and Head, Section of
Rheumatoid Surgery, Cleveland Clinic Foundation, Cleveland, Ohio,
USA

Russell E. Windsor MD
Assistant Professor, Department of Orthopaedic Surgery, Cornell
University Medical College; Assistant Attending Orthopaedic Surgeon,
The Hospital for Special Surgery and The New York Hospital, New
York, USA

Robert E. Zickel MD
Clinical Professor of Orthopaedic Surgery, Columbia University, New
York, USA

Contributing Medical Artists

G. Bartlett

L. Butler
Medical Illustrator, 46 Selworthy House, Battersea Church Road,
London SW11 3NG, UK

Laurel L. Cook
Medical Illustrator, Medical Graphics, 69 Revere Street, Boston,
Massachusetts 02 114, USA

Michael J. Courtney

Peter Cox MMAA, AIMI, RDD
Medical Illustrator/Graphic Designer, 2 Frome Villas, Frenchay,
Bristol BS16 1LT, UK

Laura Pardi Duprey
146 H. Union Avenue, Rutherford, New Jersey 07070, USA

Patrick Elliott BA(Hons) ATC, AIMI
Senior Medical Artist, Department of Medical Illustration, Royal
Hallamshire Hospital, Glossop Road, Sheffield S10 3QX, UK

D. Howat
Medical Illustrator, 688 Orrang Road, Toorak, Victoria, Australia

Mark Iley
Illustrator, 12 High Street, Great Missenden, Bucks HP16 9AB, UK

Donn Johnson
Veterans Administration Medical Center, Atlanta, Georgia, USA

T. King

The late Robert Lane
Medical Illustrator, Studio 19A, Edith Grove, London SW10, UK

Gillian Lee FMAA, AIMI, AMI, RMIP
Medical Illustrator, 15 Little Plucketts Way,
Buckhurst Hill, Essex IG9 5QU, UK

Geoffrey Lyth FA, BA, FMAA
Abbey View, Sneaton, Nr Whitby, North Yorkshire YO22 5HS, UK

Gillian Oliver MMAA, AIMI, FTF
Freelance Medical Illustrator, 15 Bramble Road, Hatfield,
Hertfordshire AL10 9RZ, UK

J. A. Pangrace AMI
Medical Illustrator, 9500 Euclid Avenue, Cleveland, Ohio 44195,
USA

R. C. Pearson
Medical Illustrator, Department of Photography and Medical
Illustration, Robert Jones and Agnes Hunt Orthopaedic Hospital,
Oswestry, Shropshire, UK

F. Price

Paul Richardson
6 Crofton Road, Orpington, Kent BR6 8AF, UK

Adrian Shaw
Medical Illustrator, 138 Penylan Road, Cardiff CF2 5RE, UK

William Thackeray
Medical Illustrator, 117 Oliphant Avenue, Dobbs Ferry, New York
10522, USA

Philip Wilson FMAA, AIMI, FTF
Freelance Medical Artist, 23 Normanhurst Road, St Paul's Cray,
Orpington, Kent BR5 3AL, UK

Anthony C. S. Yiu
Medical Illustration Unit, University of Hong Kong, Pokfulam, Hong
Kong

Department of Medical Illustration
Western Infirmary, Glasgow, UK

Contents of Part 1
Principles, Fractures and Spine

Preface   xxviii

Repair of musculoskeletal tissues   **Emergency skin cover in orthopaedics**   1
                                         M. D. Brough

                                         Tendon repair, replacement and transfer   16
                                         B. Helal
                                         S. C. Chen

                                         Repair of divided peripheral nerves   24
                                         Rolfe Birch

                                         Vascular injury and repair   39
                                         J. S. P. Lumley

Infections   **Surgical management of acute bone and joint infections**   54
                                         M. F. Macnicol

                                         Chronic infections of bone and joint   61
                                         R. A. B. Mollan

Arthropathies   **Swanson arthroplasty of the metacarpophalangeal joint for rheumatoid disease**   68
                                         James E. Culver

                                         Synovectomy of the elbow for rheumatoid disease   73
                                         Alan H. Wilde

                                         Surgical procedures in haemophilia   77
                                         R. B. Duthie
                                         I. W. Nelson

Bone biopsy   **Techniques of bone biopsy**   91
                                         Mark C. Gebhardt
                                         Henry J. Mankin

Fracture treatment

Principles of fracture management   **100**
C. E. Ackroyd

Traction treatment of fractures   **123**
John D. M. Stewart

External skeletal fixation   **145**
J. Kenwright

Upper limb fractures

Fractures of the long bones of the upper limb   **153**
Paul T. Calvert

Fractures at the elbow in adults   **165**
G. S. E. Dowd

Operative treatment of fractures of the hand   **175**
N. J. Barton

Primary treatment of the acutely injured hand   **188**
Campbell Semple

Lower limb fractures

Intracapsular fractures of the neck of the femur   **199**
C. E. Ackroyd
G. C. Bannister
V. G. Langkamer

Trochanteric fractures of the femur   **209**
G. C. Bannister
C. E. Ackroyd
V. G. Langkamer

Subtrochanteric fractures of the femur: Zickel nail fixation   **216**
Robert E. Zickel

Küntscher's closed intramedullary nailing technique for the treatment of femoral shaft fractures   **223**
Kevin F. King

Supracondylar fractures of the femur   **242**
C. E. Ackroyd

Fractures of the patella   **252**
V. G. Langkamer
C. E. Ackroyd

Tibial plateau fractures   **256**
J. K. Webb

Management of tibial shaft fractures   **268**
J. K. Webb
R. J. Langstaff

Fractures of the ankle   284
C. L. Colton
C. E. Ackroyd

Recognition and treatment of compartment compression
syndromes   295
Thomas E. Whitesides Jr
Michael H. Heckman

Fractures and dislocations in the foot   309
P. S. London

Pelvis and acetabulum

Displays, correction and fixation of stove-in hip joints   321
E. Letournel

Replacement and fixation of the posterior lip of the acetabulum   339
E. Letournel

Exposure and fixation of disrupted pubic symphysis   346
E. Letournel

Fractures in children

Operative treatment of children's fractures   351
I. J. Leslie

Delayed union, non-union and malunion

Delayed union, non-union and malunion of long-bone fractures   369
G. S. E. Dowd
George Bentley

Metastatic disease

Metastatic bone disease in the limb   384
Malcolm W. Fidler

Amputations

General principles of amputation surgery   397
J. C. Angel

Amputation through the upper limb   402
J. C. Angel

Forequarter amputation   409
Paul C. Weaver

Hindquarter amputation   414
Paul C. Weaver

Disarticulation of the hip   427
J. C. Angel

Above-knee amputation   422
J. C. Angel

Disarticulation at the knee   427
J. C. Angel

Below-knee amputation   431
J. C. Angel

Syme's amputation   437
J. C. Angel

Transmetatarsal amputation   441
J. C. Angel

Amputation of the toes   444
J. C. Angel

Cervical spine

Axillary approach for thoracic outlet syndrome   447
Robert D. Leffert

Transoral approach to the cervical spine   453
H. Alan Crockard
Andrew O. Ransford

Anterior fusion of the cervical spine   463
David L. Hamblen

Posterior fusions of the cervical spine   471
David L. Hamblen

Thoracic and lumbar spine

Halofemoral traction   482
J. C. Dorgan

The halo–body cast   486
Sean P. F. Hughes

Posterior procedures for idiopathic scoliosis   491
Michael Edgar

Anterior procedures for spinal deformity   504
T. R. Morley
P. J. Webb

Luque instrumentation for neuromuscular scoliosis   512
George Bentley
Julian Jessop

Surgical management of lumbar disc prolapses   517
H. V. Crock

Chemonucleolysis for herniated intervertebral disc   530
Michael Sullivan

Posterior decompression for spinal stenosis   534
Michael Sullivan

Posterior lumbar spinal fusion   539
E. O'Gorman Kirwan

Intertransverse fusion for spondylolisthesis and lumbar instability   545
E. O'Gorman Kirwan

Surgical reduction of severe spondylolisthesis   549
J. P. O'Brien

Operations for infections of the spine   559
John C. Y. Leong

Metastatic bone disease of the spine   571
Malcolm W. Fidler

Approaches to the spine   597
J. K. Webb

Spinal injuries   624
Sir George Bedbrook
Philip H. Hardcastle

Index   671

Contents of Part 2
Regional Elective Orthopaedics

Preface   xxviii

Shoulder   **Recurrent anterior dislocation of the shoulder**   671
                      William Angus Wallace

                      Injuries of the acromioclavicular joint   686
                      William Angus Wallace

                      Arthroscopy of the shoulder   692
                      J. I. L. Bayley

                      Rotator cuff repair   697
                      J. I. L. Bayley

                      Operations for Erb's palsy   705
                      B. Helal
                      S. C. Chen

                      Rupture of the biceps   709
                      B. Helal
                      S. C. Chen

                      Arthroplasty of the shoulder   713
                      Alan Lettin

                      Arthrodesis of the shoulder   721
                      The late Sir Henry Osmond-Clarke

Elbow   **Prosthetic replacement of the elbow**   729
                      Thomas P. Sculco
                      Philip M. Faris

                      Tendon replacement to restore elbow flexion   736
                      B. Helal
                      S. C. Chen

Forearm, wrist and hand

Tendon reconstruction in the forearm 745
B. Helal
S. C. Chen

Surgery of the wrist 765
I. J. Leslie

Tendon transfer for mobile radial deviation of the wrist 805
B. Helal
S. C. Chen

Tendon injuries in the hand 808
John P. W. Varian

Primary repair of the divided digital flexor tendon 828
Harold J. Richards

Two-stage tendon reconstruction using gliding tendon implants 836
James M. Hunter
Peter C. Amadio

Dupuytren's contracture 855
W. M. Steel

Trigger finger and thumb 865
Neil Citron

Pelvis and hip

Operations for congenital dislocation of the hip 870
A. Catterall

Innominate osteotomy 893
A. Catterall

High femoral osteotomy in childhood 900
E. W. Somerville

Slipped upper femoral epiphysis 909
M. J. Griffith

Correction of flexion contracture of the hip 921
B. Helal
S. C. Chen

Adductor release (with or without partial anterior obturator neurectomy) 926
W. J. W. Sharrard

Hip flexor release: iliofemoral approach 931
W. J. W. Sharrard

Iliopsoas tendon lengthening or recession: medial (Ludloff) approach 936
W. J. W. Sharrard

Proximal hamstring release   940
W. J. W. Sharrard

Total hip replacement arthroplasty   943
Kevin Hardinge

Girdlestone's pseudarthrosis of the hip   965
E. W. Somerville

Arthrodesis of the hip   970
J. Crawford Adams

Thigh and knee

Distal hamstring release   981
W. J. W. Sharrard

Transfer of the hamstrings to the quadriceps in the adult   985
J. A. Fixsen

Proximal gastrocnemius release   989
W. J. W. Sharrard

Supracondylar osteotomy of the femur   992
J. A. Fixsen

Rupture of the quadriceps mechanism   995
B. Helal
S. C. Chen

Quadricepsplasty in the adult   1003
J. A. Fixsen

Diagnostic arthroscopy of the knee   1007
George Bentley
Anthony J. B. Fogg

Arthroscopic surgical procedures   1019
Ian Stother

Arthroscopic meniscectomy   1043
Ian Stother

Arthroscopic meniscal repair   1056
Robert W. Jackson
Sanford S. Kunkel

Open meniscectomy of the knee   1062
Adrian N. Henry

Loose bodies in the knee   1073
Paul Aichroth

Repair and reconstruction of knee ligament injury   1079
Paul Aichroth

Recurrent dislocation of the patella   1102
Paul Aichroth

Synovectomy of the knee   1109
W. Waugh

Tibial osteotomy for arthritis of the knee   1113
J. P. Jackson

Arthroplasty of the knee   1119
Russell E. Windsor
John N. Insall

Compression arthrodesis of the knee   1131
The late Sir John Charnley

Massive replacement for tumours of the lower limb   1137
H. B. S. Kemp
John T. Scales

Leg and foot   **Treatment of leg length inequality**   1152
                          Andrew M. Jackson

                          Distal gastrocnemius release   1169
                          W. J. W. Sharrard

                          Lengthening and repair of the tendo Achillis 1172
                          B. Helal
                          S. C. Chen

                          Transfer of tibialis posterior tendon to the dorsum of the foot 1184
                          B. Helal
                          S. C. Chen

                          Multiple tendon transfers into the heel   1187
                          E. W. Somerville

                          Arthrodeses of the ankle   1191
                          E. W. Somerville

                          Arthrodeses of the foot   1199
                          E. W. Somerville

                          Wedge tarsectomy   1208
                          E. W. Somerville

                          Operations for flat foot and pes cavus   1211
                          Leslie Klenerman

                          Operations for congenital talipes equinovarus 1220
                          E. H. Bates

The Robert Jones operation for clawing of hallux   1227
B. Helal
S. C. Chen

Flexor to extensor transfer for clawing of the lateral four toes (Girdlestone's operation)   1230
B. Helal
S. C. Chen

Forefoot reconstruction   1232
B. Helal
S. C. Chen

Hallux valgus and hallux rigidus   1244
H. Piggott

Dorsal nerve transfer for plantar digital neuroma (Morton's metatarsalgia)   1255
W. N. Gilmour

Hammer and mallet toe   1259
H. Piggott

Subluxation of the lesser metatarsophalangeal joints   1263
H. Piggott

Dorsally displaced fifth toe   1267
H. Piggott

Ingrowing toe-nail   1270
H. Piggott

Index   1273

Preface

The 10 years that have elapsed since the publication of the third edition of *Orthopaedics* have seen the most exciting developments in the applied science of operative surgery. This new edition aims to reflect these changes and to present in a concise manner the indications for operative treatment of all common orthopaedic conditions that face the contemporary practising surgeon. New procedures are described to reflect the speed of change in the subject where these are considered to be established. Important non-operative techniques such as traction methods are covered also.

All the chapters have been rewritten and 31 new chapters have been added: seven on important general subjects such as musculoskeletal infections, management of primary and secondary tumours and arthritis, nine on the spine, six on the upper limb and hand, three on the knee, three on foot surgery, and three on fracture management. A few classic procedures such as arthrodesis of the shoulder and knee are retained because of their international importance and the principles they embody. Each author has presented his subject in his personal style but the form of illustrations has been standardized and improved.

The needs of the orthopaedic trainee and young consultants in practice have been foremost in preparing this edition; but the experienced surgeon will find much useful information, especially when faced with some of the less common procedures that occur in any busy practice.

The restructuring of this edition has involved many colleagues to whom we are deeply indebted. In particular Chris Russell, Julian Jessop and Chris Lavy have provided invaluable help. Mary Bramwell made the completion of the task possible. As before the staff of Butterworth–Heinemann provided their expertise and have been unfailingly helpful.

George Bentley
Robert B. Greer III

Recurrent anterior dislocation of the shoulder

William Angus Wallace   FRCS Ed, FRCS Ed(Orth)
Professor of Orthopaedic and Accident Surgery, University of Nottingham, UK

Introduction

Aetiology

Dislocations of the glenohumeral joint are common injuries and are frequently associated with a tendency to recurrence, particularly in the young. The initial episode may involve minor or major trauma, depending on the susceptibility of the individual. An indirect injury to the shoulder, with a forcible abduction and lateral rotation strain to the arm, is the most common mechanism. The risk of recurrence after an anterior dislocation depends on the initial mechanism of injury and the age of the patient.

Simonet and Cofield[1] have shown from a review of 116 cases, followed up 5 years after injury, that patients aged under 20 years at the time of their first anterior dislocation have a 66 per cent incidence of recurrent dislocation and, in addition, an 18 per cent incidence of subluxation symptoms. Patients from 20 to 40 years had a 40 per cent incidence of recurrence with a further 9 per cent having subluxation symptoms, while in their series there were *no* recurrences in those aged over 40 but 10 per cent had subluxation symptoms. If the initial dislocation had been the result of an athletic or sporting injury and the patient was aged under 30 years the prognosis was worse, with the incidence of recurrence rising to 77 per cent.

Management of the initial dislocation

The first dislocation may reduce spontaneously, but if the patient attends hospital with the shoulder still dislocated an anteroposterior and modified axial radiograph[2] is recommended. Once dislocation is confirmed, reduction may be attempted by suspension of a weight from the patient's wrist while he lies prone on a table or trolley with the arm hanging over the edge. If this fails, in dislocations treated within the first 12 hours an attempt at reduction using sedation is recommended, but only if the proximal humerus has been shown to be free of fracture lines on plain radiographs. In all other circumstances the patient should be given a full general anaesthesia with muscle relaxation before the shoulder is reduced. For manipulative reduction the Hippocratic method is the safest: the operator's unshod foot is placed in the patient's axilla and firm sustained traction applied to the arm until the humeral head suddenly jumps back into joint. Kocher's manoeuvre, which involves a forcible rotation, is no longer recommended as it has been the cause of a significant number of iatrogenic humeral neck fractures.

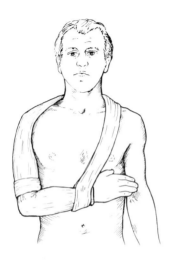

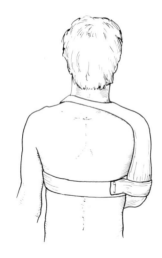

1

1

In those who spontaneously reduce and in patients who require manipulative reduction, further immobilization of the shoulder is recommended using a Gilchrist sling[3] made from a 3 metre length of stockinette. Alternatively, a broad arm sling and body bandage, or a commercially available shoulder immobilizer may be used.

The period of immobilization is currently a source of contention. Kiviluoto et al.[4] (1980) have shown, in patients under the age of 30, that there is an increased incidence of recurrence if only 1 week of immobilization is used compared with 3 weeks. However, Hovelius[5,6] has shown no difference between those mobilized early and those immobilized for 3–4 weeks. The lowest recurrence rate has been reported by Yoneda, Welsh and MacIntosh[7] who treated young university students with 5 weeks' absolute immobilization in a sling and body bandage and found their recurrence rate was reduced to only 17 per cent.

A sensible management policy would be that patients under 35 at the time of their first dislocation should be treated with strict immobilization for 5 weeks if they wish to return to active sport or for 3 weeks if they are likely to lead a less active life. In those over 35 years recurrence is rare irrespective of treatment, therefore only 1 week of immobilization is required, but no sporting activities for 6 weeks.

Preoperative

Assessment of patients
with recurrent anterior dislocations

Four questions should be asked if a patient seeks help for a recurrent anterior dislocation of the shoulder.

1. Are the symptoms severe enough to warrant surgical treatment? Normally surgery is only considered if dislocation has recurred on at least two occasions or when subluxation symptoms are significantly interfering with everyday life.

2. Is there documentary evidence of the initial dislocation and if so in which direction did the humeral head displace?
3. Is it absolutely sure that the direction of the recurrent dislocation is anterior?
4. Does the patient have a 'loose' shoulder or multi-directional instability?

If radiographs are available from the first episode then the diagnosis will be supported *but* the patient could also have a 'loose' shoulder. The direction of instability is established clinically by carrying out two tests – the anterior apprehension test and the posterior stress test.

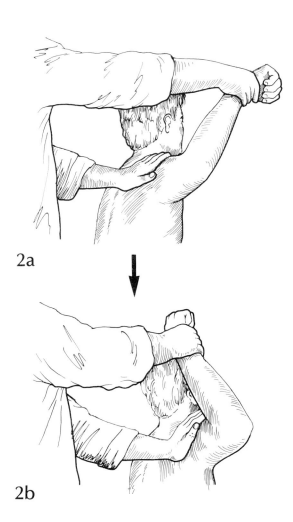

2a

2b

Anterior apprehension test[8]

2a & b

The affected arm is abducted to 90° in neutral rotation and the examiner gently rotates the arm laterally while controlling the scapula with his other hand as shown. If the shoulder is unstable anteriorly the patient will develop apprehension and the anterior third of deltoid or the subscapularis will develop spasm to protect the shoulder from dislocating.

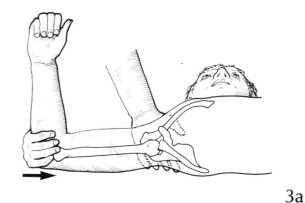

3a

Posterior stress test[9]

3a & b

The patient lies in the supine position. The examiner stabilizes the scapula by resting his hand between the scapula and the examination table. He places his fingers behind the neck of the scapula and the humeral head and moves the arm to 90° abduction in neutral rotation. The elbow is kept at 90° and the arm is brought forwards into flexion with the examiner applying firm axial pressure through the humeral shaft in order to attempt to displace the humeral head posteriorly. The examining hand will feel the humeral head sublux or dislocate in a posterior direction and this will be confirmed by then reversing the manoeuvre and extending the shoulder again when the head will be felt to 'clunk' back into joint.

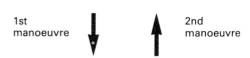

1st manoeuvre   2nd manoeuvre

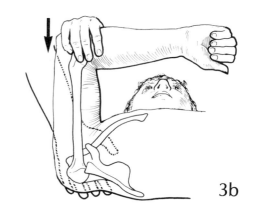

3b

Sulcus sign[10]

4

The 'loose' shoulder is identified by eliciting the sulcus sign. The patient is seated and asked to relax. The surgeon applies downward traction to the arm while observing the contour of the shoulder he is examining. If a sulcus appears just below the acromion this indicates the humeral head has subluxed inferiorly and the shoulder is 'loose'.

If a 'loose' shoulder is diagnosed, referral to an orthopaedic surgeon with a special interest in shoulder problems is recommended; these patients are particularly difficult to treat, and there is a surgical failure rate in excess of 50 per cent.

Voluntary recurrent anterior dislocation

There are a group of patients who can anteriorly sublux or dislocate their shoulder at will. A number of these patients have psychological problems. They should be managed in the first instance by advice to stop dislocating the shoulder, to avoid any activities which are known to cause the shoulder to come out of joint and to build up the rotator cuff muscles with specific strengthening exercises. The majority of patients settle using this regime and surgery is rarely required.

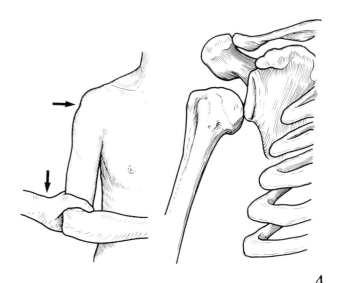

4

Pathological lesions

Carter Rowe[11] from Boston in 1978 reported his experience of surgical treatment of recurrent anterior dislocation over a period of 30 years. In 85 per cent of cases the capsule was completely avulsed or separated from the anterior glenoid rim. The glenoid labrum was absent or completely destroyed in 73 per cent, and intact but separated from the rim in a further 13 per cent of cases. Damage to the bony rim of the glenoid was present in 73 per cent of cases, with 44 per cent actually fractured. A Broca[12] or Hill–Sachs[13] lesion – a bony dent on the posterolateral aspect of the humeral head – was present in 77 per cent of cases. Rowe's failure rate using the Bankart operation was 3.5 per cent but increased to 5 per cent if a medium or large sized Broca lesion was present.

It has been shown by Pieper[14] that patients with recurrent anterior dislocation have a reduced humeral retroversion of $25° \pm 10°$ compared with the normal value of $40° \pm 6°$. This supports the concept of the Weber lateral rotation osteotomy[15] for the treatment of recurrent anterior dislocation. Unfortunately Pieper's findings have not been supported by Cyprien et al.[16] nor by Pfister and Gebauer[17] who have shown no difference in humeral torsion between normal controls and patients with anterior dislocation. Nor could they show a relationship between the glenoid version and recurrent dislocation.

Humeral rotation osteotomy will not be considered further.

Choice of operation

Table 1 shows the published success rates for different operations for recurrent anterior dislocation of the shoulder. The Putti–Platt operation is the traditional British operation but it suffers from two drawbacks – it has the highest recorded failure rate and it is usually associated with a marked loss of lateral rotation of the shoulder that limits its usefulness, particularly in sportsmen who require a good range of elevation and rotation.

The best operation is usually the operation which the operator is most acquainted with and which he therefore does the best. My own preference is for the Bankart operation, particularly if the shoulder is only subluxing in an anterior direction, but it is difficult and may be tedious to carry out. The Boytchev procedure will produce a near-normal range of movement early after the operation (often within 4 months) but there is a 30 per cent incidence of temporary musculocutaneous nerve palsy.

Table 1 Results from recurrent dislocation operations

Operation	Dislocation plus subluxation recurrence rate (%)	Number of patients	Author
Putti–Platt	5	79	Quigley & Friedman (1974)[18]
	14	132	Morrey & Janes (1976)[19]
	19	68	Hovelius (1979)[20]
Bankart	5	18	Adams (1948)[21]
	4	145	Rowe et al. (1978)[11]
	4	45	Zinnecker (1984)[22]
Bristow–Helfet	7	30	Helfet (1958)[23]
	16	31	Albrektsson et al. (1982)[24]
	13	112	Hovelius (1984)[25]
Magnuson–Stack	3	75	DePalma et al. (1967)[26]
	2	154	Karadimas et al. (1980)[27]
	3	38	Ahmadain (1987)[28]
Boytchev	0	17	Conforty (1980)[29]
	0	26	Ha'Eri (1986)[30]
	12*	17	Sugimoto et al. (1987)[31]

* 2 patients had one minor subluxation each in the early postoperative period

Structures to protect in anterior shoulder surgery

5

Operations on the front of the shoulder are carried out close to the distal part of the brachial plexus. The illustration shows the close proximity of these nerves. The nerve which is most vulnerable is the musculocutaneous nerve which lies behind the conjoined tendons of biceps and coracobrachialis and passes into the posterior aspect of the coracobrachialis muscle. This nerve is usually well protected when the conjoined tendon is attached but as soon as a coracoid osteotomy is performed it becomes vulnerable; great care must be taken to avoid a traction injury to the nerve. The nerve usually enters the coracobrachialis muscle at least 5 cm distal to the coracoid but its anatomy is very variable.

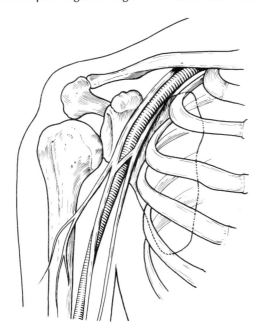

5

Operations

The approach to the front of the shoulder is similar for most of the operations. It is therefore appropriate to describe the standard approach and then the different techniques for each operation will be described in detail. The closure technique and postoperative management will finally be presented.

Position of patient

6

The patient is placed supine on the operating table with the trunk at a 45° head-up tilt. A sandbag or 500 ml infusion bag is placed behind the medial border of the scapula to throw the shoulder forward for easier surgical access. The head is supported either with a head ring or, as shown, with a neurosurgical head support. A surgical preparation of almost half the trunk and the *whole* of the affected arm is recommended. A thyroid-type double head-drape is used to isolate the patient's head and the anaesthetic equipment from the surgical field. The arm is draped separately to facilitate manoeuvrability.

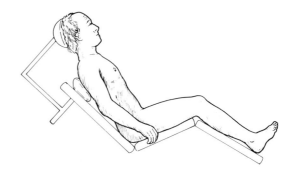

6

Skin incision

The incision varies depending on whether the patient is male or female.

7

In men the standard incision is from the tip of the coracoid vertically downwards towards the anterior axillary fold for a distance of 8 cm. This allows easy access through a large incision and provides an excellent exposure of the deeper anatomy.

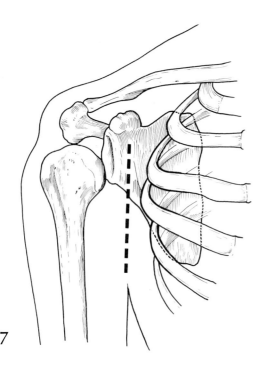

7

8

In women cosmesis is exceptionally important. Two alternative cosmetic incisions can be used – the 'bra-strap' incision or the axillary approach. In the former, the incision is hidden behind the patient's bra strap, and in order to site it correctly it is essential to mark the position of the bra strap before operation.

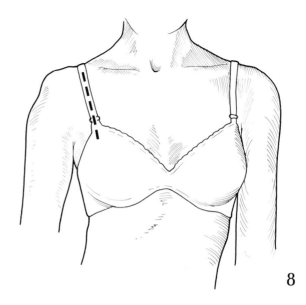

8

9

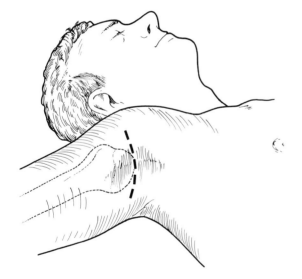

9

The axillary incision is made in the anterior half of the apex of the axilla and is extended forward as far as the anterior axillary fold formed by the pectoralis major tendon. The skin edges are then widely undermined and the lowest centimetre of the musculotendinous junction of the pectoralis major is divided. Abduction of the arm and retraction upwards of the pectoralis major tendon reveal the subscapularis tendon and conjoined tendon, and the coracoid may also be exposed. The pectoralis major should be repaired during closure. The disadvantages of the axillary approach are the more limited access and the occasional development of a thickened scar causing axillary discomfort.

Approach through the first muscle layer

10

The subcutaneous fat is divided and the deltopectoral groove is sought. This is located by identifying the cephalic vein distally and dissecting it proximally. As it passes upwards in the deltopectoral groove it dives down between the deltoid and pectoralis major. The vein is preserved but its lateral tributaries are either cauterized, or ligated between sutures, and then divided. If the main vein is damaged it may be tied off with no ill effect. The groove is then opened widely and held open with one pair of self-retaining retractors.

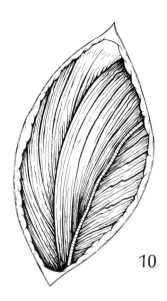

10

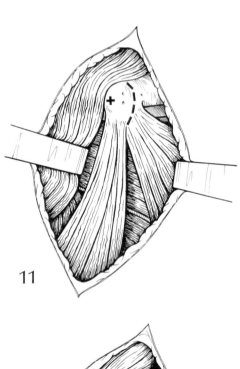

11

Approach through the second muscle layer

11 & 12

The coracoid process is now exposed in the upper part of the wound. The conjoined tendon of origin of coraco-brachialis and the short head of biceps constitute the second layer. A cruciate stab incision is made on the tip of the coracoid, and the coracoid is predrilled using a 2.5 mm drill and tapped with a 3.5 mm tap after measuring the depth of the drill hole. The periosteum approximately 1 cm from the tip of the coracoid is divided transversely and a coracoid osteotomy performed with either an osteotome or with an oscillating saw. A stay suture is then placed through the drill hole in the tip of the coracoid and the detached coracoid tip with the conjoined tendon attached is then reflected downwards. Care must be taken to avoid excessive traction on the conjoined tendon. The musculocutaneous nerve enters the deep surface of the coracobrachialis muscle and can be injured by injudicious traction. Once reflected downwards, the whole of the subscapularis muscle comes into view with the distal edge of the muscle identified by a leash of veins passing along its lower border.

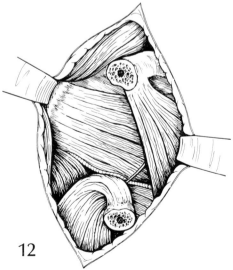

12

PUTTI–PLATT OPERATION[32]

Approach through the third muscle layer

13

The inferior border of the subscapularis is indicated by the transverse leash of anterior circumflex humeral vessels and the dissection should go no lower than this point. The vessels are now cauterized or divided between ligatures. Lateral rotation of the humerus puts the subscapularis under tension. Two stay sutures are now inserted into the subscapularis muscle 4 cm medial to its humeral attachment. These sutures are essential before dividing the subscapularis because if allowed to retract the cut muscle will come to lie dangerously close to the main nerves arising from the brachial plexus and there is then a risk of nerve injury when the subscapularis is subsequently sought. Subscapularis is now divided transverse to its fibres and 2 cm medial to its humeral attachment. The deep surface of the subscapularis is usually adherent to the joint capsule, and although it is preferable to protect the anterior capsule of the shoulder joint as a separate layer during the division, this is not essential.

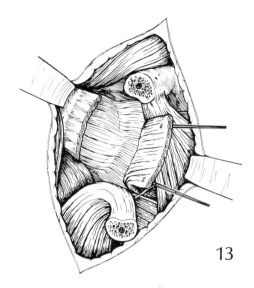

13

Entry into the shoulder joint

14

The anterior capsule of the shoulder is divided in the same line as the subscapularis tendon – 2 cm from the lateral insertion of the subscapularis. A Bankart retractor inserted into the joint will allow a good view of the anterior glenoid rim but there is no need to sublux the joint in order to demonstrate any Broca lesion.

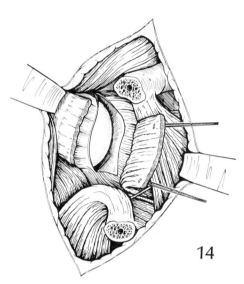

14

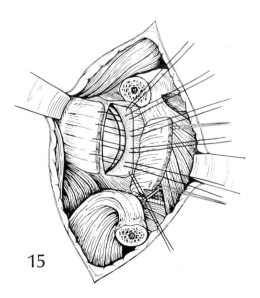

15

Attachment of subscapularis to the scapular neck

15

The lateral portion of subscapularis and the capsule are used as one flap in this operation. First the anterior scapular neck is roughened using a curette. The lateral flap is then sutured to the glenoid labrum and capsule so that it will adhere to the roughened area. Up to six braided non-absorbable mattress sutures are used and all should be inserted before they are tied as demonstrated. The humeral head should be levered backwards by the assistant as the sutures are tightened, but 45° of lateral rotation of the glenohumeral joint should still be possible at this stage.

Attachment of the medial capsular layer

16

The medial capsule is now double-breasted over the lateral subscapular layer and sutured using three braided non-absorbable sutures.

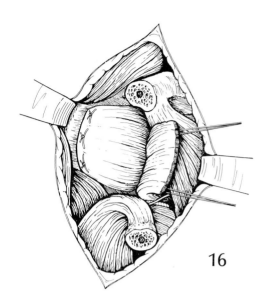

Attachment of the subscapularis layer

17

This is drawn across the deeper capsular layer and sutured with interrupted absorbable sutures to the deeper layers at a tension which will allow only 30°–45° of lateral rotation of the shoulder joint.

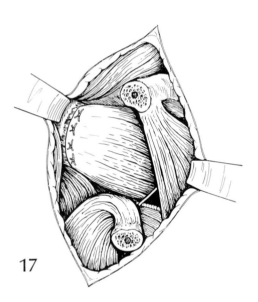

Reattachment of the coracoid

18

The coracoid is reattached with one 3.5 mm stainless steel screw of appropriate length. No washer is normally required as the screw usually settles nicely into the tip of the coracoid without cutting through.

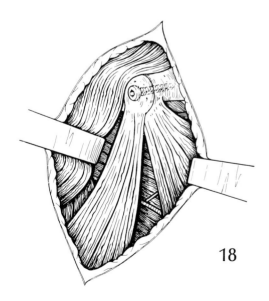

BANKART OPERATION[11]

Approach through the third muscle layer

19

This is very similar to the Putti–Platt except that the subscapularis is carefully dissected from the anterior capsule by sharp dissection as the subscapularis is divided and it is important *not* to divide the capsule at this stage. To avoid entering the joint a small amount of subscapularis tendon is often left on the anterior capsule.

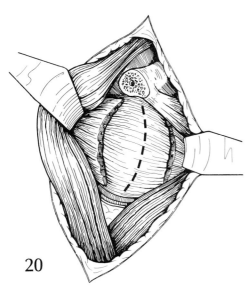

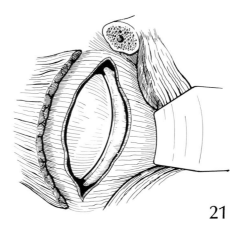

Entry into the shoulder joint

20

The arm is fully rotated laterally before a vertical incision is made into the joint just lateral to the rim of the glenoid. This ensures that the anterior flap will be of proper length to allow an adequate lateral rotation of the shoulder postoperatively.

Exposure of the anterior glenoid margin

21

The anterior glenoid rim is exposed more easily if a Bankart retractor is inserted into the joint . If the capsule is separated from the anterior glenoid rim, a Homan retractor is inserted into the glenoid neck and used to retract the medial part of the capsule. If the capsule and glenoid labrum are firmly attached to the anterior glenoid rim, these soft tissues can be used to reattach the anterior capsule and no drill holes are necessary.

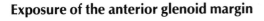

Preparing the anterior glenoid margin drill holes

22

The rim of the glenoid and the neck of the scapula can now be freshened with a curette or dental burr. Three or four holes are made through the rim using a right-angled dental drill and a strong, sharp-pointed towel clip. It is important that these holes are sufficiently deep to leave a solid anterior bridge after they have been drilled.

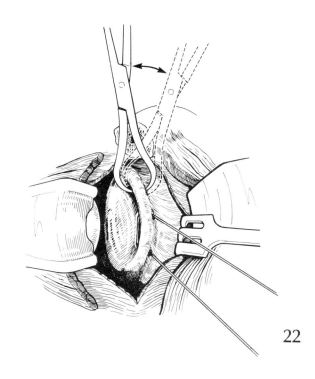

22

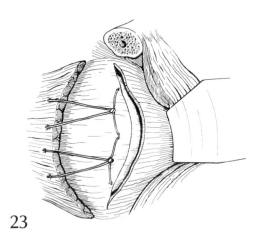

23

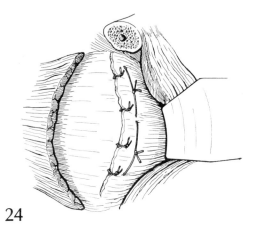

24

Attachment of the capsule to the glenoid

23 & 24

A No. 2, braided, non-absorbable suture is used. Using appropriate needles the sutures are placed through the holes as a mattress suture, with a small groove created in the articular cartilage, and then through the anterior capsular layer. *All* the sutures should be inserted before any are tied firmly with the arm in full medial rotation. The medial capsular flap is then sutured over the front of the repair using the ends of the same sutures, thus providing a solid reinforcement, and any free edge of medial capsule tacked down with interrupted absorbable sutures.

Repair of subscapularis

The subscapularis is repaired by end-to-end suture using three or four interrupted absorbable mattress sutures.

Reattachment of the coracoid

This is performed as in the Putti–Platt operation.

MODIFIED BRISTOW–HELFET PROCEDURE[25]

Technique

25

The subscapularis muscle and capsule of the shoulder are split longitudinally at a point between the middle third and the lower third of the muscle, and the gap held open with a self-retaining retractor. This gives access to the anteroinferior glenoid rim, which is roughened and drilled with a 3.2 mm drill to receive the attachment of the coracoid process. The coracoid is fixed using a 4.5 mm lag (malleolar) screw of sufficient length to engage the posterior cortex of the scapula. Hovelius[25] has clearly shown that the position of the coracoid is crucial to the success of this operation. It *must* be anchored on the inferior one third of the glenoid rim and its lateral edge should be flush with the articular surface of the glenoid with no palpable step. The conjoined tendon should be sutured to the subscapularis after removal of retractors to provide additional stability to the fixation.

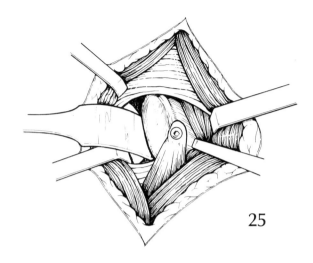

25

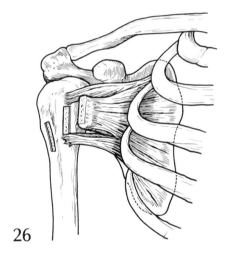

26

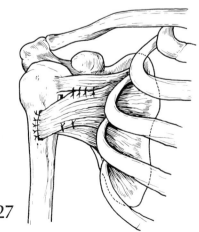

27

MODIFIED MAGNUSON–STACK PROCEDURE[26]

Technique

26 & 27

No osteotomy of the coracoid is required for this operation. The central four-fifths of the tendon of subscapularis is separated by incisions near its upper and lower margins. Its insertion is detached, taking a small wedge of bone and the capsulomuscular flap is dissected medially to allow inspection of the glenoid. The shoulder is then rotated medially and the subscapularis insertion is transplanted under reasonable tension lateral to the bicipital groove about 1 cm distal to the greater tuberosity. The bony wedge is placed in a shallow gutter and fixed either with staple or sutures. The upper and lower margins of the transferred tendon are sutured to local soft tissues.

MODIFIED BOYTCHEV PROCEDURE[30]

Technique

28 & 29

The conjoined tendons attached to the osteotomized coracoid process are retracted and freed downwards as far as the penetration of the coracobrachialis muscle by the musculocutaneous nerve. The musculocutaneous nerve must be identified either by careful dissection without undue traction or by palpation in view of the known occurrence of postoperative nerve palsies. The transverse leash of anterior circumflex humeral vessels at the lower border of subscapularis is identified and if necessary ligated. With the arm held in full medial rotation, a cholecystectomy forceps is passed between the subscapularis muscle and the capsule of the shoulder joint. A tunnel is created in this plane by opening the forceps and withdrawing the instrument. The tunnel is enlarged until the operator's little finger can be passed easily through the tunnel. The detached coracoid process with the conjoined tendons is passed through the tunnel and reattached to its original site with a 3.5 mm screw of appropriate length. It is important to check there is no tension on the musculocutaneous nerve at this stage. If there is, the lower fibres of subscapularis should be surgically divided to free the nerve.

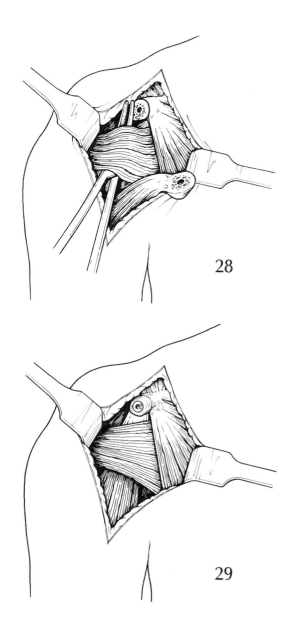

28

29

Closure

For all procedures the deltopectoral interval is loosely closed with two or three interrupted absorbable 0-gauge sutures over a suction drain. The subcutaneous fat is closed carefully with interrupted 2/0 absorbable sutures and the skin should be closed with 2/0 polypropylene continuous subcuticular suture reinforced with adhesive skin sutures. In the shoulder region there is no place for simple interrupted sutures because of the significant cosmetic deformity created by the suture holes which can be disfiguring. A simple absorbent, adhesive dressing is applied to the wound.

A Gilchrist sling (see *Illustration 1*) or a broad arm sling is applied in the operating theatre with a cotton wool axillary pad to absorb moisture.

Postoperative management

The patient remains in hospital for 24–72 hours, depending on the level of postoperative discomfort. The suction drain is removed at 24 hours after operation.

For the Putti–Platt, Bristow–Helfet and Magnuson–Stack procedures, a Gilchrist sling is recommended for 3–4 weeks. Alternatively, a broad arm sling under the clothes or a commercial shoulder immobilizer can be used for the same period. For the Bankart and Boytchev procedures a broad arm sling is required for only 10 days to 2 weeks.

No formal physiotherapy is required after any of these procedures. The patients are encouraged to 'use your arm as normally as possible'. Gentle swimming can be started from 6 weeks and a return to normal sports 3 months after operation.

References

1. Simonet WT, Cofield RH. Prognosis in anterior shoulder dislocation. *Am J Sports Med* 1984; 12: 19–24.

2. Wallace WA, Hellier M. Improving radiographs of the injured shoulder. *Radiography* 1983; 49: 229–33.

3. Gilchrist DK. A. stockinette-Velpeau for immobilization of the shoulder girdle. *J Bone Joint Surg [Am]* 1967; 49-A: 750–1.

4. Kiviluoto O, Pasila M, Jaroma H, Sundholm A. Immobilization after primary dislocation of the shoulder. *Acta Orthop Scand* 1980; 51: 915–9.

5. Hovelius L, Eriksson K, Fredin H, *et al*. Recurrences after initial dislocation of the shoulder: results of a prospective study of treatment. *J Bone Joint Surg [Am]* 1983; 65-A: 343–9.

6. Hovelius L. Anterior dislocation of the shoulder in teenagers and young adults: a five year prognosis. *J Bone Joint Surg [Am]* 1987; 69-A: 393–9.

7. Yoneda B, Welsh PP, MacIntosh DL. Conservative treatment of shoulder dislocation in young males. In: Bayley I, Kessel L, eds. *Shoulder surgery*, Berlin: Springer Verlag, 1982; 76–9.

8. Gerber C, Ganz R. Clinical assessment of instability of the shoulder: with special reference to anterior and posterior drawer tests. *J Bone Joint Surg [Br]* 1984; 66-B: 551–6.

9. Norwood LA, Terry GC. Shoulder posterior subluxation. *Am J Sports Med* 1984; 12: 25–30.

10. Neer CS, Foster CR. Inferior capsular shift for involuntary inferior and multi-directional instability of the shoulder: a preliminary report. *J Bone Joint Surg [Am]* 1980; 62-A: 897–908.

11. Rowe CR, Patel D, Southmayd WW. The Bankart procedure: a long-term end result study. *J Bone Joint Surg [Am]* 1978; 60-A: 1–16.

12. Hartmann H, Broca A. Contribution a l'etude des luxations de l'epaule. *Bulletin de la Societe Anatomique de Paris*, 5Me Serie 1890; 4: 312.

13. Hill HA, Sachs MD. Grooved defect of the humeral head: frequently unrecognized complication of dislocations of the shoulder. *Radiology* 1940; 35: 690–700.

14. Pieper H-G. Correction of pathological amount of humeral retroversion in operative treatment of recurrent shoulder dislocation. In: Takagishi N, ed. *The shoulder*. Japan: PPS, 1987: 276–80.

15. Weber BG. Operative treatment for recurrent dislocation of the shoulder: preliminary report. *Injury* 1969; 1: 107–9.

16. Cyprien JM, Vasey HM, Burdet A, Bonvin JC, Kritsikis N, Vuagnat P. Humeral retrotorsion and glenohumeral relationship in the normal shoulder and in recurrent anterior dislocation (scapulometry). *Clin Orthop* 1983; 175: 8–17.

17. Pfister A, Gebauer D. The operative treatment of recurrent shoulder dislocation dependent of the retroversion angle: a computed tomography study. In: Takagishi N, ed. *The shoulder*. Japan: PPS, 1987; 270–5.

18. Quigley TB, Freedman PA. Recurrent dislocation of the shoulder: a preliminary report of personal experience with seven Bankart and 92 Putti–Platt operations in 99 cases over 25 years. *Am J Surg* 1974; 128: 595–9.

19. Morrey BF, Janes JM. Recurrent anterior dislocation of the shoulder. Long-term follow-up of the Putti–Platt and Bankart procedures. *J Bone Joint Surg [Am]* 1976; 58-A: 252–6.

20. Hovelius L, Thorling J, Fredin H. Recurrent anterior dislocation of the shoulder: results after the Bankart and Putti–Platt operations. *J Bone Joint Surg [Am]* 1979; 61-A: 566–9.

21. Adams JC. Recurrent dislocation of the shoulder. *J Bone Joint Surg [Br]* 1948; 30-B: 26–38.

22. Zinnecker HJ, Puhringer A, Bartalsky L. Experience in the treatment of recurrent anterior dislocation of the shoulder with a modified version of Bankart's procedure. In: Bateman JE, Welsh RP, eds. *Surgery of the shoulder*. Philadelphia: Decker. St Louis: CV Mosby, 1984: 91–3.

23. Helfet AJ. Coracoid transplantation for recurring dislocation of the shoulder. *J Bone Joint Surg [Br]* 1958; 40-B: 198–202.

24. Albrektsson BE, Herberts P, Korner L, Lamm CR, Zachrisson BE. Technical aspects of the Bristow repair for recurrent anterior shoulder instability. In: Bayley I, Kessel L, eds. *Shoulder surgery*. Berlin: Springer Verlag, 1982: 87–92.

25. Hovelius L. Operative treatment of recurrent anterior shoulder dislocation with the Bristow–Latarjet procedure. In: Bateman JE, Welsh RP, eds. *Surgery of the shoulder*. Philadelphia: Decker. St Louis: CV Mosby, 1984: 87–90.

26. DePalma AF, Cooke AJ, Prabhakar M. The role of the subscapularis in recurrent anterior dislocations of the shoulder. *Clin Orthop* 1967; 54: 35–49.

27. Karadimas J, Rentis GR, Varouchas G. Repair of recurrent anterior dislocation of the shoulder using transfer of the subscapularis tendon. *J Bone Joint Surg [Am]* 1980; 62-A: 1147–9.

28. Ahmadain AM. The Magnuson–Stack operation for recurrent anterior dislocation of the shoulder: a review of 38 cases. *J Bone Joint Surg [Br]* 1987; 69-B: 111–4.

29. Conforty B. The results of the Boytchev procedure for treatment of recurrent dislocation of the shoulder. *Int Orthop* 1980; 4: 127–32.

30. Ha'Eri GB. Boytchev procedure for the treatment of anterior shoulder instability. *Clin Orthop* 1986; 206: 196–201.

31. Sugimoto Y, Nakatsuchi Y, Saitoh S, Kutsuma T, Sugiura K. Boytchev procedure for recurrent dislocation of the shoulder. In: Takagishi N, ed. *The shoulder*. Japan: PPS, 1987: 261–5.

32. Osmond-Clarke H. Habitual dislocation of the shoulder. The Putti–Platt operation. *J Bone Joint Surg [Br]* 1948; 30-B: 19–25.

Illustrations by Peter Cox

Injuries of the acromioclavicular joint

William Angus Wallace FRCS Ed, FRCS Ed (Orth)
Professor of Orthopaedic and Accident Surgery, University of Nottingham, UK

Introduction

The acromioclavicular joint is one of the most commonly injured joints of the body. The injury is usually caused by a heavy fall onto the shoulder or a blow to the top of the shoulder as occurs in a rugby tackle. The patient experiences pain on the point of the shoulder immediately after the injury, with pain clearly localized to the acromioclavicular joint area, and often bruising appears 48 hours later.

The traditional management of this injury is conservative and this has been supported by recent reports by Bannister[1] and Dias[2]. Although there has been an eagerness in recent years to operate on these patients, work by Imatani[3] and by Glick[4] has clearly shown that the majority of sportsmen do well following non-operative management of their acromioclavicular joint dislocation. However, a small group of patients would appear to benefit from early surgery and an additional small group do require late surgical treatment after a poor result from non-operative treatment.

Classification

Three categories of injury are now widely recognized and were described by Allman[5].

Grade I injuries cause local damage, usually only to the superior acromioclavicular ligament with no joint disruption; there is no deformity – only local tenderness over the joint.

In Grade II injuries there is damage to both the superior and inferior acromioclavicular ligaments and stretching of the coracoclavicular ligaments, with a minor step (less than the height of the acromioclavicular joint) seen at the point of the shoulder.

In Grade III injuries the coracoclavicular ligaments are completely ruptured or avulsed; obvious deformity is present at the point of the shoulder with a high-riding clavicle and a weak shoulder. Bannister[6] has further divided Grade III injuries into Grade III-stable and Grade III-unstable injuries, with stability assessed on special stress radiographs taken with the elbow held at 90° while a weight of 5 kg is held in the hand. An additional indication of a Grade III-unstable injury is the clinical finding that the lateral end of the clavicle lies under the skin and is separated from its enveloping muscles – the trapezius above and the deltoid below.

Although all classifications concentrate on the vertical displacement on radiographs it is important also to examine clinically for anteroposterior displacement as it is usual for the lateral end of the clavicle to be displaced posteriorly after Grade III injuries. By gentle palpation, the lateral end of the clavicle and the acromion can be identified and their anteroposterior stability can be assessed by gentle pressure.

Indications for surgical intervention

Acute injuries

There is rarely an indication for surgical treatment for Grade I and Grade II injuries. Grade III injuries may be treated conservatively as recommended by Dias[2] who considered long-term disability was rare. There is merit in identifying the Grade III-unstable injury described by Bannister[6] and performing early open reduction and internal stabilization of this injury.

Late or chronic injuries (all grades)

In this situation the patient complains of either pain or deformity.

Pain If pain is the problem, this is usually due to mechanical pain either from muscle strain or from early arthritic change in the acromioclavicular joint. The degree of joint stability must first be assessed carefully. If the joint is stable, but arthritic, excellent results with a 90 per cent success rate will be obtained by resection of the lateral 1 cm of the clavicle[7] but with careful repair of the soft tissues. However, if the joint is unstable the joint surfaces must be assessed very carefully both before and at the time of operation. If the joint surfaces are in good condition the author recommends accurate open reduction and internal stabilization of the acromioclavicular joint. However, if the joint surfaces are badly damaged or cannot be accurately reduced a Weaver–Dunn procedure[8,9] is performed.

Deformity Patients with a chronic dislocation of the acromioclavicular joint have two deformities, an obvious 'bump' caused by the prominent lateral end of the clavicle together with the appearance of a dropped shoulder. In females the dropped shoulder may cause a problem with shoulder straps tending to fall off and apparent uneven hemlines of dresses. The 'bump' may be very obvious and can be fully corrected by operation as can the dropped shoulder, but in both cases one cosmetic problem will be replaced by another, the operation scar. Unfortunately scarring in the shoulder region is unpredictable and stretched and keloid scars may occur. The wise surgeon will counsel his patient carefully on the problem before operation and will take all appropriate steps to avoid unsightly postoperative scarring.

Operations

Position of patient

1

The patient lies supine with the operating table tilted upwards at an angle of around 40° (the deck-chair position). A sandbag is placed under the medial border of the scapula and the patient's head is supported either with a head ring or a neurosurgical head support but with the neck laterally flexed to the opposite side.

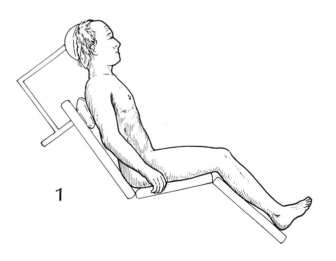

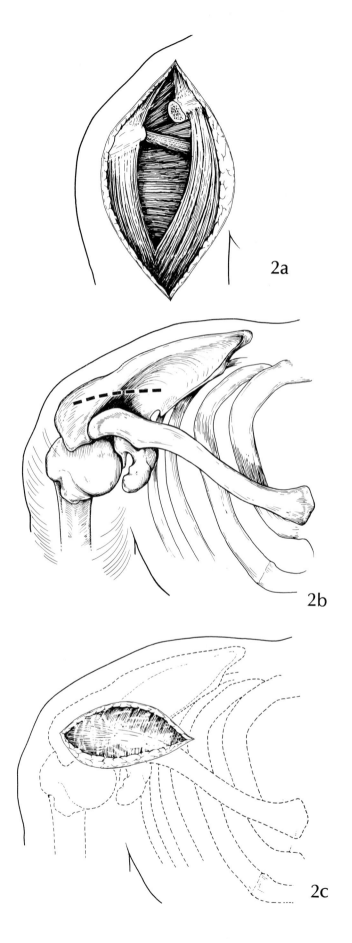

2a

Incisions

2a, b & c

The author recommends one of two incisions – either (a) a vertical parasagittal incision which provides excellent access to the acromioclavicular joint and the deltoid muscle, or (b) a posterior coronally-directed incision which lies behind the acromioclavicular joint, provides less good access but is a very good cosmetic incision for females because it lies on the top of the shoulder and is usually not visible from in front or behind. Every attempt should be made to retain the continuity of the cloak of anterior muscles – the trapezius above and the deltoid below. The deeper approach to the acromioclavicular joint is through a vertical incision in the line of the muscle fibres and then through the joint.

2b

2c

REDUCTION AND INTERNAL STABILIZATION

Open reduction

3

Under vision the acromioclavicular joint should be reduced after the necessary dissection and freeing-up of the soft tissues. Once the clavicle is fully reduced – with no step on inspection from the front and with the front edge of the clavicle matching the anterior edge of the acromion – the position should be held temporarily with one smooth K-wire inserted under power from the lateral end of the acromion, across the acromioclavicular joint into the clavicle.

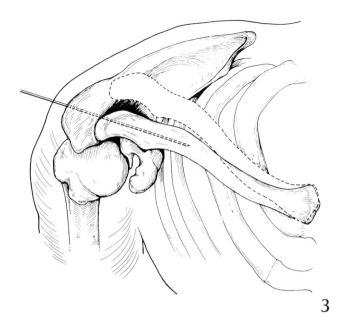

3

Stabilization with a coracoclavicular screw

4

This method is modified from the technique described originally by Bosworth[10]. The surgeon's index finger is passed through the vertical incision in the deltoid to palpate the coracoid and locate its position. The screw is to be positioned starting from the posterior part of the clavicle 4 cm from its lateral end and passing forward and downward to insert into the base of the coracoid. This is a difficult screw to position correctly and does require some experience. A 4.5 mm hole is first drilled in the clavicle and then a 3.2 mm drill is passed through this hole and the base of the coracoid is 'felt' with the tip of the drill while the surgeon's index finger again locates the tip of the coracoid manually. A 3.2 mm hole is now drilled into the base of the coracoid. A 4.5 mm AO screw of suitable length and with a large washer is now inserted through the hole and screwed into the coracoid until it starts to compress the clavicle onto the coracoid. The temporary K-wire fixation is now removed and the acromioclavicular joint inspected. The screw is adjusted and when stabilization appears satisfactory a check radiograph is taken to ensure the screw position is satisfactory and the radiological appearance is acceptable.

Soft tissue reconstruction should now be carried out around the joint, firmly repairing the superior acromioclavicular ligaments with the local soft tissues and finally ensuring a full repair of the deltoid and the trapezius with synthetic absorbable sutures.

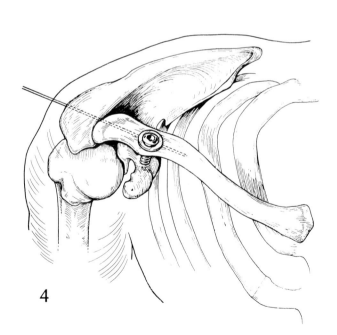

4

WEAVER–DUNN TECHNIQUE FOR CHRONIC DISLOCATIONS

5

The lateral end of the clavicle is exposed through a deep vertical incision and, after creating a soft tissue curtain of periosteum with trapezius above and deltoid below in continuity and with sharp dissection, that curtain is gradually pushed back medially from the lateral 2 cm of the clavicle. Using an oscillating saw, a bevelled cut is made, removing the lateral 2 cm of the clavicle and leaving the clavicle longer superiorly. A large (4.5 mm) drill hole is made in the lateral end of the clavicle to accommodate the coracoacromial ligament and two vertical 2 mm drill holes are inserted vertically through the superior cortex of the clavicle into the previously drilled hole. The freed acromial end of the coracoacromial ligament is now anchored with a No 2 non-absorbable suture using a Kessler or Bunnell tendon suture technique, and the suture ends passed through the 2 mm drill holes – thus opposing the coracoacromial ligament to the cut end of the clavicle. The suture is pulled tight, the lateral end of the clavicle is thus reduced and the suture tied. The deltoid and trapezius are now meticulously reconstructed using synthetic absorbable sutures.

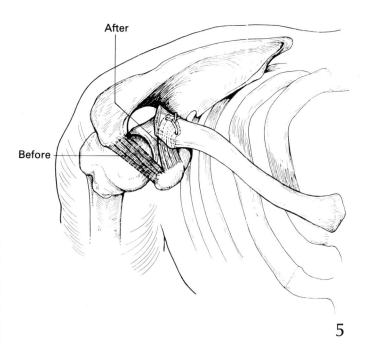

5

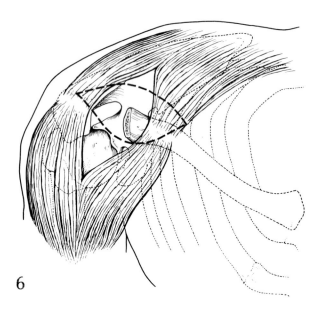

6

RESECTION OF THE LATERAL 1 CM OF THE CLAVICLE

6

The lateral end of the clavicle is exposed through a deep vertical incision and, after creating a soft tissue curtain of periosteum with trapezius above and deltoid below in continuity, the curtain is dissected back using sharp dissection to expose the lateral 1 cm of the clavicle. Using an oscillating saw with the blade parallel to the plane of the acromioclavicular joint an osteotomy is made which allows the lateral articular end of the clavicle to be removed.

Closure

For all procedures a careful and complete reattachment of the deltoid to the trapezius, with a resulting reinforcement of the repair of the new acromioclavicular joint, is essential. The subcutaneous tissues are approximated with interrupted absorbable sutures and the skin wound is closed with a subcuticular 2/0 polypropylene suture followed by adhesive wound closure strips to protect the healing wound from broadening. A broad arm sling (or Mastersling) is used for 2–3 weeks and mobilization of the shoulder carried out thereafter. For patients with a coracoclavicular screw in place, mobilization of the arm should be restricted to below shoulder level (i.e. 90° elevation) until after the screw is removed at 6–8 weeks after stabilization.

References

1. Bannister GC. The management of complete acromioclavicular dislocation: a randomised prospective controlled trial comparing early movement with coracoclavicular screw fixation. MCh Orth Thesis, University of Liverpool, 1983.

2. Dias JJ, Steingold RF, Richardson RA, Tesfayohannes B, Gregg PJ. The conservative treatment of acromioclavicular dislocation: review after five years. *J Bone Joint Surg [Br]* 1987; 69-B: 719–22.

3. Imatani RJ, Hanlon JJ, Cady GW. Acute, complete acromioclavicular separation. *J Bone Joint Surg [Am]* 1975; 57-A: 328–32.

4. Glick JM, Milburn LJ, Haggerty JF, Nishimoto D. Dislocated acromioclavicular joint: follow-up study of 35 unreduced acromioclavicular dislocations. *Am J Sports Med* 1977; 5: 264–70.

5. Allman FL. Fractures and ligamentous injuries of the clavicle and its articulation. *J Bone Joint Surg [Am]* 1967; 49-A: 774–84.

6. Bannister GC, Wallace WA, Stableforth PG, Hutson MA. The management of acute acromioclavicular dislocation. *J Bone Joint Surg [Br]* 1989; 71-B: 848–50.

7. Taylor GM, Tooke M. Degeneration of the acromioclavicular joint as a cause of shoulder pain. *J Bone Joint Surg [Br]* 1977; 59-B: 507.

8. Weaver JK, Dunn HK. Treatment of acromioclavicular injuries, especially complete acromioclavicular separation. *J Bone Joint Surg [Am]* 1972; 54-A: 1187–94.

9. Warren-Smith CD, Ward MW. Operation for acromioclavicular dislocation: a review of 29 cases treated by one method. *J Bone Joint Surg [Br]* 1987; 69-B: 715–8.

10. Bosworth BM. Acromioclavicular separation: a new method of repair. *Surg Gynecol Obstet* 1941; 73: 866–71.

Arthroscopy of the shoulder

J. I. L. Bayley FRCS
Consultant Orthopaedic Surgeon, Royal National Orthopaedic Hospital, Stanmore, Middlesex, UK

Introduction

Shoulder arthroscopy is now established as a useful diagnostic and operative technique. In resistant shoulder pain and obscure instability, the clinical diagnosis may be altered in up to half the cases depending on the type and site of the pathology. In cases of shoulder pain in which no clinical diagnosis can be made with any confidence, arthroscopy reveals the diagnosis in two-thirds. The global results of anterior repair for unstable shoulders using arthroscopic techniques have been disappointing and the method is only applicable when there is a significant Bankart's labral detachment. On the other hand the results of anterior acromioplasty by arthroscopic techniques have been generally encouraging.

This chapter will only describe the technique of diagnostic arthroscopy of the shoulder, which deserves more general application.

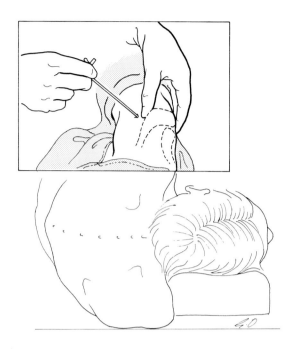

Operation

Position

1

The patient is placed in the lateral position and the arm is draped free following skin preparation. For diagnostic arthroscopy the arm is not immobilized in traction but is held by an assistant so as to allow free movement. Preparation and draping are routine.

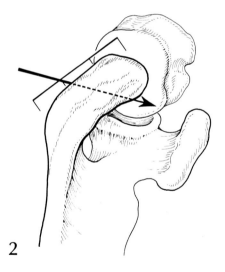

Approach to subacromial space

2

An attempt must be made in all cases to inspect the subacromial space. The arthroscope is introduced 'dry' just under the lateral border of the acromion at the junction of the posterior and middle thirds. Preinjection of irrigant should not be carried out since, if the needle does not enter the bursal space, injected fluid will collapse the walls of the bursa, making subsequent entry of the arthroscope difficult. The sharp trocar is used to penetrate the deltoid and then, using a blunt obturator, the arthroscope is advanced towards the acromioclavicular joint until a tell-tale 'give' in resistance is felt.

The telescope is introduced but irrigation is only begun under direct vision, since the arthroscope may be 'perched' at the bursal wall which can still be collapsed by fluid egress into surrounding areolar tissue. Under vision there is an opportunity to advance the arthroscope into the bursal space as irrigation begins. Using this technique it is possible, after suitable experience, to enter a defined bursal space in 80 per cent of cases. Separate irrigation for simple diagnosis is not usually required.

Arthroscopic appearances – subacromial space

The superficial surface of the supraspinatus tendon is easily seen and is usually smooth with no disruption of the bursal floor. The greater tuberosity, the deep surface of the anterior acromion and the coracoacromial ligament are all easily identified (*Plate 1**). The deep surface of the acromioclavicular joint can only be seen when the bursal cavity extends sufficiently far medially.

The superficial surface of the supraspinatus tendon and the deep surface of the anterior acromion are visibly roughened in cases of 'impingement'. Sometimes flap tears may occur. They can be assessed by probing with a needle (*Plate 2*). Subtle changes can be appreciated which defy diagnosis by available imaging techniques.

Glenohumeral appearances

Glenohumeral joint arthroscopy should be preceded by examination under anaesthetic to assess laxity of the shoulder expressed as a percentage of the humeral head diameter. However, the technique is subjective and the presence of increased humeral head glide demonstrates laxity but does not imply symptomatic instability. The arthroscope is introduced via a posterior portal after preinjection of irrigant. The portal is placed a thumb's breadth below and a thumb's breadth medial to the posterior angle of the acromion. The arthroscope is introduced into the empty space between the humeral head and the glenoid, which can be appreciated by gliding the humeral head backwards and forwards on the glenoid by the thumb and forefinger placed astride the shoulder. The instrument is advanced down to the shoulder capsule with the sharp obturator, which is changed to the blunt obturator in order to penetrate the joint. A common mistake is to skid medially off the back of the scapular neck.

If there is some doubt as to the exact position of the glenohumeral joint line, the arthroscope with the blunt obturator can be used to 'palpate' the rim of the glenoid and the humeral head. It is then a simple matter to puncture the capsule in the space between the two. Having entered the joint, the obturator is changed for a standard 30° telescope. An outflow portal is only introduced for diagnostic arthroscopy if there is troublesome bleeding. Generally the field can be kept clear using hydrostatic distension with irrigant.

The origin of the biceps tendon from the supraglenoid tubercle provides the central reference point from which the inspection is begun (*Plates 3* and *4*). The tendon can be followed over the humeral head and into the bicipital sulcus, noting any degenerative, inflammatory or mechanical changes (*Plates 5* and *6*). The deep surface of the cuff can then be scanned when any deep surface disruption will be readily apparent.

The arthroscope is next advanced into the anterior compartment and the glenohumeral ligament complex inspected (*Plate 7*). The anterior glenoid rim is easily seen and any labral detachment is readily demonstrated. If necessary a hook or probe can be inserted through the 'quiet area' of the rotator interval just in front of and below the anterior acromion.

Next the arthroscope is swept around the glenoid rim into the inferior axillary recess. An assessment is made of any anteroinferior or inferior capsular pouch and the posteroinferior glenoid rim is inspected for signs of attrition which would indicate posterior instability (*Plate 8*). The instrument is then drawn through the posterior compartment, during which process an inspection of the posterior surface of the humeral head can be made (*Plate 9*). Subtle defects in the articular surface can be seen which would not be visible radiographically but which confirm the presence of anterior instability.

Finally, an assessment is made of the articular surfaces and the synovium. Early osteoarthritis causing shoulder stiffness can be differentiated from the frozen shoulder syndrome. Localized synovitis in the superior glenohumeral joint space, apparently a 'forme fruste' of the frozen shoulder syndrome, can be readily appreciated (*Plate 10*). It does not cause limitation of movement but can present with a typical subacromial painful arc syndrome which mimics supraspinatus impingement.

Postoperative management

After removing the arthroscope, sterile wound closure strips are applied to the skin portals and covered with a waterproof dressing. These are left *in situ* for 5 days. The shoulder is rested in a collar and cuff for 24 hours before allowing unrestricted activity.

Colour plates 1–10 are on pages 695–696.

Arthroscopy of the shoulder

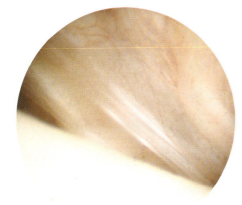

1

Plate 1. The superficial surface of the supraspinatus tendon can be seen in the lower part of the field. It is smooth and without bursal floor disruption.

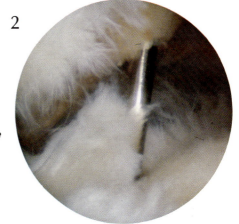

2

Plate 2. The superficial surface of the supraspinatus tendon has clearly been disrupted by impingement on the undersurface of the anterior acromion, where there are also signs of wear. There is a partial thickness flap tear of the tendon which is being examined for size and mobility using a needle probe.

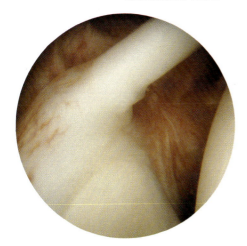

3

Plate 3. The right glenohumeral joint has been entered from the posterior aspect. The origin of the long head of biceps tendon can be seen from the supraglenoid tubercle. This is the reference point from which to begin inspection of the joint.

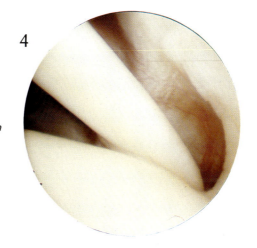

4

Plate 4. The biceps tendon has been followed through the superior glenohumeral space to the biceps sulcus, where it can be inspected in more detail by manoeuvring the draped arm.

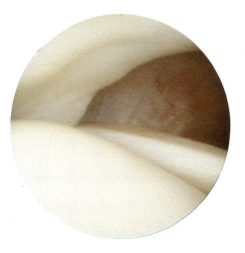

5

Plate 5. The normal deep surface of the supraspinatus tendon of the left shoulder can be seen with its insertion into the greater tuberosity just behind the biceps sulcus.

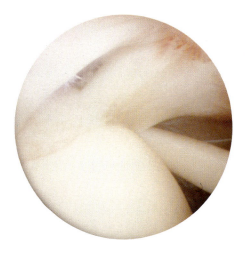

6

Plate 6. In this shoulder there is a deep surface cleft tear at the junction of supraspinatus and infraspinatus.

7

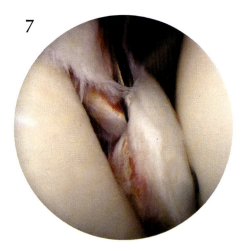

Plate 7. The right anteroinferior compartment of the glenohumeral joint is demonstrated from the posterior approach. The labrum has been detached from the rim of the glenoid and can be probed using a hook introduced through the 'quiet area' of the rotator interval.

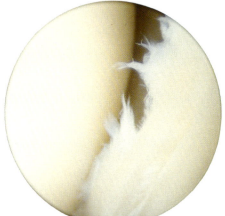
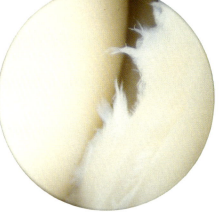

8

Plate 8. The posteroinferior glenoid rim of the left shoulder has been disrupted as a result of recurrent posterior dislocation.

9

Plate 9. There is defect in the articular surface of the posterior aspect of the humeral head – a sure sign of post-traumatic anterior instability. In this case the defect was not seen with other imaging techniques because it is very shallow and does not broach the subchondral bone plate.

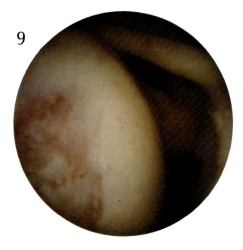

10

Plate 10. The superior compartment of the left glenohumeral joint is seen. There is a chronic low grade synovitis. The patient presented with a painful arc syndrome with no limitation of movement and elsewhere in the joint the synovium was not involved. Note the normal appearance of the humeral head and biceps tendon.

Illustrations by Gillian Oliver

Rotator cuff repair

J. I. L. Bayley FRCS
Consultant Orthopaedic Surgeon, Royal National Orthopaedic Hospital, Stanmore, Middlesex, UK

Introduction

The main aim of rotator cuff repair is to relieve pain, but operation may be indicated to restore a severe functional deficit or to preserve future function, particularly in a younger patient with an acute tear. Pain relief is generally good but restoration of function depends largely on the size and chronicity of the tear and the state of the tissues. Nevertheless, although global tears are the most taxing, repair can give surprisingly satisfactory results and is well worthwhile, provided pain and dysfunction are sufficient to justify the necessary prolonged rehabilitation.

The need for repair is determined by the extent and nature of the rupture. Longstanding attrition of the supraspinatus tendon beneath the anterior acromion may wear a small hole in the tendon with thickened margins such that rotator cuff function, though vitiated by pain, remains mechanically competent. In such cases it may suffice to decompress the tendon by anterior acromio-plasty, particularly if the procedure is carried out arthroscopically. In large ruptures, however, where a substantial segment of tendon insertion has given way as a result of trauma in the young, or avascular degeneration in the older patient, the rotator cuff is rendered incompetent and repair is required. The outcome depends upon patient selection and surgical planning. The patient must be prepared to co-operate in a carefully controlled rehabilitation regime and to wait an average of 9 months before achieving full benefit from the surgery. Surgical planning involves the design and choice of an appropriate surgical approach to the subacromial region and selection of a suitable technique of repair.

Two surgical exposures are available to address the spectrum of pathology. Small or acute defects can be repaired through an anterior deltoid splitting incision such as might be used for a simple subacromial decompression. Large or chronic retracted defects are more easily dealt with via an approach which splits the acromion in the plane of the scapula. Preoperative assessment of the size of the rupture is therefore important; loss and weakness of active lateral rotation are useful clinical indicators of a significant cuff disruption.

697

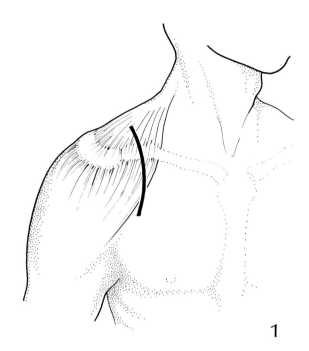

1

Operation

Surgical exposure

1 & 2

The basic principle of any approach to the subacromial space is the preservation of trapeziodeltoid continuity. In the anterior approach, the skin is incised in a line which a bra-strap might occupy and deepened to the areolar tissue over the clavicle and deltoid epimysium. A full-thickness flap is developed as far lateral as the outer border of the acromion. The deltoid is now split in the line of its fibres for a distance of not more than 5 cm from the acromio-clavicular joint.

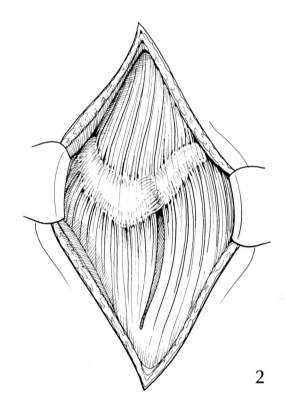

2

3

If it is intended to excise the acromioclavicular joint, the incision is extended proximally through the joint into trapezius. The acromial branch of the acromiothoracic artery requires coagulation where it runs anterior to the acromioclavicular joint deep to deltoid before exposing the coracoacromial ligament. An aponeurotic flap is now developed by sharp dissection over the acromion which carries deltoid with it and allows exposure of the anterior acromion part way along its lateral border. It is preferable to create an osteoperiosteal flap with an osteotome rather than risk compromising trapeziodeltoid continuity by tearing a thinning aponeurotic flap. A medial flap can be developed over the clavicle if excision of the acromioclavicular joint is to be carried out either for access, cuff decompression, or treatment of an associated intrinsic acromioclavicular joint osteoarthritis.

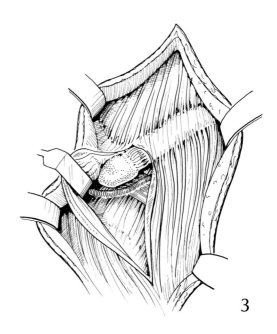

3

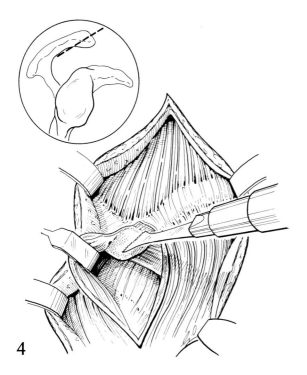

4

4

An anterior undercutting acromioplasty is now carried out with a reciprocating power saw, aiming to remove the hooked part of the anterior acromion and creating a flattened undersurface to the acromion with an upward slope from back to front.

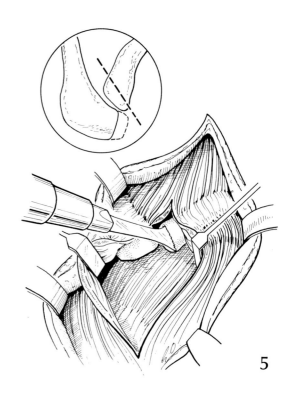

5

If the outer end of the clavicle is to be excised it should be accomplished in a line running posteromedially – in order to avoid a prominent posterolateral corner to the residual stub of clavicle – and by undercutting to create deep space for the rotator cuff whilst preserving an acromioclavicular arch for deltoid purchase.

5

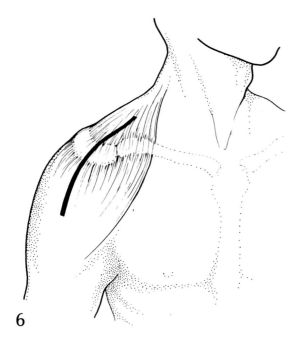

6

6

Large chronic cuff defects are better exposed through a more laterally disposed incision. The skin incision passes across the point of the shoulder in the line of the scapula and is developed to expose trapezius and deltoid.

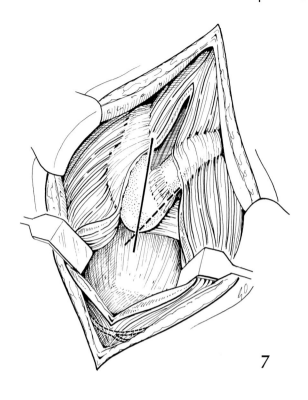

7

7 & 8

After raising osteoperiosteal flaps the acromion is divided with a reciprocating saw in the line of the scapular blade, such that the osteotomy exits on the lateral border of the acromion at the point where it is intersected by a line extrapolated along the anterior border of the clavicle. By this technique, after enucleation of the anterior fragment of acromion and closure of the aponeurosis, the soft tissues bridge between the clavicle and acromion in such a way that the mechanical leverage of deltoid is reduced by no more than the distance the anterior acromion projected forwards beyond the line of the clavicle. After splitting trapezius and deltoid in the same line over no more than a 5 cm length distally to avoid the circumflex nerve and 3 cm proximally, division of the subacromial bursa will allow the cuff defect to be defined.

Having determined by preliminary inspection that repair is possible, the anterior fragment of acromion should be enucleated in the manner of a patellectomy from its aponeurosis by sharp dissection in order to improve access and to decompress the subsequent repair. Often the outer end of the clavicle also requires undercutting.

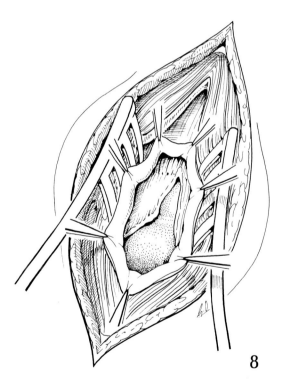

8

Repair

The principles of the repair are constant whichever approach is used. Firstly, a retracted cuff should be mobilized in order to bring it back towards its original insertion. Next, the fibrotic edges of the defect should be excised if possible to bleeding tissue, and finally the cuff should be resutured into a trough cut as close to the original insertion as possible and commensurate with allowing the arm to come close to the trunk without disrupting the repair. Associated splits are closed side-to-side.

Mobilization is usually not required in small or fresh tears but in chronic lesions there may be marked retraction. Bursal adhesions are first divided by sharp dissection whilst exerting traction on the cuff via stay sutures. Next, the coracohumeral ligament may require release from its coracoid attachment, and finally the transacromial approach allows a complete circumferential capsulotomy around the glenoid rim. Only in the presence of marked loss of cuff substance do these three manoeuvres fail to mobilize a retracted cuff sufficient to allow repair.

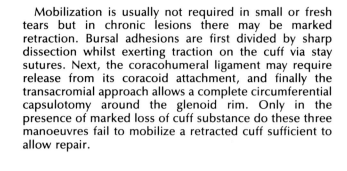

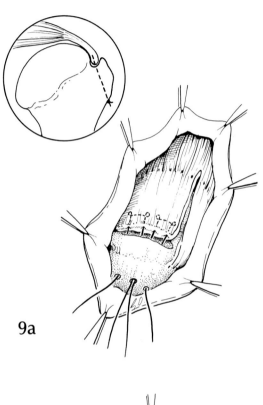

9a

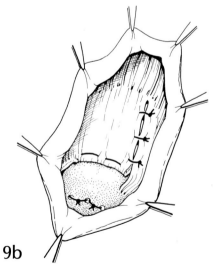

9b

9a & b

Most tears are due to a combination of disinsertion and a longitudinal split. The pattern of each lesion should be studied to decide the correct method of repair. The disinserted segment is repaired into a trough cut into the greater tuberosity at the humeral articular margin, using a braided synthetic non-absorbable suture in a Kessler pattern stitch. The sutures are passed through drill holes in the base of the trough and tied over the outer cortex of the tuberosity. Any longitudinal component is sutured side-to-side. The repair does not need to be water-tight but should be secure when the arm is brought down to within 15° of the trunk.

In chronic tears, when loss of tendon substance and length may prevent direct reinsertion into the greater tuberosity, it is a mistake to cut the trough so far medial that it encroaches into the articular surface of the humerus. In the absence of proven artificial tendon substitutes, several reconstructive procedures have been described. None has proved to be markedly superior but in general it is better to use local tissue whenever possible. Two such procedures have stood the test of time.

BICEPS TENODESIS

The intra-articular tendon of the long head of biceps is sectioned at the level of the biceps sulcus. The distal portion is tenodesed to soft tissues within the sulcus and the proximal stump, still attached to the supraglenoid tubercle, is sutured into the trough and used as a spacer between supraspinatus and infraspinatus. The procedure sacrifices the humeral head depressing action of the biceps muscle, but in extreme cases the net gain is worthwhile.

SUBSCAPULARIS AND INFRASPINATUS TENDON TRANSPOSITION

10a & b

In a proportion of cases, despite marked retraction and loss of cuff tendon superiorly, the anterior and posterior tissues remain intact. Although it is important to preserve functioning cuff at the front and back, the upper half of these cuff remnants can be spared for transfer to the superior aspect of the humeral head to distribute cuff action equally around the articular circumference. The transposed tendons are sutured as earlier described into a trough cut in the greater tuberosity. The V-shaped defect between them can often be filled with the retracted stump of supraspinatus.

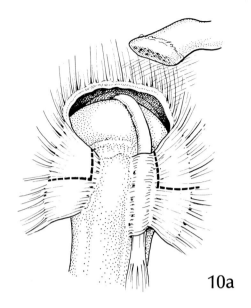

10a

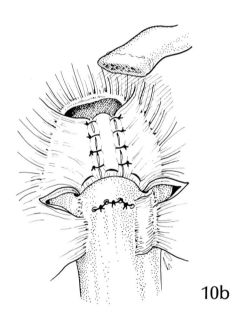

10b

Wound closure

11

The trapeziodeltoid flaps are repaired side-to-side over a suction drain. The muscle layers should be apposed with horizontal – rather than vertical – mattress sutures through the epimysial layer to avoid muscle infarction.

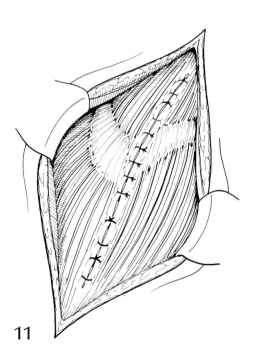

11

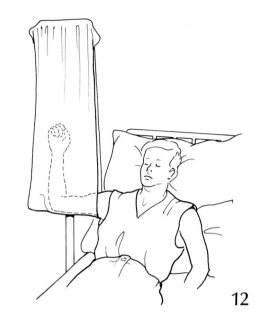

12

Postoperative management

12 & 13

Pending tendon healing, no active use is allowed for 6 or 8 weeks but shoulder mobility is preserved by passive movement. The arm should be maintained in some elevation in order to protect the repair and to encourage blood flow to the tendon. Initially, therefore, the limb is supported in a roller towel whilst postoperative discomfort settles and, after 3–5 days is placed on a foam abduction wedge with which the patient is discharged home.

Passive mobilization into elevation is continued until 6 or 8 weeks from operation, when the abduction wedge is discarded and assisted active exercises are started. Thereafter shoulder control is progressively but gradually developed over the ensuing months. It is much better to aim for slow but steady progress rather than trying to push the shoulder beyond its limits.

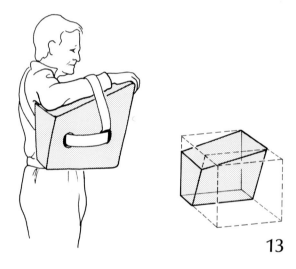

13

Illustrations by Gillian Oliver after B. Hyams

Operations for Erb's palsy

B. Helal MChOrth, FRCS
Honorary Consultant Orthopaedic Surgeon, The Royal London Hospital and The Royal National Orthopaedic Hospital, London, and Enfield Group of Hospitals, UK

S. C. Chen FRCS
Consultant Orthopaedic Surgeon, Enfield Group of Hospitals, UK

Introduction

Erb's palsy[1] is an upper brachial plexus birth palsy, in which the shoulder girdle muscles, especially the supraspinatus and infraspinatus muscles, are affected and a medial rotation and adduction deformity of the shoulder develops. The subscapularis muscle which functions normally becomes contracted as a result of its action being unopposed. There are several operations described for this condition, but the ·authors consider that Sever's modification[2,3] of Fairbank's operation[4] and the Bateman procedure[5] give satisfactory results.

Operations

SEVER'S MODIFICATION OF FAIRBANK'S OPERATION

Incision

1

An incision is made along the deltopectoral groove from the tip of the coracoid process to the insertion of the deltoid muscle.

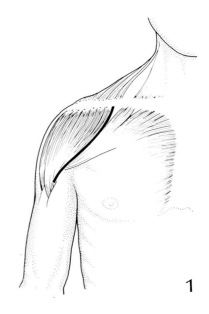

1

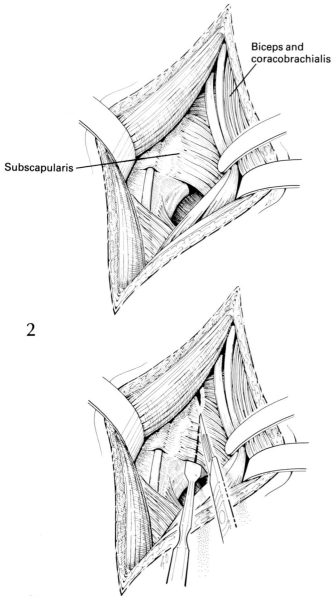

Biceps and coracobrachialis

Subscapularis

2

3

Exposure and release

2 & 3

The pectoralis major muscle is divided parallel to the humerus along the tendinous insertion. The coracobrachialis and short head of the biceps muscles are identified and retracted medially. This exposes the subscapularis muscle. The shoulder is laterally rotated and abducted and the subscapularis muscle cut without cutting the joint capsule by elevating the muscle from the capsule with a MacDonald dissector.

Postoperative management

A shoulder spica is applied with the shoulder abducted and laterally rotated, the elbow flexed to 90°, the forearm in supination and the wrist in a neutral position. The spica is removed after 2 weeks and physiotherapy started – both passive and active exercises.

MUSCLE TRANSFER FOR DELTOID PARALYSIS
(Bateman's operation)

Incision

4

The patient is placed prone. A T-shaped incision is made, the horizontal limb along the acromioclavicular arch and spine of the scapula.

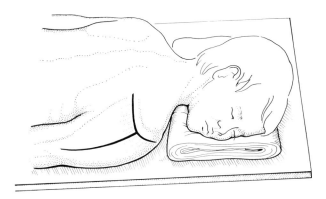

4

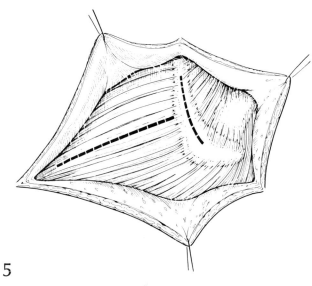

5

Osteotomy

5 & 6

The atrophied deltoid is exposed by retracting the flaps. The deltoid muscle is split longitudinally and the shoulder joint exposed. The spine of the scapula is osteotomied near its base, in a lateral direction, with the trapezius still attached to it.

The trapezius is detached from the lateral part of the clavicle avoiding damage to the coracoclavicular ligament. The shoulder is abducted to 90°. The lateral aspect of the humerus is freshened near the deltoid insertion.

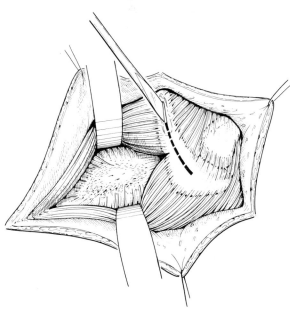

6

7

The acromion with the trapezius is pulled over the humeral head and attached with screws to the humerus as close to the deltoid tuberosity as possible.

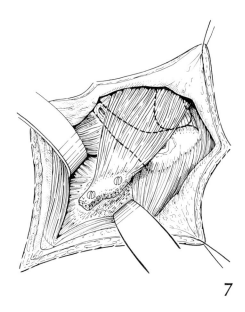

7

Postoperative management

The arm is immobilized with the shoulder abducted to 90° in a shoulder spica for 6 weeks. Gradually the arm is brought down to the side using an abduction splint. When the acromion has united with the humerus, passive and active exercises are started to re-educate the transferred muscle.

References

1. Erb WH. Ueber eine eigenthümliche Localisation von Lahmungen im Plexus brachialis. *Verh naturh-med Ver Heidelb* 1874–77; n.f., 2: 130–7.

2. Sever JW. Obstetric paralysis. *Am J Dis Child* 1916; 12: 541.

3. Sever JW. The results of a new operation for obstetrical paralysis. *Am J Orthop Surg* 1918; 16: 248–57.

4. Fairbank HAT. Birth palsy: subluxation of the shoulder joint in infants and young children. *Lancet* 1913; 1: 1217.

5. Bateman JE. *The shoulder and environs*. St Louis: Mosby, 1955.

Illustrations by Gillian Oliver after B. Hyams

Rupture of the biceps

B. Helal   MChOrth, FRCS
Honorary Consultant Orthopaedic Surgeon, The Royal London Hospital and The Royal National Orthopaedic Hospital, London, and Enfield Group of Hospitals, UK

S. C. Chen   FRCS
Consultant Orthopaedic Surgeon, Enfield Group of Hospitals, UK

Introduction

Rupture of the biceps occurs at one of two sites: rupture of the long head of biceps affects the elderly patient, while rupture of the distal tendon of biceps is a lesion of the young.

RUPTURE OF LONG HEAD

This usually causes very little disability in the elderly patient, as the short head of the biceps and the brachialis muscle are intact and can take over elbow flexion. The flexors of the forearm also contribute to this. However, there is some loss of muscle power, as about half the biceps muscle is made inactive by the rupture of the long head. There is, in addition, a slight cosmetic disfigurement as the biceps muscle becomes bunched up in the lower part of the upper arm. In patients who lead a robust life and need normal muscle power, it is necessary to reattach the long head, usually to the short head.

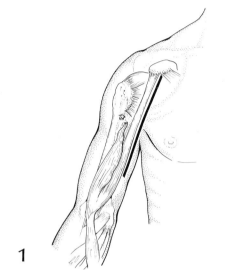

1

Operation

The elbow is kept flexed at 90° during the operation, to relax the long head of the biceps.

Incision

1

An incision is made along the medial border of the biceps muscle from the tip of the coracoid process to the middle of the upper arm.

Repair

2

The ruptured long head of the biceps is searched for and is usually found crumpled up in the lower and lateral part of the muscle belly of the biceps.

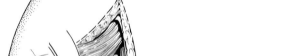

2

3

The short head of the biceps which is attached, with the coracobrachialis, to the tip of the coracoid process is identified. The long head is pulled proximally until the lateral belly feels the same in consistency as the medial belly of the biceps. The long head is anchored to the short head using three non-absorbable sutures.

3

Postoperative management

4

The arm is nursed in a loop sling for 3 weeks. Passive exercise to the shoulder and elbow is started after 1 week.

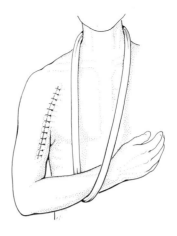

4

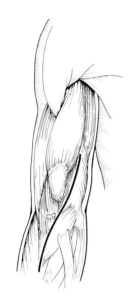

5

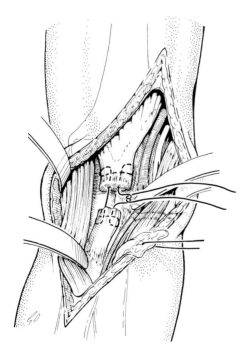

6

RUPTURE OF DISTAL TENDON

Unlike rupture of the long head, which usually occurs in the older patient and is due to some degeneration of the tendon, rupture of the distal tendon of the biceps occurs in the fit young man after strenuous activity. This lesion results in significant weakness and must therefore be repaired.

Operation

Incision

5

A lazy-S incision is made across the front of the elbow.

Repair

6

The median nerve and brachial artery must be identified. The ruptured ends of the distal tendon of the biceps are located. If these ends are not shredded, an end-to-end anastomosis of the tendons is performed with the forearm in supination to facilitate easier approximation.

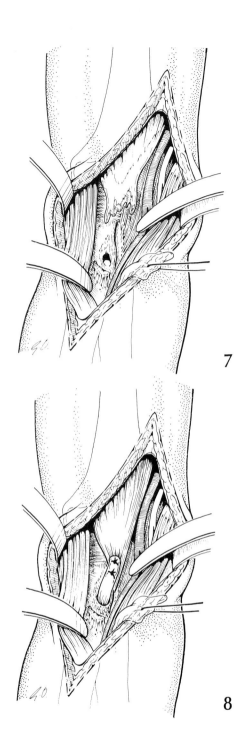

7 & 8

If the tendon ends are frayed, a drill hole is made in the upper end of the radius as near as possible to the bicipital tuberosity. The tendon is threaded through the drill hole and sutured back on itself using non-absorbable sutures.

7

8

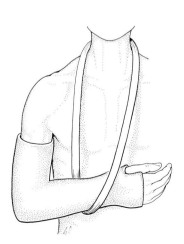

9

Postoperative management

9

An above-elbow plaster cast is applied to include the wrist and hand. This is removed at the end of 3 weeks and gentle mobilization exercises to the elbow are started.

Illustrations by Peter Cox after P. G. Jack

Arthroplasty of the shoulder

Alan Lettin MS, FRCS
Consultant Orthopaedic Surgeon, St Bartholomew's Hospital and Royal National Orthopaedic Hospital, London, UK

Introduction

Indications

Arthroplasty of the shoulder is usually performed to relieve pain and restore a functional range of movement to patients suffering from pain and stiffness of the glenohumeral joint resulting from rheumatoid arthritis, post-traumatic arthritis or primary osteoarthritis. Arthroplasty may also be performed as a primary procedure for fractures and fracture-dislocations of the head of the humerus when they are unsuited to other methods of treatment.

The proximal part of the humerus may also be replaced using a special custom-made prosthesis for resectable tumours.

There are three types of arthroplasty: (1) excision arthroplasty, (2) hemiarthroplasty and (3) total replacement arthroplasty which is either constrained or unconstrained.

Excision arthroplasty

This is occasionally performed as a primary procedure following severe fractures and fracture-dislocations of the head of the humerus, when the rotator cuff is disrupted and the fragments of bone are too comminuted to allow satisfactory reduction and internal fixation. Although an excellent range of passive movement is frequently possible after the operation, active movement is usually poor because of the lack of a stable fulcrum, and movement is frequently painful.

Excision of the head of the humerus and the glenoid may occasionally be employed in the primary treatment of arthritic shoulders, but this has the same disadvantages.

Excision arthroplasty may be necessary when a replacement arthroplasty fails. As a secondary procedure it gives more satisfactory results because the stability of the false joint is improved by the excessive fibrous tissue which forms following the failure of the primary operation.

Hemiarthroplasty

Replacement of the head of the humerus (e.g. with a Neer prosthesis[1]) is best reserved for the early treatment of severe fractures and fracture-dislocations, when the rotator cuff is intact or capable of repair. Without the stability afforded by a functioning rotator cuff, the prosthesis subluxates superiorly on the glenoid and gives a poor result. It is usually unsatisfactory in rheumatoid arthritis.

Total replacement arthroplasty

Total replacement arthroplasty was introduced into modern surgical practice in 1969[2,3]. There are now several prostheses available but basically they fall into two groups, constrained and unconstrained.

In the first group, the glenoid may be replaced by a cup and the head of the humerus by a ball which articulates in the cup (e.g. Stanmore); or the ball is attached to the scapula and the cup is contained by the upper end of the humerus (e.g. Kessel).

The unconstrained replacements (e.g. Neer II) use an anatomically shaped humeral component of appropriate size to replace the head of the humerus and a shallow saucer-shaped ultra-high molecular weight polyethylene component to resurface the glenoid.

Because of their inherent stability, constrained replacements provide a stable fulcrum for muscle action and are not dependent on the rotator cuff for stability. They are therefore more suitable for the treatment of pain and limitation of movement resulting from severe rheumatoid and other forms of arthritis, when the rotator cuff is destroyed and cannot be repaired. When the rotator cuff is intact or repairable, an unconstrained replacement is more satisfactory and is less likely to become loose.

Even without an intact rotator cuff, the pain relief and movement resulting from total replacement arthroplasty are similar for the constrained and unconstrained replacements[4,5].

Preoperative

Position of patient and towelling

The patient lies supine with the affected side towards the edge of the operating table, and a firm oblong sandbag is placed between the shoulder blades. The head is towelled separately with double towels and the trunk and legs completely covered. A separate towel is firmly bandaged around the distal half of the upper arm, forearm and hand, leaving the limb free. The remaining uncovered skin may be conveniently sealed with two medium-sized adhesive drapes, which secure the towels in place.

Operation

Incision

1

The same approach to the shoulder may be used for each prosthesis. The skin and subcutaneous fat are incised from the clavicle to the anterior fold of the axilla, crossing the tip of the coracoid process of the scapula.

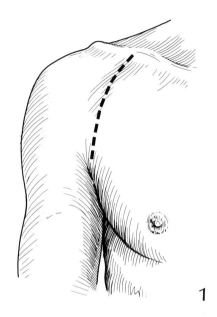

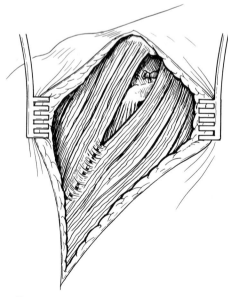

Exposure and development of deltopectoral groove

2

The subcutaneous fat is stripped from the underlying muscle by blunt dissection to expose the cephalic vein, which passes obliquely across the wound as it lies in the deltopectoral groove. This is ligated and divided at the lower margin of the wound and dissected proximally almost to the clavicle, and the tributaries are coagulated as they are divided. The proximal end of the vein is ligated and divided just below the clavicle before it disappears through the clavipectoral fascia. The free segment of the vein is removed to avoid troublesome bleeding later in the operation.

Exposure and division of coracoid process

3

The pectoralis major and deltoid muscles are separated with a self-retaining retractor. When absolutely necessary, exposure may be improved by detaching the clavicular portion of the deltoid from the clavicle as far laterally as the acromioclavicular joint, leaving sufficient muscle attached to the bone to hold sutures during closure. The coracoacromial ligament is divided. Then, after drilling a hole of 3 mm diameter along the centre of the coracoid process to facilitate later reattachment, it is resected with an osteotome or Gigli saw proximal to its muscle attachments.

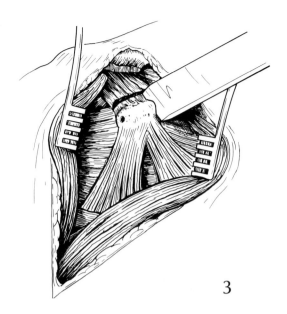

3

4

Division of subscapularis and exposure of joint

4

The upper and lower borders of the subscapularis muscle are identified and marked with stay sutures just lateral to the musculotendinous junction. The identification of the lower border is facilitated by the presence of one or more veins running parallel to it. These should be coagulated. The upper margin may be difficult to define. In rheumatoid arthritis, proliferating synovium frequently bulges over the upper border of the subscapularis. The subscapularis is divided through the tendinous part just lateral to the stay sutures and retracted medially. The underlying capsule cannot always be identified as a separate layer, but when it is a definite entity it is also divided and retracted with the muscle.

The supraspinatus or its remnants are identified. If present, they should be separated from the undersurface of the acromion by blunt dissection.

Resection of humeral head and exposure of glenoid

5

The head of the humerus is dislocated forward out of the wound and resected at the level of the articular margin with an osteotome or power saw. If the supraspinatus is intact, this leaves its attachment to the greater tuberosity undisturbed. When the head of the humerus is badly affected by disease then the articular margin may not be clear. When the Neer II prosthesis is used, the trial humeral component is laid alongside the humeral head to enable the level of resection to be marked; this lies at the maximum diameter of the bone. The bone is cut obliquely so the cut face is retroverted 30°–40° with respect to the plane of the humeral condyles and 45° to the long axis of the shaft (see *illustration 8b*). Care should be taken not to remove too much bone.

In the case of a severely comminuted fracture which cannot be reconstructed, the fragments are removed and the humerus trimmed as near as possible to the ideal plane of resection.

For excision arthroplasty no more need be done.

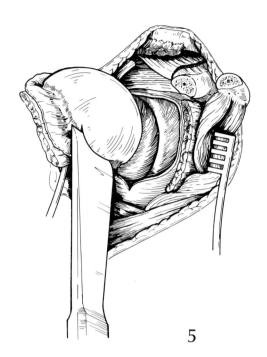

5

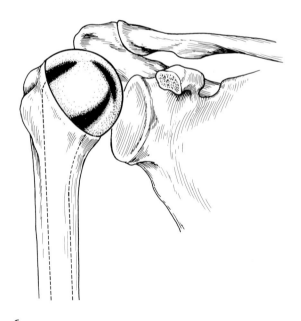

6

Preparation of the humerus and replacement of head of humerus alone

6

The medullary cavity at the centre of the cut surface is located and the loose cancellous bone removed with a curette from the upper end of the humerus; the debris is washed out. The prosthesis selected should have a medullary stem which fits the canal, and a head diameter equal to the diameter of the cut surface. After trial reduction, the prosthesis is cemented into place or left as a push-fit according to personal preference.

When a total replacement is to be used, excavation of the humerus is best left until after the glenoid has been prepared.

STANMORE PROSTHESIS

Preparation of glenoid

7

The resected humerus is returned to the wound and retracted laterally to expose the posterior capsule, which is divided along the margin of the glenoid. The tip of a Bankart retractor is slipped under the posterior lip of the glenoid to give access to the glenoid. This is much easier when the rotator cuff is degenerate or disrupted, but if intact it may be divided if exposure of the glenoid or the subsequent insertion of the prosthesis is unduly difficult.

The margins of the glenoid are defined carefully for the glenoid may appear to be much enlarged as a result of osteophyte formation. Any residual articular cartilage and the subchondral bone are carefully removed with a Capener gouge, leaving the rim of the glenoid intact. The underlying cancellous bone is removed carefully with a gouge and a sharp curette or powered burr to create as big a cavity as possible. The thick bar of bone in the lateral border of the scapula is excavated from within the inferior lip of the glenoid using Paton's burrs of increasing diameter and a small curette. The index finger of the non-dominant hand is placed on the costal surface of the lateral border of the scapula to give direction to the instrument. The cavity is made of sufficient size to take the inferior anchoring prong of the prosthesis.

The cancellous bone is removed from within the base of the coracoid process with a curette. Sometimes it is possible to create a shallow third hole in the spine of the scapula in the depth of the main cavity. These holes are to key the cement.

Trial reduction

8a & b

The inferior prong of the glenoid component of the prosthesis (right or left as appropriate) is inserted into the inferior keyhole and then the cup is tilted backwards into the cavity of the glenoid. The inferior lip of the cup should rest on the inferior margin of the glenoid, and the plane of the face of the cup should be in the line of the lateral border of the scapula. The cup cannot be completely contained by the glenoid but the upper prongs can be shortened if necessary to allow the cup to drop back into the cavity until it rests on the rim of the glenoid.

The humeral component of the prosthesis is inserted into the prepared cavity in the upper end of the humerus with the arm extended and laterally rotated. The plateau of the prosthesis rests on the cut surface of the humerus, and if the line of resection is correct, the head will be retroverted 30°–40° with respect to the humeral condyles. It is difficult to articulate the two components before they are cemented into place but it is possible to determine whether reduction will be possible without the need for resection of more bone from the upper end of the humerus.

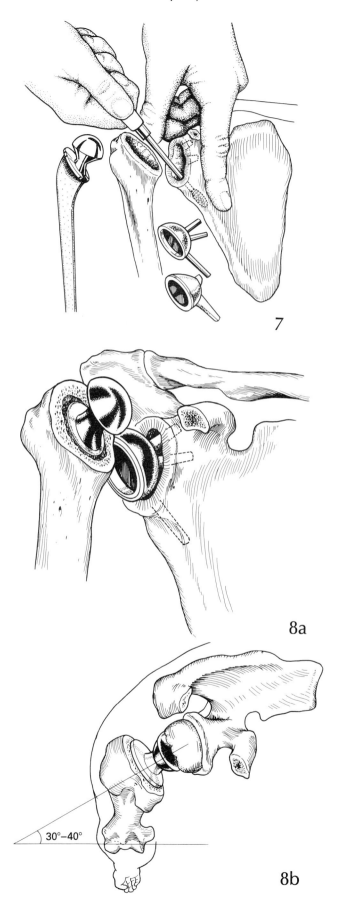

7

8a

30°–40°

8b

Insertion of the prosthesis

9

Debris is washed from the prepared glenoid cavity which should be made as dry as possible before being packed with acrylic cement. Care should be taken to ensure that the cement packs into the keyholes. The prosthesis is inserted as before, making sure that the inferior prong passes into the cavity in the lateral border of the scapula. While the prosthesis is held firmly in place with the tip of the index finger, excess cement is moulded around the cup to provide a smooth finish. The wound is flooded with cold saline until the cement is hard. Any excess cement is removed with bone nibblers. The medullary cavity of the humerus is packed with cement and the humeral component of the prosthesis is inserted; it may then be finally tapped home.

The two components can be articulated when the cement is hard by medial rotation of the arm and direct pressure on the upper end of the humerus. The components can be felt to snap together and resist distraction as the polythene retaining ring in the rim of the cup grips the head. If this is not the case it is usually due to a film of fluid or flap of soft tissue in the cup.

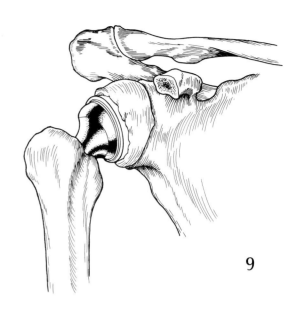

9

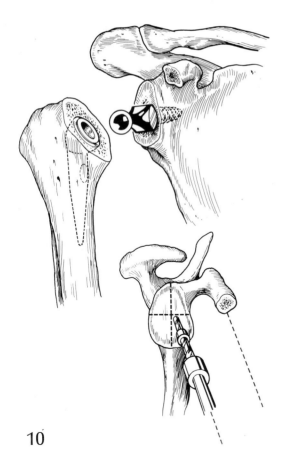

10

KESSEL PROSTHESIS

Preparation of glenoid and insertion of prosthesis

10

The glenoid is exposed as before. A hole is drilled into the scapula with a 6mm twist drill, starting at a point just anterior and inferior to the centre of the glenoid. This starting point should be located with care after defining the true margin of the glenoid. The drill is directed in a line parallel to the axis of the coracoid process and so enters the thickest part of the scapula. The entrance of the hole is enlarged with the special countersinking tool. A trial reduction is carried out with the non-threaded glenoid component and the plastic humeral component as a prelude to any final adjustments to the resected humerus. It is impossible to alter the position of the glenoid component once the hole has been drilled because of the thin cross-section of the scapula. The threaded glenoid component is screwed into place with a special spanner and the humeral component cemented into the prepared cavity at the upper end of the humerus so that the rim of the socket lies flush with the resected surface. When the acrylic cement has set the components are articulated.

NEER PROSTHESIS

Preparation of glenoid and insertion of prosthesis

11a

The glenoid is exposed taking care to preserve the supraspinatus, when present. The template is placed on the glenoid so that the longitudinal slit is in line with the lateral border of the scapula. The subchondral bone is carefully perforated with a hand drill to create a series of holes the length of the slit. The template is removed and the holes joined together with bone nibblers or a powered burr.

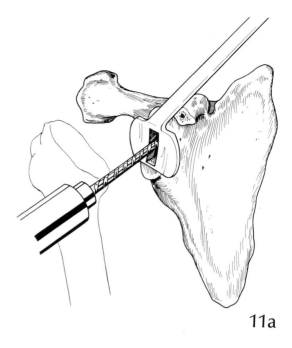

11a

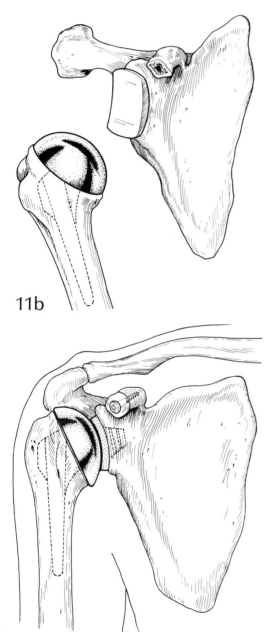

11b

11c

11b & c

The underlying bone from the glenoid is removed with a small curette or powered burr to create a cavity large enough to accommodate the keel of the glenoid component and the cement. The size of the cavity and the slit is checked with the trial prosthesis and progressively both the slit and the cavity are enlarged until the back of the trial prosthesis lies on the surface of the glenoid.

Any residual articular cartilage is carefully removed from the surface of the glenoid, leaving it roughened and irregular. The cavity is filled with cement and the real glenoid component inserted and held in place firmly until the cement sets. Surplus cement is then removed.

The upper end of the humerus is delivered from the wound and the arm is laterally rotated and extended to bring the prepared medullary cavity into view. A trial humeral component is selected with an intramedullary stem diameter which is easily accommodated and a head thickness which allows a trial reduction to be accomplished without tension on the soft tissues. The size of the prosthesis is adjusted as necessary using the larger intramedullary stems in large patients. When a satisfactory fit is achieved, the permanent prosthesis is cemented in place.

Closure

The subscapularis is repaired under slight tension with interrupted sutures. The tip of the coracoid process is reattached with a single screw or by sutures should it split. The clavicular portion of the deltoid is sutured to the clavicle if necessary and the deltopectoral groove closed before suture of the subcutaneous fat and skin. The arm is bandaged to the chest wall over a layer of cotton wool, with hand directed towards the opposite shoulder.

Postoperative management

After 24 hours the suction drains (if used) are removed. There is rarely any significant blood loss. A radiograph is taken of the shoulder through the dressing to confirm the satisfactory position of the prosthesis.

The bulky dressings are removed after 3–4 days and the arm supported in a sling. The sling is removed intermittently for pendulum exercises over the next 24–48 hours. Then passive flexion and extension exercises are begun, depending on the degree of discomfort, at first under supervision and later the patient is encouraged to use the unoperated arm to mobilize the operated shoulder. After 7–10 days isometric exercises against resistance are started to improve the tone of all muscle groups, the sling is discarded and the patient discharged from hospital. Stitches are removed after 10–14 days. Lateral rotation is avoided for 3–4 weeks. Movements slowly improve for 3–6 months after the operation with assiduous exercises, depending on the underlying condition and the state of the rotator cuff.

Complications

Dislocation

Dislocation may occur, especially whilst the muscles are atonic immediately after operation. Closed reduction is usually possible and in the case of late dislocation should be followed up by a further period of immobilization.

Loosening

If loosening of the prosthesis occurs it may be possible to replace it. The remaining bone adjacent to the glenoid usually proves inadequate for fixation, however, and coversion to an excision arthroplasty is preferable. Both components may be removed through the original incision, together with any loose cement or bone, leaving two flat surfaces. The soft tissues are carefully repaired and the abundant fibrous tissue, which is usually present, is left undisturbed. Postoperative management after excision arthroplasty is similar to that after replacement arthroplasty.

References

1. Neer CS. Articular replacement for the humeral head. *J Bone Joint Surg [Am]* 1955; 37-A: 215–28.

2. Lettin AWF, Scales JT. Total replacement of the shoulder joint. *Proc R Soc Med* 1972; 65: 373–4.

3. Lettin AWF, Scales JT. Total replacement arthroplasty of the shoulder in rheumatoid arthritis. *J Bone Joint Surg [Br]* 1973; 55-B: 217.

4. Lettin AWF. Total shoulder replacement in rheumatoid arthritis. In: Kölbel R, Helbig B, Blouth W, eds. *Shoulder replacement*. Berlin: Springer-Verlag, 1987: 103–11.

5. Kelly IG, Forster RS, Fisher WD. Neer total shoulder replacement in rheumatoid arthritis. *J Bone Joint Surg [Br]* 1987; 69-B: 723–6.

Arthrodesis of the shoulder

The late **Sir Henry Osmond-Clarke,** *KCVO*, *CBE*, FRCS(I), FRCS(Eng)
Former Orthopaedic Surgeon to Her Majesty Queen Elizabeth II; Consulting Orthopaedic Surgeon, The Royal London Hospital, London and Robert Jones and Agnes Hunt Orthopaedic Hospital, Oswestry, UK

Introduction

Indications

Arthrodesis of the shoulder is undertaken mainly for inflammatory conditions such as tuberculosis, much more rarely than formerly for paralytic lesions and rarely for osteoarthritis or rheumatoid arthritis of the shoulder, for gross injuries and after the resection of benign neoplasms.

The shoulder may be approached either from the front (or anterosuperiorly) or from behind.

Contraindications

Distraction at the shoulder joint The posterior operation should not be done for paralytic lesions of the shoulder unless it is combined with intra-articular ablation of the joint and fixation of the humeral head to the glenoid by pin or screw, otherwise the graft may act as a fulcrum about which the head of the humerus is levered out of the glenoid.

Preoperative

Position of patient

Anterior approach The patient lies on the back with a small sandbag under the scapula and buttock so that he is slightly tilted towards the opposite side.

Posterior approach The patient lies prone with the face turned towards the opposite side and the affected arm hanging over the edge of the table. The body part of a plaster of Paris shoulder spica should have been applied some days previously.

Anaesthesia

General anaesthesia with an endotracheal tube is satisfactory.

Operations

ANTERIOR OPERATION

Incision

1

The incision is like that used for recurrent dislocation of the shoulder (see p. 676) except that it is extended backwards to a point behind the posterior margin of the acromion.

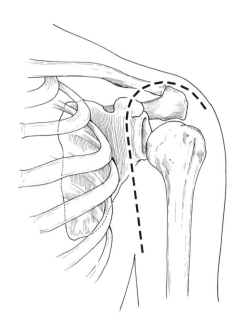

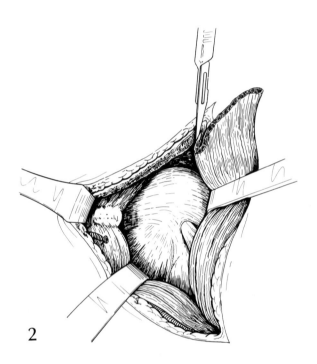

Exposure

2

The deltopectoral groove is identified and the same procedure carried out as in the similar stage of the Putti–Platt capsulorrhaphy (see p. 679). The cephalic vein is tied, and the deltoid muscle is detached from its clavicular attachment and from the anterior two-thirds of its acromial attachment. This exposes the coracoid process, the musculotendinous cuff and capsule and the long tendon of the biceps.

Division of capsule

3

The transverse humeral ligament and the capsule above it are divided longitudinally to free the tendon of the biceps.

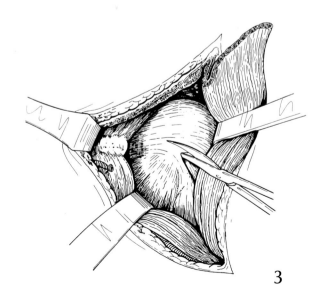

Entry into joint

4

The tendon of the biceps is retracted forwards and the musculotendinous cuff and capsule are divided transversely, opening up the shoulder joint.

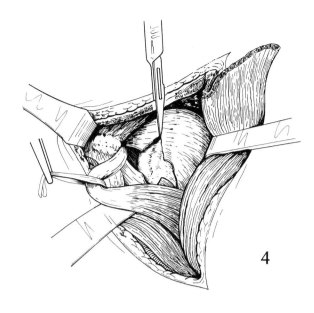

4

5

Preparation of bony surfaces

5

With a gouge the joint surfaces are thoroughly rawed, all the remains of the cartilage and sclerotic bone being removed to expose bleeding cancellous bone.

Positioning of arm

6

The humeral head is placed in contact with the glenoid and the arm is held in the position that will ensure optimum function. This is in fact the position which allows the patient to get his hand to his mouth and allows the arm to come to the side in repose. In an adult it amounts to 40° of abduction, 15°–25° of forward flexion and 25°–30° of medial rotation. An adolescent can be allowed about 50° of abduction because of the greater mobility of the scapula.

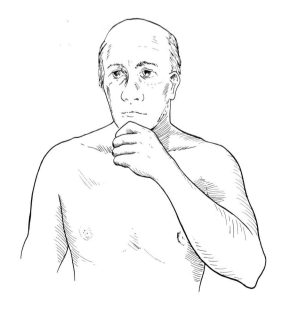

6

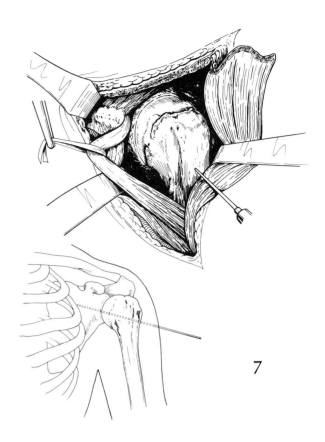

Insertion of guide wire

7

While the above position is carefully maintained by an assistant a guide wire is inserted from the outer aspect of the humerus at an angle of about 60° so that it penetrates the humeral head and the glenoid; it should be directed upwards and backwards. Its position is checked by radiographs.

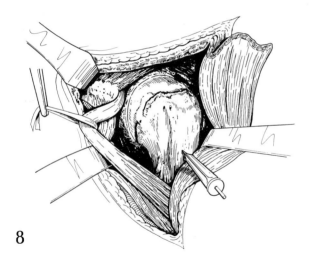

Insertion of Smith-Petersen nail

8

When a satisfactory position of the guide wire has been achieved a cannulated Smith-Petersen nail is driven over the wire and firmly impacted. Alternatively, one or two lag compression screws may be used. The wire is removed.

Reinforcement of arthrodesis

9

The arthrodesis is reinforced by bending the rawed acromion downwards and inserting it into a notch cut in the humerus.

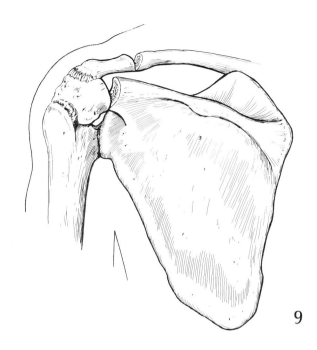

9

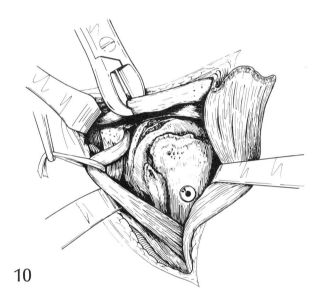

10

Mobilization of acromion

The above manoeuvre is facilitated by partly dividing the clavicle and the spine of the scapula. The soft tissue attachments should be left intact to ensure an adequate blood supply and to preserve a reasonably stable 'hinge'.

10

Part-division of clavicle   The clavicle is partially divided by means of bone-cutting forceps.

11

Part-division of scapula   The spine of the scapula is cut with bone-cutting forceps.

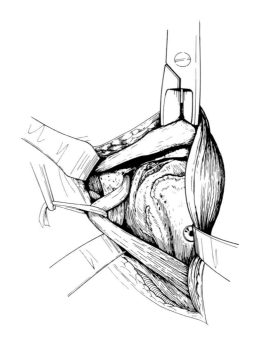

11

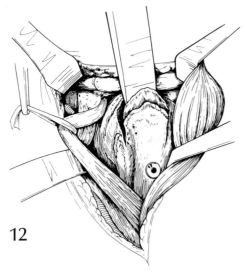

12

Formation of notch in humerus

12

The notch in the humerus is made by inserting a chisel from above downwards and fracturing the greater tuberosity outwards.

Completion

13

The outer parts of the clavicle and acromion are bent down into the gap formed by the outwardly levered tuberosity. One or two sutures keep them in snug contact. The wound is closed in layers.

Alternative techniques

Other techniques are in use. Some surgeons prefer to use a lag-screw rather than a Smith-Petersen triflanged nail. Others, notably Charnley and DePalma, describe the use of compression by Steinmann pins passed through the clavicle and acromion above and the neck of the humerus below.

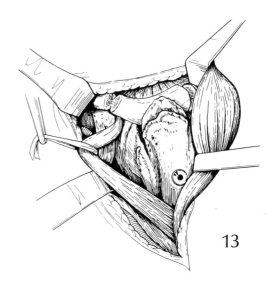

13

THE POSTERIOR OPERATION

14

The aim of the operation is to insert a tibial graft, cut as illustrated, between the scapula and the humerus about 5 cm below the shoulder joint. It has been claimed by Brittain[1], the originator of this operation, that the compression force exerted by the arm constantly tending to adduct ensures more certain union than other methods.

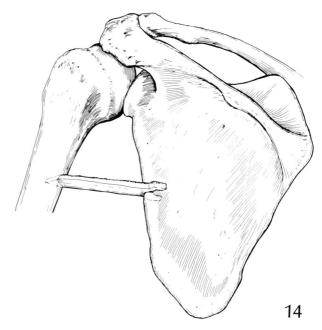

14

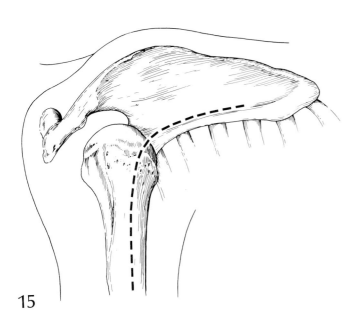

15

Incision

15

A curved incision is made, beginning near the lowest third of the scapula and extending along the axillary border and down the arm for about 10 cm.

Exposure

16

The incision is carried down through the teres minor muscle onto the axillary border of the scapula. If the circumflex scapular artery is in the way it is divided and ligated. The infraspinatus behind and the subscapularis in front are stripped from the scapula sufficiently to allow a notch to be made in the bone with nibbling forceps.

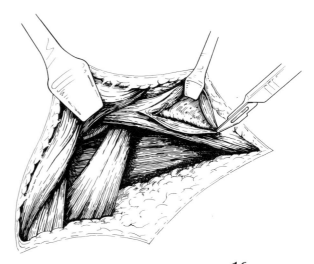

16

Notching of scapula and drilling of humerus

17

When the axillary border has been notched, the posterior border of the deltoid is retracted and the lateral and medial heads of the triceps are split to expose the shaft of the humerus just below its surgical neck. A suitable hole is drilled in the humerus; its position and direction are determined with due regard to the length of the graft (cut from the subcutaneous surface of the tibia at the beginning of the operation) and the correct positioning of the arm.

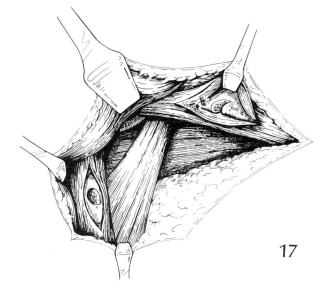

17

Insertion of graft

18

The graft is embedded firmly in both bones. It is usually easier to place it in the humerus first and then by manoeuvring the arm to coax the other end into the slot in the scapula. The wound is closed in layers.

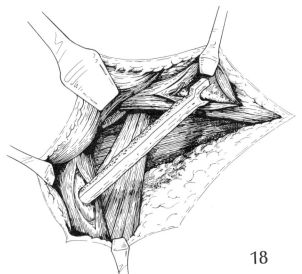

18

Postoperative management

ANTERIOR OPERATION

A plaster of Paris shoulder spica is applied; this is not easy on the anaesthetized patient, and it is therefore wise to remove the plaster and the sutures after about 2 weeks and to apply a fresh, snugly fitting spica which should be retained until union has occurred, usually in about 3–4 months. When the arthrodesis is firm the patient begins a course of exercises to mobilize the scapula on the chest wall and to restore the greatest possible function to the arm.

POSTERIOR OPERATION

The patient is carefully turned, and plaster of Paris is applied to the arm and connected with the previously applied body plaster to form a shoulder spica. Stitches are removed in about 2 weeks and a snugly fitting spica is applied; special care must be taken at this stage to avoid disturbing the attachments of the graft. The plaster must be worn for not less than 4 months because this graft takes a considerable time to revascularize.

Reference

1. Brittain HA. *Architectural principles in arthrodesis*. 2nd ed. Edinburgh and London: Livingstone, 1952: 168.

Illustrations by Peter Cox

Prosthetic replacement of the elbow

Thomas P. Sculco MD
Associate Director, Department of Orthopaedic Surgery, The Hospital for Special Surgery, New York, USA

Philip M. Faris MD
Clinical Associate Professor, Louisana State University Medical Center, USA

Introduction

The evolution of elbow arthroplasty has progressed from interposition arthroplasty to metal-to-metal uniaxial hinges to semiconstrained metal to polyethylene hinges and metal-to-polyethylene resurfacing arthroplasty[1]. Resection and interpositional arthroplasties, using organic and inorganic materials, have been attempted for degenerative disease of the elbow with varied success[2–6]. Because of this unpredictability, especially related to residual pain and instability, interposition arthroplasty has been virtually abandoned except for use in patients with haemophilia[7] and in the salvage of failed elbow prostheses.

In the mid 1950s, experimentation with hemiarthroplasty began[8–12]. The proximal olecranon, radial head, and distal humerus all were independently replaced using metal components with acrylic or metal stems. These were fixed to bone with screws, wires, or sleeves to attain mechanical fixation; results were mixed. With the introduction of methylmethacrylate, the problem of fixation to bone seemed lessened and further development ensued. In 1972, Dee[13] described a metal-to-metal hinge arthroplasty using methylmethacrylate and intramedullary fixation. Other similar hinges were developed by Scales, McKee, Shiers, and others during this period; their designs had varying success with short and intermediate follow-up[1].

As the understanding of the biomechanics of the elbow increased, prosthetic designs developed to give (1) the semiconstrained or sloppy hinge and (2) the unconstrained or resurfacing design. Examples of semiconstrained prostheses are the Coonrad, Mayo, Pritchard–Walker, Triaxial, and Volz. Examples of the unconstrained prostheses are the Ewald, London, Kudo, Liverpool, and Souter.

Biomechanics of the elbow joint

Analysis of elbow kinematics has developed slowly compared to data available on the knee and hip. Morrey and Chao[14] in 1976, presented a complex kinematic analysis of cadaveric elbows and confirmed Fisher's[15] observation that the axis of elbow flexion is fixed and localized to the centre of the trochlea. This axis must also be oriented in an oblique fashion relative to the humeral axis, allowing the carrying angle to change from approximately 10° of valgus in extension to 5° of varus in full elbow flexion. Axial rotation of the forearm occurred during elbow flexion and extension. In this study, the ulna was essentially fixed during axial rotation.

The variation in carrying angle from valgus in extension to varus in flexion was disputed by London[16] in 1981. He felt that this finding was erroneously based on an axis through the condyles at a right angle to the humeral shaft. When the axis of movement was defined as perpendicular to the plane of the trochlear sulcus, then flexion/extension of the humeroulnar and humeroradial joints is uniplanar. Instant centres were localized to the arc of the trochlear sulcus except in the last 5°–10° of extension when the instant centre moved toward the olecranon fossa, and in flexion when the instant centre moved toward the coronoid fossa. Similar variation was seen in the humero-radial joint.

The range of elbow movement required for activities of daily living has been elucidated by Morrey et al.[17] using a triaxial electrogoniometer. Ranges required varied from 15° of flexion for tying shoes to 140° for reaching the occiput. Total rotation required was 100° with 50° of supination needed for personal hygiene.

Although the elbow is not a weight-bearing joint as are the knee and hip, the forces acting across the joint are significant. Under physiological stress (i.e. lifting an 11 kg weight) forces of greater than body weight are predicted at 90° of flexion and increase to three times body weight at 20° of flexion[11]. Further increases in force occur as full extension is approached, as the forearm pronates, and as rapid acceleration is introduced. The direction of the forces applied is mostly shear at 90° of flexion and becomes more axial with increasing extension. Twisting moments about the humerus are also high, depending upon the activity for which the arm is used.

In summary, many factors must be considered in the design of an elbow prosthesis, including (1) adequate range of movement, (2) restoration of normal centres of rotation, and (3) twisting forces acting upon the joint.

Current design

The triaxial prosthesis, which has been used at The Hospital for Special Surgery since 1975, is a 'sloppy hinge' allowing 10°–12° of varus/valgus freedom and 4°–6° of rotational movement besides full flexion and extension. Some minor modifications in the original design have been made to improve its resistance to dislocation and fracture and to increase its component–bone–cement composite strength. Currently, the device consists of cobalt–chrome ulnar and humeral components with the humeral component having a built-in 7° valgus carrying angle. Articulation is via a polyethylene bearing interposed between the metallic humeral and ulnar components. The articulation, then, is a metal-to-polyethylene interaction which maintains its 'sloppiness' under a 65 newton compressive force. A distraction force of 49.5 newtons is required to disarticulate the components.

In a recent report, Inglis et al.[18] reported the 2–9 year results (mean 5 years) on 61 patients with 73 triaxial total elbow prostheses. The average arc of flexion was 28° to 125° with pronation of 68° and supination of 60°. Forty-six elbows were rated excellent, 18 good, 2 fair, and 7 were poor results. There were no cases of aseptic loosening, component migration, or circumferential progressive radiolucent lines. There were 16 major complications including infection in 3, persistent nerve palsies in 3, skin slough in 2, condylar fractures in 3, and dislocation in 5 elbow prostheses. The current design displayed a lower dislocation rate than the earlier axle design. Continuing design modifications are aimed at reducing the incidence of dislocations and improving load-transfer characteristics.

Indications

1. Pain is the chief indication for elbow arthroplasty.
2. Rheumatoid arthritis and juvenile rheumatoid arthritis are indications for which arthroplasty produces good results.
3. Degenerative, post-traumatic and ankylosed elbows give less satisfactory results.

Neither limitation of movement nor instability have shown marked improvement after arthroplasty.

Contraindications

Relative contraindications include previous elbow sepsis, severe bone loss, insufficient soft tissue coverage, absent triceps and/or biceps function, and poor wrist and hand function.

Operation

INSERTION OF THE TRIAXIAL PROSTHESIS

Position of patient

The patient is placed in a 45° lateral decubitus position with a sandbag placed beneath the ipsilateral shoulder.

Incision

1

A longitudinal incision, curved gently on the ulnar side of the olecranon, is begun approximately 7 cm proximal to the olecranon and carried 7 cm distal to the olecranon tip.

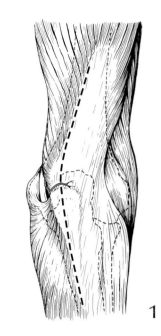

Dissection

The ulnar nerve is isolated near its exit from beneath the medial head of the triceps, dissected free from the cubital tunnel, and cleared distally to its first muscular branch. The ulnar nerve is isolated and retracted using a 6 mm Penrose drain held with a suture, not a haemostat, as this may produce undue traction on the nerve.

Exposure

2

The distal humerus is exposed subperiosteally through the medial intramuscular septum. The fascia of the flexor carpi ulnaris is incised longitudinally 1 cm medial to the ulnar crest. The fascial incision connects, in continuity, with the triceps incision. It is carried through the flexor carpi ulnaris directly to the ulna. The fascia and periosteum, along with the triceps insertion, are elevated sharply from the ulna and olecranon. Extreme care must be taken to keep the triceps muscle, triceps insertion, and ulnar periosteum in continuity. Elbow extension allows relaxation of these tissues. Further subperiosteal elevation of the anconeus provides access to the radial head, which is resected just proximal to the orbicular ligament. Because of the intrinsic stability of the triaxial prosthesis, the ulnar collateral ligament may be released from the medial humeral condyle, and the elbow will remain stable.

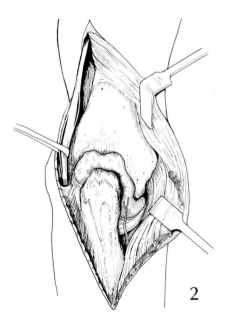

Complete capsulectomy is performed. The anterior ulna is cleared of soft tissue to the coronoid process or beyond if necessary for flexion contracture release. Commonly an osteophyte is present at the coronoid process and this is removed. It is particularly important to release soft tissue contractures from the coronoid to allow the ulna to be brought anterior to the humerus in full flexion. This is necessary to reduce the prosthetic components. The anterior humerus is likewise cleared of contracted soft tissue to allow complete elbow extension. All osteophytes are removed, especially along the medial and lateral olecranon.

Preparation for prosthesis

3a & b

Bone cuts are begun after adequate soft tissue release. The trial ulnar component is superimposed over the olecranon process and a rectangular cut is outlined using methylene blue. The ulnar intramedullary canal is located and the mouth of the canal is opened and shaped using the intramedullary broach and a high-speed burr. Trial placement of the ulnar component is performed and the olecranon is repetitively shaped until the ulnar component fit is snug and its centre of rotation corresponds with the anatomical centre.

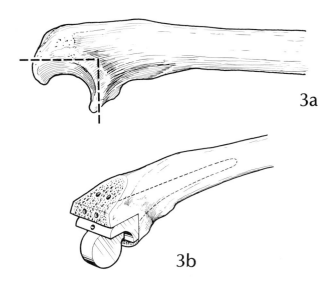

3a

3b

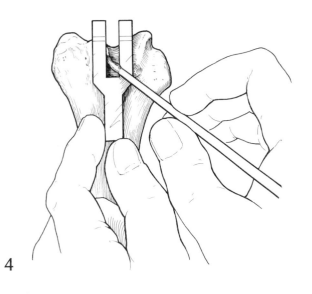

4

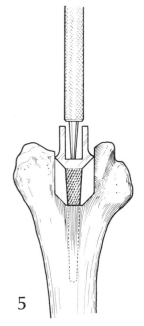

5

4

The humeral trial component is superimposed posteriorly over the humeral condyles. The posterior humeral surface must be adequately visualized. The cuts are outlined with methylene blue with the depth of cut fashioned to recreate the centre of rotation. It must be appreciated that the humeral medullary canal is slightly lateral to the centre of the trochlea and if the humeral cut is too far medial, fracture of the medial epicondyle may occur.

5

All cuts are made using a micro-oscillating saw. Broaches are provided for humeral and ulnar components. After all cuts are made and the trial components fit snugly, the trial humeral polyethylene is placed and the components are reduced in maximum flexion. Movement is tested. A full range of movement should be attained including full extension. If full extension is unobtainable, further soft tissue release anteriorly off the humerus and/or ulna is necessary. In extreme cases the humeral component may be seated more proximal in the humerus.

Insertion

The humeral and ulnar canals are plugged with bone plugs which are shaped and fitted for the canals. The canals are lavaged with pulsatile lavage and packed with methylmethacrylate. The final components are placed simultaneously and held in position. Excess methacrylate is removed and the cement is allowed to cure. The components are reduced in flexion. The elbow again is tested for stability and range of motion.

Closure

6

Three drill holes are placed in the olecranon in a medial to lateral direction and No. 1 non-absorbable sutures are placed through these holes. The triceps sleeve is reattached using the non-absorbable suture. The remainder of the fascial sleeve is then repaired over small vacuum drains. The ulnar nerve is allowed to lie in a position of least tension or compression, which may be anterior to the cubital tunnel.

Routine subcutaneous and skin closure follows and the arm is placed in 30° of flexion in a soft compressive dressing with medial and lateral plaster splints. No pressure should be allowed over the tip of the olecranon.

Postoperative management

Postoperatively, the drains are removed after 24–48 hours and prophylactic antibiotics are discontinued after 48 hours. On the fourth day, the dressing is changed and the arm is placed in a long-arm splint with a flexion-lock hinge. Movement is allowed from 30° to 90° of flexion for the first 3 weeks when the sutures are removed. The wound is watched closely and any evidence of wound inflammation, dehiscence, or necrosis requires cessation of exercises. The brace is removed at 3 weeks when strengthening and full range of movement exercises are begun.

Review of results

Semiconstrained resurfacing prostheses

To date there is a paucity of long-term clinical follow-up data available concerning resurfacing semiconstrained prostheses[19–25]. From the literature on resurfacing-type elbow replacements, the loosening rates are modest compared to hinges, pain relief is satisfactory, and restoration of function is good, but, unacceptable rates of instability, infection, and ulnar nerve palsy persist. A high proportion of these complications are soft tissue-related and, with adaptations of Bryan and Morrey's[26] triceps-sparing approach, may be diminishing.

Semiconstrained total elbow prosthesis

Beginning in 1974, several semiconstrained or 'sloppy' hinge-type prostheses were developed. Again, minimal long-term data is available concerning many of the designs currently being used (i.e. Volz, Schlein, Pritchard-Walker, Mayo, Coonrad, and Triaxial). Greater than two-year follow-up results in adequate numbers are available for the Mayo–Coonrad[27] and Triaxial[18].

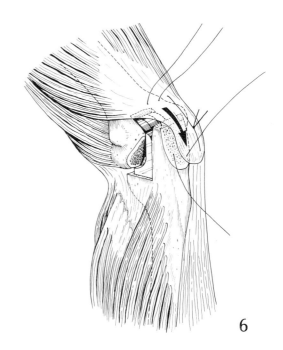

6

Complications and their treatment

Complications of elbow arthroplasty include most of those seen after other joint replacements (i.e. infection and loosening), but also include some that are more specific to elbow replacement (i.e. dislocation, skin slough, ulnar nerve neuropathy, and triceps disruption).

Infection

Overall, infections have been reported in 4–12 per cent of cases. This high rate may be due to the patient population, many of whom are steroid-dependent rheumatoid arthritics. Additionally, there is meager soft-tissue coverage at the elbow, and previously the use of the triceps tongue-type approach led to many wound problems. As in all arthroplasty surgery, deep infection carries a high morbidity. Our approach to this problem has been similar to our approach to all joint arthroplasties. We prefer implant removal, when this is possible, followed by thorough surgical debridement, 6 weeks of intravenous antibiotics (mean inhibitory concentration greater than 8:1) and reimplantation. Removal of ulnar and humeral components which are well fixed may be complex and if not performed with care may produce severe bone loss and fracture. In cases of inadequate soft tissue or bone stock, reimplantation is inadvisable and soft tissue interpositional arthroplasty is performed using external fixation. In an occasional, isolated case, when any surgical procedure might be contraindicated, *in situ* maintenance of the prosthesis using antibiotic suppression may be attempted, though is rarely successful.

Loosening

Loosening has not been a major problem with the triaxial prosthesis, occurring in only 2 per cent of cases to date. Primary revision of loose components is preferable, using custom-made long-stem prostheses. If bone stock is insufficient, then soft tissue interpositional arthroplasty is advisable. Arthrodesis is a reasonable alternative in young patients, but may be difficult to effect.

Dislocation

Dislocation of the ulnar component from the humeral polyethylene bearing may occur in two ways. It may be due to prosthetic uncoupling in extreme flexion (130°) which is rarely attained, and is treated by closed or open reduction and flexion-block orthosis. The other type of dislocation occurs later postoperatively in those very active individuals who place extreme varus/valgus rotational loads on the elbow at 90° of flexion. In this case, cold flow deformation of the polyethylene bearing progresses until the ulnar component is no longer 'captured' by the bearing and disarticulates. This complication is also uncommon and is treated by replacement of the polyethylene bearing. A yoke may be a useful addition to prevent recurrence.

Skin problems

Skin problems of major proportions have diminished significantly since development of the triceps sleeve approach. Simple areas of delayed wound healing or small eschars may be treated with changes in sterile dressing. If delay in healing persists or if skin slough is greater than 1–2 cm then skin grafting and/or muscle pedicle flap coverage may be required. Skin problems must be treated aggressively and with care as involvement deep to the prosthesis can be catastrophic and jeopardize the survival of the implant.

Neuropathy

Ulnar nerve neuropathy has been reported in 5–15 per cent of cases and most frequently is a sensory paraesthesia which resolves spontaneously. This complication is best prevented at the time of surgery by protection and gentle handling of the nerve. Anterior transposition at the time of arthroplasty is indicated if the nerve does not lie untethered in the cubital tunnel. Neurolysis and anterior transposition may be required postoperatively if symptomatic improvement does not occur over a 12-month period.

Triceps disruption

Triceps disruption, if discovered early, may be treated by extension splinting or casting for 4 weeks. When disruption is appreciated later (after 2 weeks) then reattachment or reconstruction is necessary.

Summary

Total elbow arthroplasty is an appropriate surgical procedure with good clinical results when restricted to those disease entities for which it is most successful, i.e. those patients with juvenile and adult-onset rheumatoid arthritis and osteoarthritis. All other arthropathies should be approached with caution. Current designs and techniques are improving as are the long-term results; however, the complication rate remains high. The surgical technique is demanding and attention to detail is imperative. The triceps sleeve approach, use of a prosthesis which allows the use of a soft tissue sleeve for stress distribution, recreation of the anatomical centre of rotation, and intensive postoperative rehabilitation are recommended to maximize results and minimize complications.

References

1. Coonrad RW. History of total elbow arthroplasty. In: Inglis AE, ed. *Symposium on total joint replacement of the upper extremity, New York 1979*. St Louis: Mosby, 1982: 75–90.

2. Knight RA, Van Zandt LL. Arthroplasty of the elbow: an end-result study. *J Bone Joint Surg [Am]* 1952; 34-A: 610–78.

3. Dee R, Reis M. Non-prosthetic elbow reconstruction. *Contemp Orthop*, 1987; 14(2): 37–48.

4. Murphy JB. Arthroplasty. *Ann Surg* 1913; 57: 593–647.

5. Putti V. Arthroplasty. *J Orthop Surg* 1921; 19 (old series): 419.

6. Shahriaree H, Sajadi K, Silver CM, Sheikholeslamzadeh S. Excisional arthroplasty of the elbow. *J Bone Joint Surg [Am]* 1979; 61-A: 922–7.

7. Smith MA, Savidge GF, Fountain EJ. Interposition arthroplasty in the management of advanced haemophilic arthropathy of the elbow. *J Bone Joint Surg [Br]* 1983; 65-B: 436–40.

8. Barr JS, Eaton RG. Elbow reconstruction with a new prosthesis to replace the distal end of the humerus: a case report. *J Bone Joint Surg [Am]* 1965; 47-A: 1408–13.

9. MacAusland AR. Replacement of the lower end of the humerus with a prosthesis: a report of four cases. *West J Surg* 1954; 62: 557–66.

10. Mellen RH, Phalen GS. Arthroplasty of the elbow by replacement of the distal portion of the humerus with an acrylic prosthesis. *J Bone Joint Surg* 1947; 29: 348–53.

11. Street DM, Stevens PS. A humeral replacement for the elbow: results in 10 elbows. *J Bone Joint Surg [Am]* 1974; 56-A: 1147.

12. Torzilli PA. Biomechanics of the elbow. In: Inglis AE, ed. *Symposium on total joint replacement of the upper extremity, New York 1979*. St Louis: Mosby, 1982: 150–68.

13. Dee R. Total replacement arthroplasty of the elbow for rheumatoid arthritis. *J Bone Joint Surg [Br]* 1972; 54-B: 88–95.

14. Morrey BF, Chao EYS. Passive motion of the elbow joint: a biomechanical analysis. *J Bone Joint Surg [Am]* 1976; 58-A: 501–8.

15. Fisher G, *cited by* Fick R. *Handbuch der Anatomie und Mechanik der Gelenke, unter Berichsichtigung der Bewegenden Muskeln*. 1911; 2: 299.

16. London JT. Kinematics of the elbow. *J Bone Joint Surg [Am]* 1981; 63-A: 529–35.

17. Morrey BF, Askew LJ, An KN, Chao EY. A biomechanical study of normal functional elbow motion. *J Bone Joint Surg [Am]* 1981; 63-A: 872–7.

18. Figgie HE III, Inglis AE. Current concepts in total elbow arthroplasty. *Adv Orthop Surg* 1986; 9: 195–212.

19. Ewald FC, Scheinberg RD, Poss R, Thomas WH, Scott RD, Sledge CB. Capitello-condylar total elbow arthroplasty: two to five year follow-up in rheumatoid arthritis. *J Bone Joint Surg [Am]* 1980; 62-A: 1259–63.

20. Davis RF, Weiland AJ, Hungerford DS, Moore JR, Volenec-Dowling S. Non-constrained total elbow arthroplasty. *Clin Orthop* 1982; 171: 156–60.

21. Rosenberg GM, Turner RH. Non-constrained total elbow arthroplasty. *Clin Orthop* 1984; 187: 154–62.

22. Kudo H, Iwano K, Watanabe S. Total replacement of the rheumatoid elbow with a hingeless prosthesis. *J Bone Joint Surg [Am]* 1980; 62-A: 277–85.

23. Soni RK, Cavendish ME. A review of the Liverpool elbow prosthesis from 1974 to 1982. *J Bone Joint Surg [Br]* 1984; 66-B: 248–53.

24. Pritchard RW. Anatomic surface elbow arthroplasty: a preliminary report. *Clin Orthop* 1983; 179: 223–30.

25. Roper BA, Tuke M, O'Riordan SM, Buestrode CJ. A new unconstrained elbow: a prospective review of 60 replacements. *J Bone Joint Surg [Br]* 1986; 68-B: 566–9.

26. Bryan RA, Morrey BF. Extensive posterior exposure of the elbow: a triceps sparing approach. *Clin Orthop* 1982; 166: 188–92.

27. Morrey BF, Bryan RS, Dobyns JH, Linscheid RL. Total elbow arthroplasty: a five year experience at the Mayo Clinic. *J Bone Joint Surg [Am]* 1981; 63-A: 1050–63.

Illustrations by Gillian Oliver after B. Hyams

Tendon replacement to restore elbow flexion

B. Helal MChOrth, FRCS
Honorary Consultant Orthopaedic Surgeon, The Royal London Hospital and The Royal National Orthopaedic Hospital, London, and Enfield Group of Hospitals, UK

S. C. Chen FRCS
Consultant Orthopaedic Surgeon, Enfield Group of Hospitals, UK

Introduction

Before any operation to restore elbow flexion is carried out, it is important to ensure that the hand and fingers are capable of normal function and that the muscles to be transferred have normal power. If the forearm flexor muscles are normal they can be used to restore elbow flexion. However, if they are paralysed or weak then the pectoralis major or minor, the sternomastoid, the latissimus dorsi or the triceps muscle may be used.

Operations

STEINDLER FLEXORPLASTY[1, 2]

1

To assess whether the forearm flexor muscles are capable of flexing the elbow, the shoulder is abducted to 90° and with the forearm supinated the patient attempts to flex the extended elbow. If this can be performed the muscles are strong enough for transfer.

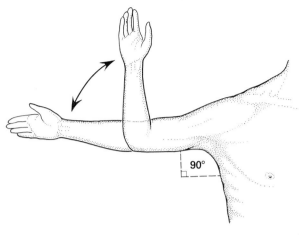

1

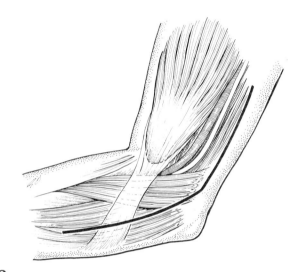

2

Incision

2

A curved incision is made over the medial side of the elbow starting from about 7.5 cm above the medial epicondyle and ending on the anterior surface of the forearm.

Mobilization of flexor muscles

3

The ulnar nerve is identified behind the medial epicondyle and it is retracted backwards. The medial epicondyle is osteotomized with the common flexor origin.

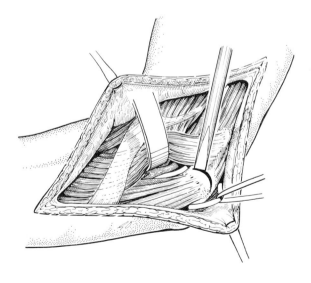

3

4

The humeral head of pronator teres, flexor carpi radialis, palmaris longus, flexor digitorum sublimis and flexor carpi ulnaris are freed for about 5 cm distally. An area of the humerus is freshened with an osteotome about 5–7.5 cm proximal to the medial epicondyle.

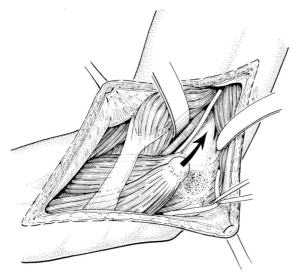

4

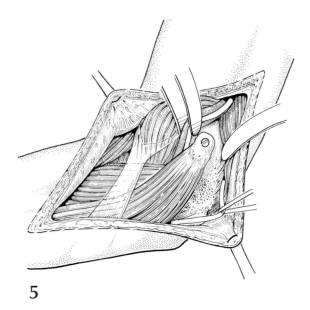

5

Reattachment of common flexor origin

5

A point on the medial side of the humerus is chosen such that, when the common flexor origin is brought up to it, the elbow will be flexed about 45°. A screw is used to fix the detached medial epicondyle onto this area of the humerus.

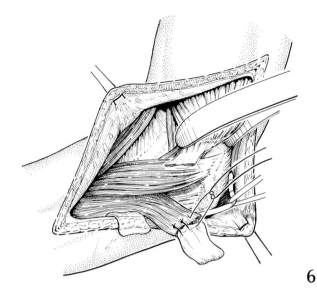

6

Bunnell's modification of Steindler flexorplasty[3]

6, 7 & 8

The main disadvantage of the Steindler flexorplasty is that the forearm becomes pronated during elbow flexion and the patient may even develop a pronation contracture of the forearm. Bunnell's modification eliminates this problem. Instead of fixing the detached medial epicondyle on the medial side of the humerus, the common flexor origin is detached without osteotomizing the medial epicondyle. The common flexor origin is lengthened with a graft of fascia lata. This is advanced 5 cm up the lateral side of the humerus. It is attached by raising an osteoplastic flap and suturing the fascia lata graft under the flap. The point of attachment should be the same as for the Steindler flexorplasty.

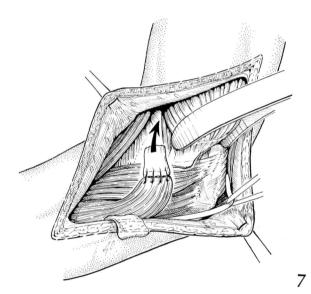

7

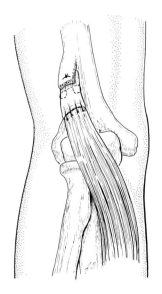

8

Postoperative management

9

An above-elbow cast is applied with the elbow in 80° of flexion and the forearm in mid-pronation. At the end of 6 weeks, the plaster cast is removed and gradual mobilizing exercises are started – both passive and active.

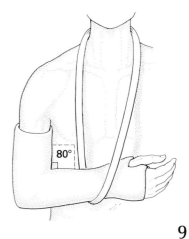

9

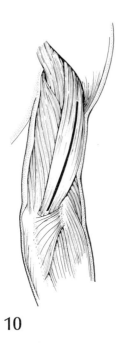

10

Mobilization and lengthening of triceps

11

The triceps tendon is detached at its insertion to the olecranon process of the ulna and dissected from the lower fourth of the shaft of the humerus. The tendon of the triceps is lengthened with a free graft of fascia lata.

ANTERIOR TRANSFER OF THE TRICEPS TENDON (Bunnell[4] and Carroll[5])

Posterior incision

10

An incision is made along the posterolateral aspect of the upper arm, and the triceps tendon exposed.

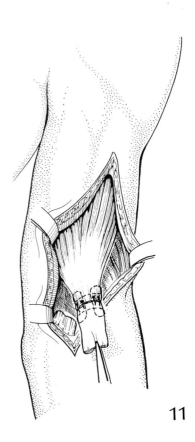

11

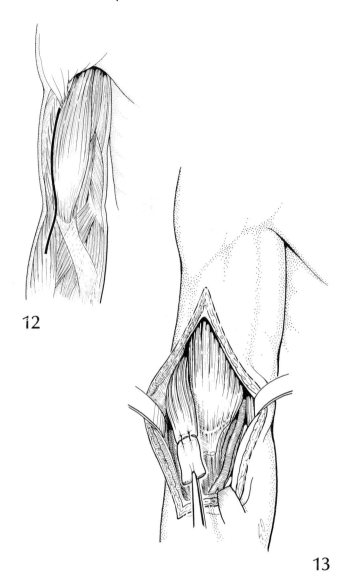

12

13

Anterior incision and tendon transfer

12 & 13

Another incision is made on the anterolateral aspect of the arm and forearm, and the lengthened tendon of the triceps brought round the lateral aspect of the humerus. The brachioradialis muscle and the radial nerve are retracted laterally and the pronator teres medially. The forearm is supinated and the biceps tendon is identified.

Attachment

14

The biceps tendon is split as near to its insertion to the radial tuberosity as possible and the lengthened triceps tendon passed through this. It is sutured to the biceps tendon using non-absorbable sutures with the elbow at 90° of flexion and the forearm fully supinated.

Postoperative management

An above-elbow plaster cast is applied for 6 weeks with the elbow acutely flexed at 80° and the forearm in mid-pronation. Passive and active exercises are started at the end of the 6 weeks.

14

TRANSFER OF THE PECTORALIS MAJOR TENDON
(Brooks and Seddon[6])

This operation to restore elbow flexion is carried out if a Steindler flexorplasty is not feasible and if the biceps muscle is completely paralysed. For the operation to be successful muscles controlling the shoulder joint must be normal; otherwise the shoulder must be stabilized by fusion.

Incision

15

An incision is made along the deltopectoral groove starting from the level of the coracoid process and extending along the upper third of the upper arm.

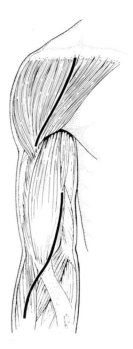

15

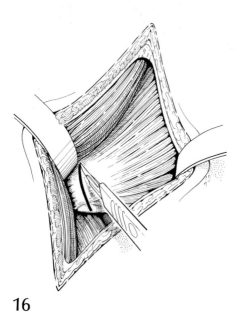

16

Dissection of pectoralis major

16

The tendon of the pectoralis major is cut as close to the bony insertion as possible. The pectoralis muscle is mobilized by finger dissection towards the clavicle, taking care not to damage the blood vessels and nerves supplying this muscle.

Mobilization of biceps

17

The long head of the biceps is exposed by retracting the deltoid laterally. This is cut as near as possible to the supraglenoid insertion without opening the shoulder joint.

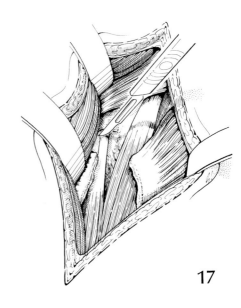

17

18

The muscle belly of the long head of the biceps is mobilized and separated from the short head. The blood vessels supplying the long head of the biceps muscle are ligated and divided.

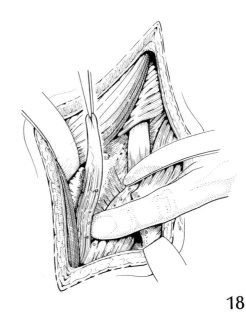

18

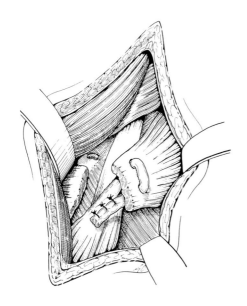

19

Transfer through anterior incision

A lazy-S incision is made on the anterior aspect of the elbow starting from the medial border of the biceps muscle to the lateral side of the forearm (see *Illustration 15*). The muscle belly of the long head is separated from the short head. Any additional nerves or blood vessels are divided and the muscle belly is freed right down to the radial tuberosity. The surgeon should ensure that the muscle belly of the long head of the biceps is completely freed by bringing it out through the elbow incision.

The muscle belly is replaced in the wound in the original position and the tendon of the long head is replaced into the proximal incision.

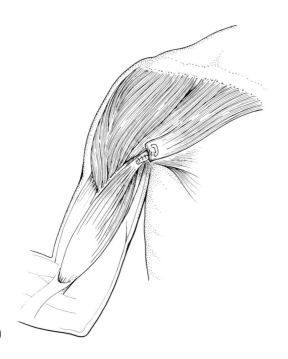

20

19 & 20

Two button-hole incisions are made in the pectoralis major tendon and the long head of the biceps is threaded through these so that it doubles back on itself. With the elbow flexed to 90° the biceps tendon is tautened and sutured to itself using non-absorbable sutures. This is further augmented by sutures placed between the pectoralis major and biceps tendons.

Postoperative management

A well-padded plaster backslab is applied with the elbow flexed to 90°. The backslab is removed at the end of 3 weeks and gradually the elbow is extended. The extension should not be too rapid, otherwise the tendon replacement will over-stretch. It usually takes about 3 months for extension to return.

References

1. Steindler A. Muscle and tendon transplantation at the elbow. *Am Acad Orthop Surg Instr Course Lect* 1944; 276–83.

2. Steindler A. Reconstruction of the poliomyelitic upper extremity. *Bull Hosp Joint Dis* 1954; 15: 21–34.

3. Bunnell S. Restoring flexion to the paralytic elbow. *J Bone Joint Surg [Am]* 1951; 33-A: 566–71.

4. Bunnell S. Tendon transfers in the hand and forearm. *Am Acad Orthop Surg Instr Course Lect* 1949; 6: 106–12.

5. Carroll R. E. Restoration of flexor power to the flail elbow by transplantation of the triceps tendon. *Surg Gynecol Obstet* 1952; 95: 685–8.

6. Brooks DM, Seddon HJ. Pectoral transplantation for paralysis of the flexors of the elbow. A new technique. *J Bone Joint Surg [Br]* 1959; 41-B: 36–43.

Illustrations by Gillian Oliver

Tendon reconstruction in the forearm

B. Helal MChOrth, FRCS
Honorary Consultant Orthopaedic Surgeon, The Royal London Hospital and The Royal National Orthopaedic Hospital, London, and Enfield Group of Hospitals, UK

S. C. Chen FRCS
Consultant Orthopaedic Surgeon, Enfield Group of Hospitals, UK

Introduction

Tendon reconstruction may be necessary in the forearm for either spasticity or paralysis. Spasticity of a muscle may be due to cerebral palsy, or could follow a cerebrovascular accident. The more usual indication is for paralysis of a muscle due to irreversible nerve injury, or a neuromuscular disease, e.g. poliomyelitis, multiple sclerosis or muscular dystrophies. It is important to determine whether the neuromuscular disorder is progressive, because the transferred tendon may later be involved in a progressive lesion.

Before surgery is undertaken, it is advisable to give the patient a course of physiotherapy or splintage in order to correct any fixed deformities and to assess the state of the affected muscles over a period of 2–3 months. In spastic paralysis it may be necessary to produce a temporary paralysis of the overactive muscles by nerve block in order to assess the strength of their antagonists. It is also important to observe the psychological make-up of the patient to assess whether he or she is well-motivated.

It is only after a period of conservative therapy that surgical treatment should be advised.

SPASTIC CONDITIONS

Pronation deformity of the forearm

Pronation deformity of the forearm is not very disabling, and is preferable to a supination deformity, as most actions of the hand are carried out with the forearm in some degree of pronation. However, a pronation defor-mity associated with a flexed and ulnar-deviated wrist, usually seen in cerebral palsy, is disabling.

There are two surgical procedures which are equally satisfactory.

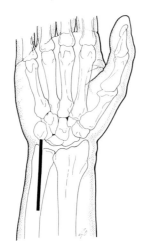

1

TRANSFER OF FLEXOR CARPI ULNARIS
(Green and Banks[1])

1

A longitudinal incision is made on the anterior aspect of the wrist, extending 4 cm proximally from the pisiform bone.

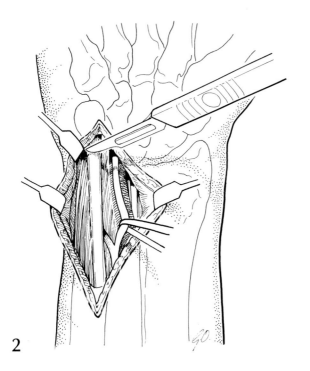

2

2

The ulnar nerve is identified and protected. The tendon of the flexor carpi ulnaris is detached from the pisiform bone and freed by sharp dissection from the ulna. A strong suture is attached to the end of the tendon.

3a & b

A second longitudinal incision is made over the muscle belly of the flexor carpi ulnaris, starting 4 cm from the medial epicondyle and extending about 8 cm distally. The tendon of the flexor carpi ulnaris is brought out through this incision. The muscle belly is dissected from the ulna and the deep fascia, taking care to protect the ulnar nerve and its branches.

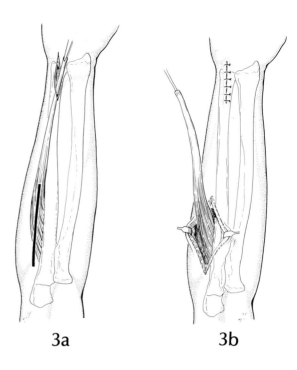

3a   3b

4

A third longitudinal incision is made on the dorsum of the wrist over the tendon of the extensor carpi radialis longus, extending from the wrist joint line proximally for about 5 cm. The tendon of the extensor carpi radialis longus is identified.

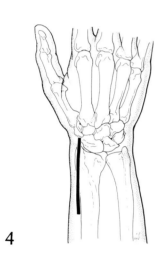

4

5

A check is made that the muscle belly and tendon of the flexor carpi ulnaris are freed along its course from its origin, and can be brought across the dorsum of the wrist. A tunnel is made from the proximal anterior incision, around the ulnar side of the forearm, to the dorsal incision.

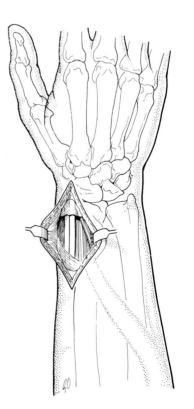

5

6

The tendon of the flexor carpi ulnaris is brought out of the dorsal incision through this tunnel. The strong suture attached to the end of the tendon greatly facilitates this manoeuvre. A check is made to ensure that the muscle belly and tendon of the flexor carpi ulnaris are in a direct line of action for attachment to the extensor carpi radialis longus.

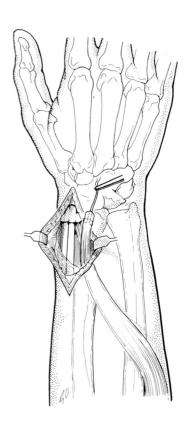

6

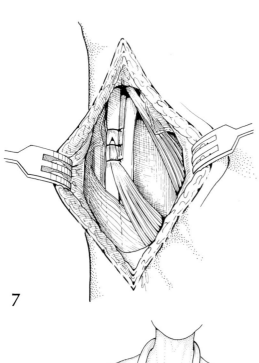

7

7

A small incision is made in the tendon of the extensor carpi radialis longus, and then the tendon of the flexor carpi ulnaris is passed through it. With the wrist in full dorsiflexion, and the forearm in supination, the tendons are sutured together.

If less supination and radial deviation are required, the tendon of the extensor carpi radialis brevis is chosen for attachment to the tendon of the flexor carpi ulnaris.

The wounds are sutured.

8

An above-elbow plaster cast is applied with the elbow flexed at 90°, the forearm in full supination and the wrist in dorsiflexion.

Postoperative management

Passive and active exercises of the fingers and thumb are carried out to maintain mobility of their joints. The plaster cast is bivalved at the end of 3 weeks and converted into a night splint. Elbow, forearm and wrist exercises are added to the finger exercises. The night splint is worn for a further 6 weeks.

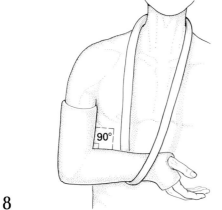

8

REDIRECTION OF PRONATOR TERES TENDON
(Sakellarides, Mital and Lenzi[2])

9

A ventral longitudinal incision is made over the radius in the mid-forearm. The lateral cutaneous nerve of the forearm and the superficial branch of the radial nerve are identified and protected from injury. The brachioradialis muscle is identified and retracted medially.

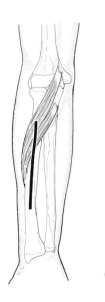

9

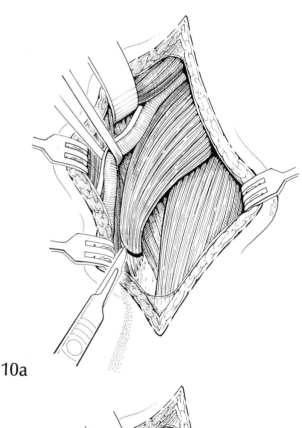

10a

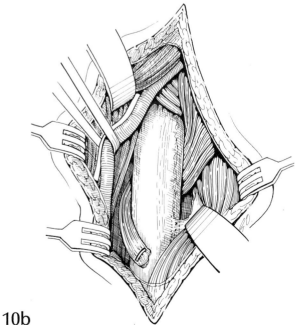

10b

10a & b

Next, the tendon of the pronator teres is identified and detached from its insertion to the radius. A non-absorbable suture is passed through the end of the tendon using a Kessler stitch.

The interosseous membrane is detached from the radius. The tendon of the pronator teres is passed through the interosseous space and around the lateral side of the radius. Using a large drill, a hole is made in the radius at the same level as the original insertion of the pronator teres. The tendon of the pronator teres is passed through the hole in the radius. With the forearm in full supination and the elbow flexed at 90°, the tendon of the pronator teres is tied to the radius. The wound is closed.

Postoperative management

An above-elbow plaster cast is applied. At the end of 3 weeks the plaster cast is converted into a night splint, and mobilizing exercises to the elbow and wrist are carried out. The night splint is used for 8 weeks.

Supination deformity of the forearm

In paralytic disorders, active pronation of the forearm may be lost. This can be disabling to the patient, as satisfactory hand function relies on the ability of the forearm to be actively pronated. However, the biceps muscle may be functioning normally, and active supination is possible. In the early stages, passive pronation is present; but in longstanding supination deformities of the forearm there may be contractures of the inferior radio-ulnar joint and the interosseous membrane, and even passive pronation may be lost.

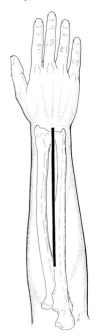

11

CAPSULOTOMY OF THE INFERIOR RADIO-ULNAR JOINT AND RELEASE OF THE INTEROSSEOUS MEMBRANE OF THE FOREARM (Zancolli[3])

11

A long dorsal incision is made in the forearm, starting from the inferior radio-ulnar joint and extending proximally three-quarters of the length of the forearm.

12

The extensor muscles are retracted medially and the interosseous membrane exposed by careful dissection. The posterior interosseous nerve is in the substance of these muscles and is therefore fairly well protected from damage. The interosseous membrane is incised at its attachment to the ulna. The inferior radio-ulnar joint is exposed and a dorsal capsulotomy is carried out. A check is made that passive pronation is possible at this stage. If not, the supinator muscle may have to be released. The wound is sutured.

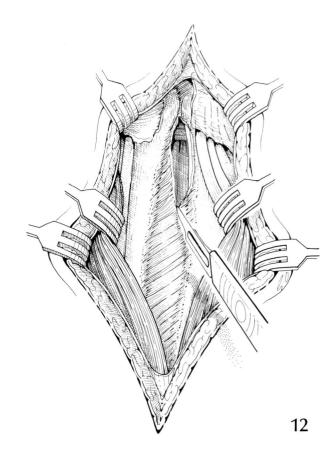

12

REDIRECTION OF BICEPS TENDON

13a & b

An S-shaped incision is made on the front of the elbow starting medially above the joint and ending over the radial head. The brachial artery and median nerve are identified and protected from injury. The biceps tendon is next identified.

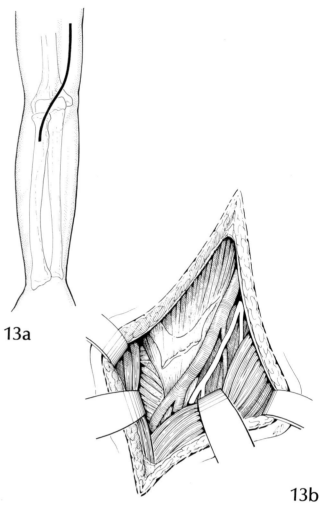

13a

13b

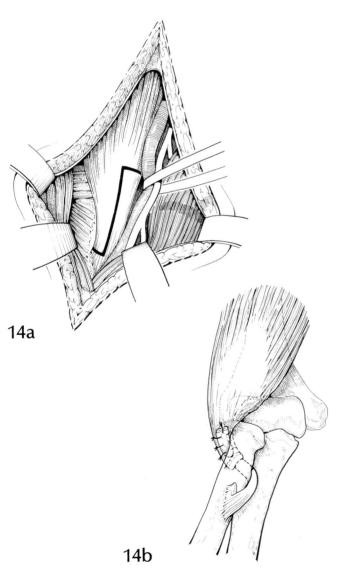

14a

14b

14a & b

A long Z-shaped incision is made in the tendon near its insertion to the radial tuberosity. The distal part of the tendon is then passed medially and posteriorly to the radius and brought out onto the lateral side of the radius. With the elbow flexed at 90°, the tendon is reattached to its proximal end under tension. The wound is closed.

Postoperative management

An above-elbow plaster cast is applied with the elbow flexed at 90°, and the forearm pronated. At the end of 3 weeks, the plaster cast is converted to a night splint, and pronation exercises are commenced. The night splint is worn for 8 weeks and then discarded.

Flexion deformity

In cerebral palsy, there may be severe flexion deformities of the wrist and fingers, which cannot be corrected passively, due to overactivity or contracture of the flexor muscles of the forearm.

By releasing these flexor muscles from their origins it may be possible to extend not only the wrist but also the fingers.

RELEASE OF THE FLEXOR MUSCLES OF THE FOREARM

15

An S-shaped incision is made, starting proximally behind the medial epicondyle and crossing the front of the elbow joint into the middle of the forearm over the ulna. The medial cutaneous nerve of the forearm is identified and protected.

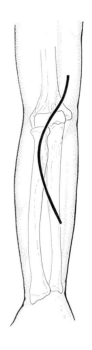

15

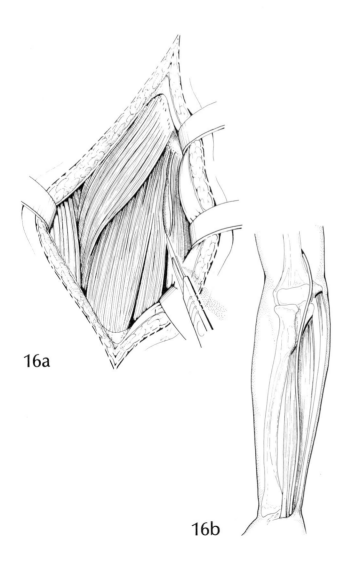

16a

16b

16a & b

The ulnar nerve is identified and dissected from its groove behind the medial epicondyle. The medial intermuscular septum is excised at this stage, to facilitate anterior transposition of this nerve at a later stage.

The fibrous arch of the flexor carpi ulnaris is incised and the branches of the ulnar nerve to the flexor carpi ulnaris and flexor digitorum profundus are identified. The origins of these two muscles are then detached and freed distally down to the middle of the ulna.

17

Next, the origins of the pronator teres, flexor carpi radialis, flexor digitorum sublimis, palmaris longus and flexor carpi ulnaris are detached from the medial epicondyle. The median nerve is now seen passing between the two heads of pronator teres. The ulnar nerve is transposed anterior to the elbow joint. The subcutaneous tissue and skin are sutured.

Postoperative management

A below-elbow plaster cast is applied with the forearm in supination, and the wrist and fingers in the extended neutral position. Flexion and extension exercises for the elbow are started early. At 3 weeks the plaster cast is converted into a night splint, and active and passive movements of the wrist and fingers are carried out. The night splint is discarded at the end of 8 weeks.

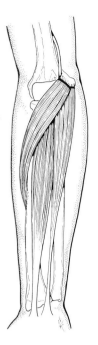

17

PARALYTIC CONDITIONS

One or a combination of the three nerves to the hand may be irreversibly damaged, by injury.

Radial nerve palsy

When the radial nerve is damaged in the upper arm, usually in the radial groove of the humerus, all the muscles in the limb supplied by it are paralysed. They are the brachioradialis and the extensor carpi radialis longus supplied by the main radial nerve; and the extensor carpi radialis brevis, supinator, extensor digitorum communis, extensor digiti minimi, extensor carpi ulnaris, abductor pollicis longus, extensor pollicis brevis, extensor pollicis longus and extensor indicis supplied by the posterior interosseous nerve. In addition, the sensory branches of the radial nerve are also damaged, and there is loss of sensation of the dorsal and radial border of the hand.

When the posterior interosseous nerve alone is damaged, the brachioradialis and the extensor carpi radialis longus are spared, and there is no sensory loss as the posterior interosseous nerve is a pure motor nerve.

In a radial nerve palsy, there is loss of dorsiflexion of the wrist, thumb and fingers, and abduction of the thumb. Three tendon transfers can provide these movements.

1. The pronator teres is transferred to the extensor carpi radialis brevis to provide wrist extension.
2. The flexor carpi ulnaris is transferred to the extensor digitorum communis to provide extension of the fingers.
3. The palmaris longus, if present, is transferred to the extensor pollicis longus to provide thumb extension; if the palmaris longus is absent, the flexor carpi ulnaris is transferred to the extensor pollicis longus (in addition to the extensor digitorum communis).

Extension of the fingers will also extend the wrist.

In a posterior interosseous nerve palsy, the pronator teres is transferred to the abductor pollicis longus, the flexor carpi ulnaris to the extensor digitorum communis, and the palmaris longus to the extensor pollicis longus (brachioradialis if palmaris longus is absent). The extensor carpi radialis longus is active, and reinforces wrist extension.

TRIPLE TRANSFER

Mobilization of flexor carpi ulnaris and palmaris longus

18

An L-shaped ventral incision is made along the lower half of the forearm on the ulnar side, with the transverse limb along the flexor crease of the wrist and its junction with the vertical limb centred on the pisiform bone.

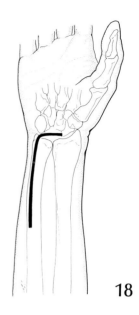

18

19

The tendon of the flexor carpi ulnaris is identified and detached from the pisiform bone, taking care not to damage the superficial and deep branches of the ulnar nerve. The muscle belly is freed from the ulna and mobilized proximally to the upper third of the forearm. If present, the tendon of the palmaris longus is also detached from the palmar fascia and mobilized.

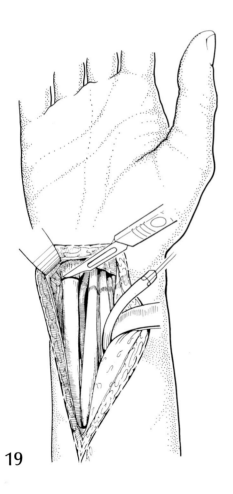

19

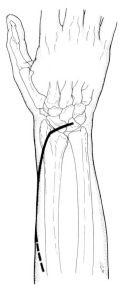

20a

Mobilization of pronator teres

20a & b

A second L-shaped incision is made on the dorsum of the forearm with the transverse limb along the dorsal crease of the wrist and the vertical limb along the distal half of the radial side of the forearm. The proximal edge of the extensor retinaculum is identified, incised across and a flap based proximally is made in the deep fascia.

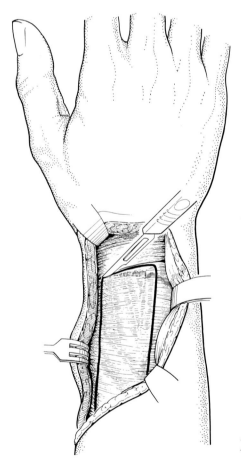

20b

21a & b

The flap is turned back and the extensor tendons are exposed. The tendons of the abductor pollicis longus, the extensor pollicis longus, the extensor digitorum communis and the pronator teres (PT) are identified. The extensor pollicis longus is freed and brought out of its groove to lie in the same plane as the tendons of the extensor digitorum communis. The pronator teres is detached from the radius and held with an end-suture.

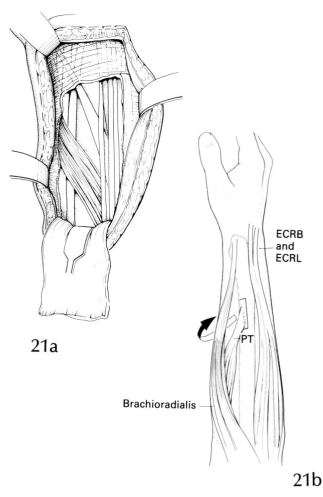

21a

ECRB and ECRL

PT

Brachioradialis

21b

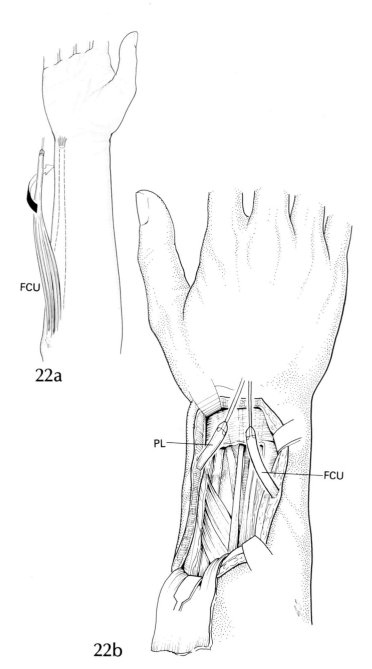

FCU

22a

PL

FCU

22b

Transfer of flexor carpi ulnaris

22a & b

Oblique subcutaneous tunnels are made on the radial and ulnar sides of the forearm extending distally from the dorsum to the ventral sides proximally. The tendon of the flexor carpi ulnaris (FCU) is passed along the ulnar side of the forearm to emerge on the dorsum. Similarly, the tendon of the palmaris longus (PL) is passed along the radial side. The positions of these two tendons are checked to make sure that their lines of pull are as near to the direction of pull of the extensor digitorum communis, extensor pollicis longus and extensor carpi radialis brevis (ECRB).

23

The wrist is held in full dorsiflexion. The fingers are held with the metacarpophalangeal joints in full extension, the proximal and distal interphalangeal joints in full flexion. The thumb is held fully extended and abducted. A thin Kirschner wire is passed through the tendons of the extensor digitorum communis and the extensor pollicis longus. The tension of each tendon is checked to make sure that the correct tension is applied to each. This is checked by extending the wrist, when full passive flexion of the fingers should be possible; and by flexing the wrist, when full extension of the fingers should occur.

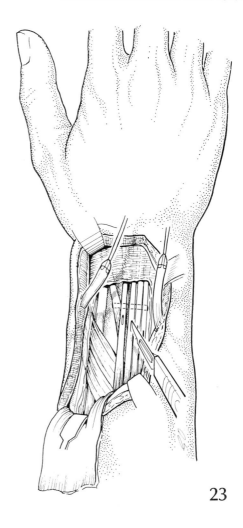

23

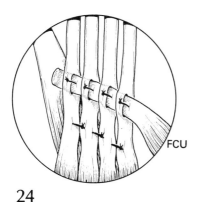

24

24

A No. 15 blade is passed through each tendon in an oblique direction, and along the line of pull of the flexor carpi ulnaris tendon. Sufficient muscle fibres are dissected away from the end of the flexor carpi ulnaris tendon to enable it to be passed through and to be sutured to each tendon with non-absorbable sutures. The Kirschner wire is now removed.

Transfer of pronator teres and palmaris longus

25a, b & c

The tendon of the extensor carpi radialis brevis is split near its insertion, and the pronator teres (PT) is passed through and sutured to it with non-absorbable sutures.

The tendon of the extensor pollicis longus is split, and the palmaris longus (PL) tendon is passed through and sutured to it with non-absorbable sutures.

If the palmaris longus is absent, the brachioradialis is used.

Closure

The flap in the deep fascia on the dorsum of the forearm is sutured back into place. The subcutaneous tissue and skin are sutured.

The L-shaped incision on the ventral surface of the forearm is then sutured in layers.

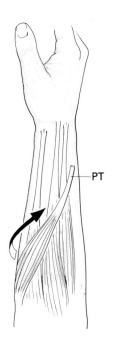

25a

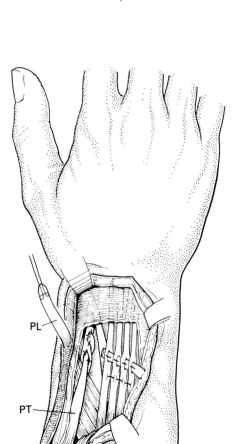

25b

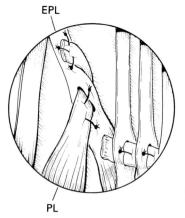

25c

Postoperative management

26

A well-padded below-elbow plaster backslab is applied with the wrist in full dorsiflexion, the metacarpophalangeal joints flexed at 90°, and the interphalangeal joints fully extended. At the end of 3 weeks the plaster backslab is removed and converted into a night splint. Active thumb, finger and wrist exercises are started. The night splint is discarded at the end of 2 weeks.

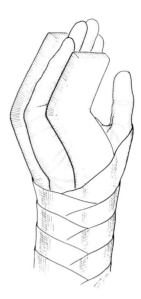

26

Median nerve palsy

When the median nerve is damaged in the arm above the elbow, the flexor group of muscles, i.e. pronator teres, flexor carpi radialis, flexor digitorum sublimis, palmaris longus, flexor carpi ulnaris, radial part of the flexor digitorum profundus, flexor pollicis longus and pronator quadratus, are paralysed leading to loss of forearm pronation, wrist flexion, index and middle finger flexion, and thumb flexion and opposition. There is also sensory loss in the median nerve distribution.

The thumb movements are restored by two reconstructions: the extensor indicis is used to provide thumb opposition; and the extensor carpi radialis longus is transferred to the flexor pollicis longus to provide thumb flexion. The muscle bellies of the flexor digitorum profundus to the ring and little fingers are innervated by the ulnar nerve which is undamaged, so they are sutured to the flexor digitorum profundus tendons of the index and middle fingers to provide a mass action in flexion. In addition, the brachioradialis is transferred to the conjoined tendons to reinforce the mass action.

Protective sensation may be restored to the thumb and index finger by transferring island flaps from the ring and little fingers.

TRANSFER OF EXTENSOR INDICIS TO THE THUMB
(Burkhalter, Christensen and Brown[4])

27

A small transverse incision is made on the dorsum of the metacarpophalangeal joint of the index finger.

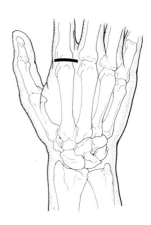

27

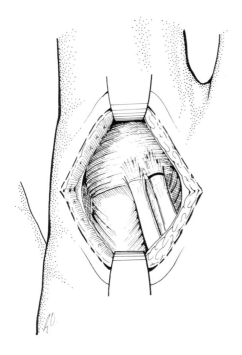

28a

28a & b

The tendon of the extensor indicis proprius is identified lying on the ulnar side of the extensor digitorum communis tendon. It is divided and the distal stump is sutured onto this tendon. The proximal end of the extensor indicis proprius is freed as much as possible with blunt dissection.

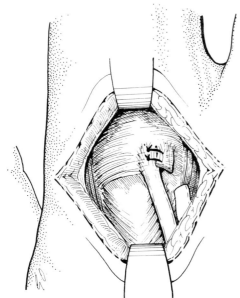

28b

29

A longitudinal incision about 3 cm long is made on the ulnar side of the forearm just proximal to the flexor crease of the wrist. The muscle belly of the extensor indicis is identified by tugging on its tendon in the distal wound. The proximal part of the tendon is freed by blunt dissection. Using a blunt hook, the tendon is brought out of the proximal wound. The distal wound is now sutured.

A tunnel is made in the subcutaneous tissue towards the pisiform bone, making sure that the tunnel is always kept in the superficial tissues, so as not to damage the ulnar nerve and its branches in this area.

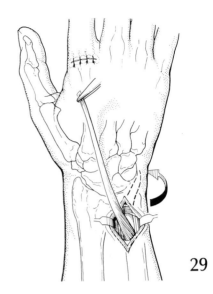

29

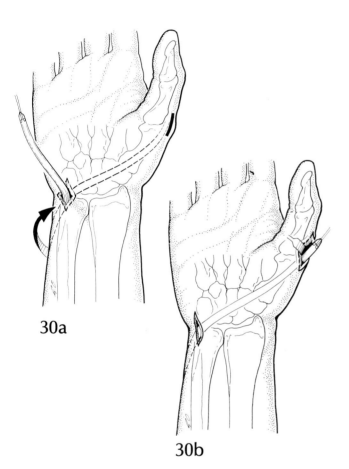

30a

30b

30a & b

A small incision 1 cm long is made just distal to the pisiform. The tunnelling is continued towards the radial side of the metacarpophalangeal joint of the thumb, where a small incision 2 cm long is made. The extensor indicis tendon is now brought out through the incision just distal to the pisiform. It is then re-routed towards the thumb, and brought through the wound on its radial side.

31

A button-hole is made in the abductor pollicis brevis tendon, and the extensor indicis tendon is passed through and sutured to it, with the thumb held in full abduction, and the wrist in 10° of palmarflexion.

Correct tension is important. If it is too tight, an abduction contracture of the thumb can occur. If it is too loose, satisfactory opposition is not possible.

The wounds are now sutured.

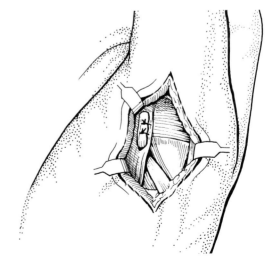

31

TRANSFER OF BRACHIORADIALIS TO FLEXOR DIGITORUM PROFUNDUS

32

An L-shaped incision is made on the flexor surface of the forearm with the transverse limb across the crease of the wrist, and the vertical limb 5 cm long on the radial side. The radial nerve and its branches are identified and protected.

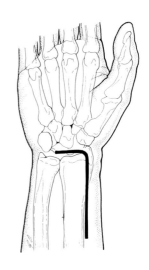

32

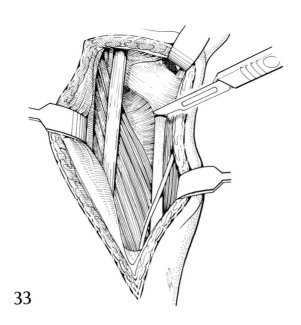

33

The brachioradialis is detached from its insertion to the lateral side of the lower end of the radius and freed, so that its direction of pull is in line with the flexor digitorum profundus tendons.

33

34

The four tendons of the flexor digitorum profundus are identified and sutured together with non-absorbable sutures. The flexor digitorum profundus tendons to the index and middle fingers are then cut proximally to free them from their paralysed muscle bellies. The brachio-radialis tendon is sutured under tension to the conjoined flexor digitorum profundus tendons on the radial side.

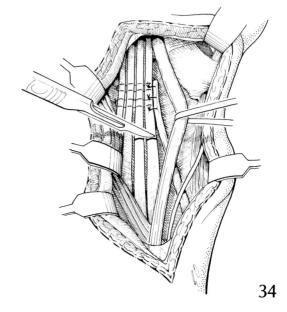

34

TRANSFER OF EXTENSOR CARPI RADIALIS LONGUS TO FLEXOR POLLICIS LONGUS

35

A transverse incision is made over the insertion of the extensor carpi radialis longus and extended to the base of the second metacarpal. The tendon is detached and freed by blunt dissection. It is brought out on the radial side onto the flexor surface of the forearm.

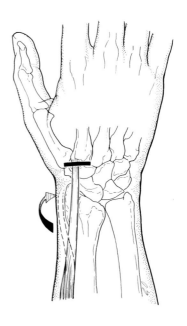

35

36

The flexor pollicis longus tendon is identified, and the extensor carpi radialis longus tendon is attached to it by interweaving the two tendons together, with the wrist in neutral position, the thumb in 20° of flexion at the interphalangeal joint, full extension at the metacarpophalangeal joint, and full abduction at the carpometacarpal joint.

The L-shaped wound on the flexor surface of the forearm and the small transverse wound on the dorsum of the wrist are now sutured.

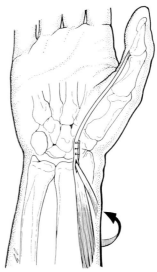

36

Postoperative management

A plaster backslab is applied with the wrist in a neutral position, the metacarpophalangeal joints of the fingers in 90° flexion, and the proximal and distal interphalangeal joints in full extension. The thumb is immobilized in full abduction at the carpometacarpal joint, in neutral position at the metacarpophalangeal joint, and in 20° of flexion at the interphalangeal joint. The Kleinert technique of early mobilization is not used, as the extensor carpi radialis longus and extensor indicis are extensors and may pull off in the immediate postoperative phase. The plaster backslab is removed at the end of 3 weeks, and passive and active thumb and finger exercises are started.

Ulnar nerve palsy

When the ulnar nerve is damaged in the arm, above the elbow, the ulnar part of the flexor digitorum profundus is paralysed, leading to loss of flexion of the distal interphalangeal joints of the ring and little fingers; the flexor carpi ulnaris is also paralysed, leading to loss of ulnar deviation of a palmarflexed wrist. In addition, the ulnar nerve supplies most of the intrinsic muscles in the hand, and paralysis of these muscles results in a weak grip. Paralysis of the adductor pollicis and the first dorsal interosseus results in a weak pinch.

Tendon reconstruction of the hand is dealt with elsewhere, but it is important to realize that combined nerve lesions can occur, and will influence tendon reconstruction in the forearm.

Combined median and radial nerve paralysis

In this situation the ulnar nerve is the only functioning nerve, and the muscles which it innervates, namely flexor carpi ulnaris and the medial part of the flexor digitorum profundus, are those available for transfer.

The flexor carpi ulnaris is transferred around the ulnar side of the forearm to the extensor digitorum communis and extensor pollicis longus, and the four tendons of the flexor digitorum profundus are joined together by non-absorbable sutures.

It is necessary to carry out an arthrodesis of the wrist as there are no functioning prime movers of this joint. The arthrodesis is always carried out after the tendon transfers.

The thumb can be flexed at the metacarpophalangeal joint by the flexor pollicis brevis which is supplied by the ulnar nerve, but it may be necessary to arthrodese the interphalangeal joint to provide a good pinch grip.

Combined median and ulnar nerve paralysis

In this situation, only the radial nerve is functioning. The palmar surface of the hand, including the finger tips, is anaesthetic. Only the extensor muscles in the forearm, namely brachioradialis, extensor carpi radialis longus, extensor carpi radialis brevis, extensor indicis, extensor digitorum communis and extensor carpi ulnaris, are active.

The extensor carpi radialis longus is transferred to the flexor digitorum profundus, and the brachioradialis to the flexor pollicis longus, to provide flexion of the fingers and thumb. A closed fist is usually associated with an extended wrist and therefore these transferred tendons are synergistic in their actions. Therefore, the wrist should never be arthrodesed.

It may be necessary to carry out metacarpophalangeal arthrodesis of the thumb, and Zancolli capsulodesis[5] of the metacarpophalangeal joints of the fingers.

Combined radial and ulnar nerve paralysis

In this situation, only the median nerve is functioning in the forearm. The muscles innervated by it, namely pronator teres, flexor carpi radialis, flexor digitorum sublimis, palmaris longus, flexor carpi ulnaris, the radial two tendons of the flexor digitorum profundus and flexor pollicis longus, are available for transfer.

Flexor carpi radialis longus is transferred around the radial side of the forearm into the extensor digitorum communis and extensor pollicis longus. If the palmaris longus is present it is transferred to the abductor pollicis longus. Clawing of the ring and little fingers is corrected by Zancolli capsulodesis[5].

It is usually necessary to arthrodese the wrist joint, but this is done only as the final stage in the treatment, after the tendon transfers have been carried out.

References

1. Green WT, Banks HH. Flexor carpi ulnaris transplant and its use in cerebral palsy. *J Bone Joint Surg [Am]* 1962; 44-A: 1343–52.

2. Sakellarides HT, Mital MA, Lenzi, WD. Treatment of pronation contractures of the forearm in cerebral palsy by changing the insertion of the pronator radii teres. *J Bone Joint Surg [Am]* 1981; 63-A: 645–52.

3. Zancolli EA. Paralytic supination contracture of the forearm. *J Bone Joint Surg [Am]* 1967; 49-A: 1275–84.

4. Burkhalter W, Christensen RC, Brown P. Extensor indicis proprius opponensplasty. *J Bone Joint Surg [Am]* 1973; 55-A: 725–32.

5. Zancolli EA. Clawhand caused by paralysis of the intrinsic muscles: a simple surgical procedure for its correction. *J Bone Joint Surg [Am]* 1957; 39-A: 1076–80.

Illustrations by Peter Cox

Surgery of the wrist

I. J. Leslie MChOrth, FRCS
Department of Orthopaedic and Traumatic Surgery, Bristol Royal Infirmary, Bristol, UK

RHEUMATOID ARTHRITIS

General considerations

Surgery of the rheumatoid hand and wrist requires careful preoperative evaluation. It must be remembered that rheumatoid arthritis is a systemic disease, and that surgery of the peripheral part of the upper limb is a single event in the long-term management of the systemic disease as well as other treatment that may be necessary in other joints of the upper and lower limbs. Careful patient selection is crucial and the decision for surgery should be taken in conjunction with the rheumatologist. Therefore, ideally, combined clinics with rheumatologists should be held and the timing of surgery, as well as the operative procedure, should be carefully evaluated at these clinics. The therapist is an extremely important member of the evaluating team and should have a particular interest in both rheumatoid disease and hand therapy.

Indications and principles in planning surgery

While there are specific indications for individual operations, it is uncommon for there to be only one particular problem which requires one operation. Surgery needs to be planned as multiple operations may well be required. Certain general principles must be taken into consideration when planning such surgery. These are detailed below.

1. An assessment of *shoulder and elbow function* is important. It is pointless reconstructing a hand when it cannot be put to any good use because of painful restriction of elbow and shoulder joint function.

2. The mere presence of a *deformity of the hand* does not necessarily mean an operation is required. Rheumatoid disease has a slow progression and patients adapt very well to a slowly progressive deformity. Surprisingly, good function can be maintained without pain in a very deformed hand. A careful functional assessment of the hand must be performed and this is best done by the therapist who will have the time and facilities available to sit down with the patient and discuss the problems and requirements. The therapist should be included in the discussion when surgery is being considered.

The cosmetic appearance of the hand is not an important indication for surgery; however, in young people with rheumatoid arthritis this may be an important factor to the patient. Considerable psychological problems may result from a deformity and the surgeon should be prepared to undertake surgery for this reason, provided that function is not compromised, and a careful discussion of this aspect should be undertaken with the patient.

3. While surgery for arthritic joints is usually undertaken because of *pain*, this may not necessarily be so in the hand and wrist. It is important to discuss with the patient the reason for operating, i.e. relief of pain, improvement of function, or both.

4. The patient with rheumatoid disease may well have significant problems with the lower limbs and for that reason may have to use walking aids. Therefore *the need to use crutches* or a walking stick may alter the type of surgery which is considered in the upper limb, i.e. a wrist arthrodesis versus a wrist arthroplasty.

5. When planning surgery of the rheumatoid hand and wrist, the general principle should be to *start reconstruction proximally and work distally*, leaving the thumb until last, e.g. metacarpophalangeal joint replacement will not work well if the patient has an unstable, painful wrist. The order of surgery should be considered along the following guidelines.

(a) Wrist joint
(b) Metacarpophalangeal joints of the fingers
(c) Proximal interphalangeal joints of the fingers
(d) Thumb (if the thumb is done last it can then be put into the best position of function to correspond to the position achieved in the fingers).

6. It is important that the surgeon gains the confidence of the patient when multiple surgical procedures may well be necessary. For this reason it is usually better to *start with a simple procedure* which has a high success rate. The more difficult procedures can then be performed at a later date when the patient understands what is required in the postoperative programme and the surgeon can assess how the patient will respond to the more complicated procedures. While the simple procedures can be performed by any competent orthopaedic surgeon, those that require more intricate work on the joints and tendons and thus carry a high risk of loss of function should be left to a surgeon who is more skilled in the atraumatic techniques that are required and who has access to the expertise available from a skilled hand therapist.

7. It is important that the *patient's expectations* of the operations are not higher than those of the surgeon. The patient must be aware of why the operation is being performed and also be prepared to undergo an extensive rehabilitation programme postoperatively.

8. It is advisable to *operate on only one hand at a time* as the patient will be extremely incapacitated if both hands are in splints or bandages. The amount of surgery performed on one hand at any one time must also be restricted as extensive operations, especially on the dorsal and palmar aspect, may result in significant swelling and subsequent stiffness.

9. *Prophylactic surgery* may be necessary and this mainly involves the preservation of tendon function, i.e. synovectomy and decompression of synovial compartments.

Operations

DORSAL SYNOVECTOMY

Synovitis of the extensor tendons, especially when tense and painful, may result in rupture of one or more of the extensor tendons. The extensor retinaculum remains intact and allows an increased pressure to develop within the dorsal compartments. Synovium will bulge at each end of the retinaculum, producing an 'hour glass' effect. Decompression is necessary to prevent tendon rupture.

Indications

Indications for dorsal synovectomy are persistent swelling of the dorsal compartments despite medical treatment and ruptured extensor tendons.

Incision

1

A straight longitudinal incision is made in line with the shaft of the third metacarpal. It extends from a point approximately 6 cm proximal to the wrist joint to the level of the mid-shaft of the metacarpal.

Approach

The incision is taken directly down to the extensor retinaculum. Veins and cutaneous nerves should be preserved. The delicate skin should be lifted by the assistant using skin hooks to avoid grasping with forceps. A scalpel is used to develop the plane between the subcutaneous tissue and the extensor retinaculum. Excessive retraction on the skin should be avoided and the skin flaps should be kept as thick as possible. On the radial side some terminal branches of the radial nerve may be seen and these should be preserved and lifted with the subcutaneous tissue.

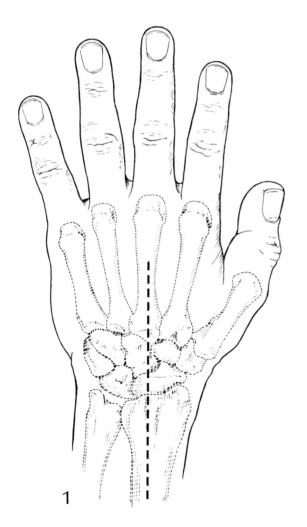

1

2

The extensor retinaculum is incised as shown and is lifted from the ulnar side towards the radial side. The extended Flap A will be used as a sling for extensor carpi ulnaris. Flap C is left attached on the ulnar side and Flap B is left attached on the radial side. Segment D is left in place to stop the tendons bow-stringing on wrist dorsiflexion. It is necessary to dissect the vertical septa off the dorsal surface of the radius, taking care not to buttonhole the retinaculum.

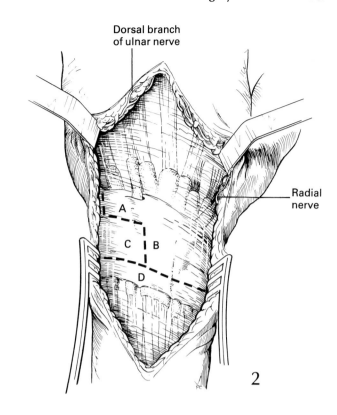

3

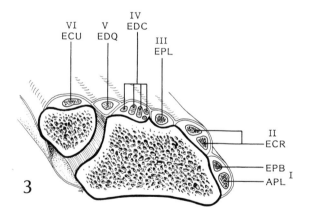

The compartments of the extensor mechanism at the wrist joint are shown. The dissection can be carried radially to expose extensor pollicis longus unless there is significant synovial involvement of the extensor carpi radialis tendons, in which case the retinaculum should be lifted to expose the next compartment.

Synovectomy and reconstruction

4a & b

The synovium is dissected off the tendons by sharp dissection with a scalpel or scissors. It can also be pulled off using a pair of curved artery forceps. A blunt hook is used to lift the tendons clear of the wrist joint. Any sharp spicules on the underlying bone should be removed. At this stage the following procedures can be carried out if necessary.

1. Synovectomy of the wrist
2. Excision of the distal end of the ulna
3. Synovectomy of the distal radio-ulnar joint
4. Repair of extensor tendons.

The terminal branch of the posterior interosseous nerve can be found on the distal radius underlying the extensor tendon to the middle finger. It is often worth dividing this with bipolar coagulation as it helps to relieve pain on the dorsum of the wrist.

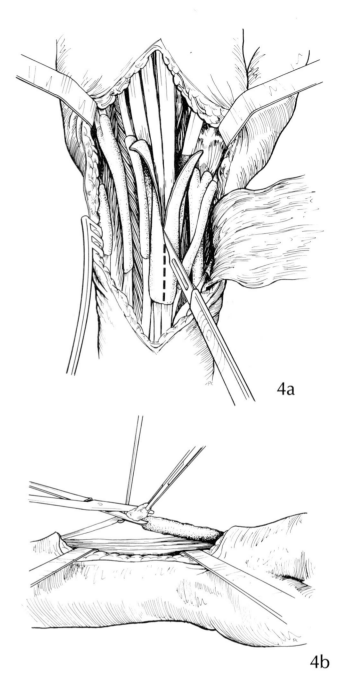

4a

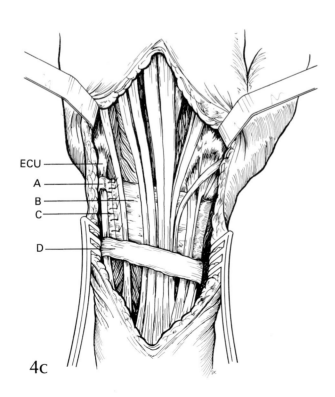

4b

4c

ECU
A
B
C
D

4c

4c

Following synovectomy, the extensor retinaculum is passed beneath the extensor tendons of the thumb and fingers and is sutured back to the ulnar flap using an absorbable suture material. Flap A of the retinaculum is passed beneath the tendon of the extensor carpi ulnaris and brought back over the top of it to create a pulley. It is sutured to Flap B using a braided polyester suture material. This reconstruction places the extensor carpi ulnaris tendon over the distal end of the ulna, reduces the ulnar deviation forces and helps to elevate the carpus.

Skin closure and postoperative management

A small suction drain is placed beneath the skin which is sutured in one layer with interrupted 4/0 nylon. A soft gauze dressing is applied followed by a soft wool dressing. A plaster slab is placed on the palmar aspect for 10 days until the wound is healed. Mobilization of the wrist and fingers is then commenced unless extensor tendon repair has been performed, in which case the fingers and wrist are immobilized for 3 weeks followed by dynamic extension splinting to the fingers.

DARRACH'S PROCEDURE (excision of the distal end of the ulna)[1]

Rheumatoid arthritis at the wrist joint level usually also involves the radio-ulnar joint. It may produce a painful synovitis, arthritis or subluxation of the distal ulna.

Indications for operation

Indications are painful subluxation of the distal radio-ulnar joint secondary to rheumatoid arthritis, osteoarthritis or old wrist fractures, and painful supination/pronation of the forearm with tenderness of the distal radio-ulnar joint.

In patients with rheumatoid arthritis, this operation is usually done in association with other wrist procedures such as a synovectomy, arthrodesis or arthroplasty. In the patient with osteoarthritis it will usually be performed as an isolated procedure.

Incision

5

When the procedure is performed in isolation, a longitudinal incision is made on the dorso-ulnar side of the distal ulna. Care is taken to preserve the dorsal branch of the ulnar nerve which crosses the ulnar border of the hand between the ulnar styloid and the pisiform. However, its position can be variable. The extensor retinaculum is incised longitudinally, leaving a flap on the ulnar side which will enable the retinaculum to be repaired at the end of the procedure. The capsule of the distal radio-ulnar joint is now exposed.

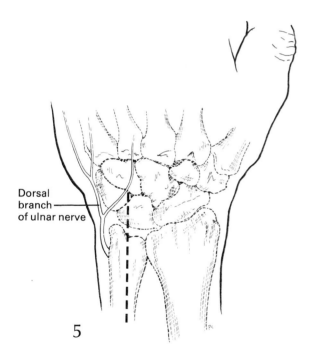

Dorsal branch of ulnar nerve

5

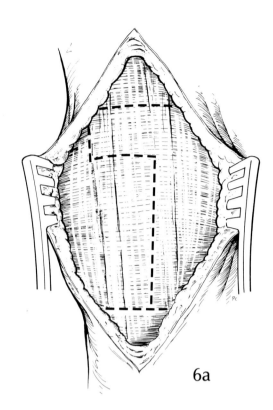

6a

Approach

6a & b

When this procedure is performed in association with other operations on the dorsum of the wrist joint, exposure through the retinaculum will be similar. The tendons of extensor carpi ulnaris and extensor digiti minimi are mobilized and retracted. A longitudinal incision is then made in the capsule from the ulnar styloid for about 3 cm proximally. The periosteum is incised and the neck of the ulna is exposed subperiosteally. The soft tissues are retracted by placing two small bone levers around the palmar side of the neck, ensuring that the tips of the retractors remain in close contact with the bone.

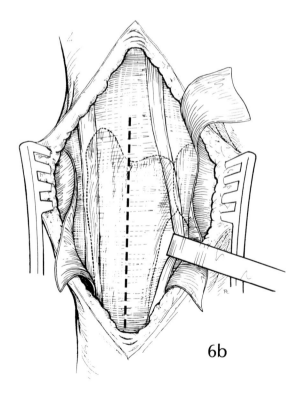

6b

7

A sagittal power saw is used to divide the bone at the level of the proximal limb of the sigmoid cavity of the radius. This is usually about 1.25–2 cm from the ulnar styloid. If more than 2 cm of ulna are resected, then the proximal end tends to sublux, creating an unpleasant prominence beneath the skin, and the tendon of extensor carpi ulnaris may click over the end. An alternative method of division of the ulna is to drill multiple holes at the level of resection and then complete the procedure with bone cutters. The distal fragment of ulna is grasped with pointed bone-holding forceps and, after rotation and elevation, sharp dissection is used to release it from its soft tissue attachments. The fragment is extracted. Excess synovium is then removed from the radio-ulnar joint.

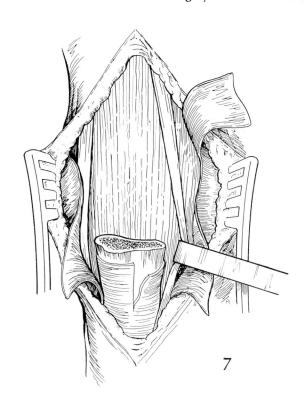

7

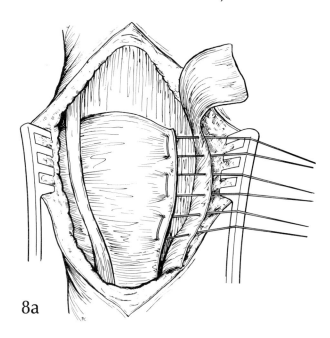

8a

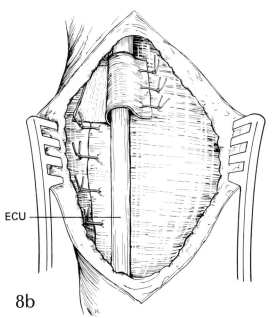

ECU

8b

Closure

8a & b

An assistant depresses the distal end of the ulna while the dorsal capsule is repaired with absorbable 2/0 suture material. The retinaculum is sutured firmly over the stump of the ulna and the flap of retinaculum is used to create a pulley for the extensor carpi ulnaris. The skin is closed with interrupted 4/0 nylon.

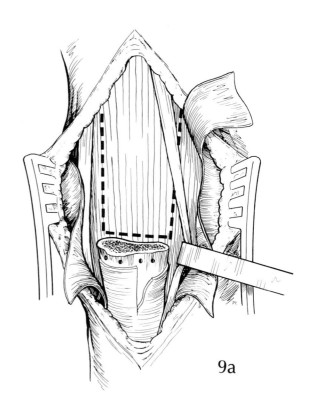

9a

9a & b

If the distal end of the ulna tends to sublux dorsally, a flap of palmar capsule can be raised on a distally based flap and sutured to the dorsal surface of the ulna via drill holes. The flap is sutured in place with the forearm supinated and an assistant depressing the ulna. The wound is dressed with cotton gauze and wrapped in wool. The forearm is supinated and a plaster slab is applied to the palmar surface of the wrist.

Postoperative management

The hand is elevated for 48 hours and then maintained in a sling, allowing movement of the shoulder, elbow and fingers, but no forearm rotation. The slab is removed at 3 weeks and a full mobilization programme followed.

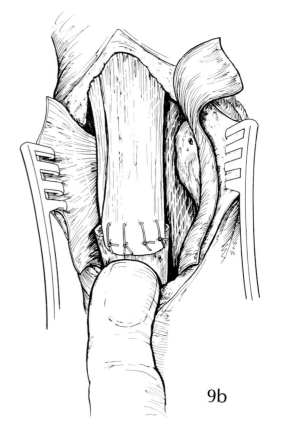

9b

THE LAUENSTEIN PROCEDURE

The potential complications of the Darrach procedure are progressive ulnar translocation of the carpus, ulnar deviation and subsequent painful instability of the wrist. The Lauenstein procedure leaves the distal end of the ulna as an articular surface for the carpus and allows mobility by creating a pseudarthrosis proximal to the head of the ulna[2].

Indications

The indication for this procedure is painful subluxation of the distal radio-ulnar joint associated with arthritic changes in those who are young, and in those who show a potential for ulnar translocation of the carpus, e.g. those in whom ulnar translocation is already present or where the 'slope' of the radius is steep towards the ulnar side.

Incision

This is the same as for excision of the distal end of the ulna as an isolated procedure.

Procedure

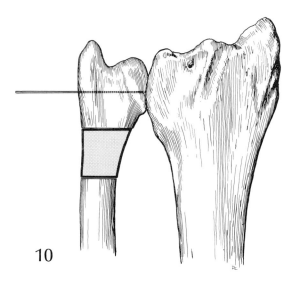

10

10

After the ulna has been exposed subperiosteally, a 2 mm Kirschner wire is drilled into the head of the ulna in the coronal plane with the wrist in neutral rotation. It will be used to manipulate the bone.

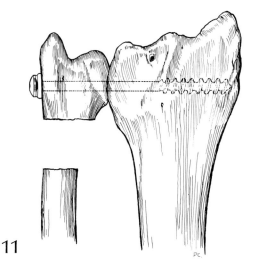

11

11

Osteotomy of the neck is performed with a sagittal power saw at a level just proximal to the radial articular surface of the distal radio-ulnar joint. A second osteotomy is made about 12–15 mm proximal to this and a segment of ulna is removed. The radio-ulnar joint is exposed by manipulating the distal fragment with the Kirschner wire. Articular cartilage is removed from the surfaces of both the distal ulna and the radio-ulnar articulation of the radius. The head of the ulna is then apposed to the distal radius and a Kirschner wire is driven across this joint. Pointed bone reduction forceps hold the position while the Kirschner wire is removed and replaced with a small-fragment AO cancellous screw.

12

Alternatively, a 1.6 mm Kirschner wire can be driven through the opposite cortex of the radius and left protruding so that it is just palpable beneath the skin. A second Kirschner wire is inserted obliquely to the first. Both are cut off flush with the ulna and will later be removed from the radial side. Bone graft taken from the excised piece of ulna can be used to augment the fusion.

The edges of the proximal ulna stump are rounded off and the dorsal capsule is sutured over this distal stump while the forearm is supinated and an assistant depresses the bone. If the shaft of the ulna tends to protrude despite this, then a palmar flap of capsule can be elevated leaving its hinge distally, as in the Darrach procedure. This is then sutured through drill holes to the distal stump.

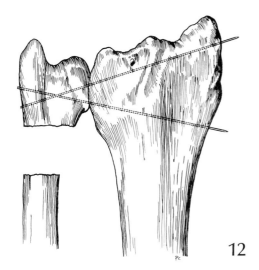

12

Closure and postoperative management

These are the same as for the Darrach procedure, except that splinting should be continued for 4 weeks.

RECONSTRUCTION OF RUPTURED EXTENSOR TENDONS

Reconstruction of one or several ruptured extensor tendons, excision of the head of the ulna or fusion of the wrist joint may be necessary during dorsal synovectomy for rheumatoid arthritis.

13

Rupture of a single tendon If only one tendon is ruptured, and this is usually the extensor digiti quinti, then a side-to-side anastomosis can be made with the adjacent extensor tendon using 4/0 non-absorbable braided suture material. Tension should be applied to the distal stump of the ruptured tendon at the time of the anastomosis. The correct tension is always difficult to achieve. However, after the anastomosis, when the wrist is fully flexed, the finger should come into full extension; and when the wrist is fully dorsiflexed, the finger should adopt a position of flexion similar to the others. With the wrist in neutral, full passive flexion should be achieved without pulling the anastomosis apart.

Rupture of two tendons The tendons to the ring and little finger are usually the two that are found ruptured. Both of these can be anastomosed to the intact tendon of the middle finger; however, it is then more difficult to gauge the correct tension. The above criteria apply in determining the correct tension.

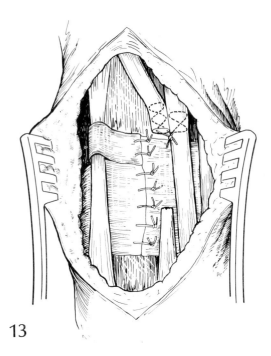

13

Transfer of extensor indicis proprius

If the extensor indicis is available then this can be used to provide active extension to the ring and little fingers.

Procedure

14 & 15

The extensor tendons at the wrist joint will already be exposed for a dorsal synovectomy. A separate transverse incision is made over the head of the second metacarpal.

The extensor indicis proprius lies on the ulnar side of the extensor digitorum communis. Prior to distal division of the extensor indicis proprius, an anastomosis with 4/0 absorbable suture is made between the indicis proprius and the communis while slight traction is applied to the proprius. This reduces the extensor lag which occurs after this procedure. The extensor indicis proprius is then divided just proximal to the anastomosis. It is pulled proximally into the wrist incision and then anastomosed to the conjoint distal ends of the ruptured extensor tendons. Anastomosis may be made end-to-end or by weaving the proprius through the other two tendons.

Postoperative management

A palmar plaster slab is applied holding the wrist in 20° of dorsiflexion and the proximal phalanx of the fingers in full extension.

At 10 days the sutures are removed and dynamic extension traction is applied to the proximal phalanges while the wrist is maintained in dorsiflexion. Active flexion against the resistance of the elastic bands is then allowed for the subsequent 3 weeks, at which time the splintage is removed. A night splint is applied for 6 weeks holding the fingers extended.

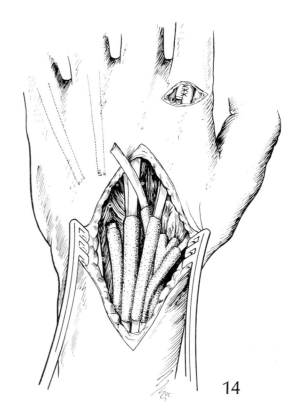

14

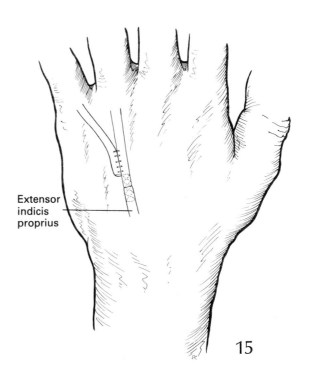

Extensor
indicis
proprius

15

Rupture of all extensor tendons

If all the extensor tendons to the fingers are ruptured, then it is necessary to transfer the flexor digitorum superficialis from the ring finger or from the ring and middle fingers. The tendons of extensor carpi radialis longus or extensor carpi ulnaris may be used but often require a bridging graft.

Procedure

16a & b

A transverse incision is made at the distal palmar crease at the base of the ring finger. The flexor digitorum sublimis (FDS) is isolated by a small incision in the distal palmar crease just proximal to the A1 pulley. The finger is flexed and the FDS is divided as distally as possible. After the tendon has been withdrawn above the wrist the wound is closed with interrupted nylon. FDS to the middle finger may be taken then if two tendons are to be used.

A zigzag incision is made over the palmar aspect of the forearm commencing approximately 2–3 cm proximal to the flexor wrist crease. Flexor digitorum superficialis from the ring finger is then withdrawn into the wound. Tendon-passing forceps are then placed subcutaneously around the radial border of the forearm to emerge in the volar incision. The tendon is grasped and delivered into the wound over the dorsal aspect. An anastomosis is made to the four extensor tendons to the fingers. If FDS from the middle finger is used as well then it is sutured to extensor digitorum communis (EDC) of index and middle fingers, while FDS from the ring finger is sutured to EDC of ring and little fingers.

If extensor pollicis longus is also ruptured, then one of the following tendons may be transferred into the distal stump: extensor carpi radialis longus, extensor pollicis brevis, flexor digitorum superficialis to the middle finger, or palmaris longus.

Postoperative management

A bulky dressing is applied with a palmar plaster slab holding the wrist in 20° of dorsiflexion and supporting the proximal phalanges. The arm is elevated for 48 hours. When the patient is comfortable at 3 to 5 days, dressings are reduced and a new splint applied. At 3 weeks dynamic extension splinting is applied to the proximal phalanx of each of the fingers. A static night splint is also used. Active flexion against resistance is encouraged for a further period of 3 weeks and then the patient is allowed free of the splints for periods during the day. The resting night splintage is continued for a total of 8 weeks.

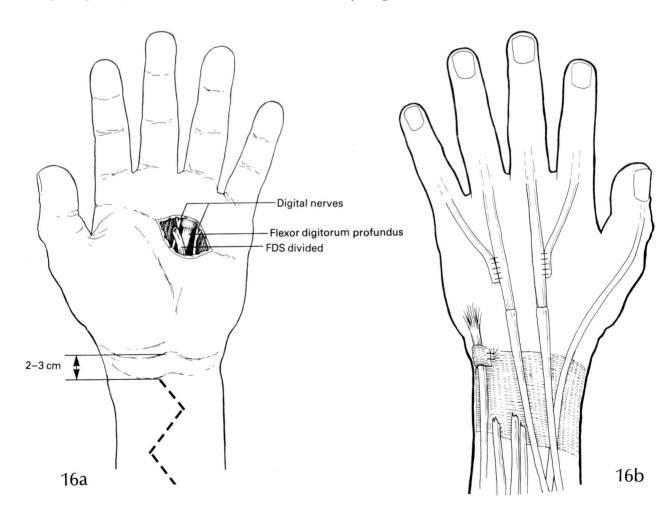

Digital nerves

Flexor digitorum profundus

FDS divided

2–3 cm

16a

16b

FLEXOR SYNOVECTOMY

Proliferative synovium around the flexor tendons at the level of the wrist joint may produce an hour-glass deformity on the palmar aspect. Swelling will appear in the palm of the hand as well as proximal to the wrist crease. Hydrocortisone injections are usually given in the early stages.

Indications

There are three indications for operation: symptomatic compression of the median nerve; rupture of flexor pollicis longus and/or other flexor tendons; and persistent swelling and pain despite medical treatment.

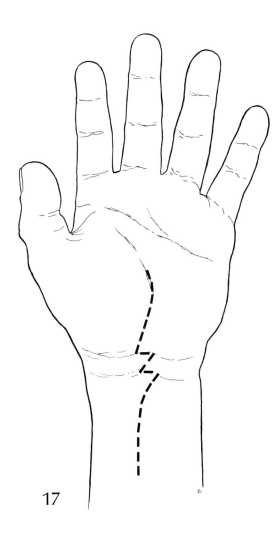

17

Incision

17

A longitudinal incision is made in the mid-palmar line which extends proximally across the wrist joint in a zigzag fashion.

Approach

18a & b

The subcutaneous fat and the palmar aponeurosis are divided by sharp dissection, maintaining traction on the skin with skin hooks. Vessels are coagulated with bipolar diathermy. A midline incision is made in the deep fascia of the forearm and the median nerve identified. A vessel loop is placed around the nerve and all subsequent dissection is performed on its ulnar side. The flexor retinaculum is divided under direct vision to expose the carpal tunnel. Care must always be taken to ensure that the motor branch of the median nerve is not divided. The median nerve is retracted to the radial side and the synovium is removed from round the flexor tendons by sharp dissection. The floor of the carpal tunnel is palpated and any sharp spicules of bone are removed with nibblers.

Closure

The tourniquet is released and the wound is packed with swabs soaked in saline while the arm is elevated for 3 minutes. Obvious bleeding points are coagulated with bipolar diathermy. A small vacuum drain is inserted. The skin is closed with interrupted 4/0 nylon. A well-padded palmar plaster slab is applied holding the wrist in approximately 20° of dorsiflexion.

Postoperative management

The arm is elevated for 48 hours and the drain is removed at 24 hours. The patient is discharged with the hand resting in a high arm sling for 3–4 days. Active finger movements are encouraged as soon as the patient is comfortable. The plaster slab and the sutures are removed at 10 days and full mobilization of the wrist is allowed.

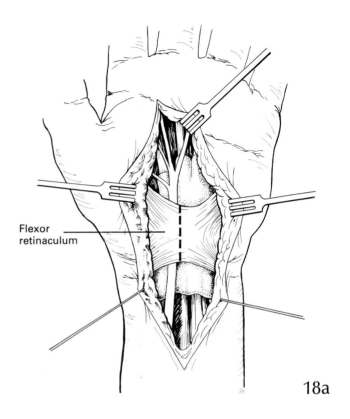

Flexor retinaculum

18a

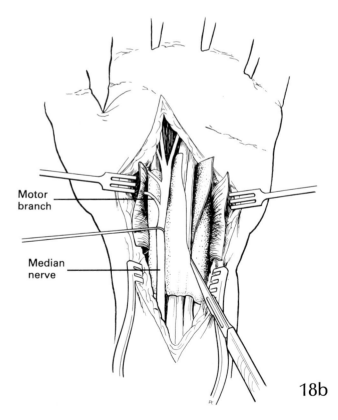

Motor branch

Median nerve

18b

ARTHRODESIS OF THE WRIST

Indications

Indications are severe pain in the wrist on flexion/extension combined with radiological changes of Grade III or IV; loss of hand function owing to volar subluxation of the carpus (volar translocation); bone destruction with ulnar translocation and loss of hand function. This may occur after a previous excision of the head of the ulna.

Before proceeding to surgery, the patient should be given a wrist splint which will provide the opportunity to see what the wrist is like after an arthrodesis. However, the splint will reduce rotation of the forearm whereas fusion will not. The splint will also give the surgeon some help in deciding if a fusion will improve the pain and/or function of the wrist joint. Careful consideration should be given before arthrodesing the second wrist in bilateral cases as an arthroplasty may give better function.

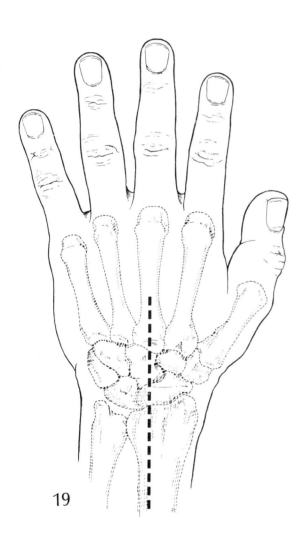

19

Incision

19

A straight dorsal incision is centred over the wrist joint and extends from a point 4 cm proximal to the wrist to the proximal third of the third metacarpal. It is important to make the incision of adequate length so that excessive traction on the skin edges is avoided during the operation.

Exposure

20

A dorsal synovectomy is usually performed as previously described. The retinacular flaps are made as before, but it is unnecessary to leave a proximal retinacular band. The dorsal capsule of the radiocarpal joint is incised transversely at the distal end of the radius. It is elevated, leaving the capsule attached distally. The distal end of the ulna is excised and the articular surface of the radiocarpal joint is exposed by flexing the wrist. Bone nibblers are used to remove synovium and remnants of articular cartilage. If the joint alignment is satisfactory, then the third metacarpal will lie in line with the radius and it is not necessary to perform an extensive dissection.

If there has been palmar or ulnar translocation of the wrist joint, then it may be necessary to release further sections of capsule on the ulnar, palmar and radial sides. When dissecting on the radial side it is essential to take care not to damage the abductor pollicis longus or the extensor pollicis brevis tendons which lie in very close apposition to the distal end of the radius. After further capsular dissection the wrist can be fully flexed to display the entire distal end of the radius as well as the carpal bones. It may be necessary to resect some bone from the dorsum of the distal radius to expose a reasonable area of cancellous bone and enable the carpus to sit on the end of the radius. The carpus and the distal end of the radius are shaped so that one fits into the other. Sometimes it is necessary to make a transverse cut with the power saw in order to achieve two flat surfaces if there has been gross erosion on the palmar aspect of the radius.

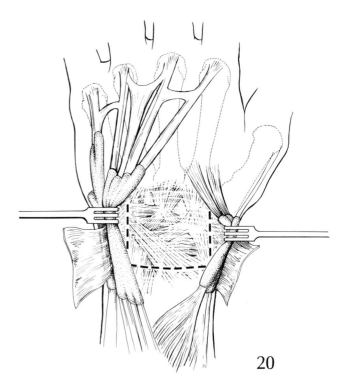

20

Internal fixation

21a & b

This is achieved by passing a Steinmann pin down the shaft of the third metacarpal, through the carpal bones and across the wrist joint into the medulla of the radius[3].

A longitudinal incision is made over the metacarpopha-langeal joint of the third metacarpal. The extensor hood is divided on the ulnar side and the extensor tendon is retracted to the radial side. The capsule and synovium are divided in the midline. A Steinmann pin approximately 15–20 cm in length is mounted on a T-handle and introduced through the head of the metacarpal. It is passed along the shaft, across the carpus until the point is seen to emerge. It is then lined up with the medullary cavity of the distal radius and driven longitudinally along

it. Care must be taken not to miss the shaft of the radius completely or to penetrate its soft cortex. Bone graft taken from the head of the ulna is packed into any available space and the hand is manually impacted against the radius. The Steinmann pin is countersunk deep into the articular surface of the metacarpal using a punch or a specially designed threaded introducer. If rotation of the carpus on the radius is a problem, then an oblique 2 mm Kirschner wire can be inserted through the radial styloid and across into the carpus. Alternatively, a bone staple can be placed across the dorsum.

If the metacarpophalangeal joint of the middle finger is not involved in the disease, then a Steinmann pin can be passed in a retrograde direction from the carpus to emerge between the second and third metacarpal heads[4]. This is then driven back down the centre of the radius.

This type of arthrodesis produces a wrist in neutral position, which would seem to be quite satisfactory for the patient with rheumatoid disease, even if both wrists are fused[5].

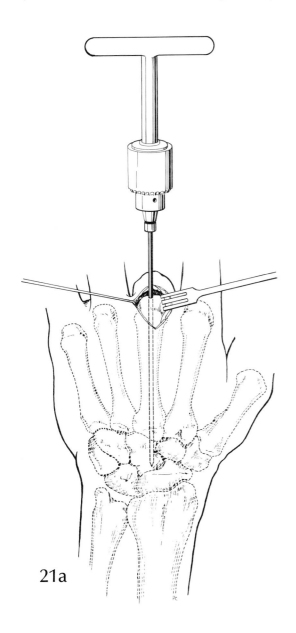

21a

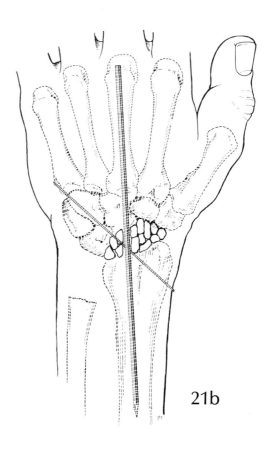

21b

Closure

The distally based flap of dorsal capsule is sutured back to the distal radius with absorbable suture material and this covers the bone graft. The extensor retinaculum is then placed beneath the extensor tendons and sutured to itself on the ulnar side, depressing the shaft of the ulna at the same time. A small vacuum drain is inserted and the skin is closed with interrupted nylon.

Postoperative management

Gauze dressings are applied to the wound and a well-padded palmar plaster slab is applied. The arm is elevated for 48 hours and the drain is then removed. At 2 weeks the sutures are removed and a complete short-arm plaster is applied supporting the wrist. This is kept in place for 8–10 weeks or until fusion is sound.

Limited wrist arthrodesis (Chamay)

If the mid-carpal joint is reasonably well-preserved the lunate and the proximal carpal row may be fused to the radius and some wrist movement will be maintained[6]. This technique should always be considered before undertaking complete arthrodesis of the wrist in rheumatoid arthritis.

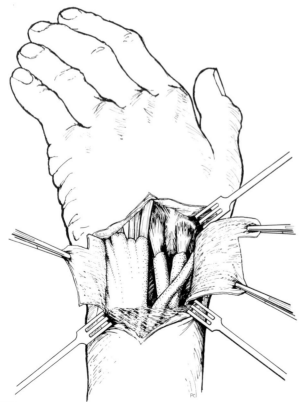

22

ARTHROPLASTY OF THE WRIST

Arthroplasty of the wrist in rheumatoid arthritis has gained popularity in recent years and the Swanson Silastic (Dow Corning, UK) prosthesis[7] is perhaps the most widely used. Since arthrodesis is such a successful operation, the role of arthroplasty is still controversial. However, when a patient requires an operation on both wrists, it is useful if one hand is fused to give good power grip and the other has a replacement arthroplasty to maintain some movement which is helpful for toilet purposes.

Contraindications

Contraindications to arthroplasty are extensive extensor tendon rupture, especially if the wrist extensors are compromised; insufficient bone stock, especially in the distal radius; a history of previous infection; and poor skin cover. An anteroposterior and a true lateral radiograph are essential in the planning of the operation.

Incision

A straight longitudinal incision is made in the line of the third metacarpal. It should extend for approximately 6–8 cm proximal to the wrist joint. Care is taken to preserve cutaneous nerves and veins.

Procedure

22

The extensor retinaculum is divided longitudinally on the ulnar side over the line of the extensor digiti minimi, leaving a longer flap on the distal edge. The retinaculum is reflected towards the radial side with its base between the first and second dorsal compartments. The retinaculum on the ulnar side is elevated to expose extensor carpi ulnaris. A narrow strip of retinaculum is left proximally to prevent bow-stringing of the extensor tendons. A synovectomy of the extensor tendons is performed.

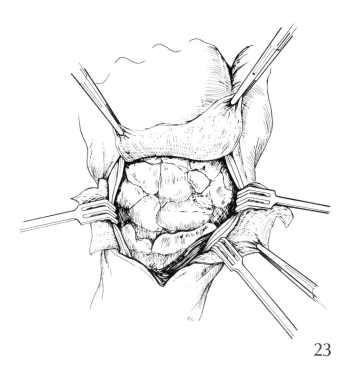

23

23 & 24

A transverse incision is made across the capsule of the wrist joint just proximal to the articular surface. This flap of capsule is reflected distally leaving it attached to the dorsum of the carpal bones. The head of the ulna is resected. The capsular attachment to the radial styloid is reflected distally, taking care not to injure the tendons in the first two dorsal compartments. The wrist is palmarflexed to expose the distal end of the radius and the carpal bones. A power saw is used to make a transverse cut across the distal end of the radius leaving, if possible, some of the subchondral bone to give support to the prosthesis. The lunate and the proximal pole of the scaphoid are removed either with a rongeur or a sagittal power saw.

The medullary cavity of the distal radius is reamed, using a broach, curette or a Swanson burr mounted on a power driver. It is reamed to take the appropriate trial prosthesis. The medullary cavity of the third metacarpal is identified. This can be done by passing a Kirschner wire through the head of the capitate and out through the head of the third metacarpal. The wire is then removed and this track is opened up, using initially a hand burr followed by a Swanson burr mounted on a power reamer.

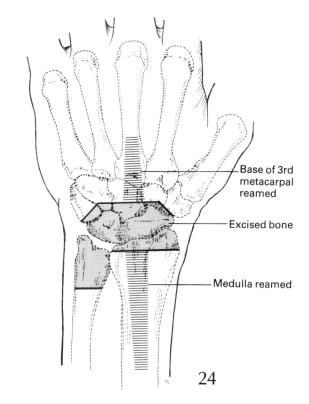

Base of 3rd metacarpal reamed

Excised bone

Medulla reamed

24

25a & b

The cavity is shaped to accommodate the distal end of the trial prosthesis which should not extend beyond the metaphysis of the third metacarpal. The trial prosthesis is then inserted into the distal radius and then the distal stem is introduced into the palmarflexed carpus as the wrist is dorsiflexed. The range of movement is tested and 30° of dorsiflexion and palmarflexion should be possible. If there is impingement on dorsiflexion, then it may be necessary to resect more of the distal end of the radius.

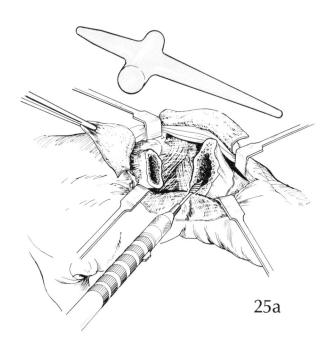

25a

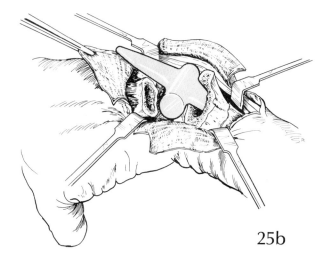

25b

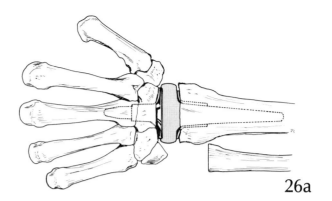

26a

26a & b

If grommets (titanium protective sleeves) are to be used then the appropriate size is inserted into the prepared cavities and further reaming may be necessary to allow these to fit well into the bone. The distal grommet is normally used on the dorsal surface and the proximal grommet on the palmar surface. The size of the grommet corresponds to the prosthesis.

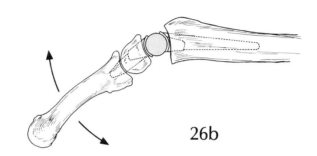

26b

27

The trial prosthesis and grommets are removed. A 1 mm round burr is used to make two holes on the palmar aspect of the distal radius, and 2/0 braided non-absorbable sutures are used to reattach the palmar capsule to the distal end of the radius. Three further holes are drilled on the dorsal surface of the distal radius and the suture material passed through the holes, leaving the needles attached to each of the three threads.

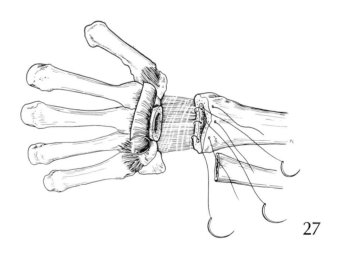

27

The bone cavities are washed out thoroughly with saline. Titanium grommets of the appropriate size are inserted into the distal end of the radius and into the carpal cavity. The definitive prosthesis of correct size is now removed from the packet and care is taken not to touch it with the gloves nor to rest it on any surface. The electrostatic charge on the Silastic material will attract foreign material and it should be handled with non-toothed forceps. The long proximal stem is inserted into the distal end of the radius, the wrist is palmarflexed and the distal stem inserted into the carpal cavity. The wrist is dorsiflexed and a stable reduction should be achieved.

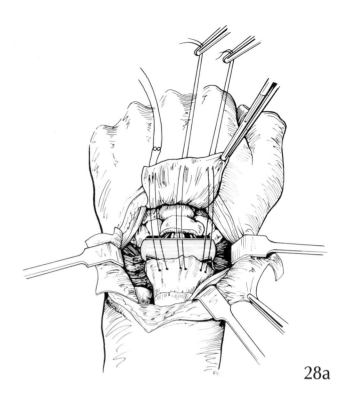

28a

Closure

28a & b

The distally based dorsal capsular flap is sutured to the distal end of the radius using the suture material previously inserted through the bone. The extensor retinaculum is passed beneath the extensor tendons and sutured as described for a dorsal synovectomy, holding extensor carpi ulnaris on the dorsum. A suction drain is inserted and the skin is closed with 4/0 monofilament sutures. A bulky dressing is applied with a palmar plaster slab holding the wrist in neutral.

Postoperative management

The arm is elevated for 7–10 days. The drain is removed at 48 hours. At 10 days the dressing is reduced and sutures are removed. A below-elbow cast is then applied to the arm for a further 4 weeks. On its removal mobilization is commenced. Sometimes it may be helpful to use a dynamic extension splint.

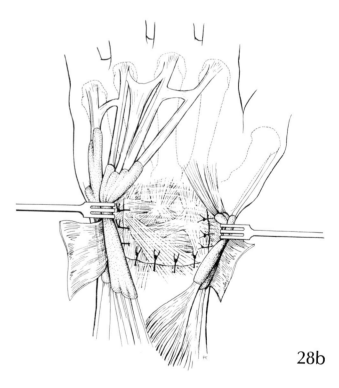

28b

DECOMPRESSIVE PROCEDURES

DE QUERVAIN'S DISEASE

This condition is an aseptic inflammation of the synovium lining the abductor pollicis longus tendon and the extensor pollicis brevis tendons as they pass over the lower end of the radius and under the extensor retinaculum. The condition is more common in women and is characterized by pain over the distal end of the radius aggravated by thumb movement. There is often local swelling and tenderness over the radial styloid area which radiates proximally along the line of the two tendons. Adduction of thumb with ulnar deviation of the wrist may produce pain (Finkelstein's test). Occasionally there is crepitus in the tendon sheath when the thumb is moved. The diagnosis can be confused with osteoarthritis of the carpometacarpal joint of the thumb.

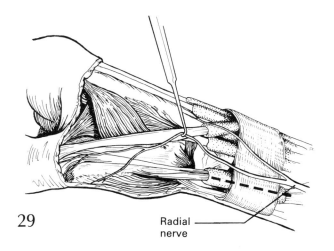

29

Radial nerve

Conservative treatment Conservative measures should be tried before surgical intervention. Repetitive use of the thumb should be avoided if it is possible and this may require a change in occupation. The thumb may be supported in a crêpe or elastic bandage and longer relief may be achieved by the application of a moulded lightweight splint which should immobilize the wrist and the thumb up to the proximal phalanx. The injection of a local steroid agent into the tendon sheath is often quite beneficial and may have a long-lasting effect. Care must be taken not to inject into the substance of the tendon.

Indications for operation

If the conservative measures fail and the patient's housework and/or occupation is being limited, then exploration is indicated.

Procedure

29

It is preferable to carry out the operation using a tourniquet on the upper arm and with regional or general anaesthesia. The local injection of an anaesthetic agent may distort the anatomy.

A longitudinal or zigzag incision is made over the tendon of extensor pollicis brevis or slightly to the dorsal side. It is possible to use a transverse incision which has a better cosmetic result but places the terminal branches of the radial nerve at greater risk.

The skin edges are elevated using skin hooks and the extensor retinaculum is exposed, taking great care to avoid damage to the terminal branches of the radial nerve. The thickened extensor tendon sheath is incised along its dorsal border and the tendons of abductor pollicis longus and extensor pollicis brevis are identified. Abductor pollicis longus may exist as more than one tendon, but this may lead the surgeon to believe that both tendons have been decompressed. It is important to identify extensor pollicis brevis separately and release it from its own subcompartment. Traction on the tendon will help to identify it. Some surgeons excise a segment of the tendon sheath to prevent recurrence.

The tourniquet is released, haemostasis secured and the skin closed with a subcuticular suture. A bulky wool and crêpe bandage is applied to restrict movement of the thumb. This is removed when the suture is taken out at 7–10 days.

Complications

Damage to the terminal branches of the radial nerve can result in a painful neuroma at the site of the operation. This may be more of a problem to the patient than the original tenovaginitis. Careful dissection in the longitudinal line is essential.

CARPAL TUNNEL DECOMPRESSION

Compression of the median nerve in the carpal tunnel produces the classic symptoms of paraesthesia in the median nerve distribution, waking the patients at night and often causing them to shake the hand in order to gain relief. The symptoms may persist during the day, causing clumsiness owing to alteration of sensation in the tips of the fingers and there may be weakness of thumb abduction. The condition occurs most commonly in women and often there is no clear aetiology. However, it is known to be associated with pregnancy, rheumatoid arthritis, myxoedema, and following a Colles' fracture.

The clinical picture can be confusing as pain can radiate proximally up the forearm and care must be taken to differentiate it from more proximal nerve lesions, especially those in the cervical spine region. Phalen's test is useful: this involves maintaining the wrist in full palmar-flexion for 1–2 minutes and, if positive, the symptoms will be reproduced. Tinel's sign may be positive over the carpal tunnel. If any doubt exists, then motor and sensory electrical studies are essential. If any skeletal abnormality is suspected, a radiograph, showing a skyline view of the tunnel, may be helpful.

Conservative treatment A splint holding the wrist in slight dorsiflexion may relieve nocturnal symptoms, and can be used as a diagnostic test. Steroids are sometimes injected into the carpal tunnel, and often produce a good response but repeated injections should not be given. Also, great care must be taken to avoid injection of the steroid into the substance of the median nerve.

Anaesthesia

The operation is generally carried out under regional or general anaesthesia using a tourniquet on the upper arm. However, it can also be performed by local infiltration of 0.5 per cent bupivacaine into the area of the incision. A high arm tourniquet can still be used as long as it is inflated just before the skin incision is made; the patient can usually tolerate the discomfort of the tourniquet for 10–20 minutes, which is sufficient time for the surgeon to expose the nerve. The tourniquet can then be released.

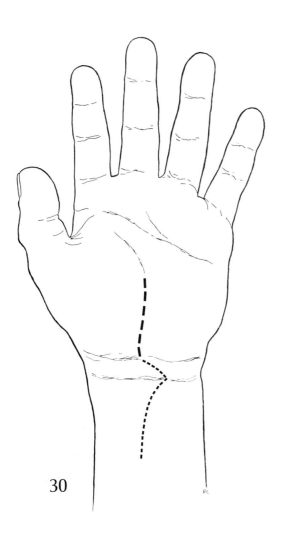

30

Incision

30

A longitudinal incision is made to the ulnar side of the midline of the palm. It commences at the distal wrist crease and extends distally for about 5 cm or to a line level with the ulnar side of the extended thumb. If it is necessary to extend the incision proximally, then the skin should be incised in a zigzag or curvilinear fashion across the wrist creases.

Exposure

31

The skin edges are elevated and retracted with skin hooks to put the underlying tissue under tension. Using sharp dissection, the palmar aponeurosis is divided longitudinally taking care not to damage the superficial palmar arterial arch which will appear at the distal end of the wound. The transverse carpal ligament is divided on the ulnar side of the midline; once an entry point has been made, a MacDonald dissector is passed proximally and distally in the carpal tunnel to clear any adhesions.

The transverse carpal ligament is then divided completely from the distal edge proximally to expose the carpal tunnel. Great care must be taken to avoid damage to the motor branch of the median nerve which in some hands may arise from the palmar aspect of the nerve and enter the transverse carpal ligament close to the midline. The edges of the ligament should be retracted; then, using a blunt dissection technique, the median nerve should be identified and, in particular, the motor branch should be sought to confirm its position and to clear it from surrounding tissue. The other terminal branches of the median nerve are carefully released.

The remainder of the carpal tunnel is inspected to exclude other space-occupying lesions, e.g. lipoma, ganglion or osteophyte. The tunnel proximal to the distal wrist crease can be inspected by elevating the skin with a retractor and, with the median nerve identified, any remaining restriction produced by the deep fascia can also be incised without extending the skin incision above the wrist. The author does not perform an internal neurolysis of the nerve at a primary operation. The tourniquet is released, the vascular flow to the median nerve is observed and haemostasis is secured.

The subcutaneous fat layer is sutured with a fine absorbable material and subcuticular polypropylene is used for the skin.

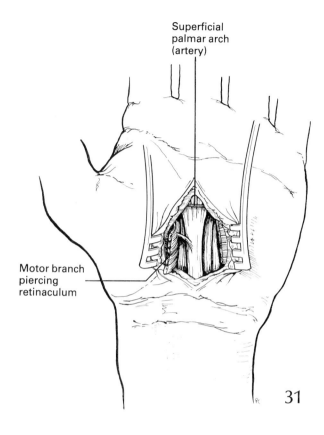

Superficial palmar arch (artery)

Motor branch piercing retinaculum

31

Postoperative management

A gauze dressing is applied to the wound, followed by a bulky wool and crêpe bandage with the wrist held in slight dorsiflexion. This is kept in place for 10 days until the sutures are removed.

Complications

Damage to the motor branch of the median nerve can produce a significant disability. It is important to identify this nerve and it is surprising how often it is seen emerging from the palmar aspect of the median nerve and penetrating the flexor retinaculum close to the longitudinal incision. If it has been divided it is important to recognize it and perform a primary repair. If the incision is continued above the wrist crease, it is important to preserve the superficial palmar branch of the median nerve. Damage to this can produce a painful neuroma.

The scar following a carpal tunnel release can be quite tender. This may be due to the formation of small neuromata in the line of the scar but can usually be well treated by desensitization exercises.

It is important to hold the wrist slightly dorsiflexed postoperatively as the tendons and nerve can bowstring across the divided flexor tunnel. This dorsiflexed position can usually be maintained by a bulky bandage, but a small plaster slab on the palmar aspect is used by some surgeons.

GANGLION AT THE WRIST

The commonest site for a ganglion at the wrist joint is on the dorsal aspect on the radial side of the common extensor tendons. It is usually more obvious on palmar-flexion of the wrist and may disappear on dorsiflexion. It may be tender, cause an ache when using the wrist or just be a cosmetic nuisance. If a ganglion is not annoying a patient in any of the above ways, it is probably best left alone as many will resolve spontaneously, particularly in children.

The next most common site is on the palmar aspect of the wrist on the radial side, in relationship to the flexor carpi radialis tendon. The radial artery is often stretched over the palmar surface of this ganglion.

EXCISION OF A DORSAL GANGLION

Procedure

32a & b

The operation should be performed using a high arm tourniquet with either general or regional anaesthesia. Local infiltration of anaesthetic usually distorts the anatomy and may make the dissection difficult.

On the dorsum of the wrist, a transverse incision is made over the ganglion. The skin edges are retracted; then, using blunt longitudinal dissection, and taking care to avoid the terminal branches of the radial nerve, the extensor retinaculum is exposed. It will be necessary to incise the extensor retinaculum, and then the ganglion with its investing fascia layers will be apparent. It is important to establish the correct plane of dissection, which is more easily done if the ganglion remains intact. The extensor tendons should be retracted to each side and care taken to avoid damage to them. The ganglion can usually be traced down to the dorsal capsule of the wrist joint. Some surgeons prefer to excise a small piece of the dorsal capsule with the ganglion while others try to ligate the neck of the ganglion and sew the dorsal capsule of the wrist joint over the top.

The tourniquet is then released and haemostasis secured. The extensor retinaculum is repaired with an absorbable suture and the skin closed with a subcuticular polypropylene suture.

Postoperative management

The wound is covered with a gauze dressing and wrapped in a bulky wool and crêpe bandage which helps to immobilize the wrist joint for the first 10 days until the suture is removed.

Complications

On the dorsal surface it is possible to damage the terminal branches of the radial nerve which may produce an area of numbness distal to the wound or may produce a painful neuroma.

The ganglion recurs in approximately 5 per cent of cases. The patient should be informed of both these possible complications before surgery.

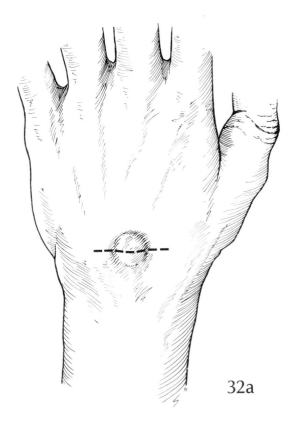

32a

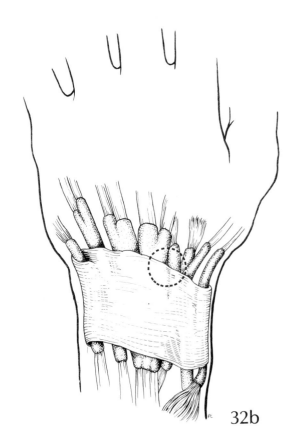

32b

EXCISION OF A PALMAR GANGLION

A longitudinal lazy-S incision is made over the ganglion. Since the radial artery often overlies the ganglion, it is important to identify this vessel proximally and dissect it free from the ganglionic tissue. Having retracted the artery, the dissection of the ganglion is carried down to the wrist joint where it is amputated and the capsule oversewn. It is important in this procedure to release the tourniquet to establish the continuity of the radial artery prior to skin closure.

The wound is closed with a subcuticular suture. Postoperative management is the same as for the dorsal ganglion, and recurrence is as frequent.

OSTEOARTHRITIS

Osteoarthritis of the wrist joint usually results from previous trauma or from Kienböck's disease of the lunate. If the osteoarthritis only involves two or even three carpal joints then a limited arthrodesis may be performed. However, if the radiocarpal and mid-carpal joints are involved then it will be necessary to perform an arthroplasty or an arthrodesis of the wrist joint. Arthroplasty of the wrist joint has not been popular in post-traumatic arthritis because such patients usually put significant forces through the wrist joint once the pain has been relieved. This is in contrast to the patient with rheumatoid arthritis who has multiple joint involvement above and below the wrist joint and therefore the forces applied are minimal.

Arthrodesis of the wrist joint allows a patient to perform most manual tasks and is therefore preferable to arthroplasty, especially in the manual worker. If mobility of the wrist joint is of utmost importance, then arthroplasty or limited arthrodesis could be considered.

In osteoarthritis advantage can be taken of the good bone stock on each side of the wrist joint which enables internal fixation to be more rigid than that which can be obtained from the osteoporotic bone of rheumatoid arthritis.

PANARTHRODESIS OF THE WRIST

While it is usual for the wrist to be fused in approximately 20° of dorsiflexion in order to aid power grip, it can be fused in a straight position with little disability. The arthrodesis can be performed using a bone graft for internal fixation, or a plate can be applied to the dorsal surface together with the bone graft in order to provide the fixation. The approach is the same for each operation.

Position of the patient

The patient lies supine with the forearm resting on a table. The tourniquet is applied to the upper arm. The patient can be slightly tilted towards the side of the operation by a sandbag placed under the opposite buttock, which will elevate the pelvis to enable a bone graft to be obtained.

Incision

A lazy-S longitudinal dorsal incision is made extending from the proximal third of the third metacarpal to 3 cm proximal to the wrist joint.

Exposure

33

The skin edges are lifted with skin hooks and the dorsal veins ligated if they are an obstruction. The extensor retinaculum is divided on its ulnar side and reflected towards the radial side. The extensor tendons are retracted to expose the distal end of the radius and the dorsal area of the carpus up to the base of the third metacarpal. If necessary, the extensor carpi radialis tendons may be detached from their insertion and reflected proximally.

The dorsal capsule of the wrist joint is incised in the shape of an I. Flaps are retracted medially and laterally. The wrist is flexed and the articular cartilage is removed from the carpal bones and from the distal radius with gouges and bone nibblers. The distal end of the ulna can be excised if it is involved in the arthritic process and can be used as a bone graft.

33

Bone graft fixation

34a

The proposed graft will be placed on the dorsum of the carpus extending from the base of the third metacarpal proximally to a point 2 cm proximal to the distal end of the radius. A trough approximately 2 cm wide should be made over the radius, carpus and the base of the third metacarpal. After cutting the edges of the trough the bone can be excavated using a chisel or a gouge.

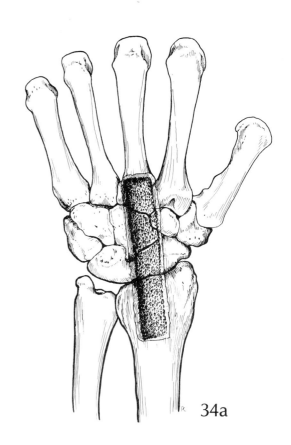

34a

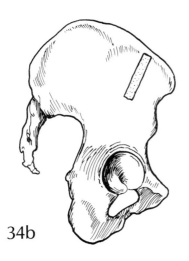

34b

34b

Bone graft is taken from the opposite ilium. The outer surface of the ilium is exposed below the iliac crest. The graft required is approximately 8 cm long and 2 cm wide and is taken in a caudo-cranial direction from the outer table of the iliac bone. The site of the graft is marked using an osteotome: the outer table and cancellous bone are penetrated but the inner table is not. A curved osteotome is then used to lift this graft, together with underlying cancellous bone, away from the inner table. It is important to take the graft from this area as it has a slight concavity which, when applied to the dorsum of the wrist, produces a slightly dorsiflexed position.

Seating of the graft

35

Prior to fixation of this graft the wrist joint is opened while in palmarflexion, articular cartilage is removed, and cancellous bone taken from the iliac crest is impacted into the joint. The wrist is dorsiflexed and the bone graft strut is placed in the trough and shaped to lie flush with the surface of the carpus. It is held in place by a lag screw which passes through the radius and a second one which passes through the base of the third metacarpal. This produces quite firm fixation of the wrist.

Plate fixation

36

The articular cartilage is removed from the joint and a trough is cut on the dorsum of the distal radius and carpus. Cancellous bone graft is packed into the joint space. The required position of the wrist is determined and fixed with Kirschner wires. A 3.5 mm cancellous screw is passed through the radial styloid to the capitate and the position is checked. A corticocancellous bone graft is placed in the trough and an 8-hole, 3.5 mm AO dynamic compression plate is then applied from the base of the third metacarpal to the distal radius. It should be contoured to produce about 20° of dorsiflexion.

Closure

It may be possible to suture the dorsal capsule of the wrist joint over the plate or the graft, but this is not essential. The extensor retinaculum is passed deep to the tendons and sutured in place over the graft or the plate. It is helpful to leave one strip of the extensor retinaculum on the dorsal surface of the tendons to limit the bowstringing, especially if there has been any degree of dorsiflexion left in the wrist.

A small suction drain is left in the wound and the skin is closed with interrupted sutures. A well-padded dressing is applied with a plaster slab on the palmar aspect of the wrist.

Postoperative management

Bone graft fixation It is advisable to leave the wrist supported in a below-elbow plaster cast for a period of 12 weeks or until fusion has been established.

Plate fixation A well-padded volar plaster slab should be left in place until the sutures are removed at 14 days. A heat-moulded splint is then applied for a period of 12 weeks. This can be a removable splint but must be left in place except for essential toilet of the skin until fusion is complete.

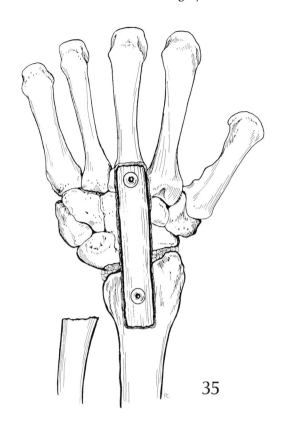

35

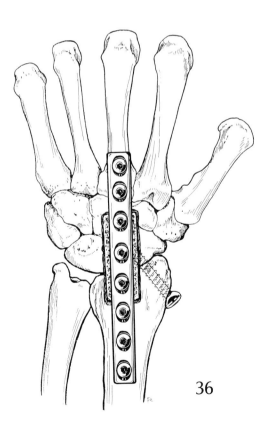

36

FRACTURES OF THE CARPAL SCAPHOID

37

Fractures of the carpal scaphoid not associated with dislocations should be treated conservatively in a plaster cast. There is considerable controversy concerning the extent of the plaster and the position of the wrist. However, a short-arm cast which encloses the proximal phalanx of the thumb in a position of function achieves a union rate of 95 per cent, and more extensive immobilization would appear unnecessary[8,9].

The duration of immobilization that is required varies with the site of the fracture. Fractures of the tuberosity and distal third require 6 weeks of immobilization. Fractures of the waist and the proximal third require 12 weeks of immobilization[8]. The plaster cast is removed after these intervals and further radiographs in four planes are necessary. It may be difficult at this stage to tell if union is complete but the patient should be allowed to mobilize the wrist and be reviewed in 4 weeks with further radiographic and clinical assessment.

Operative intervention may be necessary at this stage if radiographically there is established non-union, especially if there has been a change in position of the scaphoid since the original radiograph. Non-union occurs predominantly in fractures of the waist and the proximal pole. If, after 4 weeks of mobilization, the fracture is clinically and radiographically un-united then operative intervention is recommended. If the patient is asymptomatic yet the radiograph shows that the fracture has not yet united, then the treatment is open to controversy. London[10] recommends that the non-union be treated only if it is symptomatic, suggesting that there is a state of asymptomatic fibrous union which may never cause problems. However, other authors[11,12] suggest that osteoarthritis is the eventual outcome of an asymptomatic non-union and that operative intervention should be performed even in the absence of clinical symptoms.

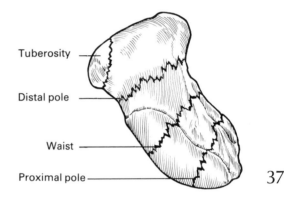

Tuberosity

Distal pole

Waist

Proximal pole

37

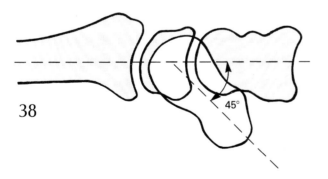

38

38

It is important to scrutinize the lateral view of the wrist carefully to detect evidence of carpal instability[13]. The normal scapholunate angle is 45°.

39a & b

A fracture of the waist of the scaphoid may cause the distal pole to tilt anteriorly, thus creating dorsiflexion of the lunate (dorsal intercalated segmental instability pattern). Disruption of the ligamentous structures may allow abnormal movement at the fracture site and therefore increase the risk of non-union. Those patients with gross instability should have a primary internal fixation of the scaphoid. In late cases it is important to recognize this anterior collapse of the carpal scaphoid which effectively reduces the overall length of the bone. The anterior collapse should be corrected by the insertion of a wedge graft which restores the scaphoid to the correct length.

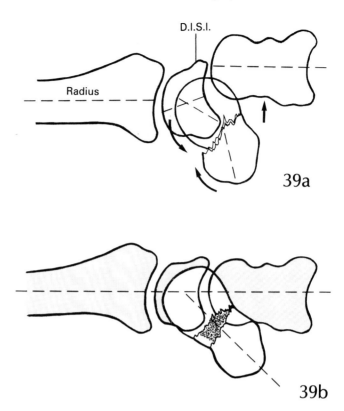

Indications for operation

Early

1. Acute trans-scaphoid perilunate dislocations of the wrist or any other dislocation of the wrist joint in which the scaphoid is fractured.
2. Displacement of the scaphoid fracture greater than 2 mm.

Late

1. If, after removal of plaster at 12 weeks, the fracture shows established non-union and early cyst formation on each side of the fracture line.
2. If, after 4 weeks of mobilization following the plaster removal at 12 weeks, the fracture remains un-united and the patient is symptomatic.

3. If, after 4 weeks of mobilization following removal of the plaster, the fracture remains un-united but the patient is asymptomatic (this indication is controversial at the present time).
4. An un-united fracture of the carpal scaphoid which presents late (often due to a further injury) and there is a carpal instability pattern.
5. If, after a fresh injury the symptoms of an old un-united scaphoid fracture are brought to light and do not settle down after a 4-week period of plaster immobilization. There is a relative indication for internal fixation if there is an instability pattern, as there would appear to be a risk of late degenerative change.
6. An established non-union of the scaphoid associated with symptomatic degenerative change of the wrist joint which may require excision of the radial styloid, limited carpal arthrodesis or a panarthrodesis of the carpus from the radius to the base of the third metacarpal.

Operations

Internal fixation of the scaphoid with or without bone graft and the Matte–Russe bone grafting procedure[14] are the two most commonly performed operations. The success rate for established non-union is similar for each procedure although the Matte–Russe bone graft procedure requires a longer period of plaster immobilization. In the acute injury internal fixation is the treatment of choice.

MATTE–RUSSE BONE GRAFT OF THE CARPAL SCAPHOID

Position of patient

After induction of general anaesthesia, the patient is placed supine and a tourniquet applied to the upper arm. A sandbag is placed under the opposite buttock to enable a bone graft to be taken from the iliac crest, and this site is then prepared.

Incision

40

An anterior approach is made to the wrist joint. A 5 cm longitudinal incision is made over the tendon of flexor carpi radialis and it is centred at the level of the tip of the styloid process. Care should be taken to identify the superficial palmar branch of the radial artery, which should be ligated.

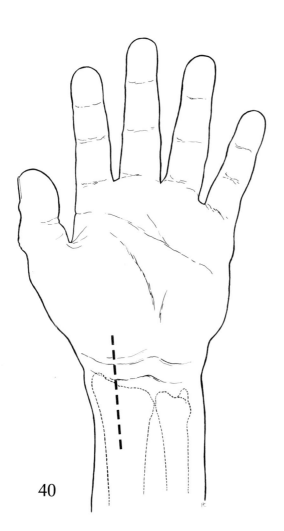

40

Approach

41

The tendon sheath of flexor carpi radialis is opened and the tendon is retracted, releasing it from its tunnel distally. A longitudinal incision is made in the base of the tendon sheath, dividing the capsule longitudinally; the joint may then be entered. The deep volar radiocarpal ligaments will need to be reconstructed at the end of the procedure.

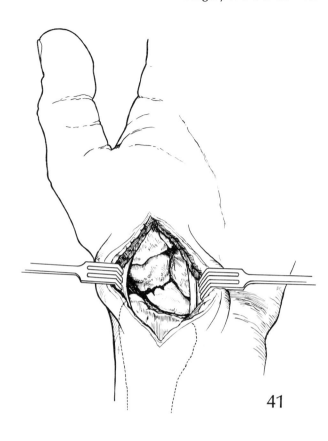

41

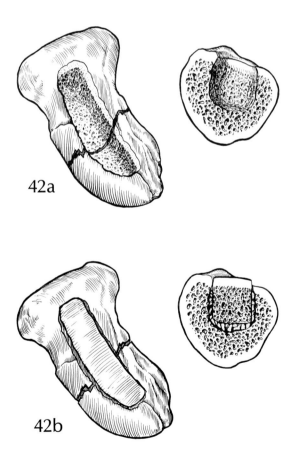

42a

42b

Procedure

42a & b

The fracture is identified and an egg-shaped cavity is created in both fragments using a small osteotome and curette. The anterior cortex is undermined distally and proximally. This creates an anterior trough in the bone.

A small corticocancellous graft is taken from the iliac crest through a small transverse incision. A small amount of cancellous bone is taken at the same time. The bone graft is trimmed to fit into the cavity. The cortex of the graft lies superficially and the fragments are distracted while the graft is pressed into the cavity. Release of the fragments should create a stable graft. The cavity around the graft is packed with small fragments of cancellous bone. If the graft is not stable then two longitudinal Kirschner wires can be used to maintain stability.

43

A modification of this technique is to use two small corticocancellous grafts, placing the cancellous surfaces face-to-face and inserting the graft on its side[15].

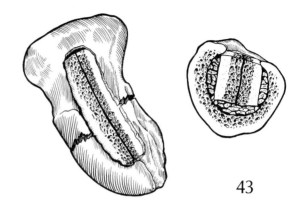

43

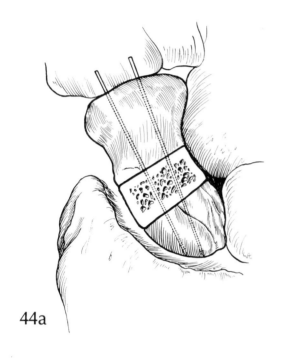

44a

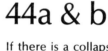

44a & b

If there is a collapse of the scaphoid bone on the lateral view then it is important to open out the volar aspect with the bone graft. The lateral view of the fractured side should be compared with the unfractured side in order to establish the correct length of the scaphoid bone. It is possible to plan the size of the wedge with preoperative drawings[16]. It is usually necessary to fix these grafts with Kirschner wires or even a screw.

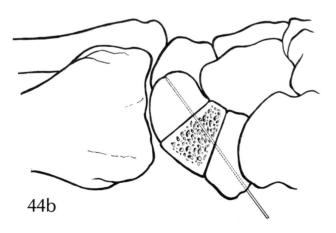

44b

Closure

The volar radiocarpal ligaments are repaired using interrupted sutures. It is easier to place all the sutures before tying any of them. The synovium is closed over the tendon of flexor carpi radialis and the skin sutured. A well-padded bandage is applied followed by a volar plaster slab with a gutter on the ulnar side.

Postoperative management

The dressing is reduced after 10 days and a below-elbow plaster applied, including the proximal phalanx of the thumb. This is left in place for 12 weeks.

INTERNAL FIXATION OF THE SCAPHOID

AO scaphoid lag screw

Position of patient

A tourniquet is applied to the upper arm and the patient's hand rests pronated on a hand table. It is necessary to have X-ray facilities peroperatively.

Incision

45

A straight incision is made over the dorsoradial side of the carpus extending from the base of the thumb to the radial styloid and then curving slightly across the back of the wrist.

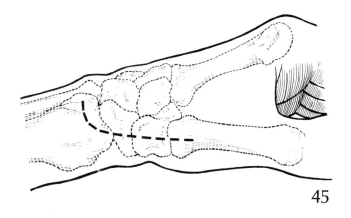

45

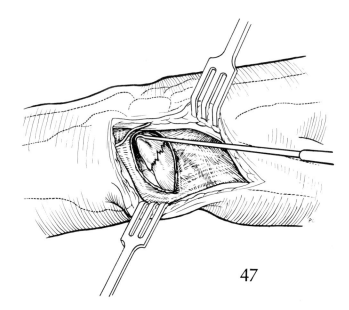

46

Exposure

46

Superficial veins may be ligated. It is important to preserve the terminal branches of the radial nerve and also the radial artery as it crosses the floor of the fossa. The tendons of extensor pollicis longus and extensor pollicis brevis are retracted. The capsule of the wrist is exposed and an oblique incision is made in line with the scaphoid.

47

The fracture is identified and a small bone hook is inserted around the proximal pole. Care should be taken not to dissect the capsule of the dorsal ridge of the scaphoid as this will influence the blood supply.

47

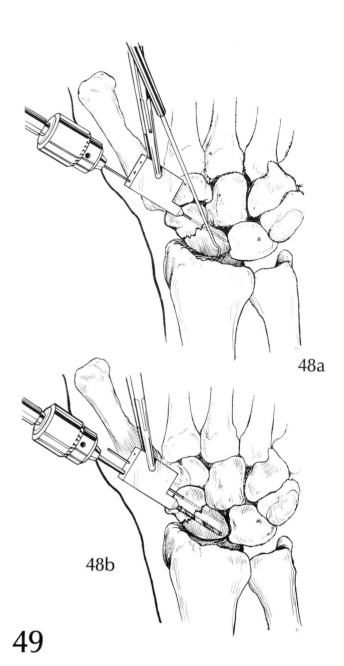

48a

48b

48a & b

Using the drill guide, the surgeon inserts a Kirschner wire along the long axis of the scaphoid. A check radiograph is taken in the posteroanterior and lateral directions. The length of the screw required is determined by measuring the length of Kirschner wire protruding from the scaphoid and subtracting that length from the total length of another similar Kirschner wire. A 2 mm drill hole is made parallel to the Kirschner wire using the drill guide. The proximal cortex is tapped using the 3.5 mm tap and an appropriate length of 3.5 mm cancellous screw is inserted into the scaphoid.

49

Compression should be observed at the fracture site. Check radiographs should be taken to ascertain the position of the screw. The Kirschner wire is removed. The capsule is closed with interrupted sutures. The skin is closed with interrupted nylon. A padded bandage is wrapped round the hand and a plaster volar slab applied with a gutter around the ulnar side.

Postoperative management

The plaster slab and bandages should be reduced at 10 days and sutures can be removed. A lightweight splint is applied for a further 2 weeks and if check X-ray films are satisfactory at that stage, total mobilization can be commenced. Full force should not be taken through the wrist for 3 months.

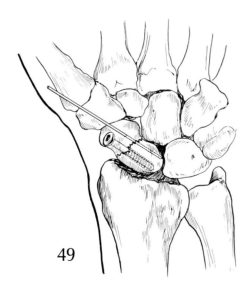

49

The Herbert bone screw

50 & 51

The insertion of a screw into the scaphoid is a difficult procedure as there is little margin for error in the alignment. A screw has been designed which overcomes some of the difficulties encountered previously. The screw does not have a head, but in its place is another thread which has a different pitch to that of the distal end of the screw[17]. Therefore the head of the screw does not protrude from the bone and compression is achieved by the differential pitch of the threads at each end of the screw. Both ends of the screw remain buried in the bone and the screw does not have to be removed. A jig is necessary for its insertion and it is essential, before commencing the operation, to make sure that all the necessary instruments and the complete range of screws are available in the set

This procedure is technically demanding and Herbert's precise instructions should be studied carefully. The jig is difficult to place in the correct position and concern about ligamentous and vascular damage to the distal end of the scaphoid has been expressed[18].

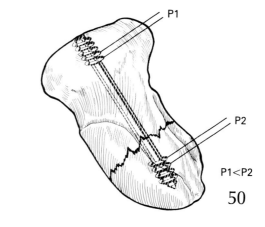

P1
P2
P1<P2

50

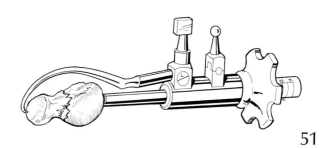

51

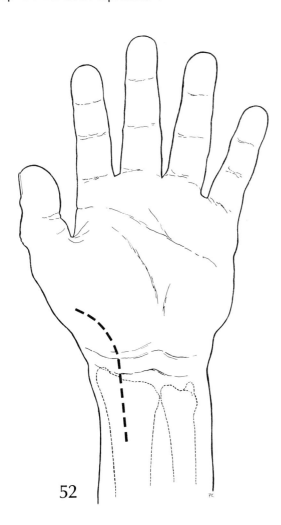

52

Preparation of the patient

The patient is placed supine on the operating table with a tourniquet applied to the upper arm and the hand resting on the table. If the screw is being inserted for an established non–union it may be necessary to take a bone graft and therefore the contralateral iliac crest should be prepared.

Incision

52

An anterior approach is made to the wrist joint. A longitudinal incision is made along the line of the flexor carpi radialis; distally it curves radially along the thenar eminence.

Approach

The superficial branch of the radial artery is ligated. The flexor sheath of flexor carpi radialis is divided longitudinally and the tendon retracted. The tendon is released from its tunnel distally. The bed of the tendon is then incised longitudinally to expose the wrist joint and the scaphoid.

Procedure

53

In the acute situation the fracture is reduced and the Herbert jig is applied. The hook of the jig must be inserted into the proximal pole. It will be necessary to dissect the ligaments between the scaphoid and the trapezium to lift the scaphoid forward so that the jig can be applied distally. The guide is then clamped to the distal pole and it should be seen to compress the fracture line.

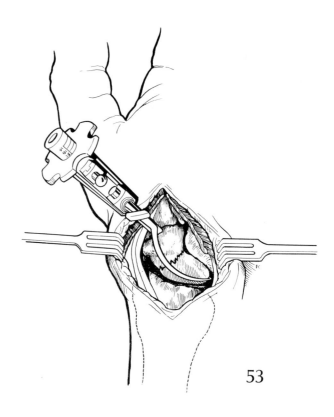

53

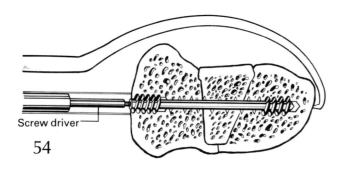

Screw driver

54

54

If the screw is being inserted into an established non-union then the fibrous tissue is removed from the fracture site and the cavity so created is packed with cancellous bone. It may be necessary to insert an anterior wedge of bone taken from the iliac crest. This should be a corticocancellous graft. The fracture is opened up, the wedge inserted and it is then held there by the compression of the jig.

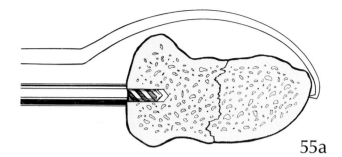

55a

55a, b, c & d

With the jig in place, a pilot drill is inserted into the proximal end for the trailing edge of the screw (a). A long drill is then inserted for the leading edge of the screw (b), the bone is then tapped and the length of the screw is measured directly from a scale on the jig (c). Insertion of all instruments is done through the jig and the instruments are so designed that the correct length of drilling and tapping is always achieved.

A screw of appropriate length is then inserted through the jig and tightened. Compression should be seen at the fracture line (d). The jig is removed and the stability of the fracture tested.

Closure

The anterior volar capsule is closed with interrupted non-absorbable sutures as described above for the Matte–Russe graft procedure.

Postoperative management

A radiograph is taken to check the position of the screw. The hand is wrapped in a well-padded bandage with a plaster cast on the volar aspect. At 10 days the cast and the sutures are removed and a light heat-moulded wrist splint is applied for a total period of 4 weeks. During this time the patient removes it for gentle mobilization.

Precautions

Care must be taken not to dissect the scaphoid too extensively from its distal pole. The jig must be applied accurately if the screw is to achieve its aim of producing compression across the fracture.

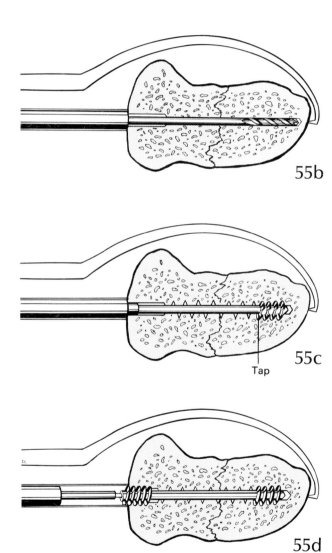

55b

Tap

55c

55d

FRACTURES OF THE PROXIMAL POLE WITH A SMALL FRAGMENT

56

If at operation the proximal pole is found to be too small or completely avascular then bone grafting procedures and fixation will not be possible. Excision of the small proximal fragment leaves a space into which the capitate may migrate and it is therefore advised that a small piece of Silastic be carved and used as a spacer. Some surgeons use the moulded Silastic scaphoid and cut off the proximal end, while others use a block of Silastic and cut it to the necessary shape at the time of the operation[19].

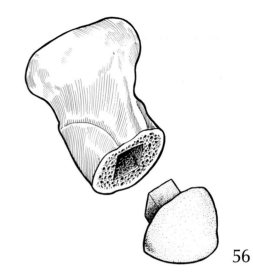

56

References

1. Darrach W. Anterior dislocation of the head of the ulna. *Ann Surg* 1912; 56: 802–3.

2. Gonçalves D. Correction of disorders of the distal radio-ulnar joint by artificial pseudoarthrosis of the ulna. *J Bone Joint Surg [Br]* 1974; 56-B: 462–4.

3. Clayton ML. Surgical treatment at the wrist in rheumatoid arthritis: a review of 37 patients. *J Bone Joint Surg [Am]* 1965; 47-A: 741–50.

4. Millender LH, Nalebuff EA. Arthrodesis of the rheumatoid wrist: an evaluation of 60 patients and a description of a different surgical technique. *J Bone Joint Surg [Am]* 1973; 55-A: 1026–34.

5. Papaioannou T, Dickson RA. Arthrodesis of the wrist in rheumatoid disease. *Hand* 1982; 14: 12–6.

6. Chamay A, Della Santa D, Vilaseca A. Radiolunate arthrodesis: factor of stability for the rheumatoid wrist. *Ann Chir Main* 1983; 2: 5.

7. Swanson AB, Swanson G de G, Maupin, BK. Flexible implant arthroplasty of the radiocarpal joint: surgical technique and long-term study. *Clin Orthop* 1984; 187: 94–106.

8. Leslie IJ, Dickson RA. The fractures carpal scaphoid: natural history and factors influencing outcome. *J Bone Joint Surg [Br]* 1981; 63-B: 225–30.

9. Taleisnik J. *The wrist.* New York: Churchill Livingstone, 1985.

10. London PS. The broken scaphoid bone: the case against pessimism. *J Bone Joint Surg [Br]* 1961; 43-B: 237–44.

11. Ruby LK, Stinson J, Belsky MR. The natural history of scaphoid non-union: a review of 55 cases. *J Bone Joint Surg [Am]* 1985; 67-A: 428–32.

12. Mack GR, Bosse MJ, Gelberman RH. The natural history of scaphoid non-union. *J Bone Joint Surg [Am]* 1984; 66-A: 504–9.

13. Fisk GR. Carpal instability and the fractured scaphoid. *Ann R Coll Surg Engl* 1970; 46: 63–76.

14. Russe O. Fracture of the carpal navicular: diagnosis, non-operative treatment and operative treatment. *J Bone Joint Surg [Am]* 1960; 42-A: 759–68.

15. Green DP. The effect of avascular necrosis on Russe bone grafting for scaphoid non-union. *J Hand Surg [Am]* 1985; 10A: 597–605.

16. Fernandez DL. A technique for anterior wedge-shaped grafts for scaphoid non-union with carpal instability. *J Hand Surg [Am]* 1984; 9A: 733–7.

17. Herbert TJ, Fisher WE. Management of the fractured scaphoid using a new bone screw. *J Bone Joint Surg [Br]* 1984; 66-B: 114–123.

18. Botte MJ, Mortensen WW, Gelberman RH, Rhoads CE, Gellman H. Internal vascularity of the scaphoid in cadavers after insertion of the Herbert screw. *J Hand Surg [Am]* 1988; 13A: 216–20.

19. Zemel NP, Stark HH, Ashworth CR, Rickard TA, Anderson DR. Treatment of selected patients with an ununited fracture of the proximal part of the scaphoid by excision of the fragment and insertion of a carved silicone-rubber spacer. *J Bone Joint Surg [Am]*; 66-A: 510–7.

Illustrations by Gillian Oliver

Tendon transfer for mobile radial deviation of the wrist

B. Helal MChOrth, FRCS
Honorary Consultant Orthopaedic Surgeon, The Royal London Hospital and The Royal National Orthopaedic Hospital, London, and Enfield Group of Hospitals, UK

S. C. Chen FRCS
Consultant Orthopaedic Surgeon, Enfield Group of Hospitals, UK

Introduction

In rheumatoid disease the inferior radio-ulnar joint is often involved early. The synovitis around the ulnar head results in inhibition of the ulnar carpal muscles. This, in turn, encourages ulnar deviation at the metacarpophalangeal joints[1]. While there is passive mobility in an ulnar direction this can be corrected by tendon transfer. Ferlic and Clayton[2] have carried out tendon transfer of the extensor carpi radialis longus to the extensor carpi ulnaris. In our experience much of the power is dissipated in extending the wrist. Helal[3] modified this transfer by splitting the transferred extensor carpi radialis longus and implanting half into the flexor carpi ulnaris and half into the extensor carpi ulnaris. This transfer has proved an effective ulnar deviator of the wrist. There is an added bonus, as the limb passing to the flexor carpi ulnaris stabilizes the ulnar shaft as the procedure is usually combined with ulnar head excision.

Operation

Incisions

1

Three skin incisions are made on the dorsum of the forearm and wrist:

1. Over the insertion of extensor carpi radialis longus
2. In line with this tendon in the lower third of the forearm
3. On the ulnar side, over the distal end of he ulna.

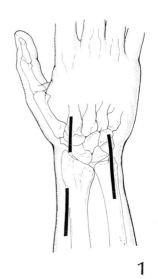

1

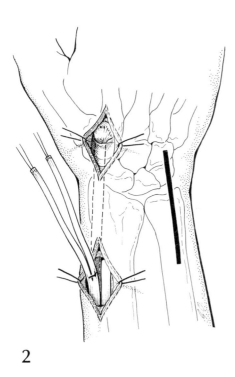

2

Transfer

2

The tendon of extensor carpi radialis longus is detached from its insertion and brought out through the proximal incision. It is split and a suture placed through the bifurcation to prevent further separation.

3

The split tendon is tunnelled through subcutaneous tissue to the ulnar side.

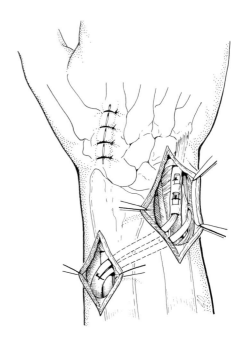

3

Exposure of ulnar tendons

4

The tendons of extensor carpi ulnaris and flexor carpi ulnaris are identified. In isolating the flexor carpi ulnaris care must be taken to protect the ulnar nerve which is close by.

Attachment

One limb of the split transferred tendon is woven into each of the ulnar carpal tendons with the wrist held in full ulnar deviation.

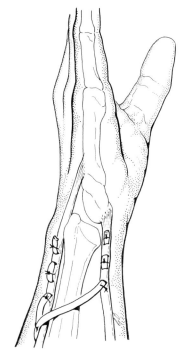

4

Postoperative management

A below-elbow plaster cast is applied with the wrist in ulnar deviation for a period of 4 weeks.

References

1. Stack HE, Vaughan Jackson OJ, The zig-zag deformity in the rheumatoid hand. *Hand* 1971; 3: 62.

2. Ferlic DC, Clayton ML. Tendon transfer for radial rotation in the rheumatoid wrist. *J Bone Joint Surg [Am]* 1973; 55-A: 880–1.

3. Helal B. The flexor tendon apparatus in the rheumatoid hand. *Clin Rheum Dis* 1984; 10: 479–500.

Tendon injuries in the hand

John P. W. Varian FRCS, FRACS(Orth)
Consultant Hand Surgeon, Blackrock Clinic, Dublin, Ireland

Much of the text in this chapter remains unchanged from the previous edition and is the work of the late Mr. R. Guy Pulvertaft. The present author has amended and expanded it in the light of his experience and some of the changing trends in tendon surgery.

Introduction

The problems set by tendon divisions in the hand are complex and their treatment varies with the site of injury, but the following observations have a general application.

1. A tendon heals readily when held in apposition and the union is sufficiently strong at 3–4 weeks to withstand slight strain.
2. Damaged tendons have a marked tendency to become adherent to the surrounding tissues, limiting their gliding movement.
3. A gentle and precise technique is essential and necessitates the use of the finest instruments and a suture material which does not provoke a tissue reaction.
4. A bloodless field, using a tourniquet, is necessary. Most surgeons remove the tourniquet and secure haemostasis prior to closure. Others, including the author, prefer to use meticulous haemostasis throughout the operation, especially during the early dissection, and then close prior to tourniquet release. The essential objective is the prevention of postoperative haematoma and the surgeon should use the technique which suits him best in attaining this objective.

Indications for operation

EXTENSOR TENDONS

Distal interphalangeal joint (mallet deformity)

1

Rupture or division of the extensor attachment to the distal phalanx is best treated by splintage in extension for 6–8 weeks or longer if the treatment has been delayed. The splint needs to be tolerable to the patient and effectively maintained. Several patterns of splint have been described; the one illustrated (devised independently by Parker and by Stack) is suitable and preferred to plaster or internal fixation.

Operative treatment is reserved for those cases in which conservative treatment has failed or which are seen late. The choice lies between arthrodesis of the distal joint or repair of the tendon. The former is often difficult to achieve and the latter tends to give poor results. Most patients are therefore advised against secondary surgery. Where tendon repair is undertaken there must be a full passive range of movement in the terminal joint.

Secondary repair is possible where there has been open severance of the tendon. In closed rupture the tendon ends are difficult or impossible to identify and tendon plication as described by Vilain[1] is preferable. Iselin[2] has reported satisfactory results excising a wedge of skin and tendon, and including both tissues in the repair suture. Operative treatment is also advisable when a considerable fragment of bone has been avulsed with the tendon and especially when this is accompanied by subluxation of the main fragment. In these circumstances the operation becomes very difficult if there is delay after injury and should not be attempted if the delay exceeds 3 weeks.

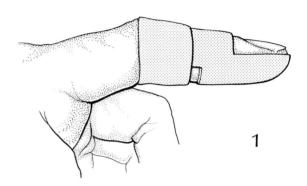

Proximal interphalangeal joint (boutonnière deformity)

The extensor tendon divides over the proximal phalanx into a central band which is attached to the base of the middle phalanx and into two lateral bands which bypass the proximal interphalangeal joint and join to be inserted into the base of the distal phalanx. Division of the central band allows the proximal joint to flex and the distal joint is drawn into hyperextension. The lateral bands migrate forwards and act as flexors of the proximal joint. Secondary ligamentous contractures lead to a fixed deformity of both joints.

2, 3a & b

When a rupture or division of the central band is seen within 5 or 6 weeks after injury, a good result can usually be obtained by splintage in extension for a period of 4–6 weeks, followed by protective mobilization in a dynamic splint. A suitable static type is the Bunnell splint which is fitted as illustrated to permit flexion of the distal joint. The Capener dynamic splint is recommended for the mobilization phase. It may also be used to correct a moderate flexion contracture.

Operative treatment is reserved for those cases which fail to respond to conservative measures and for those that are manifestly unlikely to do so. Secondary repair by simple scar excision and end-to-end suture is usually possible up to 3 months after injury but once secondary contractures develop it may not be possible to reconstitute the normal anatomy. Matev[3] corrects the deformity by transposing one of the lateral bands to the base of the middle phalanx and lengthens the other band to overcome the hyperextension of the distal phalanx. Littler and Eaton[4] centralize the lateral bands over the proximal joint, relying on the oblique retinacular ligament of Landsmeer and the lumbrical muscle to extend the distal joint.

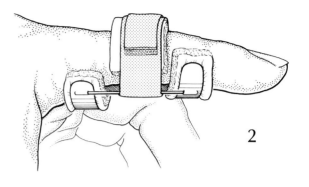

2

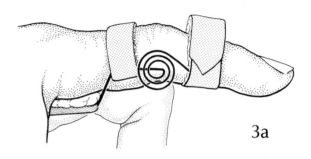

3a

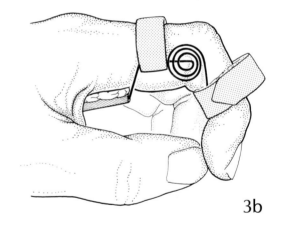

3b

Hand and wrist

Tendon retraction after division over the metacarpophalangeal joint is usually slight and an early case may be treated successfully by splintage in extension. If there is any doubt, and always in later cases, surgical repair is advisable. Tendons divided in the central and proximal parts of the hand and over the wrist joint always require repair. In late cases it may not be possible to obtain apposition of the tendon ends and a tendon graft or a tendon transfer may be needed.

FLEXOR TENDONS

Flexor digitorum profundus in the finger

When the profundus tendon alone is divided beyond the superficialis attachment, good results can be obtained by immediate suture. Delayed suture is possible if the vincula are intact and retraction has been prevented. This is likely if the laceration occurred when the profundus muscle was relaxed. (Remember that this is the case in the finger during strong pulp-to-pulp pinch against the thumb.) In these circumstances end-to-end repair is often possible up to 6 weeks after the injury, bypassing the distal pulley.

If the tendon retracted into the palm, as commonly occurs in tendon avulsion, direct repair becomes impossible after only a few days as the tendon becomes too swollen to be threaded back through the pulleys and superficialis decussation. Consideration should then be given to tendon grafting which should be delayed for 4–6 months to allow the hand to settle after the original injury. A thin tendon, preferably plantaris, is used and reaches from the proximal palm to the distal phalanx. The undamaged superficialis tendon is not disturbed. This

operation is justified for someone whose occupation demands fingertip action and for children. The purpose is to achieve perfection and, as the possibility of disturbing superficialis function exists, the operation should only be undertaken when the indications are clear and the surgeon is experienced in tendon grafting[5].

The alternative procedure is fixation in suitable flexion of the distal joint by arthrodesis or tenodesis. This should be postponed for at least 6 months as in the author's experience most patients become accustomed to the loss of flexion in the terminal joint and do not want surgery.

Flexor digitorum profundus and superficialis in the finger

During recent years there has been a movement towards the wider use of primary suture of flexor tendons divided within the digital theca, the technique of which is described in the chapter on 'Primary repair of the divided digital flexor tendon' (*see* pp. 828–835). *It must be stressed that the results are likely to be disappointing unless the facilities and the technique are of the highest order; failure will foul the ground for subsequent tendon grafting.* Neither primary suture nor tendon grafting are recommended unless the surgeon has studied the subject fully and has had adequate training in the exacting technique. When these conditions are not satisfied, it is wiser to do no more than clean and suture the wound and refer the case for tendon grafting later. The tendons are replaced by a graft when the digit has recovered from the initial trauma and all reaction has resolved, which may take 4–6 months. Apart from the inconvenience to the patient there is no inherent harm in the delay for excellent results can be achieved even after a lapse of years, provided that the digit is in good overall condition[6]. It is useless to expect tendon grafting to succeed in the presence of severe scarring, contracture or complete sensory loss. If these conditions prevail, consideration should be given to the two-stage operation described on pp. 836–854.

Flexor pollicis longus

Division of flexor pollicis longus in the distal part of the thumb should be treated by immediate suture. In the region between the metacarpophalangeal joint and the wrist the tendon is in close relationship to the sensory nerves of the thumb and the motor branch to the thenar muscles. These structures are at risk during a tendon repair and, if injured, lead to a worse disability than the lack of distal joint flexion. If the surgeon is inexperienced, it is better to perform skin suture only, with a view to tendon grafting later. However, in experienced hands, primary repair produces better results than in the finger because there is only one flexor tendon to the digit and less risk of adhesion.

In general, function can be restored in all late cases by tendon grafting. However, it must be remembered that a thumb lacking flexion at the interphalangeal joint produces little disability in many individuals, whereas a severe flexion contracture in this joint which may result from a tendon graft, can be disabling. It is advisable therefore to avoid splinting the interphalangeal joint in full flexion in the postoperative period.

Palm

Suture of the superficialis and profundus tendons divided at the same level in the palm is apt to be followed by cross-union which limits the flexion action to superficialis. Meticulous suture of sharp-cut tendons will avoid this complication, but when the tendon ends are ragged it is advisable to cut back superficialis and restrict the repair to profundus. Superficialis to the ring and little fingers should always be sacrificed in the palm. Superficialis to the index and middle fingers has an important action in strong pulp-to-pulp pinch and should be repaired if possible. Appropriate posturing of the finger in the postoperative period will separate the two tendon repairs and reduce the risk of cross-union. Secondary suture may be practicable if the proximal end is held by the lumbricalis muscle but in late cases end-to-end contact may not be obtainable and the gap should be closed with a free graft taken from superficialis.

Wrist

Tendons divided at the wrist level retract severely and their muscles shorten and prevent apposition even in a fairly recent case, which necessitates the use of multiple bridge grafts for reconstruction. It is imperative, therefore, to perform immediate suture of tendons in this region if the wound conditions permit. End-to-end suture of all the tendons is performed, using the more rapidly applied Bunnell double right-angle stitch[7] which saves time especially when repair of associated nerve injury is carried out at the same operation.

ANAESTHESIA

In Great Britain general anaesthesia is used unless there is some special indication for plexus or local nerve block anaesthesia. However, regional anaesthesia is the more common choice in many countries where general anaesthesia is not so readily available. With the advent of neurotracers and longer acting anaesthetics the techniques are becoming easier. Many would consider it an advantage to have the limb paralysed in the immediate postoperative period, avoiding the uncontrolled movements often seen during the recovery from general anaesthesia, which increase the risk of haematoma formation and the risk of dehiscence of the repair[8].

Operations for individual tendon injuries

TENDON JUNCTIONS

Suture material

Stainless steel wire causes no tissue reaction and has proved a most satisfactory suture material. Care must be taken to avoid kinking; a reef knot is tied and the wire may be cut off flush with the knot leaving no protruding ends. Monofilament wire (British wire gauge 40) can be obtained swaged to 2.5 cm bayonet-ended malleable needles which were specifically developed for tendon surgery. Synthetic fibres (4/0) are also widely used. Material should always be non-absorbable. The two junctions most commonly used in primary repair are shown in *Illustrations 4* and *5*. Other techniques have been described[9, 10, 11].

Bunnell criss-cross stitch

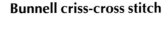

This stitch used to be the commonest method used in end-to-end tendon repair. As the result of claims that it causes ischaemia of tendon ends it has now become less popular than the Kessler stitch[12] (*see below*).

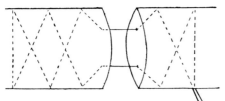
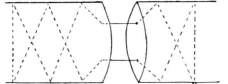

4

Kessler grasping stitch

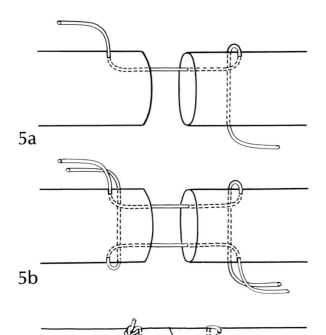

5a

5b

5c

5a, b & c

This stitch has the advantage of requiring fewer penetrations of the tendon and it is claimed that is has less tendency to compress the tendon ends and embarrass the blood supply. It has been modified by many surgeons who now no longer tie a half-knot at each corner as described by Kessler but insert the suture as shown. It is also easier to insert the suture into each tendon end in turn and tie the knots at the tendon junction, especially during primary repair when flexor sheath is being preserved.

Bunnell double right-angle stitch

6

This stitch can be inserted rapidly and is a convenient and adequate technique to use when many tendons are divided at the wrist level, especially when time is of the essence, as during a replantation.

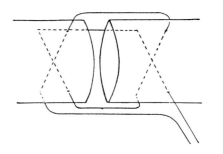

6

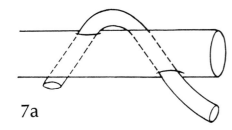

7a

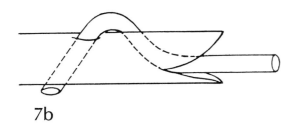

7b

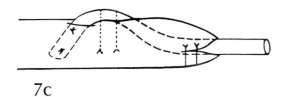

7c

Pulvertaft interlacing method

7a, b & c

The interlacing and fishmouth technique[13] is recommended when a slender tendon needs to be joined to a larger tendon and is suitable for the proximal attachment of a graft. It combines the neatness of an end-to-end junction with the strength of an interlacing suture.

Attachment of graft to distal tendon stump

8a-d

Several methods of attachment of the distal end of a tendon graft have been described but a simple one is as follows. The graft is taken through the fingertip with a Reverdin needle (Downs Surgical, Mitcham, UK) as described by Pulvertaft[13]. This gives good control of the graft beyond the tendon stump leaving the wound clear of instruments to facilitate suturing. It also allows tension adjustment at the distal junction. Sutures of 6/0 material are then inserted at three points as shown (b and c). The stump is then turned back and a further three sutures are inserted (d). Finally the stump is tacked down to the volar surface of the graft with a single suture. It is important to ensure that this tendon stump is short enough to lie distal to the distal interphalangeal joint.

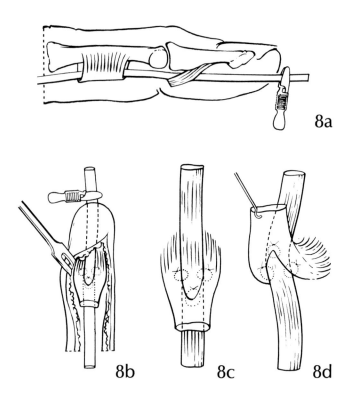

8a

8b   8c   8d

Bunnell withdrawal stitch

9

The Bunnell withdrawal stitch[7] is a neat method of attaching the distal end of the tendon or tendon graft, where there is inadequate profundus stump. The wire is passed through the phalanx to emerge on the nail where it is tied over a dental wool roll. The tendon end is snugged into a drill hole made in the volar cortex of the base of the distal phalanx. The accurate passage of each wire can be facilitated by the use of hollow needles, through which the wire is passed (see *Illustrations 13* and *14* and accompanying text). A simple wire loop is left around the proximal end of the suture and taken through the volar skin. This is then used to pull out the suture after division of the suture at the dental roll.

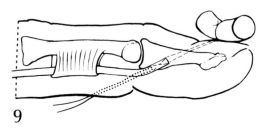

9

REPAIR OF MALLET FRACTURE

(Repair of tendon rupture is as that for boutonnière deformity – *see Illustrations 16–19*).

Incision

10

The incision is angled. The transverse arm is placed midway between the distal interphalangeal joint and the nail fold. The longitudinal arm follows the midlateral line to midway between the interphalangeal joints.

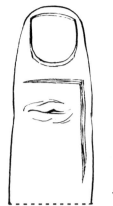

10

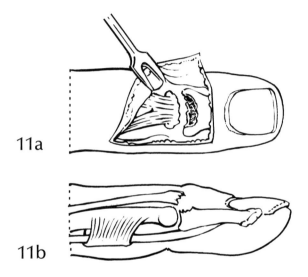

11a

11b

Exposure of extensor tendon

11a & b

The flap is raised exposing the extensor tendon. The two lateral bands are seen joining to form the single tendon which is inserted into the dorsal surface of the base of the distal phalanx. The fracture with haematoma around it is seen here.

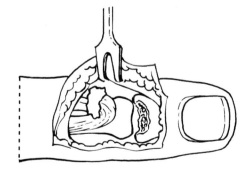

12a

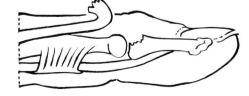

12b

Display of fracture surfaces

12a & b

The avulsed fragment of distal phalanx is reflected proximally with the insertion of the extensor tendon. The bone surfaces are cleared of haematoma but no bone is excised. At this stage the joint is open and the articulation clearly visible.

Passage of needles

13a, b &c

A large needle (18 gauge) is passed through the fracture surface in the main fragment and on through the fingertip to appear on the volar surface of the skin. This is used to railroad (c) a small hypodermic needle (25 gauge) back so that the point appears at the fracture site. This is repeated with a second pair of needles.

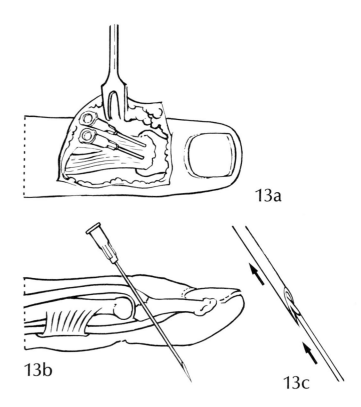

13a

13b

13c

Insertion of suture

14a & b

A stainless steel wire suture is passed through the small bone fragment or around it if the fragment is too small or comminuted. The suture should pass through the extensor tendon at its insertion. Each end of the wire is then passed down one of the needles. Stainless steel 4/0 wire is adequate for simple avulsion but where there is subluxation of the joint 2/0 wire should be used.

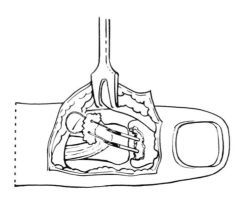

14a

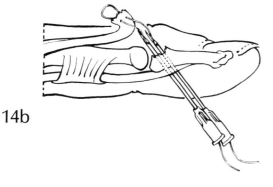

14b

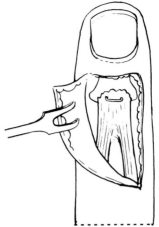

15a

Reduction of fracture and tying of suture

15a–e

The suture is pulled tight to approximate the fragments and can be tied over a dental roll on the volar surface of the finger. A pull-out suture is unnecessary as simple removal is possible as for a skin suture (b). Alternatively the dissection can be carried around the side of the distal phalanx to the flexor aspect and the suture tied over the bone (c). This is more difficult but ensures a tighter, more secure repair. Where there has been subluxation a fine Kirschner wire may be passed across the joint for added security after the suture has been tied (d and e).

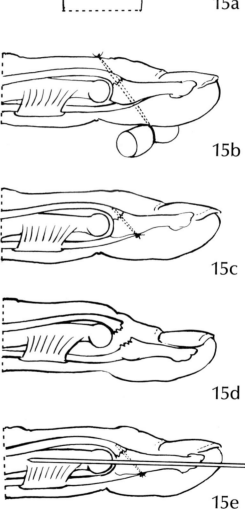

15b

15c

15d

15e

SECONDARY REPAIR OF BOUTONNIÈRE DEFORMITY

Incision

16

A curved incision is used which passes anteriorly almost as far as the midlateral line of the joint. The transverse crease lines over the dorsal surface of the joint are avoided.

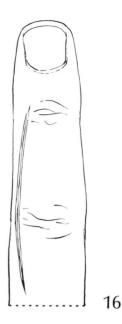

16

Exposure of extensor tendon

17

The skin and subcutaneous tissue are turned back revealing the extensor tendon. Here is seen the severed central band which is white and the scar tissue in the gap which is opalescent. The two lateral bands pass by the side of the joint to become one tendon over the middle phalanx. In a longstanding case they will have slipped forwards and release of the transverse retinacular ligaments on their flexor aspect will be necessary. It may also be necessary to release the oblique retinacular ligament (Landsmeer) to permit recovery of flexion at the terminal joint.

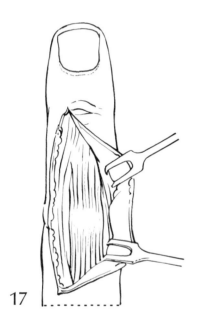

17

Removal of scar tissue

18

The scar tissue is removed and the joint opened. At this stage it is advisable to separate the central band completely from the lateral components. The central band is usually found to be adherent to the neck of the proximal phalanx. These adhesions must be freed so that the tendon moves easily when drawn in the distal direction.

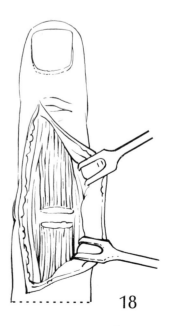

18

Suture of central band to distal remnant

19

The central band is sutured to the distal remnant with a Kessler stitch combined with a few small approximating stitches or, if the distal stump is very short, several small horizontal mattress sutures may be used. The lateral bands are held in contact with the sides of the central band with a few fine stitches (not illustrated). The final tension should allow the finger to lie in the correct position relative to the other fingers.

A similar technique may be used in the secondary repair of mallet deformity, using the incision shown in *Illustration 10*. Where there is an evulsion fracture causing the boutonnière deformity, the technique described for mallet fracture should be used (*see illustration 10–15*).

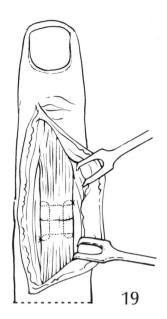

19

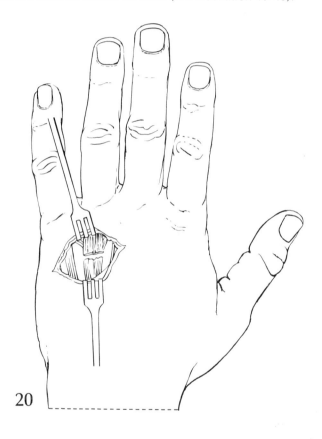

20

21

Suture of the tendon

Where it is ragged the tendon is tidied up by excising the tags. A clean severance (as with glass) requires no further excision of tendon tissue. The Kessler stitch is used and the tendon ends drawn together. This stitch is ideally suited to this situation as it grips the tendon fibres, which tend to be easily frayed at the ends, and it does not bunch up the flat tendon.

REPAIR OF TENDONS ON THE BACK OF THE HAND

Incision

20

Often the existing laceration allows adequate visualization of the tendon ends as shown but if necessary one end of the wound may be extended proximally to permit retrieval of the retracted proximal tendon stump. Dorsal digital veins should be preserved where possible. Division of cutaneous nerve branches may lead to painful neuroma formation.

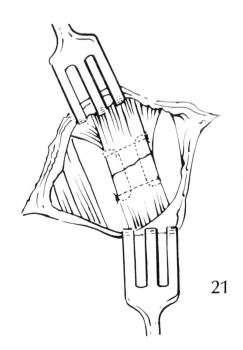

21

Flexor tendon divisions showing suitable method of repair

22

Zone 1: beyond superficialis

Primary suture should be performed if wound conditions are satisfactory; otherwise the skin is sutured and secondary suture or a tendon graft is performed later.

Zone 2: 'no man's land'

Primary suture or secondary graft depending upon the circumstances.

Zone 3: the palm

Primary suture should be performed if wound conditions are satisfactory; otherwise the skin is sutured and secondary suture or bridge graft performed later.

Zones 4 and 5: carpal tunnel and wrist

Primary suture is highly desirable. Delay necessitates bridge grafting (see *Illustration 31*).

In Zones 2 and 4, superficialis to the ring and little fingers should not be repaired, in order to avoid cross-union to the profundus repair, except where, in Zone 2, the laceration is distal to the intact vinculum longum. In these circumstances, the pull of the unrepaired superficialis puts tension on the vincular artery and compromises the blood supply to the profundus tendon. Both tendons should therefore be repaired in spite of the increased risk of cross-union.

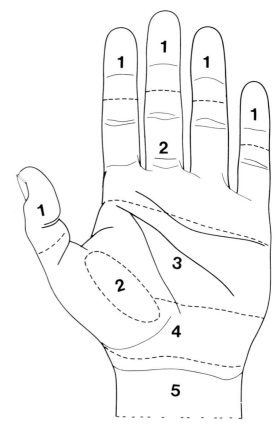

22

PRIMARY REPAIR IN THE FINGER

This is often the procedure of choice and is fully described in the chapter on 'Primary repair of the divided digital flexor tendon' (pp. 828–835).

TENDON GRAFT OPERATION

Graft source

Palmaris longus, plantaris and extensor digitorum longus are suitable. Flexor digitorum superficialis is ideal for a short bridge graft but is less suitable to use as a full-length graft. Palmaris muscle occasionally extends down the tendon too far to leave sufficient length of pure tendon. It is exposed through a short transverse incision above the

wrist and a similar incision in the mid-forearm and drawn out. Plantaris is sufficiently long to serve as two grafts and is of appropriate size; occasionally it is very thin and should not be used. Its presence cannot be determined until the first incision is made on the medial border of the tendo Achillis. A second incision is made in the midcalf, three fingers'-breadth behind the medial border of the tibia. The gastrocnemius muscle is retracted and the plantaris is seen on its deep surface; it is divided in the distal wound and drawn out of the proximal wound. Although a tendon stripper is commonly used, it has been found more satisfactory to remove these tendons in the manner described. A toe extensor tendon is best removed through a full exposure and is of ample length if divided above the extensor retinaculum. A leash of four tendons may be taken if required, but it must be remembered that the fifth toe does not possess a short extensor muscle and will drop into flexion if its sole extensor tendon is removed.

Incisions

23

In the case of the index finger, the incision (A) is made in the exact midaxial line from the nail root to the thenar crease, which it then follows to the proximal part of the palm. A similar incision is used for the little finger, but the palmar incision follows the distal crease for about 3 cm and then is continued into the proximal palm parallel to the thenar crease. For the middle and ring fingers, separate palmar incisions (B) are made in the appropriate crease lines; these may be joined to the finger incision if it is found necessary to expose the base of the finger.

The thumb requires three separate incisions: midaxial in the thumb, the thenar crease and above the wrist just medial to the tendon of flexor carpi radialis.

The Bruner zig-zag incision[14] is commonly used for the finger and gives an excellent exposure but the midaxial approach is more suitable for the operative technique to be described. The latter approach is also preferable when performing a tenolysis which may be indicated later. It cannot be used for a tenolysis once a Bruner approach has been used for the first operation without incurring the risk of delayed skin healing.

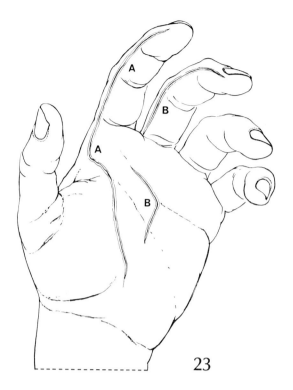

23

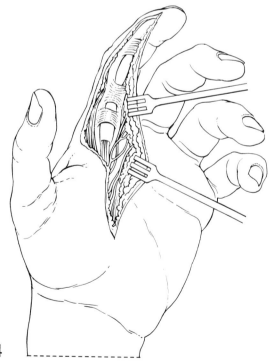

24

Exposure of the digital theca

24

The incision is deepened, passing posterior to the digital vessels and the digital nerve which are carried forwards in the flap. Care must be taken not to injure these structures which are shown crossing the operative field. The dorsal branch of the digital nerve arises just beyond the base of the proximal phalanx (not illustrated). It is not always possible to preserve this small nerve, but it should be looked for and retained if it does not unduly embarrass the exposure. This sensory branch assumes particular significance when the digital nerve has been injured more distally. The digital theca containing the tendons is fully exposed. The lumbrical muscle is seen on the radial side of the finger.

Selective excision of the digital theca and insertion of the graft

25

The theca is cut away leaving three bands to serve as pulleys. These are situated in front of the metacarpophalangeal joint and the midparts of the proximal and middle phalanges. The two proximal pulleys are essential to prevent bowstringing and should be reconstructed if adequate pulleys cannot be fashioned from a damaged and fibrosed theca. The profundus tendon and the proximal part of the superficialis tendon are completely removed. The distal part of the superficialis tendon is not removed if it is firmly adherent and its excision would leave raw tissue along the course of the graft.

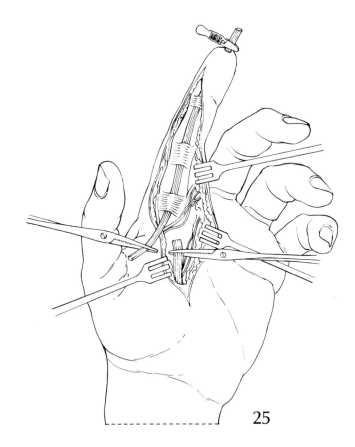

25

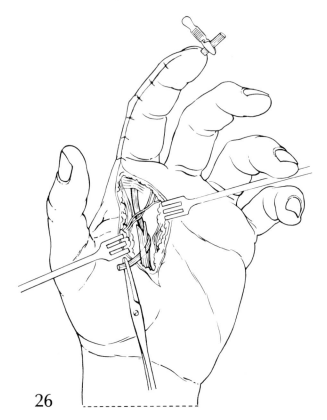

26

26

The graft is inserted and its proximal end attached to the profundus or the superficialis tendon, whichever is found to possess the better amplitude of movement. The fishmouth technique (see Illustration 7) is used. When the graft is attached to profundus, the junction is covered by the lumbricalis muscle provided that this muscle is not fibrosed resulting in a 'lumbrical plus' syndrome. The superficialis of the little finger is a weak muscle and is not suitable to use as a motor tendon. It is helpful to hold the proximal part of the motor tendon by a transfixation needle during this stage of the operation. Note the illustration shows the proximal junction being performed after the distal junction and closure of the finger. This is the author's preference.

Distal attachment of the graft

The graft is attached to the stub of the profundus tendon by the technique described (*see Illustration 8*) or by the Bunnell method (*see Illustration 9*).

Tension of the graft

27

The tension must be carefully adjusted until the finger lies in a slightly more flexed position than would appear correct in relation to the other fingers. The finger posture should be observed while moving the wrist through its full passive range. The patient has had tendon grafts for the middle and ring fingers. Tension can be adjusted at either junction. The author prefers to use the proximal junction for this as it is easier to suture the distal junction with the finger straight before tension is adjusted.

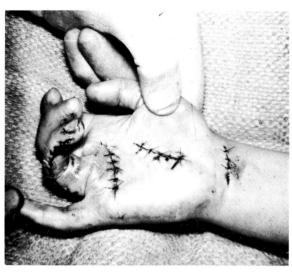

27

(*Reproduced from* Hand Surgery, *Figure 13, p. 305, by courtesy of J. E. Flynn and Williams and Wilkins Co, 1975*)

Completion of the operation

28

If it is felt necessary to secure haemostasis, the hand is covered with a moist dressing and held well elevated, combined with tilting of the table, and the tourniquet is removed from the arm. This position is maintained for 8–10 minutes by which time it is not unusual to find that bleeding has ceased. Any persistent haemorrhage is controlled by bipolar coagulation or ligation. Perfect haemostasis is essential and the wound is washed clear of blood before being closed.

The wound is dressed with tulle gras. A little fluffed dry gauze is placed between the fingers and the palm is filled with cotton gauze. Other materials can be used such as polyurethane foam, wire wool or real wool. Wool substitutes which are made from paper become moistened by sweat and wound exudate in the palm and rapidly lose their resilience. They should not be used. It should be noted that the palmar concavity is triangular and the dressing should be shaped accordingly. Rolls of bandage or wool should not be used as they tend to hold the metacarpophalangeal joints straight and allow the fingers to flex at the interphalangeal joints. The optimal position of wrist in half flexion, metacarpophalangeal joints fully flexed, and interphalangeal joints slightly flexed is held most easily by a dorsal plaster of Paris hood, which should be extended above the elbow in young children. Other surgeons splint the interphalangeal joints in flexion arguing that it is easier to recover extension with splints than to recover flexion. The author finds that splinting the interphalangeal joints in flexion produces an unacceptable number of uncorrectable flexion contractures. The limb is held elevated for 48 hours.

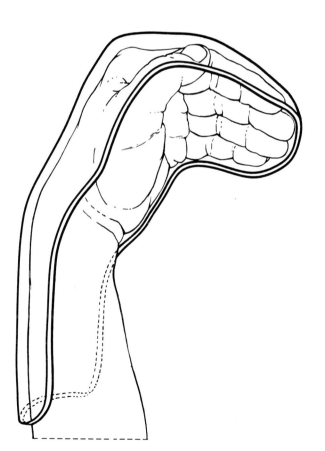

28

TENDON GRAFT FOR FLEXOR POLLICIS LONGUS

29a & b

The three incisions are: midaxial in the thumb reaching from the base of the nail to just proximal to the metacarpophalangeal joint; almost the full length of the thenar crease; and above the wrist medial to the flexor carpi radialis tendon. Through the thenar crease incision, the palmar aponeurosis is incised to expose the first lumbrical muscle, the digital nerve to the radial side of the index finger, both digital nerves to the thumb and the flexor pollicis longus tendon lying between these two nerves. The distal tendon junction is performed as in the fingers. The proximal junction is a fishmouth at the wrist proximal to the carpal tunnel.

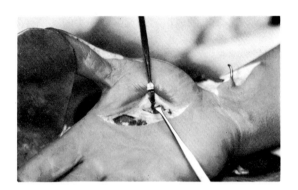

29a

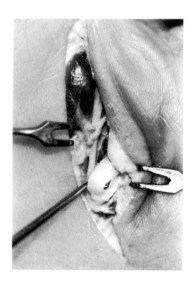

29b

(*Reproduced from the* American Journal of Surgery *1965; 109: 350, Figure 18 by permission of Dunn-Donnelly Publishing Co.*)

TENDON DIVISIONS IN THE PALM

Suture

30

The incision is determined by the position of the existing wound or scar, bearing in mind that a wide exposure is needed to repair nerves in addition to the tendons and that the tendon is likely to be divided at a more distal level than the wound would suggest. In a secondary repair one can expect to find considerable scar tissue which demands a painstaking dissection. The superficialis and profundus tendons are both sutured when conditions are suitable, but if there is a risk of cross-union it is wiser to cut back superficialis and suture only the profundus tendon as illustrated (see Introduction). Tendons severed in the distal part of the palm are considered to be in Zone 2 (see Illustration 22) and treated accordingly.

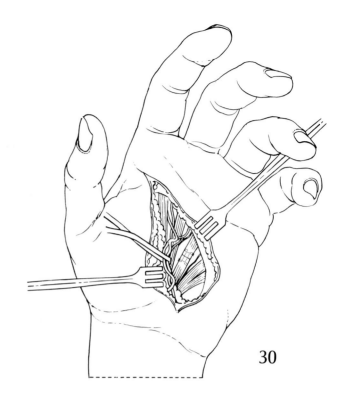

30

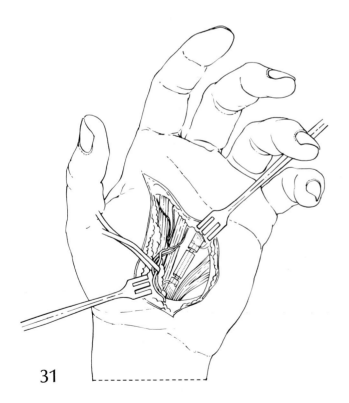

31

Bridge graft

31

In cases where there has been a delay of some months it may be difficult or impossible to bring the tendon ends into apposition. An effective repair may be performed by using a short superficialis graft to bridge the gap in the profundus tendon. The suture passes through the graft in the manner shown; in this illustration the wire has not yet been drawn tight and knotted.

TENDON DIVISIONS AT THE WRIST

32

The first step in dealing with a major injury of this kind is to enlarge the wound in distal and proximal directions and indentify the structures. Respect should be paid to the angles of the flaps which should if possible be greater than 90°.

There are 12 tendons, two main nerves and two main arteries on the flexor aspect of the wrist and two tendons – abductor pollicis longus and extensor pollicis brevis – on the radial aspect. All may be divided and it is not surprising that confusion arises when searching for the corresponding ends. Once the anatomy is clearly seen, the surgeon can proceed confidently with the repair work which may take several hours to complete. Although many hands have survived the loss of both main arteries, this cannot be taken for granted, particularly in older persons, and in any case problems associated with vascular insufficiency may arise later. Both arteries should be anastomosed. All tendons, with the possible exception of palmaris longus, should be sutured when they are divided proximal to the carpal tunnel. It is probably wiser to ignore the superficialis tendons when they are divided within the tunnel.

Opinion differs about the wisdom of primary or secondary suture of nerves divided under these circumstances; if a formal suture is not performed the nerves should be held together to prevent shortening and to preserve the orientation.

In a later reconstructive operation it is not possible to bring the tendon ends together without excessive positioning of the joints. Continuity can be restored to the essential tendons by the interposition of bridge grafts taken from superficialis when the conditions are favourable. The alternative procedure is tendon transference.

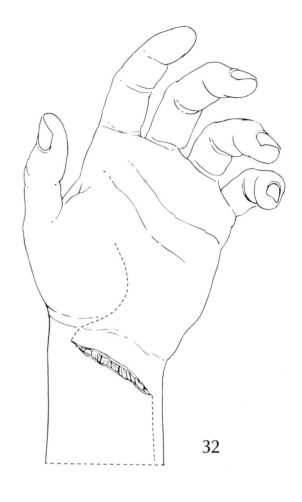

32

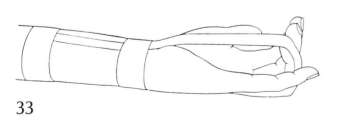

33

Postoperative management

33

At this stage – some 3–5 weeks after tendon suture – when it is customary to permit movements, there is a special risk of the tendon junction giving way for two reasons: the union is immature and adhesions limit the free gliding of the tendon which in a normal hand allows the strain to be taken up gradually. It is therefore unwise to allow complete freedom immediately after the primary splintage has been removed. Some form of protective splintage is advisable such as a check-rein strap or elastic, or a spring device.

Movements return slowly and the patient requires constant encouragement. He should be kept under personal supervision until the final state is reached which may not be for 6–9 months after operation. Occasionally, the operation of tenolysis is indicated for cases in which the active range fails to attain the passive range of movement. The temptation to try early tenolysis should be resisted. The operation is best carried out about 12 months after repair.

EXTENSOR TENDONS

Mallet deformity

The finger is splinted with the distal interphalangeal joint extended, leaving the proximal interphalangeal joint free for 5 weeks followed by 3 weeks of spring splintage (long Capener splint).

Boutonnière deformity

The finger is splinted with the proximal interphalangeal joint extended for 4 weeks followed by 3 weeks of spring splintage (short Capener splint). The distal joint may be left free.

Back of the hand

The forearm, wrist and fingers are splinted with the wrist in extension and the metacarpophalangeal and interphalangeal joints in slight flexion for 3 weeks. The fully extended position of the fingers is unnecessary and can lead to joint stiffness. During the following 2 weeks, flexion of the fingers is limited by a pad of steel wire or a volar slab bandaged into the palm against which the fingers can squeeze.

FLEXOR TENDONS

Fingers, palm and wrist

The wrist and hand are held in a plaster hood in the position described (see *Illustration 28* and accompanying text) for 3 weeks. After the removal of splintage, digit extension is limited for the further week (2 weeks in children, for whom a plaster cast is used in the first stage) by the use of an elastic check-rein strap. This strap allows flexion exercises to be practised but prevents excessive extension. Passive extension by the patient or physiotherapist should be discouraged until 6 weeks after the operation.

Physiotherapy

There can be no denying that a good physiotherapist markedly increases the quality of the results. It is important for the therapist to know how much to strain a tendon repair with passive exercises during the early stages of rehabilitation. Later, tenodesis can be cleared especially on the extensor aspect of the hand by skilled deep friction massage and ultrasonics. Many patients are afraid to attempt active exercises for fear of 'doing damage' and it is in these cases that supervised active exercises are useful, particularly in young children.

However, the patient's own intelligent cooperation is the most important factor in the aftercare and if this is lacking a good result is rarely achieved. It is for this reason that flexor tendon surgery in children under 5 years frequently gives disappointing results. As tendon union becomes stronger more active work in the occupational therapy department is given and in most hospitals this department is responsible for producing the vast range of heat-malleable plastic splints that can be so useful in rehabilitating the injured hand.

References

1. Vilain R. Repair of the extensor of the finger at its distal end. In: Stack HG, Bolton H, eds. *Proceedings of the Second Hand Club, 1956–1967*. London: The British Society for Surgery of the Hand, 1975: 155–6.

2. Iselin F, Levame J, Godoy J. A simplified technique for treating mallet fingers; tenodermodesis. *J Hand Surg* 1977; 2: 118–21.

3. Matev I. Transposition of the lateral slips of the aponeurosis in treatment of longstanding 'boutonnière deformity' of the fingers. *Br J Plast Surg* 1964; 17: 281–6.

4. Littler JW, Eaton RG. Redistribution of forces in the correction of the boutonnière deformity. *J Bone Joint Surg [Am]* 1967; 49-A: 1267–74.

5. Pulvertaft RG. The treatment of profundus division by free tendon graft. *J Bone Joint Surg [Am]* 1960; 42-A: 1363–71, 1380.

6. Pulvertaft RG. Flexor tendon grafting after long delay. In: Tubiana R, ed. *The hand*. Vol 3. Philadelphia: W. B. Saunders, 1988: 244–54.

7. Bunnell S. Tendons. In: *Bunnell's surgery of the hand*. 5th ed. Rev. by J. H. Boyes. Philadelphia: Lippincott, 1970: 393–409.

8. Rank BK, Wakefield AR, Hueston JT. *Surgery of repair as applied to hand injuries*. 4th ed. Edinburgh: Churchill Livingstone, 1973: 84.

9. Shaw PC. A method of flexor tendon suture. *J Bone Joint Surg [Br]* 1968; 50-B: 578–87.

10. Tsuge K, Ikuta Y, Matsuishi Y. Intra-tendinous tendon suture in the hand: a new technique. *Hand* 1975; 7: 250–5.

11. Becker H, Orak F, Duponselle E. Early active motion following a beveled technique of flexor tendon repair: report on fifty cases. *J Hand Surg* 1979; 4: 454–60.

12. Kessler I. The grasping technique for tendon repair. *Hand* 1973; 5: 253–5.

13. Pulvertaft RG. Tendon grafts for flexor tendon injuries in the fingers and thumb. *J Bone Joint Surg [Br]* 1956; 38-B: 175–94.

14. Bruner JM. The zig-zag volar digital incision for flexor tendon surgery. In: Stack HG, Bolton H. eds. *Proceedings of the Second Hand Club, 1956–1967*. London: The British Society for Surgery of the Hand, 1975: 423–4.

Illustrations by Adrian Shaw

Primary repair of the divided digital flexor tendon

Harold J. Richards FRCS
Formerly Consultant in the Surgery of Orthopaedics and Trauma, University Hospital of Wales and Prince of Wales
Orthopaedic Hospital, Cardiff, UK

Blood supply of flexor tendon

The maintenance of a good blood supply to the divided and repaired digital flexor tendon is the single most important factor in obtaining good healing and return of function in the repaired tendon.

Blood is supplied to the digital flexor tendon via fragile vincula, which run to the dorsal surface of the tendon from the adjacent underlying phalanges.

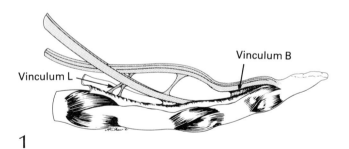

1

1

The vincula are of two types: the short (VB) and the long (VL). The short runs to the flexor tendon near its insertion and is only occasionally ruptured or damaged as when a spontaneous rupture of the long flexor occurs.

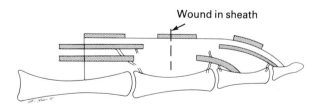

2

2

The vinculum longus, however, ruptures easily if it is attached to the proximal divided end of the tendon, which then retracts towards the palm.

3

The vinculum carries not only the blood supply (B) to the tendon but also the nerve supply (N) as shown in a section of the vinculum 6 hours after division of the flexor tendon.

When the blood supply is adequate the digital flexor tendons have the ability to heal by means of their own cells[1-6].

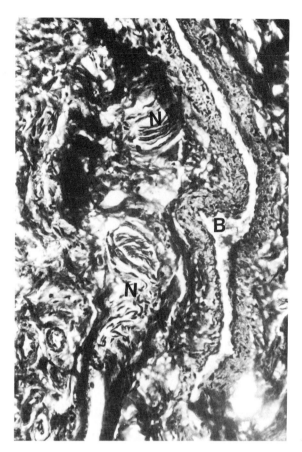

3

4 & 5

Within the flexor tendon the blood vessels run longitudinally at various depths, but they intercommunicate[7,8]. The richest blood supply is near the point of entry of the vinculum and in the central area of the tendon whilst the peripheral areas, particularly the volar aspect, have the poorest blood supply. It is essential that the suture used for repairing the tendon should interfere with the blood supply as little as possible.

The suture should, therefore, take hold of the tendon along its periphery and when running across the tendon should go through the volar half of the tendon only. The worst type of suture is a constricting one going through the full thickness of the tendon, such as a figure of eight.

Impairment of blood supply which occurs when the proximal end of the divided tendon retracts, rupturing the vinculum and its blood vessels and nerves, leads after suture of the tendon to considerable adhesion formation during healing, particularly if a constricting suture is also used. The adhesions result from connective tissue penetrating the healing tendon carrying an essential new blood supply, but the penalty for this assistance is the formation of massive adhesions which result in loss of function of the tendon after healing has taken place.

4

5

Preoperative

Indications for operation

Primary repair of the divided digital flexor tendon should be undertaken when the following conditions are met.

1. There is no extensive loss of soft tissue.
2. There is no gross contamination of the wound.
3. There are no fractures which cannot be immobilized.
4. The divided tendon ends can be approximated.
5. Adequate skill and facilities are available. These are difficult operative procedures and experience in tendon surgery is necessary. A bad result from primary repair makes any further salvage operation more difficult and impairs the final level of function of the hand.

Initial treatment

The wound should be cleaned, dressed or closed.

6

The wrist should be put in a position of full flexion and maintained in this position by splintage, usually a plaster of Paris cast or slab, supported by a non-elastic bandage. This will prevent or limit the retraction of the cut proximal end of the divided flexor tendon and protect its blood supply.

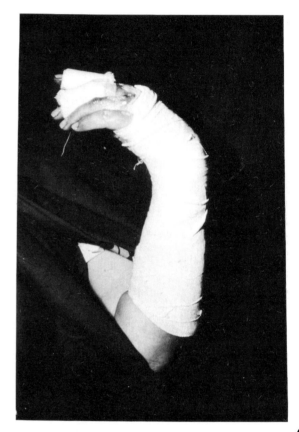

6

Technique of repair

Under general anaesthesia, without the application of a tourniquet and with the wrist held in full flexion, the original wound is explored. Flexing the finger usually brings the distal cut end of the tendon into the wound. Full flexion of the wrist usually does not bring the proximal cut end into the wound, but in most cases this can be achieved by massaging the digit from the palm distally. If the latter manoeuvre fails a delicate artery forceps can be passed proximally along the fibrosynovial sheath and the tendon grasped and pulled distally.

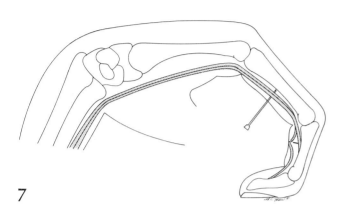

7

7

Once in the wound it can be maintained in this position by passing a hypodermic needle through the skin, fibrosynovial sheath and tendon. A non-reactive suture (3/0) can then be inserted as shown in *Illustrations 4* and *5*. The suture should run at least 1 cm along the length of the tendon before running transversely. At this point and beyond there is less softening of the tendon during healing than at the area around the site of the tendon division. The suture should be securely tied and cutting out is prevented by positioning of the wrist, hand and fingers in flexion after repair. If the tendon ends are poorly coapted, a running suture through the epitenon and outer margin of the tendon may be used (6/0 or 7/0 nylon is suitable).

8

Where there is difficulty in approximating the cut ends, or bringing them into the original wound, the latter will have to be extended as shown. The wound in the fibrosynovial sheath will have to be enlarged in a similar fashion. Where both tendons have been divided, both should be sutured, as the long vinculum runs to both tendons and the repair of one only would allow the other to retract proximally with rupture of the vinculum, blood and nerve supply. It may not be possible fully to close the fibrosynovial sheath when both tendons have been sutured.

After repair of the tendon or tendons, the fibrosynovial sheath is repaired using a non-reactive suture (5/0). Divided digital nerves, and at least one artery, are also sutured (see Chapter on 'Microsurgical techniques', *The Hand*, pp. 242–247). Where there is difficulty in getting the cut tendon into the wound and the latter has to be extended, it may be necessary to apply a tourniquet to control bleeding, but once the ends have been isolated the tourniquet should be removed as this makes it much easier to get the proximal cut end into the wound. If a pneumatic cuff type of tourniquet is applied to the upper arm following elevation of the limb and without preliminary use of an Esmarch bandage, the tourniquet can be retained, as this method does not lead to difficulty in getting the proximal cut tendon end into the wound.

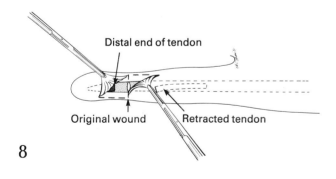

Distal end of tendon

Original wound   Retracted tendon

8

Delay in primary repair

Usually it is possible to approximate the divided cut ends of the flexor tendon at up to 2 weeks in an adult and 4 weeks in a child after the date of the injury. However, the following problems are encountered.

1. The proximal end of the divided tendon will have retracted with rupture of the vinculum and impairment of blood supply.
2. Adhesions form, making it difficult to get the distal end into the wound.

These difficulties can be overcome as far as isolation of the tendon ends is concerned by using a radiological investigation known as a tenogram[9]. A tenogram is obtained by injecting a radiopaque material (25 per cent Hypaque, Stirling Research, Guildford, UK) into the fibrosynovial sheath.

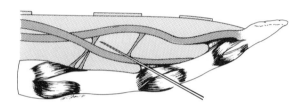

9

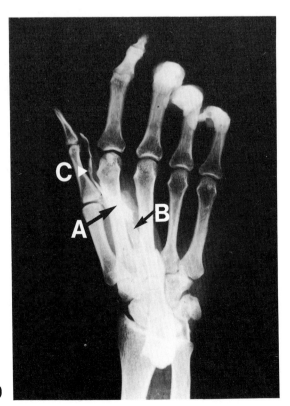

10

TENOGRAPHY TECHNIQUE

Any non-irritable opaque medium can be used for outlining the digital flexor tendon sheath but 25 per cent Hypaque is suitable. The normal closed digital flexor tendon sheath will accommodate 2 ml of this fluid, but if the sheath is connected to the common sheath (see *Illustration 10*) then more fluid can be injected as it will travel up and fill the compound flexor sheath. Five millilitres of Hypaque are drawn up into the syringe to which a fine hypodermic needle is attached.

9

The needle is then inserted obliquely into the lateral aspect of the finger and directed towards the proximal end of the digit. When the needle strikes the fibrosynovial sheath some resistance is felt but with a little firm pressure the needle passes through the sheath. The opaque medium is injected and if the needle is within the sheath, then the fluid passes easily out of the syringe. The patient can usually feel the fluid passing into the sheath and frequently will indicate accurately in which direction the fluid is flowing. A finger placed on the sheath will also detect the flow of the opaque medium along the fibrosynovial sheath. If no adhesions are present then the sheath will accommodate approximately 2 ml, but if there are adhesions, then only a limited amount of fluid will pass into the sheath, the amount depending on the degree of adhesion formation. The needle is passed into the lateral aspect of the finger so that it will slip between the tendons; if pushed into the sheath from the front of the finger, the needle is likely to penetrate the flexor tendon and prevent the opaque fluid from passing into the sheath[9].

TECHNIQUE OF DELAYED REPAIR

10

The finger is then opened at the site of the original wound (A) and over the proximal (B) and distal (C) ends of the tendon. The latter (B and C) are then threaded along the fibrosynovial sheath into the original wound and sutured. In order to approximate the cut tendon ends, both the wrist and finger may have to be flexed and postoperatively held in this position for 3 weeks. If the blood supply has been impaired then the tendon will heal with adhesions and the finger will be in a fixed flexion position. The patient should be warned of this before operation and also told that a further operation, a tenolysis, will be necessary in a year's time to restore function.

The long flexor tendon is most difficult to repair between its insertion and the insertion of the short flexor, particularly if repair is attempted 48 hours or more after injury. The distal fibrosynovial sheath is flat and small and the cut tendon tends to swell; if the sheath has been widely opened it is almost impossible to resuture it. An alternative technique of inserting a suture using a 3/0 non-reactive suture with a straight needle at either end is employed.

11

The needle is introduced as previously described into the proximal end of the divided long flexor tendon. It is then inserted into the cut distal end of the tendon and passed throughout its length and out through the pulp at the tip of the finger.

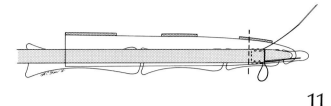

11

12

The other straight needle is passed in a similar direction.

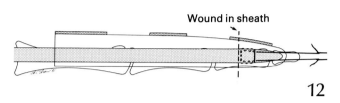

Wound in sheath

12

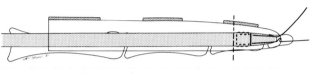

13

13

An incision is then made into the pulp tissue along one of the natural creases and the insertion of the long flexor tendon is exposed. The two sutures passing out through this insertion are isolated. The straight needles are then cut off and the sutures are drawn back into the pulp area.

14

The retracted suture ends are then threaded on to a curved needle and passed through the insertion of the long tendon to take a firm hold of it. The sutures are then tied.

Alternatively the sutures are tied at the tip of the finger over a button. This procedure has the disadvantage that the suture will probably have to be removed by a further operation.

Division or spontaneous rupture of the long flexor tendon, where the vinculum is intact, presents no difficulties as the tendon does not retract and can be repaired without difficulty, generally with an excellent functional result, as the blood supply is good. It may, however, be necessary to use a tenogram to isolate the proximal cut end.

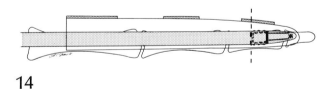

14

Postoperative management

The wrist is immobilized in full flexion using a plaster of Paris cast and the finger is allowed to take up its physiological position. The plaster cast extends from below the elbow to the tips of the fingers, except in a young child up to the age of 6, where the plaster extends above the elbow joint. The forearm is held in supination, with the elbow flexed to 100°, as this gives the best position for venous drainage from the fingers and minimizes swelling of the digit. The plaster cast is removed after 3 weeks and active exercises started. Each individual joint is mobilized separately, as well as in conjunction with the other joints. Maximum recovery of movement usually occurs within 3 months of the operation.

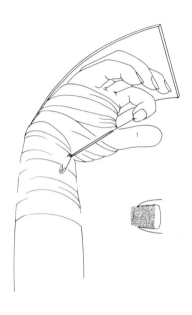

15

15

Kleinert[10] has advocated guarded extension exercises using rubber bands which hold the finger in flexion for the first few weeks after operation.

An elastic band is secured to the nail by adhesive or to a nylon loop passed through the nail tip. The insert shows the method favoured by the author: a strip of ordinary zinc oxide strapping is folded onto itself, sticky sides together, and shaped as shown; a hole is cut in the distal end for attaching the traction apparatus and the strapping is then stuck onto the nail using one of the superglues.

The band is secured to the splint so that the tension on the digit maintains it in greater flexion than its fellows. It is important that the proximal interphalangeal joint is not flexed to over 70° or fixed flexion deformity may occur, impairing the result. The patient is encouraged to extend actively the digit from the first postoperative day. The flexor muscles are inhibited by active extension, effectively reducing tension across the suture line. Close supervision is necessary if this technique is adopted.

TENOLYSIS

16

Where, after a flexor tendon repair, function is very limited or the finger is in a position of fixed flexion deformity, tenolysis should be undertaken, but not until 1 year after the operation and the tendon has had time to re-establish a normal blood supply. A tenogram may be helpful in outlining the area of adhesion.

A lateral incision is made in the finger over the area of adhesion and the skin, subcutaneous tissue and fibro-synovial sheath are raised in one flap. The adhesions are all divided so that the tendon moves freely and the skin only is sutured. As soon as the patient recovers from the anaesthetic active movements are commenced.

Where the adhesions involve the tendon sheath in its proximal end the incision has to be extended into the palm so that this part of the sheath can be explored and the adhesion divided.

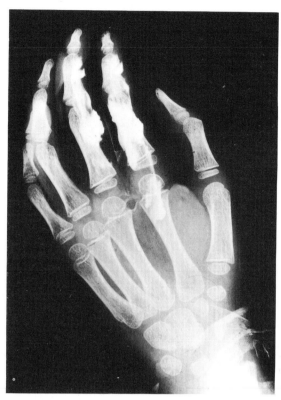

16

References

1. Matthews P, Richards H. The repair potential of digital flexor tendon: an experimental study. *J Bone Joint Surg [Br]* 1974; 56-B: 618–25.

2. Matthews P, Richards H. Factors in the adherence of flexor tendon after repair: an experimental study in the rabbit. *J Bone Joint Surg [Br]* 1976; 58-B: 230–6.

3. Richards HJ. Primary and delayed repair of flexor tendons in the fingers. *J Bone Joint Surg [Br]* 1964; 46-B: 571.

4. Richards HJ. Digital flexor tendon repair and return of function. *Ann R Coll Surg Engl* 1977; 59: 25–32.

5. Richards HJ. Factors affecting the healing and return of function in the repaired digital flexor tendon. *Aust NZ J Surg* 1980; 50(3): 258–63.

6. Richards HJ. Repair and healing of the divided digital flexor tendon. *Injury* 1980; 12: 1–12.

7. Edwards DAW. The blood supply and lymphatic drainage of tendons. *J Anat* 1946; 80: 147–52.

8. Brockis JG. The blood supply of the flexor and extensor tendons of the fingers in man. *J Bone Joint Surg [Br]* 1953; 35-B: 131–8.

9. Richards HJ. Radiographic localization of severed tendons and of adhesions within a synovial sheath. *J Bone Joint Surg [Br]* 1962; 44-B: 744.

10. Kleinert HE, Meares A. The quest of the solution to severed flexor tendons. *Clin Orthop* 1974; 104: 23–9.

Two-stage tendon reconstruction using gliding tendon implants

James M. Hunter MD
Clinical Professor of Orthopedic Surgery, Thomas Jefferson University, Philadelphia, Pennsylvania, USA;
Chief, Hand Surgery Service, Department of Orthopedics, Thomas Jefferson University Hospital

Peter C. Amadio MD
Assistant Professor of Clinical Orthopedics, SUNY, Stony Brook, New York, USA;
Active Staff, St John's Episcopal Hospital, Smithtown, New York

Introduction

Following mutilating trauma to the hand, the early priorities of treatment should emphasize the maintenance of good circulation, protective skin coverage, proper alignment of the bones and joints and the restoration of a soft bed for tendon gliding. Damaged tendons may be taught to glide again by supervised exercises. Often, however, in spite of careful primary treatment, the tendon and tendon gliding bed have been so damaged that a healing complex of scar develops and function is lost. It is the purpose of this chapter to outline the techniques of two-stage tendon reconstruction using a gliding tendon implant to assist organization of a new tendon bed prior to tendon grafting.

Implants

1

Twenty-five years of experimental and clinical research have resulted in the evolution of both a passive and an active implant gliding programme for two-stage tendon reconstruction. The implants are designed to provide firmness and flexibility to permit secure distal fixation and minimize buckling during the passive push phase of gliding. This is achieved by combining an inner woven Dacron (du Pont, USA) core for strength and an outer sheath of silicone rubber for inertness and low-friction gliding.

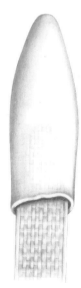

1

Passive gliding programme and implant

2

This programme implies that the distal end of the implant is fixed securely to bone or tendon while the proximal end glides free in the proximal palm or forearm. Movement of the implant is produced by active extension and passive flexion of the digit.

The passive implant is available commercially as a silicone-coated woven Dacron tape in widths of 3, 4, 5 and 6 mm with two different distal fixation possibilities. The blunt tip passive implant can be fixed by suture. A passive implant with a metal plate for distal screw fixation is also available.

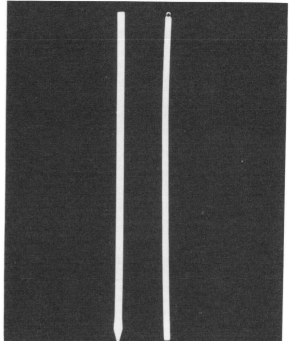

2

Active gliding programme and implant

3

The active tendon implants are fixed at the distal end to the distal phalanx or middle phalanx of the finger by either a screw twist wire or a Dacron weave through bone. Implants are fixed proximally in the forearm to the motor tendon by either a loop-to-loop technique or by suturing the Dacron weave into the motor tendon in the forearm. These methods permit the Stage I period to be extended indefinitely. The patient could have function for months or years before implant replacement by a tendon graft or another implant.

The active tendon implants that are currently available are constructed with special porous weaves of Dacron that will permit tissue ingrowth as well as permit enhanced flexibility of the constructed tendon. The length of the tendons may be changed by peeling the silicone from the Dacron and gently opening the two woven Dacron cords with a scalpel.

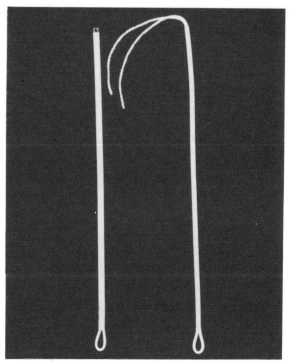

3

Care of tendon implants

Silicone rubber is highly electrostatic and, as a result, attracts airborne particles and surface contaminants. For this reason, once the implants have been removed from their sterile packets, they should be kept moist at all times. Gloves and instruments which contact the implants should always be wet. Attention to these details will minimize the risk of synovitis postoperatively.

Indications for surgery

More than 25 years of surgical experience have shown the two-stage technique of tendon reconstruction to be useful in cases of both chronic and acute tendon injuries. The basic indication is a scarred soft tissue bed which could compromise gliding after tendon graft or transfer. It has been shown experimentally that a fine, glistening, fluid-secreting sheath is formed about the gliding tendon implant, which, after removal of the implant, provides a more suitable bed for gliding of a tendon graft or transfer than the scarred tissue initially present at the time of Stage I.

By improving the quality of the tendon bed, the surgeon capable of achieving a good result with flexor tendon grafting in a finger with minimal scarring may now see similar results in initially poorer grade cases when using the two-stage method. Candidates for tenolysis and tendon grafting should also be considered candidates for two-stage reconstruction since only at the time of surgery can the surgeon truly assess the extent of tendon-bed injury.

A second indication for two-stage tendon reconstruction would be the necessity for concurrent surgery which might compromise the usual rehabilitation pattern for one-stage tendon reconstruction, repair or transfer. Simultaneous pulley reconstruction makes rehabilitation after tenolysis or one-stage tendon grafting difficult; combining pulley reconstruction with two-stage grafting allows the active movement to be deferred until pulley healing is completed. Similarly, after tendon repair, nerve injuries or concomitant fractures, particularly those of the proximal phalanx which violate the fibro-osseous canal, may require immobilization to the detriment of tendon rehabilitation. In these predictably poor situations, the use of a tendon implant can again maintain a gliding bed until later tendon reconstruction is possible. Earlier use of a tendon implant on the flexor surface may simplify replantation surgery by allowing, for example, concentration on active movement of repaired extensors in a Zone II level amputation.

Contraindications to two-stage reconstruction

Acute infection is the only absolute contraindication, as with all reconstructive surgery involving implants. Some relative contraindications should also be considered. Formation of a good gliding bed for tendon function following finger injury is a dynamic metabolic process which requires a certain minimal level of tissue viability for support. The stiff, scarred finger with destroyed joints, damaged nerves and vessels cannot be expected to support the necessary nutritional requirements for suc-

cessful healing following extensive reconstruction of any kind and will usually be served best by amputation.

Even more important to consider preoperatively is the level of patient cooperation and motivation available. Considerable therapy will usually be required to convert the potential gains made at Stage I surgery into actual ones after Stage II. If the patient is unable or unwilling to cooperate or to attend frequently enough for the surgeon to detect trouble spots early, complex reconstructions should not be undertaken. Prior to surgery, all patients should have hand therapy designed to mobilize stiff joints and to improve to the maximum the condition of the soft tissues. The timing of surgery should finally combine the judgment of surgeon, hand therapist and patient. Again, patient input and motivation are the keys to a successful result.

Antibiotic therapy

As with other orthopaedic implants, preoperative broad-spectrum intravenous antibiotics are recommended, beginning just prior to surgery and continuing for 48 hours postoperatively. The use of antibiotics containing irrigation solution is also advised.

Anaesthesia

If a passive implant reconstruction is definitely to be performed, either general or axillary block anaesthesia is recommended to control operative and tourniquet pain, as dissection and reconstruction may be extensive. If consideration is being given to tenolysis versus staged grafting or if the active implant programme is elected, local anaesthesia (1 per cent lidocaine infiltration) is recommended, to be supplemented with intravenous fentanyl and droperidol (Innovar) or meperidine and diazepam to control tourniquet pain and patient restlessness. This technique allows the surgeon to assess completeness of the tenolysis and also is helpful both in checking active amplitude of potential donor motor units and in setting proper tension to either the active implant or tendon graft. The anaesthetist should be experienced with the technique as often a very fine balance must be struck to provide sufficient sedation on the one hand, and a patient awake enough to cooperate when active movement is required, on the other. With the local sedation technique, the tourniquet is intermittently deflated at roughly half-hour intervals to prevent tourniquet paralysis and to evaluate function if appropriate. This anaesthetic technique is well tolerated by most patients and can be used for procedures lasting as long as 4 or 5 hours.

PASSIVE PROGRAMME

Stage I

Preoperative assessment of active and passive range of movement

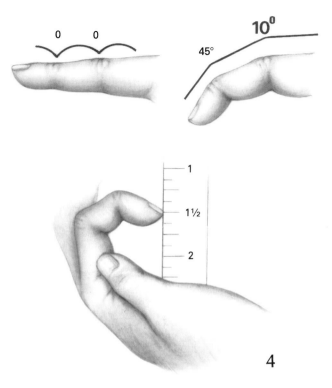

4

The angular movement of each joint in degrees and the distance that the finger pulp fails to touch at the distal palmar crease are recorded and made a part of the permanent record of each patient for progress comparison and follow-up, typically: (1) before Stage I; (2) 6 weeks after Stage I; (3) preferably active movement during Stage II surgery after graft juncture with appropriate tension; and (4) monthly after Stage II.

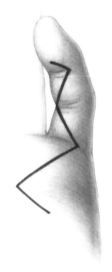

5

THE OPERATION

Incisions for flexor tendon reconstruction

5

The damaged flexor tendons and scarred sheaths are exposed through the volar zig-zag incisions popularized by Julian Bruner. The skin flap should be full-thickness, with the apices overlying the neurovascular bundles. Longer flaps may develop marginal necrosis. The neurovascular bundles must be carefully protected.

6

A separate curved incision is made in the distal forearm to expose the finger flexors and the plane between the profundus and superficialis where the implant will lie.

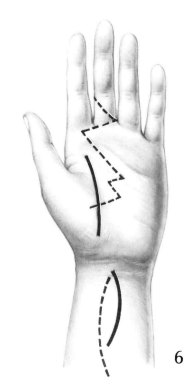

6

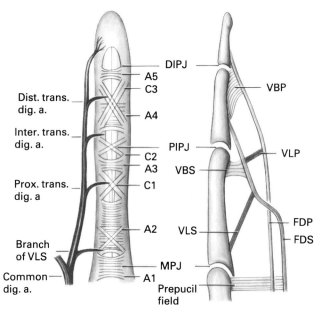

7

DIPJ, distal interphalangeal joint
PIPJ, proximal interphalangeal joint
MPJ, metacarpophalangeal joint
VPB, vincula brevia profunda
VLP, vincula longa profunda
FDP, flexor digitorum profundus
FDS, flexor digitorum superficialis
VBS, vincula brevia superficialis
VLS, vincula longa superficialis
A1-5, annular pulleys 1–5
C1–3, cruciform pulleys 1–3
VF, variable fibre

7

At the level of the cruciate pulleys, the digital arteries give four transverse tributaries which supply the synovial bed and vincular system. If possible, these should be preserved.

8

All undamaged segments of the pulley system should be preserved. Typically, transverse window incisions are made to expose the damaged tendons:

1. between A1 and A2 in the variable fibre (VF) area;
2. at the mid A2 level;
3. at the level of the cruciate pulleys C1, C2 and C3.

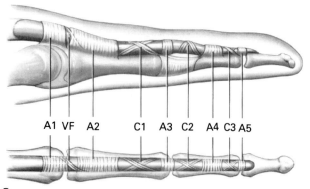

8

A1 VF A2 C1 A3 C2 A4 C3 A5

Excision of damaged tendons

9

This portion of the operation must be done carefully to avoid further injury to the tendon bed and will often be very time-consuming. A generous stump of profundus tendon, at least 1 cm, should be left attached to the distal phalanx. It is usually necessary to sacrifice the A5 pulley to perform this adequately.

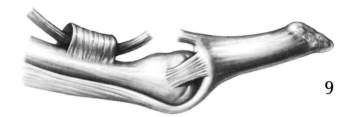

9

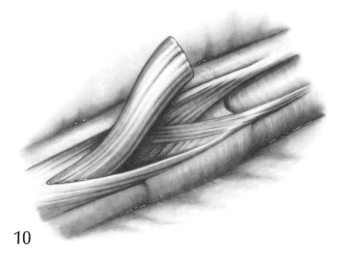

10

10

If the superficialis tendon bed has not been injured, it is left intact over the proximal interphalangeal joint. Scarring of the tendons at the proximal interphalangeal joint level is often responsible for flexion contracture. Meticulous dissection of mature scar here will permit increased range of movement later. Care must be taken to preserve the volar proximal interphalangeal joint capsule.

11

Severely scarred segments of sheath should be removed and later replaced with new pulleys. Collapsed annuli may be dilated with fine haemostats.

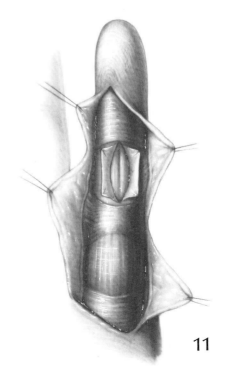

11

Division of flexor tendons in palm and excision of lumbrical muscle in palm

12

After the scarred tendons have been pulled proximally through the A1 pulley, they are transected in the palm. Scarred lumbrical muscle is resected. If the palm is uninjured, the lumbrical and profundus complex with surrounding mesotendon is carefully preserved for Stage II juncture. Usually, however, when staged tendon reconstruction is planned, scarring is present at this level and proximal juncture is planned in the distal forearm.

If more than one implant is to be used and crowding is noted in the carpal canal, the sublimi may be pulled through the carpal canal and excised in the forearm.

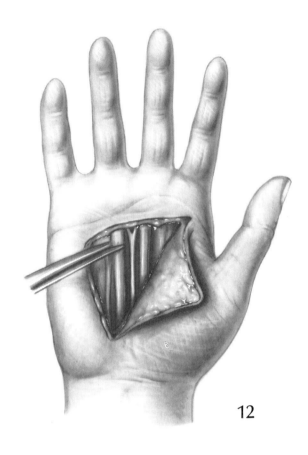

12

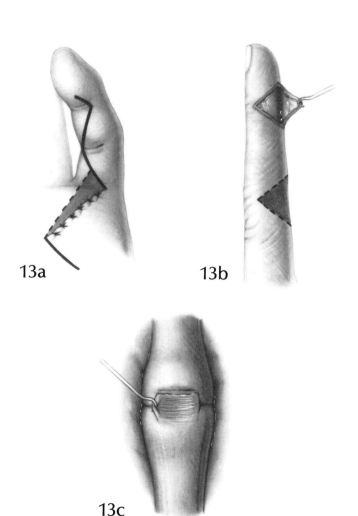

13a

13b

13c

Release of skin and joint contractures

13a–c

Finger joints should be left undisturbed if all contractures can be released by tendon removal and incision of contracted cutaneous ligaments of Cleland or the oblique retinacular ligament of Landsmeer. Shifting or advancement of skin flaps may be necessary (a). The Y-V advancement technique may be applied to release skin tension (b).

Persistent joint contracture can be released by capsulotomy of the accessory collateral ligaments and volar plate (c). If volar capsulotomy is performed, the proximal interphalangeal joint should be immobilized postoperatively by a transarticular smooth Kirschner wire for approximately 10 days, then splinted in between therapy sessions afterwards. These procedures will be most effective when the vascular status of the finger is unimpaired. In all instances of contracture release, the tourniquet should be deflated and the vascularity of the finger inspected frequently. In poor situations, arthrodesis or amputation may be indicated.

Contractures which are not fully released at the time of surgery cannot be expected to resolve during postoperative therapy. The goal of therapy should be to maintain the movement obtained at surgery.

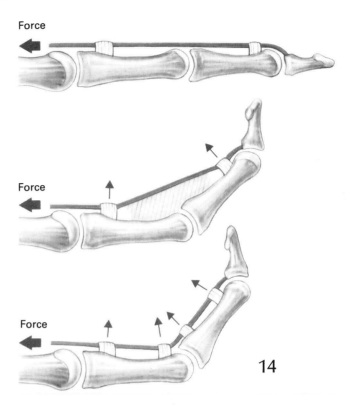

Pulley reconstruction

14

Normal active flexion cannot be expected with a deficient pulley system. Mechanically, the pulleys serve to hold the tendons close to the axis of movement of the joint. This produces a maximum angular movement for each unit of tendon excursion. Thus, bowing must lead to diminished active range, regardless of the passive potential of the joint. In the already injured finger, scarring may form below the bowed tendon, further limiting function.

14

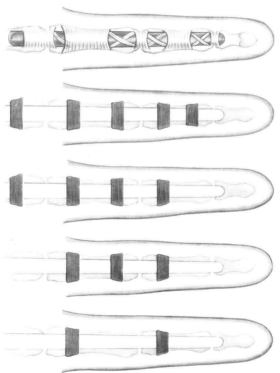

15

15

In order to preserve normal movement, therefore, it is imperative to conserve or reconstruct as many functional pulleys as possible. For purposes of reconstruction, it may be better to think of the long A2 pulley as performing two separate functions: a distal restraint for the metacarpophalangeal joint and a proximal one at the proximal interphalangeal joint.

In reconstruction, a four-pulley system is preferred. The diagram shows the anatomical situation (top) and, in decreasing preference from top to bottom, four experimentally tested pulley reconstruction possibilities.

16

Portions of excised sublimis and profundus tendons are excellent for pulley building. Several basic principles should be kept in mind. As stated above, the closer the reconstruction comes to the anatomical situation, the greater the potential for excellent active movement after the tendon grafting. Pulleys should be wide and sturdy. We prefer passing the pulley graft completely around the bone extraperiosteally but beneath the extensor tendon on the proximal phalanx and around the extensor tendon on the middle phalanx. The pulley graft should be passed around the bone twice, then sutured to itself at the remaining rim of fibro-osseous canal. We have found a Mixter haemostat helpful in passing the graft around the phalanx. Care must be exercised to retract the neurovascular bundle on each side of the finger so the graft may be passed close to bone without compromising the bundles.

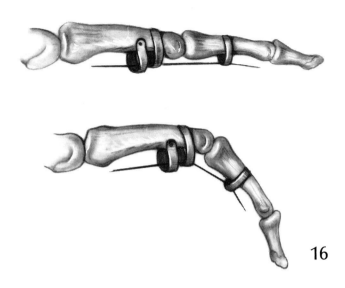

16

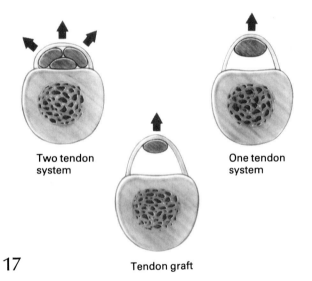

Two tendon system

One tendon system

Tendon graft

17

17

The pulleys should conform to the implant but not bind it. In this regard it is important to remember that the eventual tendon graft will be much smaller than the two-tendon system it replaces; reconstructed pulleys do not need to be as roomy as normal ones. Indeed, there may be an element of bowing in even normal pulleys after grafting, as shown in the diagram. For this reason, we currently recommend using the smaller implants, 3–4 mm in women and 4–5 mm in men, when reconstructing the pulley system.

The reconstructed pulley should be close to the joint for the reasons mentioned above but must not be so close or so bulky as to be a mechanical impediment to flexion.

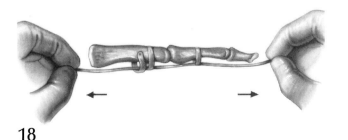

18

18

Tendon implant sizers are placed through the pulley system. With the finger held extended, the moistened implant is pulled gently back and forth to check for binding. Overly tight pulleys may lead to buckling and synovitis later.

19

Through the forearm incision, the superficial and deep flexors are identified and a preliminary selection of a Stage II motor tendon unit is made. A malleable blunt tendon carrier is passed from distally through the carpal canal to present in the forearm, between the superficialis and the profundus. The instrument is passed gently, seeking the soft mesotendon spaces. The proximal end of the implant is pulled into the forearm through the eye of the passer. The distal end is threaded through the pulley system to the fingertip. The implant should be long enough to extend proximal to the carpal canal in full finger extension. Excess length can be trimmed sharply at this time.

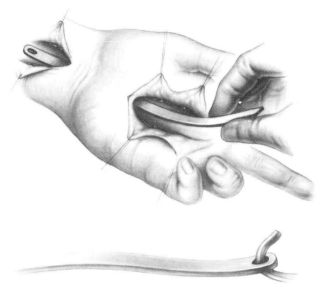

19

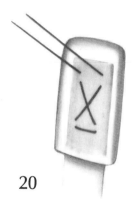

20

20

Distal end fixation will depend on the type of passive implant chosen. In any case, the flexor profundus stump should be freed to its distal attachment fibres in the distal phalanx. For the blunt tip implant, sutures should be placed in the implant as shown, being careful to keep the suture in the more central area to gain purchase in the Dacron tape. Suture placed only in the silicone rubber will not hold – the implant will loosen postoperatively and synovitis will develop. We prefer a 4/0 monofilament wire suture with a taper cut needle to minimize damage to the implant.

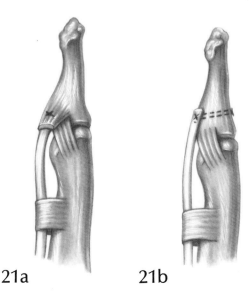

21a   21b

21a & b

Depending on the quality of the profundus stump, the blunt tip implant may be sutured directly to the profundus or fixed to the distal phalanx by passing the implant wire suture through two drill holes in the base of the phalanx. The implant is snugged against bone and the sutures tied on the dorsum of the distal phalanx through a separate incision. With either fixation technique, laterally reinforcing sutures of 5/0 monofilament wire are recommended as well.

22

If the screw-fixation passive implant is chosen, the implant must be threaded from distal to proximal through the pulley system and palm as the metal end-plate is bulkier than the implant itself and has sharp seating spikes which could damage the tendon bed. The plate is placed on the distal phalanx and a guide hole is made with a 11 mm (0.45 inch) Kirschner wire proximal to the nailbed. A self-tapping 2 mm Woodruff screw is then inserted to fix the plate securely to the phalanx. The screw should just penetrate the distal cortex of the phalanx. If too distal on the phalanx, it may damage the germinal matrix of the fingernail. Usually, the 6, 8 or 10 mm screw is used.

The alternative technique for fixing the metal plate to bone is by twist-fixing metal wire around the plate through drill holes in the bone.

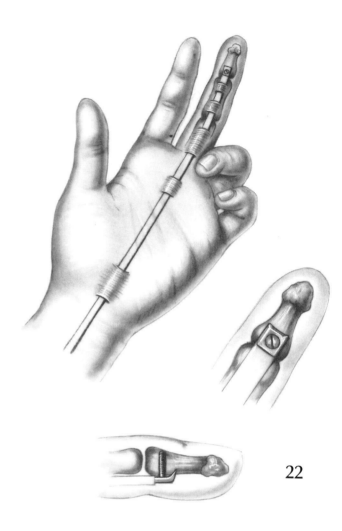

22

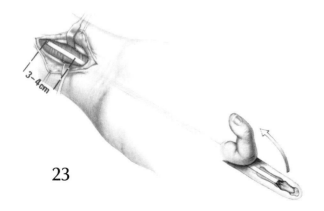

23

23

Passive gliding of the implant is tested by moistening the implant bed with saline, and holding the wrist and finger in neutral while passively flexing and extending the finger. Movement should be free, with a measured amplitude of implant movement between 3 and 4 cm at the proximal end. Any buckling must be corrected before closure or synovitis will develop between Stage I and Stage II.

Testing pulley system and recording range of movement

24

This is the important last manoeuvre of Stage I before wound closure. The free proximal end of the implant is grasped and pulled, bringing the finger from extension to maximum flexion. The following are recorded.

1. The predicted active range of movement versus the passive range of movement.
2. The measured distance of the proximal end necessary to produce the active function. This will assist in selection of the Stage II motor tendon.
3. The attitude of the finger in relation to the pulley system. Is another pulley necessary to improve function? Should a sagging pulley be snugged down closer to the bone? A pulley may rupture during this manoeuvre, requiring resuture or a tendon graft.
4. Finally, after these forceful manoeuvres the security of the distal end attachment of the tendon implant should be carefully checked.

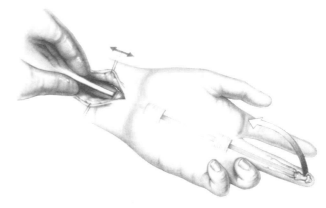

24

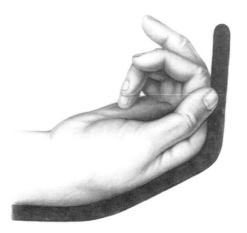

25

25

The wound is closed from distal to proximal and finally the soft tissue recess for the implant in the forearm is checked with a moistened gloved finger and passive gliding is reviewed. The hand is positioned with the wrist and metacarpophalangeal joints in flexion for closure and final dressing. This position after Stage I permits the proximal sheath to form in the long position.

POSTOPERATIVE MANAGEMENT

During the first 3 weeks, the patient is kept in the dorsal splint between therapy sessions. All therapy should be initially performed under the supervision of a hand therapist and the patient closely monitored for the development of synovitis. During the first week, gentle passive movement is started. If a flexion contracture was present preoperatively, extension splinting of the affected joint may also begin at this time. Regular passive stretching under the supervision of the hand therapist is begun during the third week and the patient is taught to flex the finger passively both with the opposite hand and by trapping or taping with an adjacent finger. Joint movement should be recorded regularly. When the patient has a soft supple finger with movement equal to that obtained in the operating room at the time of Stage I surgery, he is ready for the second stage.

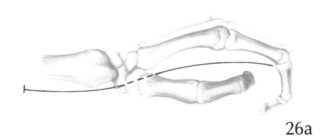

26a

26a & b

Between Stage I and Stage II, the movement and position of the implant should be checked radiographically in extension and flexion – at 6 weeks and on the day prior to Stage II are suggested.

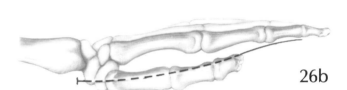

26b

Complications

If good judgement in patient selection and exact surgical techniques have been followed, complications after Stage I surgery should be rare. A complication that may occur is synovitis about the implant, which may be of two types. The most common situation is an aseptic synovitis secondary to mechanical irritation about the implant, which is characterized by pain, swelling and perhaps erythema but no signs of systemic illness. This problem is best treated by prevention. Synovitis can be minimized by careful handling of the implant to minimize accumulation of foreign particles by electrostatic attraction. Careful construction of the pulley system to avoid bowing and buckling will also do much to eliminate this problem. Distal juncture disruption is the most common cause of synovitis; again, careful attention to the details of the implant fixation are the best prevention. Finally, over-vigorous therapy may also result in synovitis.

Purulent synovitis is almost always due to contamination of the implant secondary to postoperative wound breakdown. Typically, this occurs over the distal phalanx in the region of initial injury in Zone II. Such fingers may be better treated initially by special salvage procedures, discussed below. If purulent synovitis does occur, early drainage and antibiotic irrigation may save the situation; if not, the implant should be removed and after adequate healing, the patient re-evaluated for repeat Stage I surgery.

Whatever the cause, aseptic synovitis once diagnosed is treated first by rest. If the symptoms do not resolve within 1 week, consideration should be given to early Stage II surgery. By 3 weeks after Stage I, sufficient neosheath is usually present to support Stage II surgery. Continued mobilization of the finger in the face of synovitis will result in a thickened sheath which will not support gliding or nutrition of the Stage II graft.

Stage II

THE OPERATION

Replacement of implant with a tendon graft

27

On the operating table, the passive range of movement is recorded to be compared with the Stage I range of movement. Improvements are frequently noted after Stage I hand therapy. Distal and proximal incisions are made to identify the sheath and implant. Distally, the implant is left attached to the tendon stump. Proximally, the implant is identified and the sheath at the site of the juncture is carefully examined. Portions of soft sheath may be retained at the surgeon's discretion; however, if synovitis has been present, any thickened sheath must be completely removed from the area extending from the proximal juncture site as far as the wrist flexion crease. The potential active range of movement is recorded starting with the hand and finger flat on the table. The measured rule is held by the proximal end of the implant. The implant is pulled firmly and the surgeon should note: (1) the excursion of the implant to produce the range of movement from maximum extension to maximum flexion; (2) the distance the finger pulp rests from the distal palmar crease; (3) joints with restricted movement; (4) the gliding of the implant and the fluid lubrication system of the tendon bed.

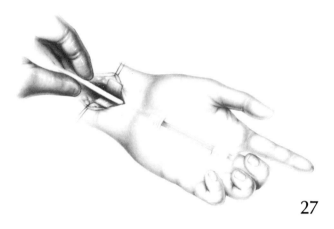

27

28

The motor tendon is selected and grasped with a small haemostat. The hand is elevated and the tourniquet is released while the lower leg is prepared to remove a long plantaris tendon graft. The technique is that described by Paul Brand.

A long toe extensor tendon may be used when the plantaris is absent. This technique uses the Brand type stripper and two incisions; (1) distally over the metatarsal joint of toe 3 or 4 and; (2) proximally at the retinacular level of the ankle. The fifth toe often has only one extensor tendon and should not be used as a donor for tendon grafting.

The graft is freed in the distal segment, passed through the proximal incision and stripped to the muscle attachment. Excellent long grafts have been removed by these techniques. Shorter tendon grafts such as palmaris longus, extensor indicis, extensor digiti minimi and segments of superficialis are removed by a standard technique and may be used for: (1) thumb, little finger and superficialis fingers with the juncture in the forearm; or (2) index, long and ring fingers to a tendon junction in the uninjured palm.

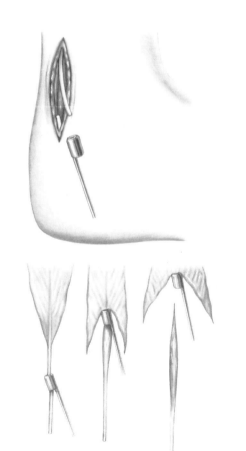

28

Removal of tendon implant and insertion of tendon graft

29

The tendon graft, carefully stripped of peritenon, is sutured to the proximal end of the implant and pulled through the new tendon bed. The implant is detached from the distal phalanx and discarded.

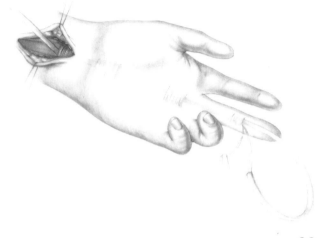

29

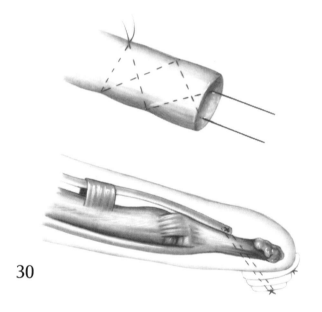

30

30

The tendon graft is secured distally by a Bunnell type suture technique to bone with monofilament 4/0 wire using a button dorsally on the fingernail. A pull-out wire is no longer used; if only one or two weaves are used in the tendon, the wire suture can be easily removed later by traction distally after the knot over the button has been cut.

The distal juncture should be carefully prepared to minimize the risk of rupture. The drill hole at the base of the phalanx should be enlarged so that the distal portion of the graft seats within the bone. Lateral reinforcing sutures of 3/0 braided polyester complete the juncture. An ophthalmic S-1 needle has been found helpful in placing these sutures in the confined space of the fingertip.

After the distal juncture is completed, the skin there should be closed since closure will be awkward after graft tension has been set.

Selection of a tendon motor

31

The tendon motor must supply the same excursion as that required to flex the finger fully with traction on the tendon graft. Selection of an appropriate motor unit, particularly in the previously traumatized extremity, is greatly facilitated by having the patient sedated but awake and cooperative at the time of Stage II surgery, as previously described.

Patient cooperation also eliminates the guesswork inherent in setting proper graft tension.

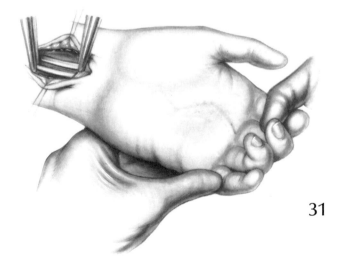

31

32a & b

When the tension is correct, the graft tendon is sutured to the motor tendon using the Pulvertaft end-weave technique. Interrupted monofilament 35 gauge wire is our suture of choice. It is extremely important to be sure that the suture passes through both the motor and graft tendon to prevent subsequent slipping of the proximal juncture. The juncture is more bulky than the implant so that proximal sheath may need to be excised at this point to permit free excursion of the juncture region.

After wound closure, a dorsal plaster splint is applied with the wrist flexed 30°, the metacarpophalangeal joints 70° and the proximal interphalangeal joints slightly flexed. A suture of 2/0 nylon may be placed through the fingernail at this time and fashioned into a loop for attachment of postoperative elastic band control.

POSTOPERATIVE MANAGEMENT

Postoperative tendon gliding requires close supervision of the patient by the therapist. Rubber band elastic flexion used early helps to protect the new tendon junctures and is applied either in the operating room or the next day. The patient is instructed to extend the finger actively against the rubber band and to allow the band to flex the finger passively, in a scheme similar to that recommended by Kleinert and others for rehabilitation after acute flexor tendon repair. It is important that the tension on the rubber band be minimal when the finger is flexed; otherwise, early proximal interphalangeal joint contractures may develop. The hand therapist should begin instructing the patient in passive movement of the interphalangeal joints during the first week. Passive flexion beyond the degree created by the rubber band is encouraged and active extension with the metacarpophalangeal joints flexed is allowed. The extension block splint is discontinued during the fourth week and a wrist cuff to which the rubber band is attached is substituted. This allows the patient to spend more time on wrist and metacarpophalangeal joint extension. The dorsal splint can be eliminated sooner if there has been difficulty in obtaining good graft sliding and active movement or if there has been a flexion contracture; later, if active movement has returned quickly. The rationale for the latter recommendation is the assumption that easy early movement implies fewer adhesions to the graft and, consequently, slow vascular ingrowth and presumably slower juncture healing. Conversely, stiffness and poor gliding would imply a greater vascular contribution to the healing process and more rapid healing.

During the sixth week, the button and distal wire suture are removed and light passive stretching may begin. Active flexion is encouraged with use of the Bunnell wood block and similar training techniques to develop supple gliding planes of connective tissue around the graft. At 8 weeks light resistive activities are begun and at 12 weeks heavy resistance and work therapy can be introduced.

Complications

The most common complications after Stage II are adhesions and rupture of the tendon graft junctures. Restrictive adhesions are most common at the proximal juncture site but may occur anywhere. They are particular-

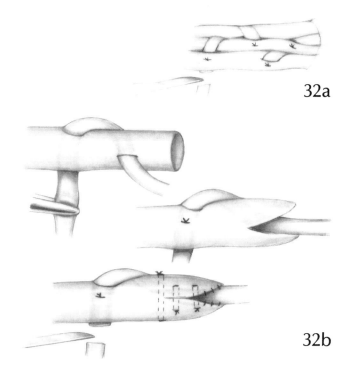

32a

32b

ly likely to develop where tight pulleys bind the graft, where inadequate pulleys allow the graft to bowstring and scar to deposit beneath the bowed graft, or in areas with poor overall tissue nutrition with consequent inadequate fluid nutrition to the graft.

If at the completion of Stage II rehabilitation adhesions are significantly restricting movement, tenolysis should be performed. Sedation combined with local anaesthesia is preferred for tenolysis since only by observing active tendon movement can all the restricting adhesions be identified. Adhesions which do not limit movement should be looked upon as providing nutrition to the graft and should not be disturbed.

Tenolysis should begin at the region of the proximal juncture; extensions may be necessary proximally as well as distally, as intermuscular scar may also limit active movement. Early movement after tenolysis is essential if the gains achieved at surgery are to be maintained. An indwelling silicone rubber catheter through which 0.5 per cent bupivacaine hydrochloride (Marcain) can be injected prior to therapy sessions has been found to be extremely helpful in controlling pain during the first postoperative week. The patient should be encouraged to take the finger through a full range of active movement several times each hour. Careful supervision by a hand therapist is required.

Rupture of the tendon graft is usually due to faulty technique in preparing junctures initially. So-called 'stretching' of the graft is probably an incomplete manifestation of this problem.

Occasionally late rupture may be due to a combination of increased activity level and incomplete juncture healing. Typically, these patients have regained movement quickly after Stage II, presumably having fewer vascular adhesions as mentioned previously. The best treatment is prevention through awareness of the situation; however, often these grafts may be salvaged by early exploration and graft reattachment.

Special indications

THE SUPERFICIALIS FINGER

33

The two-stage technique may be indicated in special circumstances to reconstruct severely damaged fingers with poor distal skin. The implant may be carried distally to the superficialis and fixed by any of the techniques described above. The distal joint can be amputated, fused or tenodesed as necessary. Stage II techniques for superficialis finger reconstruction are identical to those for standard Stage II surgery.

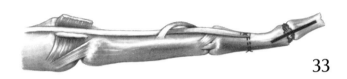

33

THE SUPERFICIALIS FINGER BY TENDON GRAFT RECESSION

34

After Stage II tendon grafting, a pulley rupture, distal or proximal to the proximal interphalangeal joint, may result in a bowed finger. A useful result may be salvaged by detaching the tendon graft distally and attaching the graft to the base of the middle phalanx. Tenodesis or arthrodesis of the dorsal interphalangeal joint completes the procedure.

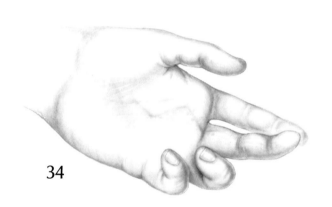

34

EXTENSOR TENDON RECONSTRUCTION

35

In some cases of extensor tendon injury, a dorsal scar may restrict the movement of a primary graft or transfer. The two-stage technique may be used to good advantage in these patients, suturing the implant distally to the dorsum of bone of either the proximal or middle phalanx and extending it proximally into the forearm.

A pulley to help centralize the implant is essential and may be made from available extensor tendon or free graft material. The lateral band system should be functional on at least one side.

Requirements for tendon excursion on the extensor side are considerably less than for flexors, particularly when intrinsics are available to extend the interphalangeal joints, and the reconstruction need only extend to the metacarpophalangeal joint. Often sufficient action is provided by the neosheath between the forearm musculature and the phalanx so that active movement is possible through this connection even prior to Stage II grafting. If the implant is then removed and no graft inserted, the sheath will collapse and form a strong fibrous band – a sort of neotendon which eliminates the necessity for grafting. This is particularly helpful in a hand which otherwise could require multiple tendon grafts, such as a replanted hand.

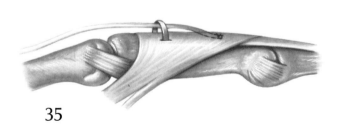

35

ACTIVE PROGRAMME

Stage I

The surgical principles of Stage I surgery for the passive programme apply equally to the active programme. Local anaesthesia should be used to facilitate selection and testing of the motor unit. Specific technical points which will be covered here relate to implant fixation and selection of a motor unit.

The active programme generally shares the same indications as the passive programme. Situations in which poor finger nutrition might limit neosheath formation and healing after Stage II may be better candidates for the active than the passive programme, for example, the older patient. Factors which would weigh against the active programme include: necessity for tenolysis in adjacent digits, since the splinting necessary to protect the active implant junctures would compromise rehabilitation for the tenolysis; and simultaneous multiple pulley reconstructions, since the immobilization required to protect the pulleys would compromise early active movement of the implant.

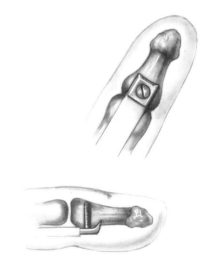

36

Stage I

THE OPERATION

Distal fixation

36

The implant* should be threaded from distal to proximal through the reconstructed tendon bed. With the finger extended, the proximal loop should be just proximal to the carpal canal so that the fixation can be to the tendon rather than to the muscle belly of the motor unit. The distal screw-fixation device is similar to that in the passive implant. If the braided cord implant is used, the cords can be separated distally until the implant is of the desired length. The braided cord may be sutured into tendon or bone.

Proximal juncture

37

The motor unit is selected from those available as in Stage II of the passive programme, attempting to make the best possible match between required excursion of the implant and available amplitude of the motor. The motor unit tendon is passed through the implant loop and sutured to itself with a Pulvertaft weave technique. Free ends of Dacron braid may be woven into the tendon for suture fixation as an alternative technique.

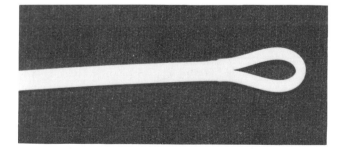

37

* Active Tendon Implant for Total Tendon Replacement – The Holter Housner International Co., Bridgeport, PA, USA

POSTOPERATIVE MANAGEMENT

Rehabilitation after the Stage I active implant is similar to that after Stage II in the passive programme, except that it may progress more quickly, as the healing which must occur is from well-vascularized tendon to itself rather than from well-vascularized tendon to avascular graft and from avascular graft to bone. The wrist cuff is usually employed after the third week and light resistive exercises begun after the sixth week.

Complications

In addition to the complications of the passive implant, both proximal and distal implant juncture rupture is a potential hazard of the active programme. Unlike the passive programme, however, in which juncture separation is detected only indirectly – by fortuitous radiography or with the development of synovitis – active implant rupture is immediately evident by sudden loss of active flexion. If the distal juncture fails, Stage II tendon grafting should be considered, since the implant will retract and the distal sheath will close. If the proximal juncture fails, however, the active programme can be simply converted to the passive programme and rehabilitation continued, with elective Stage II grafting at the appropriate time.

Stage II

THE OPERATION

If the active implant is functioning well, Stage II surgery may be delayed indefinitely. When, either electively or because of juncture separation, State II grafting is indicated, the technique is similar to that for Stage II of the passive programme. Since the motor has already been selected and prepared, the proximal end of the tendon graft is passed through the loop in the motor unit and woven to itself by the Pulvertaft technique (*see Illustration 32*) or the graft may be woven into the tendon and sutured. Again, the proximal juncture is bulky so that sheath may need to be excised in the forearm to allow for maximal amplitude of the juncture region.

POSTOPERATIVE MANAGEMENT

Stage II postoperative therapy and complications are identical for the active and the passive programmes with the exception that in Stage II gliding movement occurs rapidly and special precautions are necessary.

Summary

Flexor tendon reconstruction through the two-stage programme is a proven, useful method to restore function to the injured hand. The active implant, currently in the clinical experimental stages, has the potential to incorporate the benefits of active movement even earlier in the rehabilitation course. As research makes the tension interface between living tissue and synthetic materials more durable, a true artificial tendon will also be developed.

Illustrations by Paul Richardson

Dupuytren's contracture

W. M. Steel FRCS (Ed)
Consultant Orthopaedic Surgeon, Department of Postgraduate Medicine, University of Keele, Hartshill, Stoke-on-Trent, UK

Introduction

Aetiology

Dupuytren's disease is inherited as a dominant gene. It becomes increasingly prevalent in the older population and is much commoner in men than women. Epileptics have a 15 times higher incidence of the disease than the normal population, suggesting a genetic linkage but many of these also have a history of treatment with drugs such as phenytoin. Chronic alcoholics and patients whose hands are immobilized are also prone to the disease. Dupuytren's contracture has been called 'the Viking's curse', since its geographical incidence corresponds to the Viking homelands and the spread of Viking invaders at the beginning of the second millennium. However, studies in Japan from old people's homes have shown an incidence not dissimilar from that noted in Caucasian surveys. There have been numerous studies on the relationship to manual labour, but although the disease can follow a single traumatic incident, there seems no definite linkage with repetitive hand trauma.

Pathology

Despite interesting microscopic studies and detailed collagen analysis, the pathological mechanism is still unknown. What stimulates fibroblasts to hyperplasia and new collagen production is uncertain. The presence of an increased amount of Type III collagen in Dupuytren's tissue is probably a reflection of the production of new relatively immature collagen by active fibroblasts. The formation of the nodule seems to be the primary process whilst the development of cords is a secondary phenomenon resembling work hypertrophy. There have been several elegant studies of the anatomy of the diseased fascia which help in the understanding of the pattern of the contracture and provide an essential anatomical basis for surgical dissection.

Dupuytren's diathesis

Several factors are known to have an adverse influence on the prognosis of the disease and, if they are present, the patient should be warned of the possible gloomy outlook. These are a definite inheritance, bilateral involvement, the presence of ectopic lesions (knuckle pads, plantar nodules, penile lesions of fibrosis of the corpus cavernosum – Peyronie's disease), associated diseases (epilepsy, alcoholism), and an early onset. In patients with such a diathesis, surgery may well have to be repeated frequently as the condition progresses to involve the palm and digits of both hands. Recurrence, as well as extension of the disease, will be common.

Clinical features and natural history

Nodules are often seen in the earlier stage of the condition and are sometimes painful and tender when they first appear. They generally occur in the line of the finger rays. Skin pits are usually found in the palm, often at the distal palmar crease. They are said to arise when adhesions develop between the longitudinal and vertical fibre systems. The most frequently observed feature is the cord, extending across a joint and producing a flexion contracture. The cords may be entirely palmar, causing a metacarpophalangeal contracture, entirely digital or, more usually, involving both areas. Although most often seen in the little and ring rays, cords are not uncommon in the radial fingers and thumb. Even the terminal interphalangeal joints are occasionally involved. The progression of contracture is extremely variable and is not linear.

In a study of a series of patients with very early Dupuytren's contracture, after only one year 9 per cent had progressed, after 3 years 22 per cent had deteriorated and at 6 years 48 per cent. In the patients with a diathesis, contractures develop with great rapidity, whilst in the elderly patient with involvement of a single ray the process may take many years. Prolonged contracture leads to permanent joint stiffness causing considerable disability.

Prognosis

The overall risk of recurrence and/or extension is 34 per cent but this figure rises to 78 per cent in the patient with a diathesis and falls to 17 per cent in the elderly, slowly progressive case. The ability to correct a contracture is to some degree unpredictable. It can generally be said that metacarpophalangeal flexion deformities can always be corrected. Interphalangeal contractures may be fully correctable, partially correctable or quite incorrigible. A short history of contracture of less than 6 months is a favourable factor, whereas dense skin involvement is not. The patient should be warned that correction is unlikely to be complete but an attempt is always worthwhile.

Preoperative

Timing of surgery

With general practitioners and the lay public becoming increasingly aware of the condition, patients are presenting more frequently with early disease. The presence of a palmar nodule, skin pit or simple cord without any joint contracture does not usually warrant surgery but occasionally nodules require removal for pain. The patient should be given an explanation of the disease and advised to return at the first sign of deformity. A simple test is the inability to place the hand flat on the table, palm down. When contractures are present, surgery should be considered and the appropriate operation selected. There is seldom extreme urgency to operate for Dupuytren's disease, but the patients should be seen every 3 to 4 months and surgery brought forward if there is progression of the deformity. The exception is the patient with an occupation involving manual skills who should be treated at the first sign of contracture. In some elderly patients with very mild contractures, it may be reasonable to observe the condition without resorting to immediate surgery. Where two hands are involved, it is not always appropriate to operate first on the worst hand. If the contracture on the most seriously affected side seems irremediable, the best choice is often to correct the other hand which is still salvageable. Dominance and the patient's requirements for work and recreations influence the choices. Clinical photographs should be taken.

Selection of operation

In the absence of deformity, or in an elderly patient well-adjusted to a virtually static flexion deformity, no operation is necessary.

Fasciotomy

This is a good procedure for the elderly patient with a single, well-defined band, deep to mobile skin, and causing only a metacarpophalangeal contracture. The morbidity is trivial but there is a risk of recurrence. It is also a useful preliminary operation in very severe Dupuytren's contracture, where skin toilet is impossible, prior to the major operation. Fasciotomy plus skin graft has been suggested as an option, but it is not necessary to close skin in the palm and an 'open-palm' fasciotomy is quite satisfactory.

Limited fasciectomy

There is no longer any place for the extensive fasciectomy which was once preferred, in which attempts were made to excise all the palmar aponeurosis in an effort to prevent extension of the disease. The morbidity from this procedure was unjustified and there is no evidence that prophylactic excision of the palmar fascia prevents extension or recurrence. The current practice is to limit fasciectomy to the area of diseased tissue in the palm and digits. Moreover, it is now felt that as little normal tissue as possible should be removed, the diseased fascia should be painstakingly dissected out, preserving not only the neurovascular bundles but also as much as possible of the palmar and digital fat.

Dermofasciectomy

Replacement of involved skin is the only known method of preventing local recurrence of Dupuytren's disease. It is used in the treatment of recurrence, almost entirely in the digits, but there have been advocates for its use in the anticipation and prevention of recurrence in those patients with a diathesis where extensive skin involvement is noted at the primary operation.

Amputation

There is a definite place for the removal of digits with troublesome interphalangeal contractures which have proved incorrigible at primary or secondary operation. Often the patient will suggest amputation rather than have a useless protruding finger.

Other measures

Very occasionally proximal interphalangeal contractures, which do not correct during fasciectomy, may be relieved by careful and judicious capsulotomy, but the surgeon should be wary of embarking on heroic release of the collateral ligaments and volar plate as not infrequently this results in an even more vicious contracture. Surgical trauma to the flexor mechanism and to the interphalangeal joints should be kept to an absolute minimum during surgery if rapid return of function is to be achieved. Arthrodesis of the proximal interphalangeal joints in semi-flexion may be employed but is seldom an appropriate choice in the ulnar two digits. The success rate of interphalangeal joint arthroplasty in arthritis is so poor that its use in Dupuytren's disease should be discouraged.

Operative principles

Whether general or regional anaesthesia is used is a matter for the preference of individual surgeons and anaesthetists; either is appropriate. As in all hand surgery, certain requirements are essential, namely good lighting, a comfortable seat with arm support, good position of the hand, quiet, unhurried conditions, fine instruments, a bloodless field and adequate assistance. Incisions are planned to permit maximum exposure of the fascia to be dissected, but with the minimum risk of skin flap ischaemia and necrosis. They are placed so as to reduce the possibility of scar contracture across joints. Delicacy in handling the tissues and the avoidance of clumsy blunt dissection reduce postoperative oedema and fibrosis. Ideally the tourniquet should be released at the end of the dissection in order to achieve good haemostasis. This can be rather time-consuming and equally satisfactory prevention of haematoma can be obtained by elevation of the limb for 24 hours immediately after surgery or by using the 'open-palm' technique.

DISEASE INVOLVING ONE RAY

1 & 2

A longitudinal approach to the digit offers the most satisfactory exposure for fasciectomy and avoids the problem of dissecting the difficult area at the base of the finger through transverse incisions. Various techniques are used to prevent skin contracture and marginal wound necrosis. The most widely used is a longitudinal incision over the diseased cord, broken up by appropriate Z-plasties at the transverse skin creases. Its advantage is the direct exposure of the diseased tissue with excellent access. The disadvantage is that quite often the skin flaps are of poor quality and may slough.

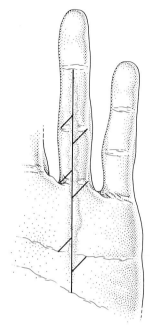

1

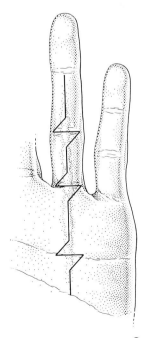

2

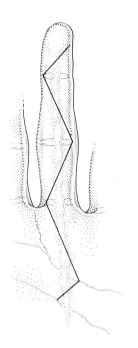

3

The Bruner zigzag approach avoids the need for Z-plasty but affords no skin lengthening at closure. Large flaps raised across densely involved dermal areas may be at risk.

3

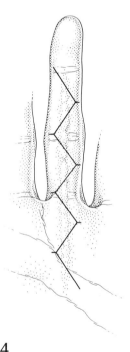

4

4

A third compromise is the multiple V–Y technique. Some skin lengthening is achieved and Z-plasty planning and manipulation is avoided.

5

In occasional circumstances, particularly the ulnar border of the little finger, a sinuous digito-palmar incision can be used.

The incision should be planned so that it extends to the interphalangeal crease beyond the last flexed joint, thus permitting access to the distal attachments of the cord. The first and often most difficult step is the dissection of the skin from the diseased nodule or cord. The dermis is often very adherent to the involved tissue and separation is tedious. Damage to the dermal circulation at this stage will carry the risk of skin necrosis. Sharp scalpel dissection is essential and magnification can be helpful. As the band is defined, the skin flaps become more secure. Frequent changing of the scalpel blade is necessary. Once the skin has been completely isolated from the diseased tissue, resection can then commence. It is wise to work from proximal to distal. After careful transverse incision of the fascial cord in the proximal palm, the involved tissue is separated from the transverse palmar ligament and paratendinous fibres. At the level of the mid-palm, the nerves and vessels are much more deeply situated than the cord and need not be disturbed. At the level of the metacarpophalangeal joint the deep vertical fibres are seen and can be divided without deeper dissection. At this stage the neurovascular bundles must be isolated and preserved. The cords are then traced to the finger and the neurovascular bundles carefully protected.

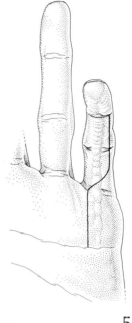

5

6

Detailed anatomical studies have increased our understanding of the pattern of involvement in the digit. The three types of cord, which should be recognized, are the central pretendinous cord, the spiral cord and the lateral cord. The central cord is comparatively easily dissected away from the flexor tendon sheath and the neurovascular bundles. The lateral cord usually lies lateral and deep to these structures, the fibres are attached to skin and seldom distort the neurovascular bundle; they are often continuous with the natatory ligament which may also be involved in the Dupuytren's process. This cord seldom contributes much to the proximal interphalangeal contracture. The most troublesome cord is the spiral, which as its name implies spirals around the neurovascular bundles, lying first deep and then superficial to these structures.

Knowledge of the anatomy is the key to safe dissection. The cord is never attached to nerves and vessels which pass through a tunnel on their way to a lateral and more superficial position. By defining the tunnel and dividing the cord carefully, the neurovascular bundle can be isolated and the cord removed in two parts. The cord's distal attachment is to the base of the middle phalanx and it is often necessary to retract the nerves and vessels to reach the distal insertion. On the ulnar side of the little finger, the spiral cord usually emanates from the tendon of abductor digiti minimi, and is continuous with that structure.

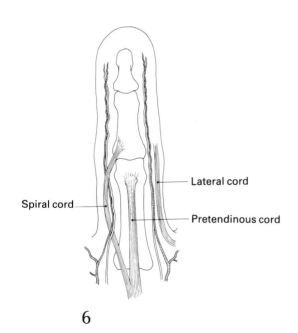

Lateral cord

Spiral cord

Pretendinous cord

6

DISEASE INVOLVING MORE THEN ONE RAY

7

The advantages of a longitudinal approach to digital dissection can be combined with Skoog's approach to palmar disease and the 'open-palm' technique. This combination has an advantage over a strictly longitudinal approach in allowing good access for the removal of widespread disease. The use of the 'open-palm' technique reduces the risk of haematoma following palmar dissection, permits early mobilization of the hand and reduces tension in the longitudinal digital incisions. The digital approach may be a midline vertical incision broken by Z-plasty, particularly when the band is central, or by the Bruner incision, which can be so planned as to give good access to laterally placed disease.

Skoog technique

Skoog emphasized the need to separate and preserve intact the transverse palmar ligament which is never involved by Dupuytren's disease. The transverse incision is made over the extent of the palmar disease, a vertical extension is made proximally, and distal longitudinal incisions fashioned over the cords extending to the digits. These incisions can be parallel or Y-shaped. The triangular skin flaps over the proximal palm need only be developed to expose the borders of the involved aponeurosis. Distally, the flaps are raised only as far as the limits of the disease. The fatty tissue in the web space outlined by the quadrilateral or triangular flap is not disturbed and there should be no problem in the blood supply of the skin. Skoog emphasized a conservative excision in the palm; the longitudinal diseased fascia is separated from the transverse palmar ligament and removed. The paratendinous septa are not disturbed and it is quite unnecessary to dissect out and isolate the neurovascular structures. By leaving the delicate connective and fatty tissues, bleeding in the palm is reduced and swelling is minimal. Function is rapidly restored.

Having isolated the involved palmar tissue, the base of the triangle which it forms is divided carefully and, working distally, is dissected away by scalpel from the underlying flexor tendon, paratendinous fibres and transverse palmar ligament. There is no need to isolate the neurovascular bundles in the mid-palm. As the dissection proceeds into the distal palm, the deep connections will be seen and must be carefully isolated from the neurovascular structures. The vertical septa are divided just deep to the plane of the fascia. There is no need to remove them at a deeper level as they are not diseased nor do they lead to recurrence. Further dissection in the finger proceeds as outlined earlier.

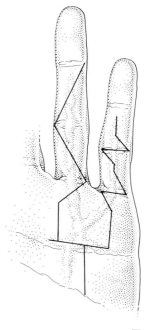

7

'Open-palm' technique (McCash)

8 & 9

The 'open-palm' technique recognizes that the blood supply of the palmar skin is so good that healing will occur regardless of wound suture. The technique can readily be combined with the Skoog approach. All the longitudinal wounds are closed but the transverse palmar wound is left open. Since there has been only a selective aponeurectomy in the palm, the dead space is minimal. A single layer of paraffin gauze is applied to the open wound, followed by fluffed gauze, wool padding and a crêpe bandage. At 5–7 days, the wound is examined and the patient instructed in active flexion and extension exercises. If necessary, the hand therapist can assist. Since there is no tension of the wound, the patient need not fear disrupting the sutures. The open wounds are remarkably pain-free and comfortable. Dressings thereafter are changed once or twice a week and the patient seen weekly in the hand clinic. No haematoma ever develops and no wound has ever failed to heal within 4 weeks. Infection is unknown. The postoperative regime is not tedious and is amply rewarded by the freedom from complications.

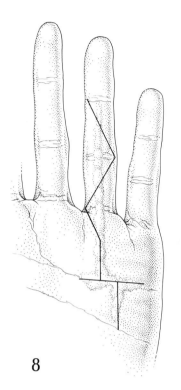

8

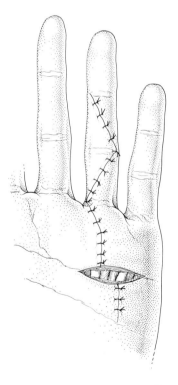

9

Joint contractures

At the end of the dissection the skin flaps are carefully palpated between finger and thumb to detect any residual nodules or Dupuytren's tissue. Palpation is the most sensitive method of detecting residual cords in the finger which may lie undetected. If there has been incomplete correction of a proximal interphalangeal contracture, it is permissible to divide the fibrous flexor sheath and the check-rein ligaments. Open capsulotomy, though favoured by some, carries a definite risk of loss of flexion, a more serious handicap than loss of extension. Accurate recording of the preoperative and residual flexion contracture is essential.

Haemostasis

Haematoma formation has been greatly reduced since the demise of extensive radical fasciectomy. The use of longitudinal incisions minimizes the risk of a palmar dead space, whilst the 'open-palm' technique completely eliminates the possibility of palmar haematoma. Bleeding can be reduced further by the use of bipolar diathermy during the operation, facilitated by allowing a little blood to remain in the vessels. Release of the tourniquet is widely practised and allows inspection of skin flaps as well as good haemostasis. A firm pad of wire wool or fluffed gauze is packed into the palm and bandaged firmly but not tightly. Forcible extension of the whole hand is to be avoided. Elevation of the limb from the moment of tourniquet release can be extremely effective in preventing haematoma and should be continued for at least 24 hours. Suction drainage is used if extensive palmar dissection has been necessary.

Skin closure

The wounds are closed with 4/0 nylon interrupted sutures, tension must be avoided and it is preferable to leave small gaps rather than to suture tightly. The 'open-palm' technique helps to reduce tension in the longitudinal finger wounds. Where Z-plasties are used, the skin is rearranged with regard to the principles of that technique.

DERMOFASCIECTOMY

Fasciectomy combined with excision and grafting of skin is frequently used in recurrent Dupuytren's contracture, and by some surgeons as a primary procedure in severe Dupuytren's disease. In patients with a strong diathesis in whom there is obvious skin involvement, it may be appropriate to anticipate recurrence by dermofasciectomy as a primary procedure. Skin proximal to the distal palmar crease need not be excised since it will not cause contracture.

The fasciectomy is carried out in the usual way through a midline incision. Particular care must be taken to avoid opening the fibrous flexor sheath, since leakage of synovial fluid will float off the graft. If the sheath is just slightly nicked it may be closed. Similarly, the proximal interphalangeal joint must not be opened. These strictures are easily met in primary fasciectomy but more difficult in recurrent disease. The area to be grafted must extend to the mid-axial line of the digit at the finger creases, but need not necessarily at points between. After fasciectomy and skin excision, a graft is cut to a pattern and sutured in place with a tie-over dressing. It is preferable for cosmetic reasons to take a full-thickness graft, using the inner arm or groin as the donor site.

RECURRENT DISEASE

When previous surgery has been carried out, dissection is considerably more difficult. The planes between normal and diseased tissue are lost and there is no longer separation between the cords and the neurovascular bundle. Careful exposure of the nerves and vessels is essential. The fibrous flexor sheaths may well be transgressed and, if joint contracture is not relieved by fasciectomy, then further capsular dissection will be necessary. If there is a need to replace involved skin there must be no synovial leakage from flexor sheath or proximal interphalangeal joint. That may limit the extent of the correction or, if synovial leakage does occur, skin grafting is precluded.

FASCIOTOMY

10

This procedure is often appropriate in elderly patients with metacarpophalangeal contractures, caused by single cords under mobile skin. The closed technique is easily performed under local anaesthesia. The skin overlying the cord and the tissues deep to the cord are infiltrated with 1 per cent local anaesthetic. A number 15 scalpel blade is inserted between skin and cord and, whilst tension is applied, the blade is rotated so that its cutting edge is applied to the cord. Without pressing on the knife, the cord is forced against the blade until the cord is fully divided. Fasciectomy at two levels in the palm is advisable to prevent recurrence.

Fasciotomy in the finger carries a considerable risk of damage to digital nerves and vessels. It should never be done closed but a small open fasciotomy is permissible, provided the neurovascular bundle can be seen and isolated. Following operation a simple dressing is applied but it is advisable to splint the hand and fingers in the corrected position to prevent relapse and recurrence.

AMPUTATION

The general principles of digital amputation are followed with one addition, the dorsal skin of the amputated digit should be filleted and used to replace involved skin in the palm or proximal finger. Thus, scarred adherent skin can be replaced by supple uninvolved dorsal skin. The only disadvantage is the appearance of hair in the palm of hirsute individuals.

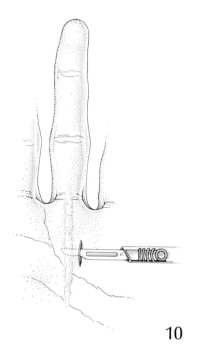

10

Postoperative management

Careful postoperative care and close supervision are the keys to the avoidance of complications. The limb is elevated for at least 24 hours after operation. The patient may then mobilize with the arm in a high sling and be discharged from hospital. At the first postoperative visit 5 to 7 days after operation, the wound should be inspected. At this stage haematoma can be recognized and released; infection, which should be extremely rare, can be treated; marginal skin necrosis, if less than one centimetre in extent, will usually heal without difficulty but larger areas should be excised and grafted before scarring and contracture spoil the operative result. When no complications have occurred the patient is encouraged to commence active flexion of the fingers. If there is any difficulty or reluctance, the aid of a hand therapist is enlisted.

Swelling of the hand should be minimal, provided the surgery has been gentle, the dressings properly applied and haematoma prevented. If there is evidence of swelling or oedema this must be treated vigorously as it is often the first sign of impending reflex sympathetic dystrophy. If the swelling is serious, the patient should be readmitted for elevation of the limb, ice packs and hand therapy. Lesser degrees may be supervised as an outpatient with similar treatment.

Open wounds are dressed at the first visit and at weekly intervals thereafter. The patient is instructed to ignore the wound and move the fingers freely. By the second week there should be sufficient wound healing to permit more vigorous exercises by the patient and, where necessary, with the help of the therapist. Sutures should be left for at least 14 days before removal. Once sound wound healing has occurred, paraffin wax may be used as a preliminary to exercise periods. Bouncing putty and other aids can be introduced to assist in building up hand strength. Occupational tasks and a programme of home activities are used at this time.

The use of splintage following Dupuytren's surgery is not universally accepted but it certainly has a place in the maintenance of the operative correction and the prevention of relapse. Splints must be individually designed, changed regularly as the contracture improves, and supervised daily by the therapists. They may be introduced as early as 1 week or as soon as the wound permits. Splintage must be intermittent and interspersed with an active exercise programme. Night splintage for several months after operation is often useful.

Recurrence

The development of further Dupuytren's disease in the area of operation is termed recurrence. It may occur within a few weeks of surgery or be delayed for years. Patients with a diathesis and those with dense skin involvement are most prone to this complication. Recurrence and/or extension has been noted in 78 per cent of patients with a strong diathesis, compared with 17 per cent in the unilateral late-onset case with no family history. Further contracture will take place if the recurr-ence affects the digital tissues. Second operations should be delayed until scars are mature, and revisions should be accompanied by skin excision and replacement whenever it is involved. The prospect of correction diminishes in these patients.

Extension

The development of further Dupuytren's disease outside the area of primary operation is termed extension and is not infrequent, particularly in those with a diathesis. Patients should be warned of this possibility. The treatment of the extension follows the lines of primary disease and offers no special difficulties.

Further reading

Egawa T, Horiki A, Senrui H. Dupuytren's contracture in Japan. In: Hueston JT, Tubiana R, eds. *Dupuytren's disease*, 2nd ed. Edinburgh: Churchill Livingstone, 1985: 100–3.

Hueston JT, Tubiana R. *Dupuytren's disease*, 2nd ed. Churchill Livingstone, 1985.

Hueston JT. The control of recurrent Dupuytren's contracture by skin replacement. *Br J Plast Surg* 1969; 22: 152–6.

Hueston JT. *Dupuytren's contracture*. Edinburgh: Livingstone, 1963.

King EW, Bass DM, Watson HK. Treatment of Dupuytren's contracture by extensive fasciectomy through multiple Y-V-plasty incision: short-term evaluation of 170 consecutive operations. *J Hand Surg* 1979; 4: 234.

Ling RS. The genetic factor in Dupuytren's disease. *J Bone Joint Surg [Br]* 1963; 45–B: 709–18.

Lubahn JD, Lister GD, Wolfe T. Fasciectomy in Dupuytren's disease: a comparison between the open palm technique and wound closure. *J Hand Surg [Am]* 1984; 9–A: 53–8.

Luck, JV. Dupuytren's contracture: a new concept of the pathogenesis correlated with surgical management. *J Bone Joint Surg [Am]* 1959; 41-A: 635–64.

McCash CR. The open palm technique in Dupuytren's contracture. *Br J Plast Surg* 1964 17: 271–80.

McFarlane RM. Patterns of the diseased fascia in the fingers in Dupuytren's contracture: displacement of the neurovascular bundle. *Plastic Reconstr Surg* 1974; 54: 31–44.

McGrouther DA. The microanatomy of Dupuytren's contracture. *Hand* 1982; 14: 215–36.

Mikkelsen OA. Dupuytren's disease: the influence of occupation and previous hand injuries. *Hand* 1978; 10: 1–8.

Millesi H. The clinical and morphological course of Dupuytren's disease. In: Hueston JT, Tubiana R, eds. *Dupuytren's disease*, 2nd ed. Edinburgh: Churchill Livingstone, 1985: 114–21.

Skoog T. The transverse elements of the palmar aponeurosis in Dupuytren's contracture: their pathological and surgical significance. *Scand J Plast Reconstr Surg* 1967; 1: 51–63.

Trigger finger and thumb

Neil Citron   MChir, FRCS
Consultant Orthopaedic Surgeon, St Helier's Hospital, Carshalton, Surrey, UK

Introduction

This common condition usually occurs in middle age and affects women more often than men. The patient complains of a digit which intermittently 'snaps', 'locks', or 'dislocates' on active movement. Closer questioning elicits a history of pain over the volar aspect of the metacarpophalangeal joint and on examination a nodule may be felt on the flexor tendon, especially in the thumb. Most cases are due to stenosis of the entrance to the fibrous flexor tendon sheath at the level of the A1 pulley, due to a chronic inflammatory tenosynovitis of unknown aetiology. This narrowing causes the development of a localized thickening of the flexor tendon, and as this passes to and fro beneath the pulley it gives rise to a momentary pain and feeling of resistance.

As the condition progresses, the tendon nodule size increases and triggering becomes constant. In severe cases the nodule can occasionally jam distal to the constriction in the sheath and the patient is unable to flex the digit. More often, in severe cases, there is limitation of extension as the nodule cannot pass distally. If this is prolonged, secondary flexion contracture of the proximal interphalangeal joint may ensue.

It is common to have more than one finger involved in the condition, often sequentially. This is especially so in diabetic patients and those with renal failure.

Rheumatoid tenosynovitis of the flexor tendons can cause triggering owing to masses of synovial proliferation on the tendon. Diagnosis of the condition is important as surgical treatment is different and more extensive than the idiopathic type[1] and will not be discussed here.

Conservative treatment

If triggering is of relatively short duration, the tendon sheath can be injected from proximal distally with local anaesthetic and steroid. A wide (21-gauge) needle should be used to obtain a good 'feedback' of the fluid pressure in the synovial sheath: injection should be without resistance, whereas if the needle has been advanced into the tendon itself a greater resistance is felt. Injection of steroid into tendons causes damage and predisposes to their rupture.

Preoperative

Rheumatoid disease should be excluded by clinical examination. Local sepsis is an absolute contraindication.

Anaesthesia

The operation may be performed under local or general anaesthesia. Where local anaesthesia is chosen, the skin in the web spaces around the finger is cleaned with 70 per cent ethanol. This is then allowed to evaporate. A 5 ml syringe filled with 1 per cent lignocaine without adrenaline is used with a 23-gauge needle. This is introduced deep into the web space parallel to the palm of the hand and aspiration attempted to avoid inadvertent intravascular injection. Then 2.5 ml of 1 per cent lignocaine without adrenaline is slowly injected deep into the web space on either side of the finger concerned. While waiting for the anaesthetic to take effect, the preparations for surgery continue.

A padded pneumatic tourniquet is placed around the forearm at its point of maximal circumference just distal to the elbow. This is more comfortable for the patient than an upper arm tourniquet. The hand and distal forearm are cleaned and draped in the usual manner. The hand is exsanguinated by elevation for 3 minutes. The patient then clenches his fist, including the thumb, and the tourniquet is rapidly inflated before he releases again.

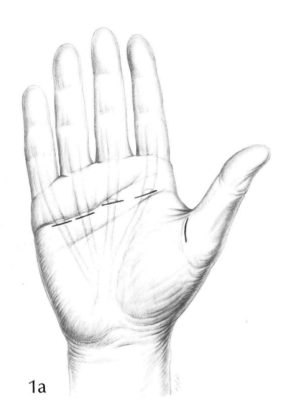

1a

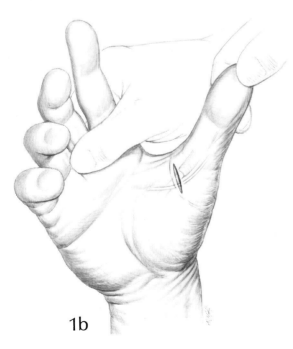

1b

Operation

Incision

1a

A small transverse incision using a No. 15 blade is made at the base of the finger just proximal to the distal transverse palmar crease for the ulnar three fingers and just distal to the proximal palmar crease for the index finger. Placing the incision next to a skin crease has two advantages.

1. Sweat and dirt do not collect in the wound as they do in the crease.
2. The effect of the crease is to evert the edge of an incision adjacent and parallel to it, so facilitating skin closure.

One way of checking the correct site of the skin incision is by the fact that the skin crease of the proximal interphalangeal joint is equidistant from the centre of the finger pulp and the proximal edge of the A1 pulley.

1b

For surgery on the thumb, an assistant holds the hand with the wrist flexed 90° so the surgeon can be face-on to the true volar surface of the digit. The incision is on this surface, just distal to the metacarpophalangeal joint crease. This avoids danger to the radial digital nerve which is very superficial at this point. Care should be taken here to ensure that the incision is through skin only, as both digital nerves are very superficial at this level.

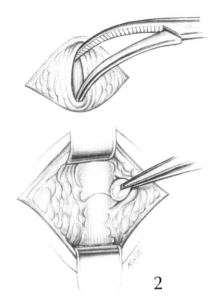

2

Dissection

2

A path is cleared down to the tendon sheath by blunt dissection and the sheath then defined on its volar aspect and the lateral sides.

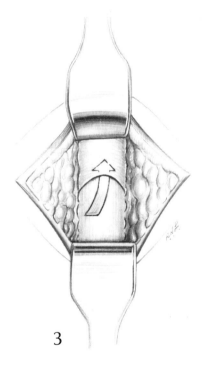

3

3

There is no need formally to dissect the digital nerves and vessels as they lie in a fibrofatty sheath and are pushed away *en bloc* during the dissection. The edge of the tendon sheath, the A1 pulley, will now be visible as a whitish crescentic edge whose position can be confirmed by moving the finger to and fro and seeing that it does not move, unlike the tendons. The position of the edge can be confirmed by introducing the flat edge of a MacDonald dissector between the sheath and the tendon. A local tenosynovitic reaction may be evident.

Release

4

Using a No. 15 blade with the sharp edge always turned *towards* the tendon, a 0.5 cm strip of the pulley is resected. Alternatively, the tendon sheath is divided longitudinally for 1 to 1.5 cm. The running of the flexor tendons is again checked and if the nodule is still snagging on the edge of the pulley a little more tendon pulley can be resected to enlarge the aperture further or the central slit extended by 0.5 cm. Care is taken to ensure that the tendon nodule does not impinge on the intact edge of the pulley when the finger is in full extension at all joints simultaneously, otherwise there is a risk of a contracture developing of the proximal interphalangeal joint.

In the index finger, special care should be taken to ensure that only a minimum of pulley is removed, or else a bow-stringing effect of the long flexor tendons can occur across the palm, rotating the finger into ulnar deviation. On no account should the nodule in the tendon be touched. Surgery is confined to the sheath! The patient is then asked to straighten the finger *fully*, maximally extending all the joints simultaneously, and confirm the free movement of the digit. A local synovectomy may be undertaken and is said to reduce the amount of postoperative tenderness.

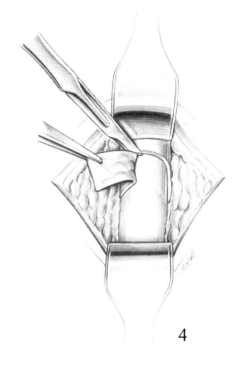

4

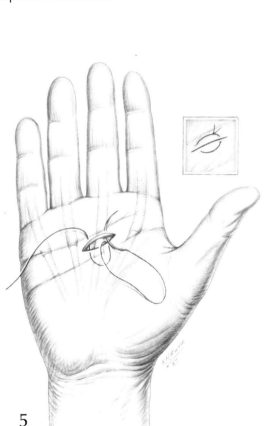

5

Closure

5

The skin is closed with one or two sutures, taking care to evert the wound edges. A single horizontal mattress suture is often all that is required. No subcutaneous sutures are used. An airstrip dressing is applied to the wound followed by an elasticated, gently compressive bandage. The tourniquet is now released and removed completely from the arm and the patient rests with his hand elevated for at least half an hour before going home in a high sling.

Postoperative management

The compressive dressing is removed on the next day by the patient himself. He is instructed to move his finger normally, beginning on the day after the operation, in order to maintain a full range of movements. After 10 days the sutures can be removed and any residual flexion deformity of the proximal interphalangeal joint corrected by dynamic extension splinting.

TRIGGER THUMB IN INFANCY AND CHILDHOOD

In infancy the thumb is usually locked in flexion because the nodule cannot pass into the narrowed sheath. The condition should be distinguished from other conditions presenting as a thumb flexion deformity.

Thirty per cent of cases presenting at birth will recover spontaneously and so operation can be deferred. Twelve per cent of those presenting at 6–24 months will have spontaneous recovery so that operation can be deferred for them also.

Operation should be undertaken if the condition persists until the child is 2 years old or else irreversible contracture of the interphalangeal joint will occur. Those cases presenting over the age of 2 years require immediate surgery.

Details of operative technique are similar to that in adults except that some form of magnification is usually used. General anaesthesia is required. Special care should be taken to avoid cutting the digital nerves to the thumb. Care should be taken to make the initial incision through the skin only and no deeper: the digital nerves should be positively identified.

Acknowledgements

I would like to thank Dr G. Foucher MD, of Strasbourg, France, for his valued instruction and comments.

Reference

1. Ferlic DC, Clayton, ML. Flexor tenosynovectomy in the rheumatoid finger. *J Hand Surg* 1978; 3: 364–7.

Further reading

Clark DD, Ricker JH, MacCallum MS. The efficacy of local steroid injection in the treatment of stenosing tenosynovitis. *Plast Reconstr Surg* 1973; 51: 179–80.

DeHaan MR, Wong LB, Petersen DP. Congenital anomaly of the thumb: aplasia of the flexor pollicis longus. *J Hand Surg* 1982; 12A: 108–9.

Dinham JM, Meggitt BF. Trigger thumb in children: a review of the natural history and indications for treatment in 105 patients. *J Bone Joint Surg [Br]* 1974; 56-B: 153–5.

Fahey JJ, Bollinger JA. Trigger fingers in adults and children. *J Bone Joint Surg [Am]* 1954; 36-A: 1200–18.

Froimson AI. Trigger thumb and fingers. In: Green DP, ed. *Operative hand surgery.* Vol. 2. Edinburgh: Churchill Livingstone 1982: 1510–3.

Uchida M, Kojima T, Sakurai N. Congenital absence of flexor pollicis longus without hypoplasia of thenar muscles. *Plast Reconstr Surg* 1985; 75: 413–6.

Illustrations by Philip Wilson

Operations for congenital dislocation of the hip

A. Catterall MChir, FRCS
Consultant Orthopaedic Surgeon, Royal National Orthopaedic Hospital, Stanmore, UK

Introduction

A decision to operate on a child with congenital dislocation of the hip is not taken in isolation but within the framework of a protocol of management in which the aim of treatment is to produce a congruous concentric reduction of the femoral head within the acetabulum by conservative means if possible.

There are four stages in this protocol:

1. Correction of any soft tissue contracture.
2. Reduction of the femoral head into the acetabulum.
3. Maintenance of the reduction until the hip is stable.
4. Follow-up to assess the subsequent development of the hip joint.

In the management of this protocol it must be emphasized that it is not wise to proceed from one stage to the next without radiological confirmation that the previous stage has been achieved.

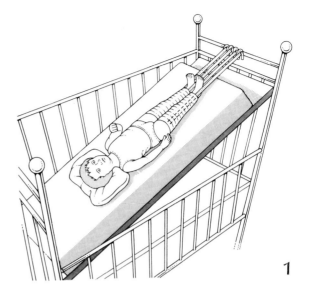

1

1 & 2

In the younger child it is usually possible to overcome the soft tissue contracture by traction of the Pugh's type for a child under the age of 1 year or by using an overhead frame between the ages of 1 and 3 years. Over the age of 3 years the incidence of avascular necrosis increases the risks of conservative treatment and makes open reduction a better option. Where the soft tissue contracture is being corrected by the use of gallows traction, skin traction is applied to the leg and allowed to set for 1 to 2 hours before the legs are suspended by fixed traction to the overhead loop. The legs are progressively abducted over 2 weeks and the child encouraged to move actively within the bed.

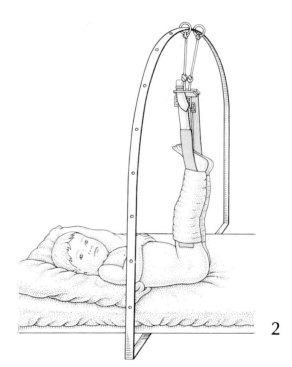

2

3

When approximately 60° of abduction has been obtained on each side, usually at 2 weeks, radiographs are taken to see if the femoral head remains high; if this is confirmed, cross-traction is applied. If during the course of this progressive abduction the adductors become unduly tight, an adductor tenotomy is performed under general anaesthesia (see below).

Once the femoral head has been brought opposite the acetabulum and this has been confirmed radiologically, the hip is examined under anaesthesia. The object of this examination is to decide whether the femoral head will engage the acetabulum, and determine the position in which it is most stable. A plaster is now applied with the leg in this position (usually 90° of flexion, 40°–60° abduction). The knees are allowed free. This plaster is retained for a total of 6 weeks and during this time the child is encouraged to mobilize. This period may be thought of as the 'trial of closed reduction', as reduction of the dislocation is not a sudden incident as it is in traumatic dislocation but an evolving process.

At the end of the 'trial of reduction' the child is readmitted and again examined under anaesthesia. If the hip is now stable and the radiographs show a concentric reduction then the trial is regarded as successful and the conservative treatment in plaster continued for a further 6 months. If there is doubt about the congruity of the hip joint an arthrogram is performed.

On occasions the adductors remain very tight and unyielding after 2 weeks of traction. In these circumstances a subcutaneous tenotomy may allow conservative treatment to continue.

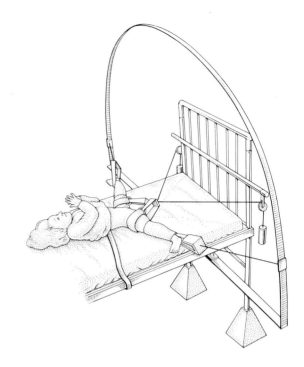

3

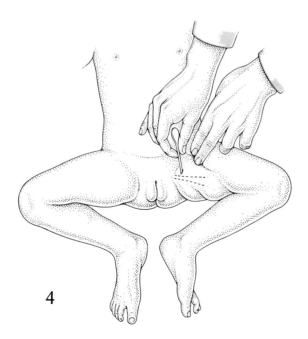

4

CLOSED ADDUCTOR TENOTOMY

4

This operation is performed under general anaesthesia with the child temporarily removed from the frame but with the traction maintained in position. The legs are placed with the hip in 90° of flexion and in abduction without undue tension. The tendon of the adductor longus is palpated and its attachment to the tibial pubic tubercle identified. The femoral artery is now palpated and a finger placed medial to this to protect the femoral vein. A tenotome is now inserted percutaneously 1 cm from the attachment of the adductor longus and medial to the finger protecting the femoral vein. The tendon is divided. A full release of all the adductors is not performed as this may produce unnecessary bleeding.

OPEN REDUCTION

Indications

Within this protocol of management the indications for open reduction of the hip are relatively simple.

1. Failure to correct the soft tissue contracture.
2. Failure of the hip to engage at the time of the examination under anaesthetic.
3. Failure of the 'trial of reduction' to produce a concentric reduction.
4. A child over the age of 3 years at presentation. There is an increased risk of avascular necrosis in these children.

Position of patient

For open reduction, Pemberton acetabuloplasty or the lateral shelf acetabuloplasty the patient is placed on the operating table with the affected hip and buttock supported on a sandbag so that a half-lateral position is achieved.

Incision

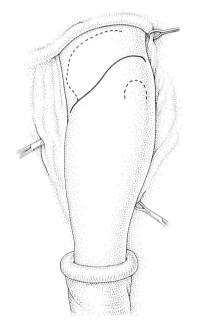

5

5

The same incision and approach is used for all operations on the hip joint. Whereas in the younger child the iliac apophysis is split in order to obtain access to both sides of the wing of the ilium, in the adult the muscles are detached from the iliac crest for the same purpose.

The incision is made half-way between the greater trochanter and the iliac crest, parallel to the iliac crest and curved downwards at its distal medial end. It is deepened through the superficial fascia and the bleeding controlled. The proximal flap is now retracted over the iliac crest and the remaining fat and fascia incised in the line of the iliac crest.

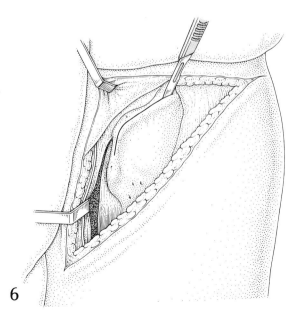

6

Fascia lata and iliac crest

6

The interval between the sartorius and the tensor fasciae latae is identified by a dense white area starting from the anterior superior iliac spine. As this is incised care must be taken to identify and preserve the lateral cutaneous nerve of the thigh on the medial side of the incision. The interval is deepened and extended up to the anterior superior iliac spine. Small bleeding vessels from the transverse circumflex iliac vessels must be controlled. The iliac apophysis is now split in the line of the crest and detached from it. The bulbous end of this apophysis passes deeply downwards towards the anterior inferior iliac spine. The apophysis will not detach from the bone until this bulb has been divided. The wing of the ilium is now exposed subperiosteally.

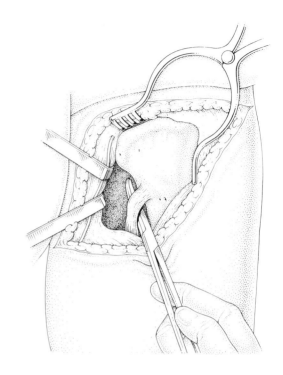

7

Detachment of the rectus femoris and dissection of the psoas

7 & 8

The rectus femoris is now identified and its straight and reflected head dissected from the underlying capsule. The straight head is divided at its attachment at the anterior inferior iliac spine and the reflected head from its distal attachment of the capsule. There is always bleeding from the superior gluteal artery at this point and this must be controlled. The rectus femoris is turned down distally and held with a stay suture. The psoas muscle covering the medial capsule is identified and dissected down to its attachment at the lesser trochanter. As the dissection proceeds medially the tendon of the psoas will be demonstrated and it is detached as near to the lesser trochanter as possible. This is facilitated by flexing and laterally rotating the leg.

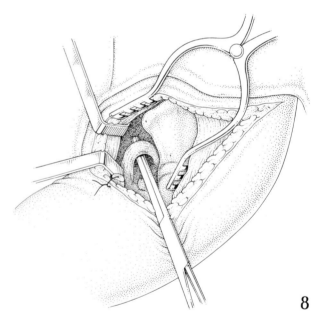

8

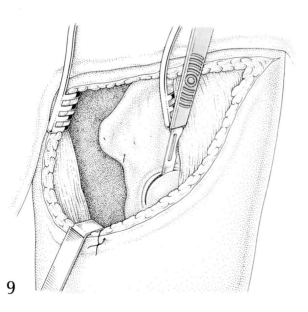

9

Dissection and incision of the capsule

9

The remaining portions of the capsule are now dissected cleanly superiorly, inferiorly and laterally so that the true and false acetabula are identified. The capsule is now opened by an incision parallel to its capsular attachment to the pubes and 1 cm distal to it.

Assessment of stability

When the capsule is opened the hip joint is inspected and this is facilitated by extending the capsular incision medially towards the transverse ligament and laterally by a vertical incision in the false capsule. The possible intracapsular obstructions to reduction are:

1. The ligamentum teres.
2. The inturned acetabular labrum or limbus.
3. The capsule.
4. The transverse ligament of the acetabulum.
5. Fatty tissues on the medial wall of the acetabulum or pulvina.
6. The shape of the acetabulum.

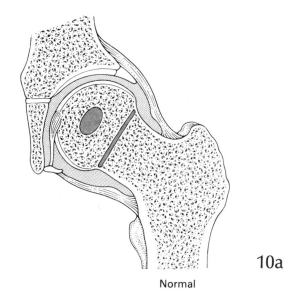

10a

Normal

10a, b & c

In true congenital dislocation the shape of the acetabulum is relatively normal with the labrum inverted, while in acetabular dysplasia with subluxation the anterolateral aspect is deformed and the labrum everted producing the double-diameter acetabulum. In the older child and those with a neurological defect this may be an indication for a Pemberton acetabuloplasty.

All these structures must be inspected. If possible the lateral acetabular labrum should be preserved as it represents the lateral growing point of the acetabulum margin. Its obstructing value to reduction may be overcome by full release of the inferior capsule and division of the transverse ligament which converts the cavity of the acetabulum from a cone to a cup-shape.

The open reduction may be considered adequate when on returning the femoral head to the acetabulum it appears fully contained or covered and is stable to axial pressure with the leg in flexion, abduction and medial rotation. If this degree of stability cannot be achieved an acetabuloplasty of the Pemberton type is required.

On occasions the soft tissues are excessively tight on attempted reduction of the femoral head. Forced reduction at this stage will result in avascular necrosis of the femoral head. This may be prevented by shortening the femur by 1–2 cm. The operation should be performed through a separate incision (see femoral osteotomy p. 884).

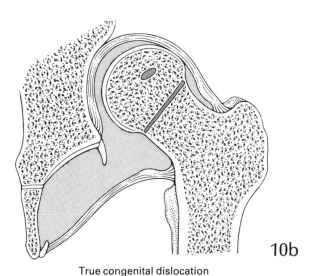

10b

True congenital dislocation

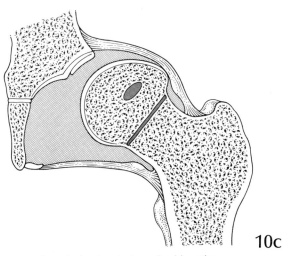

10c

Acetabular dysplasia and subluxation

Test of stability

11a, b & c

The stability of the joint to axial loading is now assessed in (a) flexion, abduction and medial rotation; (b) abduction and medial rotation; and (c) medial rotation alone. If flexion is required for stability, an innominate osteotomy is indicated and may be performed at the same time as the open reduction (*see* chapter on 'Innominate osteotomy' pp. 893–899). Where abduction and medial rotation alone are required the realignment is more conveniently obtained by a femoral osteotomy which will also correct the persisting femoral anteversion. This is best under-taken at a later stage because of the risk of avascular necrosis.

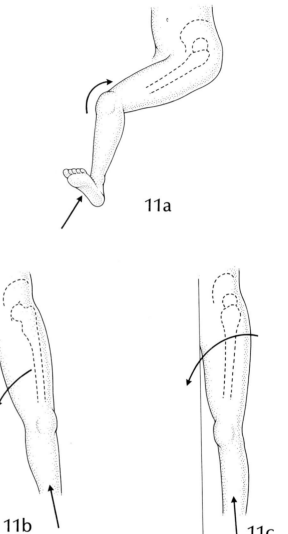

11a

11b

11c

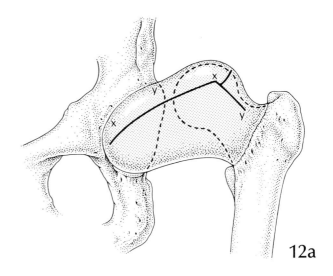

12a

Reduction of the femoral head and repair of the capsule

12a & b

The vertical incision made in the capsule of the false acetabulum is now extended down to the base of the femoral neck at its superior point. This creates a flap of anterior capsule which may be advanced medially providing good cover for the femoral head as it is reduced and also a factor preventing redislocation. In repairing the capsule three sutures are usually used. The first is placed from the region of the anterior inferior iliac spine and passes to the base of the flap at the lateral border of the femoral neck. The remaining two sutures are placed in the capsule medial to this and what was previously the anterior capsule is plicated over them. The leg is placed in the position of maximal stability while this repair is being performed. The rectus femoris is reattached to the anterior inferior iliac spine. If after the repair of the capsule there is no lateral rotation of the hip, a realignment osteotomy of the femur will be required. This is ideally performed 2 weeks after operation.

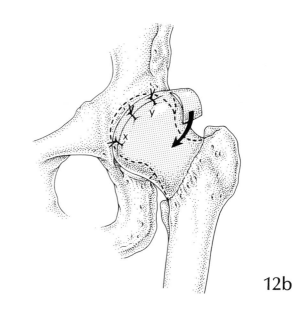

12b

Closure

13

Once the capsule has been repaired and the rectus femoris reattached, the iliac apophysis is then repaired with three sutures. The incision in the fascia lata is closed. The subcutaneous tissues and skin are closed. Where possible a subcuticular stitch should be used as this produces a neater scar than interrupted sutures.

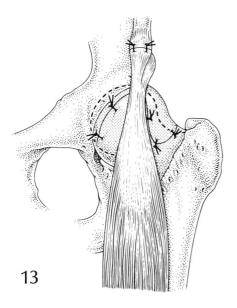

13

THE PEMBERTON ACETABULOPLASTY

The object of this procedure is to improve the stability of the femoral head at the time of open reduction when it can be shown that the anterosuperior part of the acetabulum is deficient, and there is a 'double-diameter acetabulum'. The acetabular labrum is usually found everted and adherent to this portion of the acetabulum. These circumstances are found in acetabular dysplasia with subluxation, either primary or secondary to previous surgery or neurological disease such as cerebral palsy. The hip is approached as for an open reduction.

Technique

14a, b & c

Once the need for acetabuloplasty has been demonstrated the extent of the hip capsule is identified, particularly posteriorly, so that the bony section can be made parallel to the acetabular margin. An osteotomy is performed approximately 0.5–1 cm above the capsular attachment. The osteotomy is made under radiological control, directing the line towards the triradiate cartilage. When the osteotome is just short of the triradiate cartilage the acetabular roof is displaced downwards and laterally, restoring the normal contour of the acetabulum. The position is checked radiographically. Once a satisfactory displacement has been obtained, two triangular bone grafts from the iliac crest are inserted into the defect. They do not usually require fixation and are stable once inserted.

Test of stability

The same tests of stability as were previously applied during the process of open reduction are now repeated to check that the femoral head is stable within the new acetabulum and that realignment procedures such as a femoral osteotomy are not required (see p. 884).

Capsular repair and closure

These are the same as for open reduction.

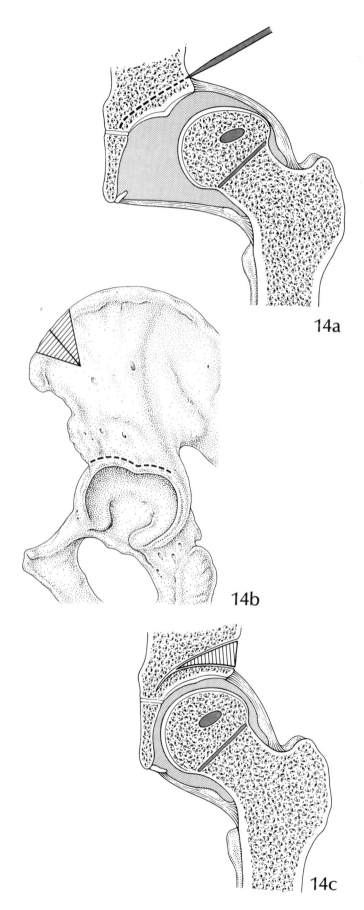

14a

14b

14c

PELVIC OSTEOTOMY

Indications

The operations to be described here are the Chiari and lateral shelf acetabuloplasty, which have similar indications. (The technique of innominate osteotomy is described separately on pp. 893–899.) These two operations are used where there is evidence of disproportion between the femoral head and acetabulum with uncovering of the anterolateral segment of the femoral head. This may be observed in the following clinical situations.

1. Primary acetabular dysplasia with fixed subluxation over the age of 7 years.
2. Following primary treatment of congenital dislocation, either by conservative or operative methods, in which a concentric congruous reduction has not been maintained and a fixed subluxation with anterolateral uncovering of the femoral head has occurred.
3. In cases of Perthes' disease presenting over the age of 9 years, with disease in the early stages. Femoral osteotomy is often associated with residual shortening; lateral shelf acetabuloplasty will reduce the forces through the hip joint by enlarging the acetabular surface and prevent further subluxation from occurring. Where there is marked uncovering late in the disease process, Chiari osteotomy may be required as part of a reconstructive procedure.
4. In conditions producing avascular necrosis of the femoral head where flattening and overgrowth of the anterolateral segment has produced uncovering. Clinically, this uncovering can be felt as 'the lump sign'. Here the Chiari procedure, possibly associated with realignment femoral osteotomy, may be indicated for persisting symptoms.

The lateral shelf acetabuloplasty is a simpler procedure but cannot be expected to produce the same degree of lateral cover as the Chiari. In addition, where there has been a lateral displacement of the femoral head away from the midline, the advantage of the Chiari operation with its medial displacement is to bring the femoral head back into a more normal load-bearing position. The ideal indication for the lateral shelf, therefore, is an unstable lateral acetabular segment with moderate uncovering of the femoral head, or as an augmentation to the lateral segment of the femoral head at the time of the Chiari procedure. Where possible the Chiari operation should be reserved for the adolescent or older patient in view of the possible damage to the lateral acetabular epiphysis.

CHIARI OPERATION

Position of the patient

The patient should be lying flat either on a Hawley table or on a radio-translucent table so that an image intensifier may be used.

Approach

This is similar to the approach for congenital dislocation of the hip but in the older patient, where the iliac apophysis is fused, the muscles need to be detached from the iliac crest. Gluteus medius and minimus are detached posteriorly from the wing of the ilium all the way back to the sacroiliac notch so that the level of the osteotomy posteriorly may be easily identified.

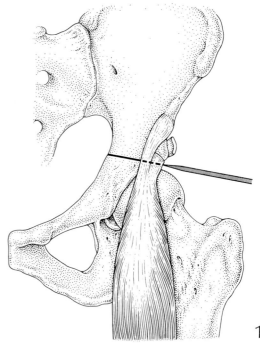

15a

Dissection of the rectus femoris

15a & b

The rectus femoris is identified and the lateral margin dissected proximally in order to demonstrate the straight and reflected heads. The reflected head is dissected from the underlying capsule and detached medially from the point where it is attaching to the straight head.

Determination of the osteotomy level

The anterolateral uncovering of the femoral head (the lump sign) is noted, as it is this portion of the femoral head which must be covered by acetabular displacement. A 2 cm osteotome is inserted in the bone at the superior margin of the capsule to determine the level of the osteotomy. This is checked radiologically and the osteotome repositioned if necessary so that it is exactly at the superior and lateral point of the acetabulum. A careful dome-shaped osteotomy is performed. It is sometimes necessary to use a Gigli saw to complete its posterior part.

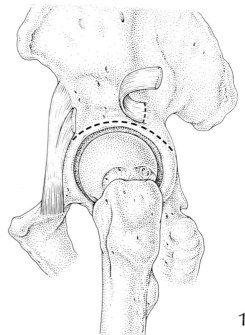

15b

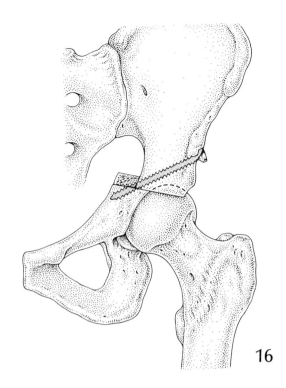

Displacement

16

It is the objective of the operation to produce cover of the anterolateral portion of the femoral head. The acetabular displacement is therefore medial and posterior. This is made easier by abducting the leg. The displacement is checked visually, by palpation, and image intensifier. If necessary the cover may be increased by the addition of a cancellous bone graft placed laterally.

16

Fixation

A drill is inserted from above the osteotomy through the wing of the ilium into the cut surface of the lower fragment and checked radiologically. A cortical screw of suitable length is inserted.

The wound is closed in layers using strong sutures to reattach the tensor fasciae latae, and gluteus medius. Suction drainage is always required.

Postoperative management

The patient is nursed in bed for 2 weeks while the wound is healing on 'slings and springs'. Slings under the thigh and calf are suspended from springs and hold the hip at approximately 40° of flexion. Active extension and flexion exercises commence on the day after operation. Once the wound is healed the patient is mobilized on crutches, bearing no weight for 10 weeks.

LATERAL SHELF ACETABULOPLASTY

Position of patient

The same position is used as for the Chiari procedure.

Approach

This is similar to the Chiari procedure but the posterior mobilization of gluteus medius and minimus is not quite so extensive as it is not necessary to reach the sacroiliac notch.

Dissection of the rectus femoris

This is similar to the Chiari procedure except that the rectus femoris is detached from the straight head and reflected posteriorly, separating it from its capsular attachment to the extent that is necessary to enable the bone graft to be applied to the capsule. It is carefully preserved as it will have to be reattached.

Identification of the lateral margin of the acetabulum

17

The capsule attachment to the lateral margin of the acetabulum is carefully identified, if necessary with the use of an image intensifier. Drill holes are made in the ilium directly above the acetabulum and directed parallel to the line of the capsule. An osteotome is then used to cut a slot on the superior margin of the acetabulum without deforming this margin; into this slot bone graft will subsequently be inserted. An osteotomy is now performed in a 'U'-shaped fashion on the outer table of the iliac bone directly above the hip joint and the flap created is hinged laterally on its proximal point. Care must be taken not to fracture this attachment. (N.B. If this fragment fractures and becomes unstable it is removed, the operation continued, and then the fragment is reattached with a single screw to hold the subsequent bone graft in position.) Bone graft is now obtained in corticocancellous slivers from the lateral table of the ilium and as much cancellous bone as possible obtained for use as a bone graft.

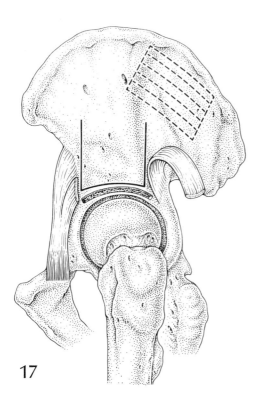

17

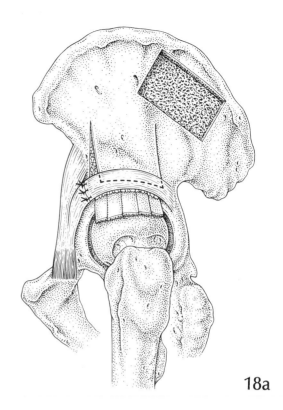

18a

Bone graft

18a & b

Strips of corticocancellous bone are now inserted into the slot that has been cut in the ilium, are contoured to the capsule to which they are applied, and brought laterally to produce the cover required. They are trimmed at this point. The position of these grafts and the extent of the cover produced is checked by image intensifier. The remaining portions of bone are applied into the gap between the everted section of the lateral table of the ilium and the bone graft that has already been applied; this bone will be held in position by the rectus femoris.

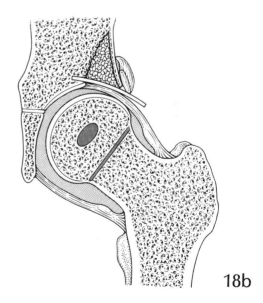

18b

Reattachment of rectus femoris

The rectus femoris is reattached to the straight head. As it is reattached the slightly unstable bone graft placed laterally over the femoral head will be stabilized into position and this stability can be further increased by accurately reapplying the anterior margin of gluteus minimus and suturing it, partly to the straight head of the rectus femoris and partly to the anterior inferior iliac spine.

Closure

The wound is closed in layers using strong sutures to reattach the tensor fasciae latae, and gluteus medius. Suction drainage is usually applied.

Postoperative management

A one-and-a-half hip spica is applied postoperatively and retained for a total period of 6 weeks to allow revascularization and incorporation of the bone graft. Then the plaster is removed and active mobilization started, initially with the use of crutches for a period of 6 weeks to allow consolidation of the graft. Once this has been confirmed radiographically, active free mobilization is encouraged.

FEMORAL OSTEOTOMY

Upper femoral osteotomy has been performed over many years for the correction of residual deformities of the proximal femur and also in an attempt to stabilize the hip after operative procedures on the joint. Previously it had been thought that the operation itself would reduce a hip but it is now recognized that it is largely a realignment procedure for a position that has already been achieved by open reduction of the joint or other procedures.

Indications

Femoral osteotomy is indicated for a number of different conditions and circumstances. These indications may be considered under a number of headings.

1. A correction of pre-existing deformity: coxa vara, coxa valga, or persistent anteversion of the femoral neck.
2. At the time of open reduction for a congenital dislocation of the hip where soft tissue tightness prevents easy reduction of the femoral head (see p. 875).
3. Realignment to stabilize a known position of the hip (a) after open reduction of congenital dislocation; (b) after containment of the femoral head in abduction in Perthes' disease or late in the disease process where hinge abduction is present to reverse the process of hinging; (c) after correction of acetabular dysplasia where adequate realignment cannot be obtained as the result of innominate osteotomy.

Technical considerations

After union of the osteotomy there will be considerable remodelling of the upper femur in response to the new position. As the result of this there is a tendency of varus position of the femoral neck to remodel into valgus, particularly when the operation has been performed under the age of 4 years. In view of this overcorrection into valgus, additional varus should be always added to a position of realignment in the young child. By contrast, in the child over 8 years the potential for remodelling is reduced and a normal neck–shaft angle of approximately 130° should be created at the time of operation.

In positioning the femoral shaft under the upper fragment it must be remembered that varus osteotomy displaces the greater trochanter laterally and the distal shaft must, therefore, be placed medially to restore Shenton's line of the neck; and when a valgus osteotomy is being performed, the shaft must be placed laterally.

Types of fixation

Where the femoral osteotomy is being performed as part of an operative procedure for which a hip spica will be required postoperatively, it is convenient to use a four-hole plate positioned anteriorly to stabilize the osteotomy and use an opening wedge technique. When, however, extension or flexion are required in addition to varus and rotation or if no plaster spica is to be used, a more secure method of fixation is required and a nail-plate, commonly 'Coventry' type, will allow early mobilization.

Operations

For all the operations to be described in this section a standard approach to the upper femur is used.

Position

The patient lies flat on his back so that the leg can be placed in the position from which realignment is to be made; no sandbag is used.

Incision

19

The incision is made obliquely forward from the posterior margin of the greater trochanter. It allows the fascia lata to be incised posteriorly to the tensor and avoids the bleeding associated with incision into this muscle.

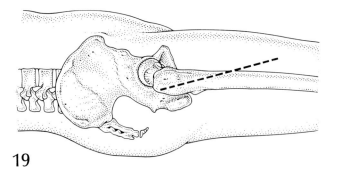

19

Division of muscle

20

The fascia lata is split in the line of its fibres and separated by a self-retaining retractor. The tissue of the trochanteric bursa is incised in the mid-lateral point and reflected forwards to reveal the attachment of gluteus medius and the vastus lateralis. The lowest fibres of gluteus medius are incised to identify the attachment of vastus lateralis.

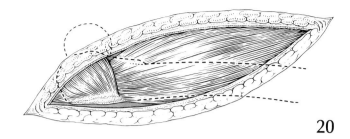

20

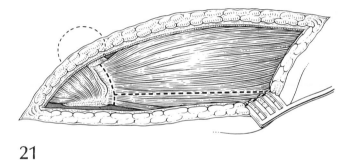

21

21

The vastus lateralis is incised parallel to its attachment on the inter-trochanteric line and a few millimetres distal to it. A longitudinal incision is made in the line of its fibres as posteriorly as possible. Both incisions divide the periosteum so that a clean edge is produced.

22

The femur is now exposed subperiosteally, elevating the vastus lateralis medially. Four Trethowan spikes are inserted, the most proximal of which should be placed at the junction of the femoral neck and shaft so that the medial border of the femoral neck may be identified. The anteversion of the femoral neck is now noted.

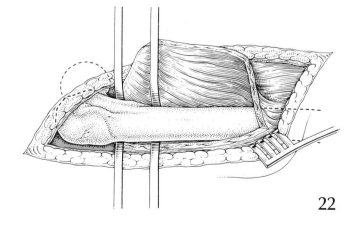

22

OSTEOTOMY USING A FOUR-HOLE PLATE

23

The leg is positioned so that the femoral head is in the desired position in relation to the hip joint and a small guide wire is inserted through the flat lateral cortex of the upper femur below the trochanteric growth-plate. The guide wire runs parallel to the inferior margin of the neck; and with the leg in the desired position for realignment, the guide wire is parallel to the floor. (At the end of the realignment osteotomy the guide wire in the upper fragment will still be in this position, but the distal femur and leg will be parallel to the opposite one and the patella will be pointing upwards.)

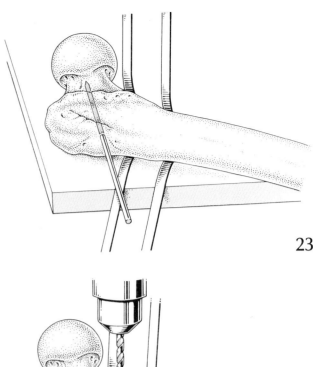

23

24

A drill hole of suitable size to accept the screw used to secure the osteotomy is now drilled in the anterior shaft just above the proposed line of osteotomy. This will be the second hole of the four-hole plate and is drilled at right angles to the floor and tapped if necessary.

The bone is now divided transversely to the axis of the shaft just below the screw hole previously made, and the periosteum is elevated from the medial and posterior surfaces of the distal fragment to allow rotatory alignment.

An osteotome is now inserted between the cut surfaces to act as a skid between the upper and lower fragments, and the leg now brought to the neutral position with the patella pointing upwards. The distal shaft is displaced slightly medially on the upper shaft to allow for the lateral displacement of the trochanter. When valgus osteotomy is performed, lateral displacement of the distal shaft is necessary.

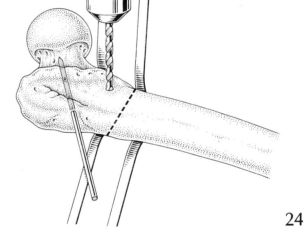

24

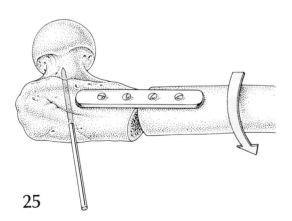

25

25

Once the desired position of the bones have been achieved, a four-hole plate is inserted by securing the second screw on the plate to the hole that has been drilled on the proximal fragment. The two holes on the distal fragment are now made with the drill at right angles to the floor and with the knee in the neutral position. Suitable screws are inserted.

The rotational element of the osteotomy is now fixed but the valgus/varus osteotomy may be altered by levelling the Steinmann pin and checking that the knee is in the neutral position. The top screw hole is now drilled and the screw inserted. The Steinmann pin is removed.

Closure

The vastus lateralis is reattached with a purse-string suture at the point of incision into the muscle. The fascia lata and subcutaneous tissues are closed in layers and a subcuticular polypropylene suture inserted into the skin.

COVENTRY SCREW AND PLATE FIXATION

26

A Kirschner wire is inserted through the same point as the Steinmann pin and passed up the femoral neck. Its length is measured.

The cortex is reemed and a screw of appropriate length inserted and tightened into position. The Kirschner wire is removed.

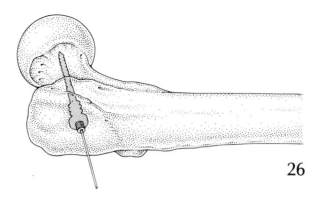

26

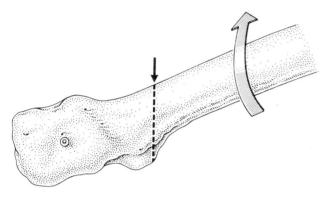

27

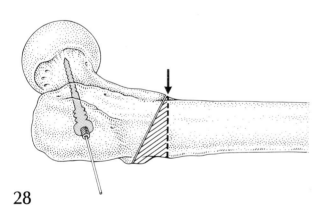

28

Osteotomy

27 & 28

In any femoral osteotomy whose aim is to realign the leg to a known position of the femoral head, an osteotomy of the femur is made with the leg held in the position from which realignment is required. Then the saw cut is made at right angles to the patient and vertical to the floor. This osteotomy is made at the level of the lesser trochanter and should not be complete. The leg is now turned to the neutral position and a second osteotomy performed at right angles to the distal shaft; this will result in a wedge of precisely the correct amount. Both osteotomies are now completed and the wedge of bone removed. Due to the plain surface of the distal fragment, any rotational correction is easily performed by bringing the patella to the neutral midline position.

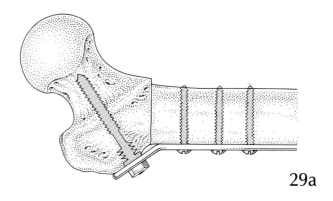

29a

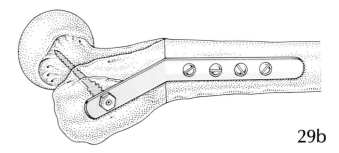

29b

29a & b

Once the necessary position has been obtained the Coventry plate is bent to fit and secured to the upper fragment by a nut and to the lower fragment with screws.
    The wound is closed in layers.

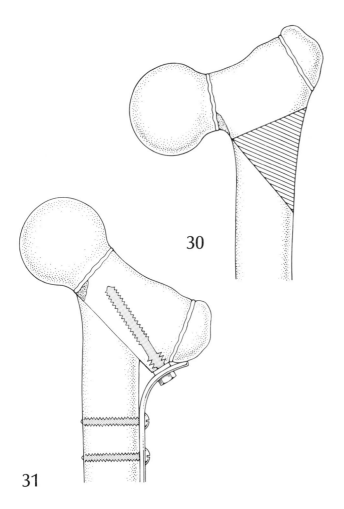

30

31

FEMORAL OSTEOTOMY FOR COXA VARA

30 & 31

For this condition the displacement described by Pauwels is used. The wedge to be removed is usually between 60° and 90°. The proximal level of osteotomy must reach the base of this femoral neck. The distal osteotomy is oblique to the shaft, in the line of the femoral neck. This produces a long line of osteotomy distally and allows the medial spike to be displaced under the medial fragment of the metaphysis. Fixation is usually by a Coventry screw-plate fixation.

The use of this operation in other conditions will be found in the chapter on 'High femoral osteotomy in childhood' (see pp. 900–908).

THE COLONNA OPERATION

This operation, which was initially described by Hey Groves[1] and subsequently reported in detail by Colonna[2] and Trevor[3], is a capsular arthroplasty and should always, therefore, be looked upon as a salvage procedure.

Indications

The indications for this operation have always been few and limited to the management of the older child with the high dislocation, particularly following previous surgery. With the advent of the new techniques of open reduction with femoral shortening the indications for the capsular arthroplasty are few; primary dislocation in the older child may now be treated by open reduction whereas previously it was treated by a Colonna operation. It is now possible to obtain a concentric reduction without undue pressure and the consequent risk of avascular necrosis.

There are at present two good indications for the Colonna operation.

1. Patients over the age of 8 years with a primary dislocation of the hip or dislocation secondary to acetabular dysplasia where there is gross deficiency of the acetabulum, particularly in its anterolateral segment. These cases are unsuitable for open reduction with femoral shortening.
2. Patients over the age of 7 years with residual dislocation following surgery, where both acetabulum and femoral head are abnormal and a concentric reduction is therefore impossible to obtain.

It should be, however, stressed that this operation is not for the surgeon performing occasional surgery on the child's hip joint.

Anaesthesia and position

The operation is performed under general anaesthesia with an intravenous infusion running, as blood loss may be great during this procedure. The patient is positioned in the full lateral position with the dislocated hip upwards.

The incision

32

The operation is most easily performed through a curved transverse incision. This starts at the anterior superior iliac spine and passes obliquely down to cross the femur approximately 3–4 cm below the tip of the greater trochanter and then passes upwards and backwards in the line of the fibres of gluteus maximus. The superficial fascia and the fascia lata are divided transversely at the level of the incision. The gluteus maximus is split in the line of its fibres.

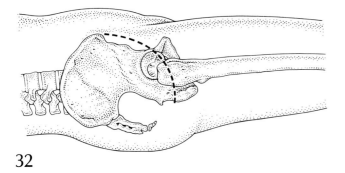

32

Dissection of muscle and capsule

33

The interval between the gluteus medius and the tensor fasciae latae is identified and dissected. At the femoral attachment the anterior fibres covering the attachment of the vastus lateralis are released and posteriorly the piriformis is identified. The greater trochanter is detached using an osteotome, dividing through the epiphysis not the growth-plate. Gluteus medius with its bony attachment is then mobilized and retracted proximally.

The gluteus minimus is now identified and dissected from the capsule so that the latter is now visible anteriorly, superiorly and posteriorly. The object of this part of the dissection is to obtain sufficient capsule to cover the entire femoral head completely. The deficiency is usually on the superior medial aspect of the femoral head; and here, as the capsule is mobilized from the edge of the acetabulum, sharp scissors are used to detach the capsule with the underlying articular cartilage. The remainder of the capsule is then freed from its acetabular attachments, the most difficult aspect of this problem being the posterior inferior aspect of the mobilization.

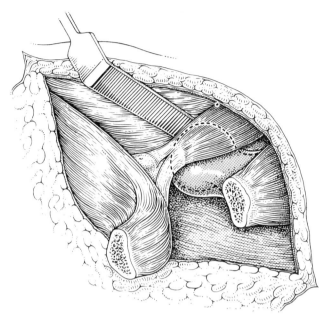

33

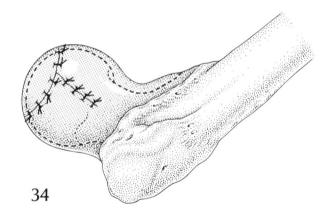

34

34

The cut surfaces of the capsule are now sutured over the femoral head so that it is covered completely.

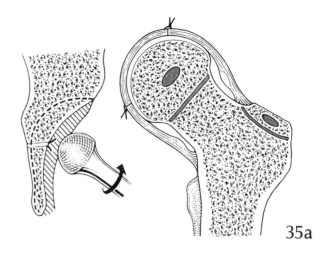

35a

Reaming of the acetabulum

35a & b

To obtain a good view of the acetabulum the leg is flexed to 90°, adducted and laterally rotated. By the use of curved gouges and small reamers the acetabulum is enlarged. As this enlargement commences the level of the acetabulum may be judged by noting the presence of the triradiate cartilage which should lie in the centre of the floor of the new acetabulum.

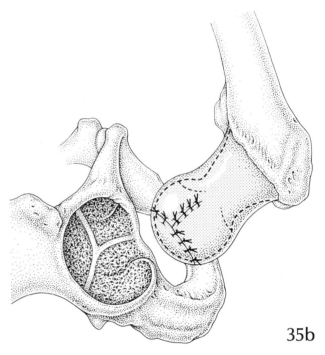

35b

36

When an adequate size of the new acetabulum has been obtained the femoral head, covered by its capsule, is reduced into it and the position of maximum stability assessed. In the majority of cases stability of the femoral head in the neutral position is present but on occasions abduction and medial rotation are required to compensate for persisting anteversion and valgus in the femoral neck. If this is present, a subsequent realignment femoral osteotomy is indicated. The ideal timing for this is 2 weeks later. The capsular repair is then reinspected to be sure that the stitches remain intact and that the femoral head covered by its capsule is placed in the acetabulum.

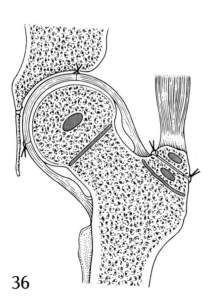

36

Reattachment of greater trochanter

Holding the femoral head reduced in the position of maximum stability the greater trochanter is reattached with sutures to the upper shaft in its anatomical position.

Closure

The fascia lata is closed with particular attention to good sutures in the midline. The subcutaneous tissues and skin are closed in the usual way. A one-and-a-half hip spica is applied.

Postoperative management

Routine postoperative management is undertaken. In many of these children blood loss has been excessive and a careful check must be made to be sure that they do not become anaemic. Where a femoral osteotomy is indicated this is performed at 2 weeks after the Colonna operation.

The plaster is removed at 4 weeks and mobilization is started, initially on traction and subsequently with the use of a hydrotherapy pool. When the patient has obtained greater than 60° of flexion and 15° of abduction he may be mobilized on crutches without bearing weight. It is important for good long-term function[4] that the child should remain without weight-bearing for a period of 6 months. In many cases a raise will be required for the opposite shoe. Provided the radiographs are satisfactory at 6 months and show no evidence of avascular necrosis, progressive weight-bearing may be encouraged. Abductor exercises may be required at this stage.

References

1. Hey Groves EW. Reconstructive surgery of the hip. *Br J Surg* 1927; 14: 486–517.

2. Colonna PC. Capsular arthroplasty for congenital dislocation of the hip: indications and technique: some long-term results. *J Bone Joint Surg [Am]* 1965; 47-A: 437–49.

3. Trevor D. The place of the Hey Groves–Colonna operation in the treatment of congenital dislocation of the hip. *Ann R Coll Surg Engl* 1968; 43: 241–58.

4. Pozo JL, Cannon SR, Catterall A. The Colonna–Hey Groves arthroplasty in the late treatment of congenital dislocation of the hip: a long-term review. *J Bone Joint Surg [Br]* 1987; 69-B: 220–8.

Acknowledgement

Illustrations 2 and 3 are drawn after G. Lyth, and 5–9 and 11 after A. Barrett.

Illustrations by Philip Wilson

Innominate osteotomy

A. Catterall   MChir, FRCS
Consultant Orthopaedic Surgeon, Charing Cross Hospital, London, and Royal National Orthopaedic Hospital, Stanmore, UK

Introduction

Indications

1. *During open reduction for congenital dislocation of the hip*   Open reduction is indicated in the management of congenital dislocation of the hip when either the femoral head cannot be brought opposite the acetabulum by traction or when a concentric congruous reduction cannot be obtained by conservative means. At the time of open reduction a unique opportunity exists to assess the stability of the hip joint to axial load. Innominate osteotomy is indicated where a position of hip flexion is required to maintain the stability of the hip joint (*see* test of stability in the chapter on 'Congenital dislocation of the hip', p. 876).

2. *In acetabular dysplasia with subluxation, when acetabular realignment is indicated*   Innominate osteotomy is indicated as a realignment procedure where arthrography has established a reducible subluxation, with flexion required for stability of the hip joint.

3. *In selected cases of Perthes' disease.*

Contraindications

Before an innominate osteotomy is performed the following requirements or prerequisites must be established.

1. A concentric position must be present between the femoral head and acetabulum.
2. There must be a free range of movement in the hip.
3. There should be no fixed deformity in the hip joint.

The operation is therefore contraindicated in the absence of concentricity or in the presence of fixed deformity or restricted movement.

Special requirements

The following equipment will be needed.

   A Gigli saw
   Two long periosteal elevators
   Two deep retractors
   O'Shaughnessy forceps
   One pair of bone cutters
   Two pairs of large towel clips

Operation

When the procedure is being performed as part of an open reduction, access to the hip joint will have already been obtained prior to the innominate osteotomy. Where the operation is performed without other procedures the following procedure is appropriate.

Position of patient

1

The operation is performed under general anaesthesia. The patient is placed with the operation side uppermost in the half-lateral position. A sandbag is placed under the buttock on the operation side.

Incision

The incision is made half-way between the greater trochanter and iliac crest, parallel to the iliac crest and curved downwards at its medial end. It is deepened through the superficial fascia, and the bleeding is controlled. The proximal flap is now retracted over the iliac crest and the remaining fat and fascia incised in the line of the iliac crest. The medial end of the distal flap is freed from the fascia lata.

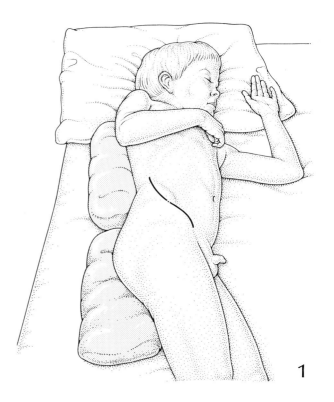

1

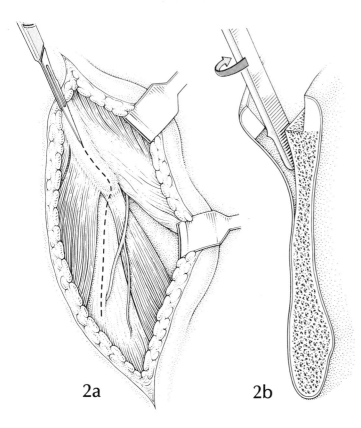

2a   2b

The fascia lata and iliac crest

2a & b

The interval between the sartorius and tensor fasciae latae is identified by a dense white area starting from the anterior superior iliac spine. This is incised and care must be taken to identify and preserve the lateral cutaneous nerve of the thigh. This is retracted medially. The interval is deepened and extended up to the anterior superior spine and the bleeding in the area controlled. The iliac apophysis is now split in the line of the crest and detached from it. The bulbous end of the apophysis passes down deeply towards the anterior inferior iliac spine. The apophysis will not detach from the bone until this has been completely divided. Some prefer to separate the whole apophysis to avoid the possibility of growth disturbance. In the adult, the muscles are detached from the iliac crest. The wing of the ilium is now exposed subperiosteally as far back as the sciatic notch.

Release of the capsule

3

Gluteus minimus is elevated from the capsule so that the attachments of the capsule, particularly posteriorly, can be identified. This allows the level of the osteotomy to be identified.

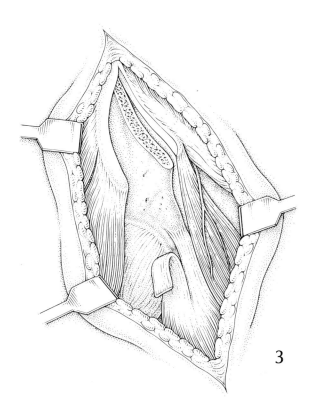

3

4

Release of the tendon of the psoas

4

The elevated periosteum from the medial side of the ilium is now incised to allow mobilization of the psoas muscle. Once the muscle has been mobilized a finger is passed under its deep surface and the tendon of the psoas identified by extending and medially rotating the hip. The hip is now flexed and a retractor placed under the deep surface. The tendon which lies in the substance of the muscle is now divided leaving the remainder of the muscle intact. Care must be taken not to damage the femoral nerve which is in a direct anterior and medial position to the psoas. When the hip is now brought into full extension no tightness can be felt in the deep surface of the muscle.

The stability of the joint to axial loading is now assessed. As the hip is flexed and abducted the prominence or lump of the anterolateral aspect of the femoral head can be felt to reduce into the acetabulum confirming that a reducible subluxation is present.

Dissection of the sciatic notch and passage of Gigli saw

5a, b & c

The sciatic notch is approached subperiosteally from the medial and lateral aspects. On the lateral side it may be visualized. A clean dissection is obtained by advancing the long periosteal dissector and then rotating it through 90°. The point of the O'Shaughnessy forceps is now passed from medial to lateral through the sciatic notch and then opened to receive the end of a Gigli saw. Care must be taken to ensure that there is no soft tissue between the forceps and the bone as the Gigli saw is passed through the sciatic notch.

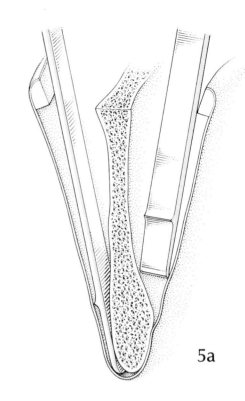

5a

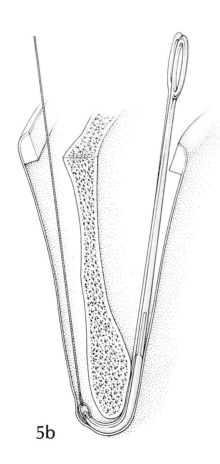

5b

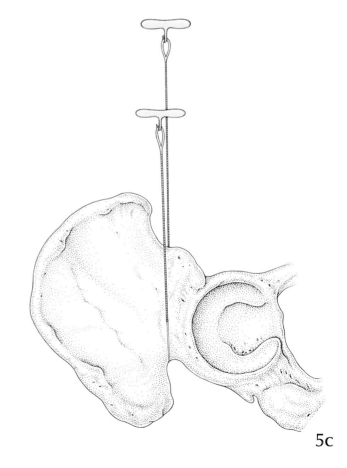

5c

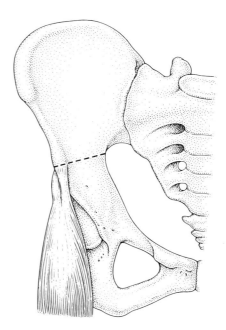

6a

Osteotomy

6a & b

The pelvis is now divided in a line from the sciatic notch to the anterior inferior iliac spine.

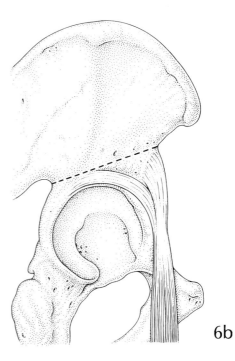

6b

Displacement

7a, b & c

The object of the realignment is to produce an anterolateral buttress to prevent further subluxation or uncovering of the femoral head. This is achieved by rotating the acetabular fragment forward and laterally with the centre of the rotation at the posterior margin of the sciatic notch (arrowed in the illustration) and the symphysis pubis. The graft to fill the defect produced by the displacement is obtained from the iliac crest. This is best cut by large bone cutters before displacing the fragment.

Towel clips are secured into both fragments, the upper one to hold the wing of the ilium still while the lower acetabular fragment is moved. The lower fragment is now rotated forward and laterally; this process is facilitated by flexing, abducting and laterally rotating the leg. This is achieved by placing the foot of the operated leg on the opposite knee and then extending and abducting the hip by pressing down on the ipsilateral knee. As the displacement occurs care must be taken not to allow the acetabular fragment to slip backwards. The two pelvic fragments must be in contact at the sciatic notch. The position is stabilized by one or two Kirschner wires, or thin Steinmann pins.

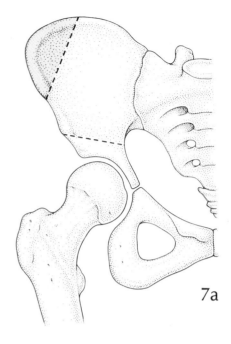

7a

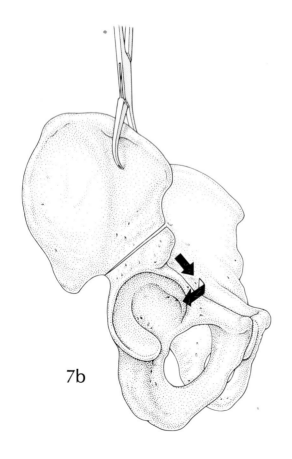

7b

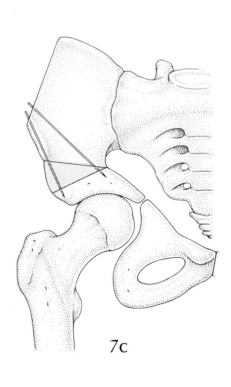

7c

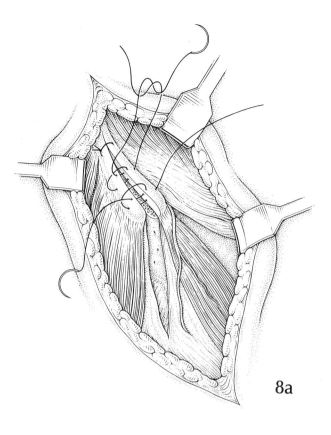

8a

Closure

8a & b

When the osteotomy has been performed as part of an open reduction the capsule is repaired as described in the chapter on 'Congenital dislocation of the hip' (pp. 870–892). The iliac apophysis is approximated by strong interrupted sutures. The hip is flexed to reduce the tension as the layers are approximated. As the fascia over the thigh is repaired care must be taken not to include the lateral cutaneous nerve of the thigh in the sutures. The subcutaneous tissues are sutured and the skin closed, either with interrupted sutures or a continuous subcuticular wire stitch.

Postoperative management

In the younger child it is convenient to immobilize the child in a plaster hip spica as this results in less pain and an early discharge from hospital. At 6 weeks the child is readmitted for mobilization, usually for 3–5 days. In the older child, if adequate fixation has been obtained by the Kirschner wires or Steinmann pins, the patient may be nursed on 'slings and springs' until the wound is healed. Mobilization is then permitted, initially on crutches without weight-bearing for 6 weeks. After this time partial weight-bearing is permitted for 3–4 weeks. Provided that radiographs at this stage show union of the osteotomy and incorporation of the graft, full mobilization is then permitted.

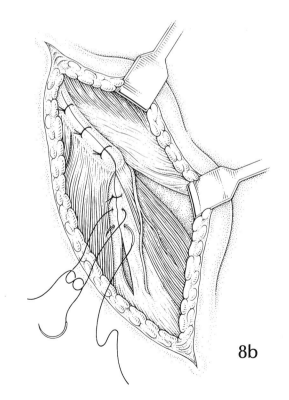

8b

Illustrations by Paul Richardson after J. M. P. Booth

High femoral osteotomy in childhood

E. W. Somerville FRCS (Ed), FRCS
Emeritus Consultant Orthopaedic Surgeon, Nuffield Orthopaedic Centre, Oxford, UK

Introduction

During the past 20 years the importance of the shape of the upper end of the femur and the femoral head in relation to the development of the hip joint has become increasingly apparent. The object of the operation is to correct any faulty mechanics which may be present so that the hip joint may be allowed to develop normally. For this reason the operation is carried out in children, sometimes very young children, because it is only when growth is rapid that it can provide the maximum benefit.

Indications

Persistent fetal alignment of the hip (persistence of an excessive degree of anteversion of the neck of the femur)

In this condition, because of the excessive anteversion, there will be 90° of medial rotation but minimal or no lateral rotation when the hip is in extension. This may lead to secondary deformities of lateral tibial torsion and valgus foot, which are ugly and may cause clumsiness. It is not yet certain whether or not this condition predisposes to osteoarthritis. The object of the operation is to restore a normal arc of rotation, i.e. 45° medial rotation and 45° lateral, preferably before the secondary deformities have developed. The operation is therefore a simple rotation osteotomy.

Congenital dislocation of the hip

In this condition anteversion plays some part in the actual initial displacement and following the dislocation it increases still further. A not uncommon cause for gradual redisplacement is a recurrence of anteversion and the development of a valgus deformity. Even if there is no valgus deformity, creation of some varus improves the stability of the joint.

Details of the specific use for this condition will be found in the chapter on 'Congenital dislocation of the hip' (pp. 870–892).

Perthes' disease

In this condition there is no anteversion and no coxa valga but a small rotation and varus osteotomy will provide better cover of the femoral head, allowing early mobilization and weight-bearing instead of a prolonged period of splintage.

Congenital coxa vara

In this condition there is a congenital abnormality of the upper end of the femur which leads to a progressive varus deformity due to growth. This condition will not correct spontaneously and will need surgical correction in all cases.

900

Operations

ROTATION OSTEOTOMY

This operation is performed for persistent fetal alignment of the hip, congenital dislocation of the hip and Perthes' disease.

1

The child is placed on the operating table in the supine position without a sandbag under the hip. The limb is held in medial rotation by an assistant and a straight incision is made on the outer side of the thigh with its upper limit just below the prominence of the great trochanter. It is about 8 cm long and is slightly oblique forwards from above downwards so that when the rotation has been carried out the incision will become vertical. The degree of obliquity will be determined by the amount of rotation obtained at the osteotomy.

The iliotibial band is split in line with its fibres, exposing the fibres of the vastus lateralis. The fascia overlying the posterior part of the muscle belly is divided in length over the posterior fibres close to the linea aspera. The muscle fibres are separated by blunt dissection. This does less damage to the small blood vessels, reducing the amount of bleeding and thereby producing less ischaemia as compared with sharp division. The periosteum is exposed and is divided in length with a knife; small bone levers are introduced anteriorly and posteriorly to the bone inside the periosteum. There may be some difficulty with the posterior lever because of the linea aspera, which may need separating from the bone with a knife.

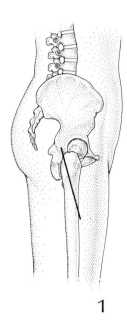

1

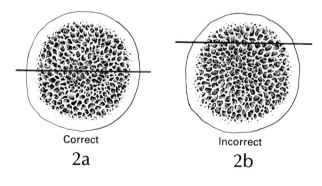

Correct
2a

Incorrect
2b

2a & b

A Steinmann pin is introduced into the lateral aspect of the upper femur just below the greater trochanter. It must traverse the diameter of the bone and penetrate through the opposite cortex.

3

To prevent sudden penetration of the pin it is wise to place over it a simple guard made from a metal tube of the appropriate length. A small Venable plate is slipped onto the pin through its upper hole and the plate laid along the bone. A second pin is introduced anterior to the plate and in line with the uppermost of the lower two holes and at the angle required for rotation. (In persistent fetal alignment 45°, in congenital dislocation of the hip 70° and in Perthes' disease 30°). Again it is of great importance that the pin traverse the diameter. The angle is checked by an assistant standing at the foot of the table in line with the femur with a goniometer set at the appropriate angle.

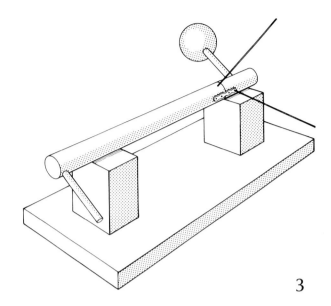

3

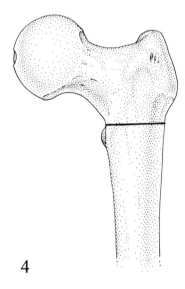

4

4

The plate is removed. A broad bone lever replaces the small one posteriorly and is rotated through 90° to ensure complete separation of the soft tissues so that they will not interfere with rotation. The small lever anteriorly is also turned on edge and the bone is divided with a saw. The division of the bone must be at right angles.

5

The distal fragment is then rotated until the pins are parallel. If there is difficulty in doing this it will be found that the pin has penetrated too far into the soft tissues on the medial side; if the lower pin is withdrawn a little the rotation can be performed easily. The plate is slipped back onto the pins.

The lowest hole is drilled first and screwed, which will ensure that the plate is properly placed. The lower hole in the upper part is similarly treated. The lower pin is removed and if the pin was of the right size it will not be necessary to drill the hole before the screw is inserted. Lastly the upper pin is removed and that hole screwed. The wound is closed in layers with care to put the minimum of stitches in the muscle and not to tie them tight to avoid ischaemia.

The operation can easily be performed bilaterally when necessary, but in a child under the age of 2 years it is better to operate on the two legs at an interval of 1 or 2 weeks.

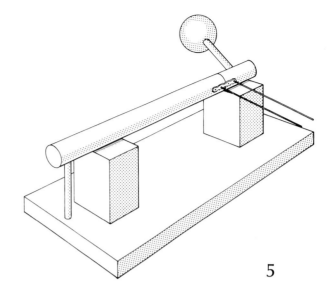

5

Postoperative management

A long hip spica is applied with the leg abducted 45°. In the small child the other leg should always be included down to the knee to prevent it adducting and being damaged.

The length of immobilization will depend on the age of the child. Under 6 or 7 years it will take 6 weeks, up to 12 years 8 weeks and after that 10 weeks to 3 months. As soon as the plaster is removed mobilization can be started, at first in the therapy pool then on dry land. Progress can be as rapid as the child can tolerate. After these operations the child will limp and it is always wise to warn the parents of this in advance so that they will not be disappointed. In a small child the limp will last only a few weeks but in a teenage child it may last many months and sometimes even as long as a year.

Prevention of complications

This is an operation which has no important complications provided it has been performed properly, but the following points are essential. The pins must pass through the diameter of the bone. The bone must be divided at a right angle. The lower screw must be inserted first to ensure the position of the plate, and if the bone is porotic, as is sometimes the case in the very young child, the screws should be introduced at different angles and not parallel to each other. While the operation can be performed at any age it is wise not to do it under 9 months of age since the bone is too small.

ROTATION OSTEOTOMY COMBINED WITH VARUS

This operation may be required in the treatment of congenital dislocation of the hip and in Perthes' disease with the signs of a 'head at risk'.

In the younger child

The exposure and preliminary part of the operation are as described for rotation osteotomy, but special care must be taken to ensure that the top pin is introduced accurately into the lateral side of the femur and as near to the epiphyseal plate as is consistent with safety. In the upper part of the wound the white cartilaginous epiphysis of the greater trochanter will be visible and the pin is introduced immediately below this. The plate is slipped onto this pin and the second pin is introduced as previously described. The bone is divided as high as possible, allowing room for the introduction of the second screw. The end of the lower fragment is drawn out of the wound by adducting the leg and using the pin as a lever.

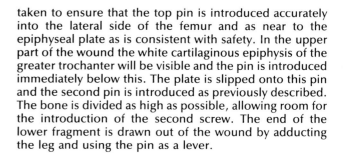

6

Using gouge-ended nibblers, a suitable amount of cortex is removed from the side of the bone where the point of the pin emerges, which when the lower fragment has been rotated will become the medial side. It is usual to remove sufficient bone to allow a varus angulation of 10° or 20°. The displacement is reduced, the pins held parallel to each other in the horizontal plane and the plate slipped on to the pins as previously described for rotation osteotomy.

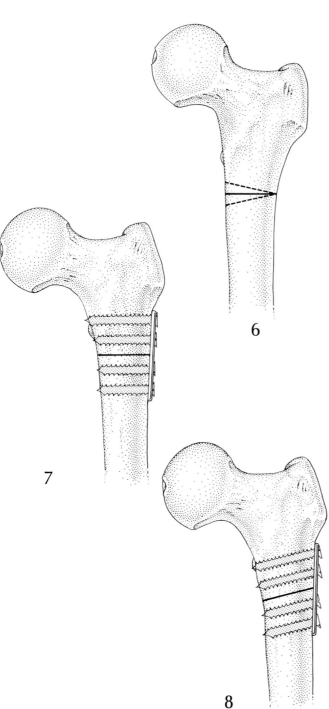

7 & 8

There is often a flare of the greater trochanter sufficiently great so that when the necessary angulation has been achieved the outer side of the femur will be straight and it will be unnecessary to bend the plate.

If this can be done it gives a much better result cosmetically but if it is not possible the plate must be bent to the appropriate angle to fit accurately.

Although the production of varus by the removal of a wedge adds an extra manoeuvre, it makes the application of the plate and the introduction of the screws simpler than in a straight rotation osteotomy. This is because the fragments are more stable and there is little or no risk of losing or increasing the amount of rotation. Fixation and closure are the same as already described.

In the older child

This operation is a modification of the previous procedure which is employed in the relapsing congenitally dislocated hip.

Leg length must be taken more seriously into account. The production of varus will cause some shortening and a medial wedge will increase the shortening even further. In most cases this is of no great importance because the leg will be too long initially and it is desirable in these cases for the leg to be a little too short rather than a little too long. However, there are some cases where it is desirable to reduce the shortening to a minimum.

The preliminaries of the operation are as already described but in the older child the bone is often too hard for the wedge to be removed with nibblers and a saw must be used.

The pins are introduced as already described, preferably by hand, because they will get a much better grip on the bone than if they are introduced with a drill and this may be helpful in subsequent manipulations. If varus without rotation is required the pins are placed parallel and in the same plane; otherwise the manoeuvres are exactly the same as described below.

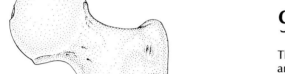

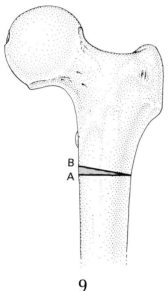

9

Removal of a medial bone wedge with rotation

9

The site of the osteotomy is selected as high as possible and a cut is made with the saw transversely half-way through the bone at A. This will be the lower cut. The upper cut is made at the required angle and is carried right through the bone at B. The angle of the wedge will be the angle of varus to be obtained. The lower cut is completed and the wedge is removed. If the lower cut is completed first it will be very difficult to control the upper fragment while completing the upper cut. The medial gap produced by removal of the wedge can then be closed, using the pins as levers, and the lower fragment can be rotated on the upper without further altering the angulation because the lower cut was made transversely. The plate, which in the larger child will need to be somewhat bigger, is applied in the manner described.

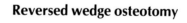

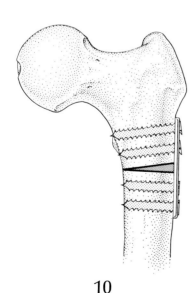

10

Reversed wedge osteotomy

10

If it is desirable to reduce the amount of shortening which will occur, a bone wedge as already described is removed in one piece from the medial side, is reversed and placed in the lateral side of the osteotomy, thus obtaining twice the angulation with half the wedge.

Opening wedge osteotomy

11

The degree of shortening can be reduced still further by not removing any wedge but opening the osteotomy on the outer side. A simple transverse cut is made as high as possible and the necessary degree of rotation obtained. The pins are separated to the required angle and the plate, bent as required, is applied to the pins and screwed in position.

In this operation and the previous one described, when angulation has been achieved the distance between the pins will have been increased and this increase must be allowed for when the screws are being introduced.

Up to the age of 12 years it is unnecessary to place any bone in the gap produced as it will fill in spontaneously. After this age it is probably wise to introduce a wedge of bone taken from the iliac crest.

Level of osteotomy

12

It is desirable, when producing varus, to make the osteotomy as high as possible. In many patients this can be done as described but in some it is difficult. In these cases the anterior surface of the upper end of the femur, including the base of the neck, is cleared. The angulation and rotation are obtained as described using the pins, but instead of the plate being threaded on to the pins it is placed anteriorly as high as possible with the upper screw passing through the base of the neck anteroposteriorly. Not infrequently the osteotomy can be carried out as much as 2 cm higher.

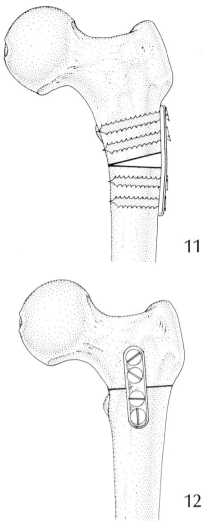

11

12

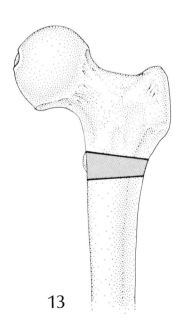

13

Shortening osteotomy

13

Occasionally the leg will have overgrown to a degree which makes it necessary to shorten it deliberately by more than will result from the varus and the wedge together. In such a case further shortening can be obtained by removing a trapezoid, with the base medial. The length of the opposite limb determines the degree of shortening to be obtained.

Other forms of internal fixation

Other forms of internal fixation have been described such as the Coventry plate and screw and the miniature nail–plate of Blundell-Jones. These have the advantage of making it possible to do the osteotomy a little higher but they are bulkier and, in the auther's opinion, the insertion of the appliance up the neck of the femur creates the risk of damage to the growth-plate if not placed with great accuracy.

Correction of congenital coxa vara

Congenital coxa vara is a growth defect of the upper end of the femur. In the most severe types complete absence of the upper end of the femur is simulated for a time after birth. In the less severe types growth of the capital side of the metaphysis is severely interfered with while the greater trochanter continues to grow normally. This results in an increasing varus deformity, the severity of which depends on the severity of the growth disturbance. Since this is a growth disturbance spontaneous correction will not occur and corrective osteotomy, which may have to be repeated, will be required. For this reason the initial osteotomy should not be performed too early.

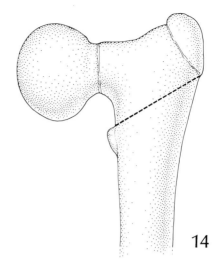

14

ROBERT JONES VALGUS OSTEOTOMY

The child is placed on the operating table with a small sandbag under the hip to be operated on. An incision is made from above the tip of the greater trochanter along the line of the femur for about 10 cm. The anterior and lateral aspects of the greater trochanter and the upper end of the femur are exposed subperiosteally.

14

With a hand saw the bone is divided from just below the prominence of the greater trochanter downwards and medially to just above the lesser trochanter, strictly in the anteroposterior plane.

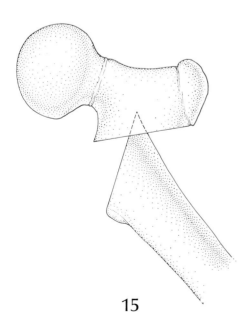

15

15

Posteriorly the periosteum is divided so that the lower fragment may be pulled downwards and angled so that the sharp spike can be driven into the medullary cavity in the proximal fragment below the midpoint of the neck.

This will permit the upper fragment to tilt downwards, allowing the wide abduction which is an essential part of the operation. Obtaining the necessary degree of abduction may be very difficult. In this case the introduction of a Steinmann pin into the upper fragment to stabilize it may help, but it may be necessary to tenotomize the adductors. This must be done with great care because if it is overdone all stability may be lost and it will be very difficult to maintain the required position. Rather than risk this it is better to shorten the bone by removing just enough of the spike to allow abduction with a tight fit. In this operation the use of internal fixation is difficult and unsatisfactory and is better avoided.

Postoperative management

A plaster spica is applied enclosing both legs in wide abduction even if only one side is being treated. It is difficult to achieve too much abduction. Union is usually sound in 2–3 months in the older child and sooner in the younger.

When union has occurred mobilization in bed and in a therapy pool can be started at once but, because of the wide abduction, may at first be slow; weight-bearing cannot be begun until adduction is almost complete.

Since this is a growth deformity some recurrence is inevitable (the younger the child at the time of operation the greater the recurrence). The parents must be warned in advance of the risk that the operation may need repeating when the child is older. By performing two operations rather than waiting until the deformity is very great before operating for the first time, the final deformity will be less.

WEDGE OSTEOTOMY

16

An alternative operation is carried out through the same incision, exposing the anterolateral aspect of the upper end of the femur. With a mechanically operated reciprocating saw, an incomplete oblique cut is made from the prominence on the lateral aspect of the greater trochanter downwards towards the calcar but not extending through the calcar. A step is then cut. A wedge is removed as indicated by the shaded area.

The cuts are all completed, the periosteum is divided posteriorly and the wedge is closed with wide abduction.

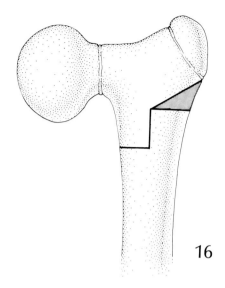

16

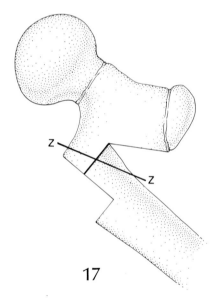

17

17

This operation usually retains a good degree of stability so that internal fixation should not be necessary, but it is not difficult to place a screw across the osteotomy if it is considered advisable (Z–Z).

In this operation the osteotomy is more difficult to cut and there is no increase in length, but in spite of this it is the simpler procedure and less prone to complications such as displacement.

Postoperative management

A plaster spica is applied enclosing both legs in wide abduction (90° between the two). Union usually occurs in 2–3 months. A check anteroposterior radiograph is taken to verify the position of the osteotomy. After 2 months the plaster is bivalved and a check radiograph out of plaster is taken.

If union is commencing, mobilization under physiotherapy supervision in hospital with daily pool therapy will rapidly restore the patient to normal activity. Weight-bearing begins when adduction is normal.

Slipped upper femoral epiphysis

M. J. Griffith   MChOrth, FRCS, FRCS(Ed)
Consultant Orthopaedic Surgeon, West Wales General Hospital, Carmarthen, UK

Introduction

The treatment of slipped upper femoral epiphysis is a controversial topic. Many questions remain unanswered. Surgical treatment will, at best, be misguided unless the surgeon has a clear three-dimensional concept of the deformity. An understanding of the surgical anatomy is an essential prerequisite to surgical intervention.

Surgical anatomy

1, 2, 3 & 4

The epiphysis slips backwards and downwards following the curved surface of the adolescent growth-plate. The slipped epiphysis lies directly behind the neck of the femur so that the appearance on routine anteroposterior radiographs is influenced by the effect of parallax. Radiographs taken with the leg in lateral rotation will show the epiphysis lying medial to the neck (varus). With the leg in medial rotation the epiphysis appears to lie lateral to the neck (valgus)[1].

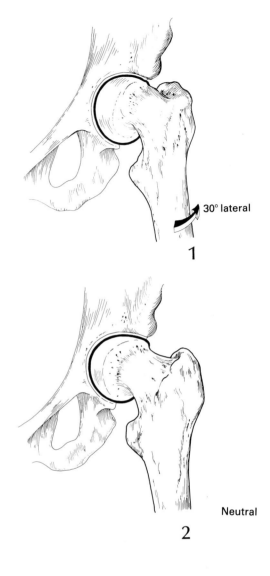

30° lateral

1

Neutral

2

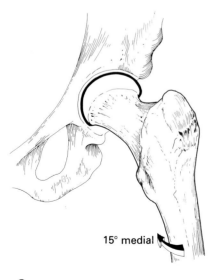

15° medial

3

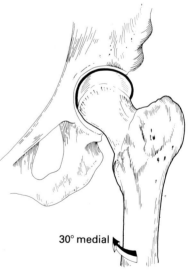

30° medial

4

5 & 6

As the epiphysis slips backwards it strips the periosteum on the posterior aspect of the neck. New bone is laid down beneath the stripped periosteum, forming a bony beak at the back of the metaphysis. The exposed anterior aspect of the neck almost always resorbs. The only significant residual blood supply to the epiphysis is through the retinacular vessels that run in the periosteum on the back of the neck; any surgical intervention must preserve these vessels.

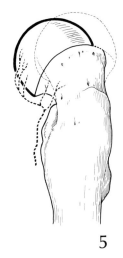 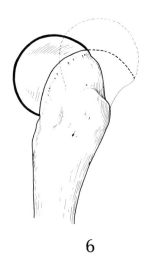

5   6

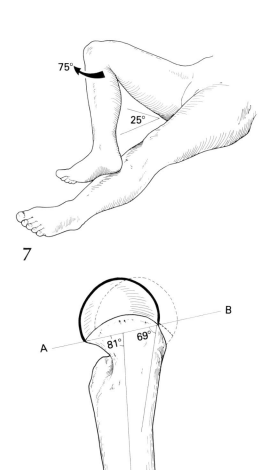

7

8

7 & 8

The severity of the slip is determined on frog lateral views of the hip. The patient lies supine and the X-ray tube is centred on the hip joint. The femur is laterally rotated 75° (90° minus anteversion angle) and elevated at an angle of 25° from the table (plane of inclination of the epiphysis on anteroposterior film), the knee is flexed to 90° and the lateral edge of the foot rested on the contralateral leg. The angle between the base of the epiphysis (A-B) and both the neck and the shaft of the femur are measured. In the normal hip the mean of these two angles is 90°. Subtracting the measured mean angle from 90° gives an accurate measure of the degree of slip[2]. Thus in *Illustration 8* the degree of slip is $90° - \dfrac{81° + 69°}{2} = 15°$.

CHOICE OF TREATMENT

A number of factors determine the choice of treatment.

Severity of slipping

The functional result in patients with slight slipping does not deteriorate with the passage of time whereas those with severe slipping will show progressive impairment of function due to osteoarthritis[3]. Patients with up to 30° (about one-third diameter) slip do not require correction of the deformity and are regarded as acceptable (*see Illustration 8*). Patients with over 50° (about half diameter) slip have permanent restriction of movement and tend to develop premature osteoarthritis. They require correction of the deformity which is regarded as unacceptable. Between these two extremes there is a grey area where the treatment will depend on the existing functional disability and the individual surgeon's experience. The premature onset of osteoarthritis is a lesser evil than iatrogenic avascular necrosis or chondrolysis. The author is reluctant to correct deformities of less than 50° slip[4].

State of the growth-plate

The need for internal fixation and the choice of osteotomy depends on whether the growth-plate remains open or closed. An open growth-plate carries the risk of further slipping.

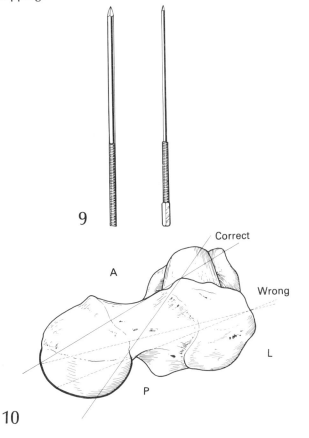

Presence of an acute component to the slip

This increases the vulnerability of the blood supply to the epiphysis.

Special considerations

Treatment may have to be modified if the patient has avascular necrosis, chrondrolysis, osteoarthritic changes, renal failure or gross hormonal imbalance.

Specific treatment will be considered under four broad categories depending on whether the severity of the slip is acceptable or unacceptable and whether the growth-plate is open or closed.

Acceptable deformity with growth-plate open

Irrespective of whether the slip is gradual or acute these patients should be treated by urgent internal fixation to prevent further slipping. Bone graft epiphysiodesis[5] is equally effective and should be considered when rapid closure of the growth-plate is required. The reader should consult the original paper and that of Melby et al[6].

TECHNIQUE OF PINNING *IN SITU*

9 & 10

The procedure is performed on a radiotranslucent operating table. The patient lies in the prone position and the affected leg draped to allow its free movement. An image intensifier is placed so as to give an anteroposterior picture of the hip.

Through a lateral approach the femur is exposed immediately below the greater trochanter. A fine threaded pin in which the thread stands proud of the wire, such as a Moore's (left) or Crawford Adams pin (right), is recommended as it is easier to remove at a later date. The pin is introduced through the anterolateral cortex just below the trochanteric ridge and drilled towards the epiphysis. Once the pin just crosses the growth-plate on the anteroposterior radiograph, the leg is placed in the frog lateral position and a true lateral radiograph of the neck and epiphysis obtained. Provided the pin lies in a suitable direction it can then be advanced to lie just below the articular cartilage.

Two further pins are then introduced in the same manner so that the tips of the pins engage different segments of the epiphysis. The hip should then be screened with the image intensifier to ensure as far as possible that pin penetration of the joint has not occurred.

Common errors of technique

1. The use of a fracture table. It is impossible to obtain true lateral radiographs with the shoot-through technique which is done on a fracture table. This makes pin placement even more difficult and increases the risk of pin penetration of the joint. There are also theoretical risks to blood supply of the epiphysis in the use of a fracture table.
2. Failure to appreciate that the epiphysis slips behind the neck. The technique is quite different to that used for a femoral neck fracture. The pin should be introduced from the anterolateral cortex (see *Illustration 10*); and if the slipping is severe, from the anterior aspect of the femur.
3. Multiple entry holes. These should be avoided as far as possible because they may so weaken the femur as to result in a subsequent fracture.
4. Pin placement in the distal one-third of the epiphysis may endanger the retinacular vessels in moderate or severe slipping.

Postoperative management

When the slipping is gradual the patient may be allowed up, with partial weight-bearing, in 2–3 days and resume full weight-bearing in 10–14 days. When the slipping is acute, the patient should rest in bed for 10 days and then avoid weight-bearing for 4–6 weeks. Patients should remain under surveillance and avoid contact sports or strenuous activities until the growth-plate is closed.

Acceptable deformity with growth-plate closed

No treatment is required and the patient is reassured.

Unacceptable deformity with growth-plate open

It is generally agreed that the more severe degrees of slip require correction of the deformity. Closed reduction, either by manipulation under anaesthesia or traction, carries an unacceptable risk to the blood supply of the epiphysis and should not be undertaken[1]. Some improvement in the range of hip movement is achieved by removal of the exposed anterior surface of the metaphysis (osteoplasty). In the author's experience this part of the neck almost always absorbs spontaneously, rendering the procedure unnecessary. In the rare cases where this does not occur, as judged on a true lateral radiograph, an osteoplasty as described by Heyman, Herndon and Strong[7] may be indicated in patients with moderate slipping (30°–50°).

Anatomical reduction is most accurately achieved by open replacement of the femoral epiphysis[8]. The initial results included a significant incidence of avascular necrosis but more recent results[9] have shown a very low incidence of complications.

The procedure demands meticulous attention to detail and should only be undertaken if the surgeon has a clear understanding of the deformity to be corrected and is confident that he can protect the residual blood supply to the epiphysis. The procedure should not be attempted if the growth-plate is closed or nearly closed as the retinacular vessels then become inseparable from the femoral neck and part of the blood supply to the head is across the old growth-plate[10]. In the author's opinion this is the procedure of choice provided these criteria are met.

Many surgeons are fearful of open replacement and prefer a corrective subcervical osteotomy for severe gradual slipping. The biplane trochanteric osteotomy[11, 12] is a well-established procedure for severe gradual slipping. It is free of risk to the capital blood supply and gives good early clinical results. Nevertheless, it is a difficult operation with a tendency to overcorrect the varus and undercorrect the posterior tilt. The procedure may be complicated by chondrolysis or significant shortening, and there are doubts about the long-term results[13].

The severe acute or acute-on-chronic slip is fraught with dangers. Closed reduction either by gentle manipulation or traction is associated with an unacceptable incidence of avascular necrosis. If the surgeon considers open replacement too hazardous then the epiphysis should be carefully pinned *in situ* and a definitive subcervical osteotomy either by the biplane or geometric technique deferred until the growth-plate is closed.

OPEN REPLACEMENT OF FEMORAL EPIPHYSIS[8]

11

The patient lies on his side with the affected leg uppermost. The hip is exposed through a lateral incision made over the proximal femoral shaft and then curving into the buttock.

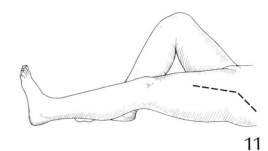

11

12

The greater trochanter is divided from below up through its growth-plate and with the attached abductors retracted proximally.

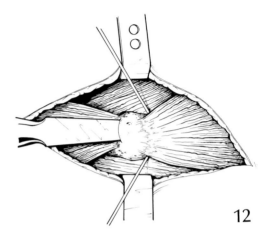

12

13

13

A T-shaped incision is made in the capsule down its lateral aspect and round the acetabular rim. The blood supply to the femoral head runs on to the femoral neck through the base of the posterior flap into the neck.

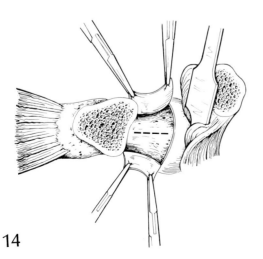

14

14

The periosteum of the neck is incised along its lateral margin between the pale avascular anterior part and the red vascular posterior surface, and round the anterior edge of the neck–head junction.

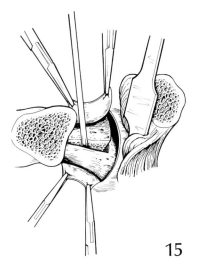

15

15 & 16

The posterior periosteum carrying the capital blood supply is carefully stripped from the back of the neck, preserving its attachment to the rim of the head proximally and the capsule distally. Using a wide gouge as a shoehorn through the remains of the growth-plate, the head is gently prized backwards off the neck, exposing the posterior beak of new bone.

The first osteotomy cut is made in the long axis of the neck to remove this beak.

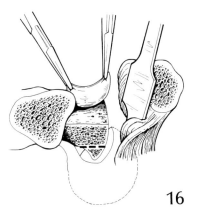

16

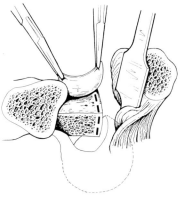

17

17

The second osteotomy cut curves across the metaphysis to remove the remains of the growth-plate and shorten the neck by 3–4 mm.

The inside of the epiphysis is gently curetted to remove the rest of the growth-plate.

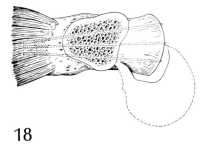

18

18

Three Crawford Adams pins are drilled up the neck to present at the metaphysis. The head is reduced and the pins driven home.

19 & 20a & b

The head should sit squarely on the neck in the lateral view, and with about 20° of valgus to the neck on the anteroposterior view.

The trochanter is reattached with a screw.

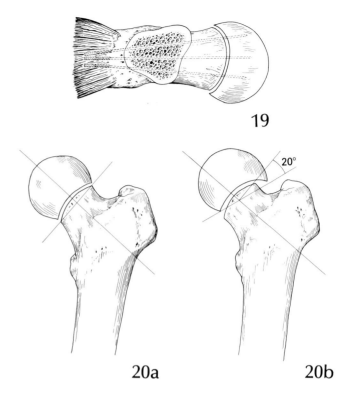

19

20a   20b

Postoperative management

Light skin traction is applied to the leg for 1 month and immediate hip flexion encouraged. After 1 month the patient is allowed up without bearing weight until radiographs show bony union of the epiphysis, usually about 3 months after operation.

BIPLANE TROCHANTERIC OSTEOTOMY[11, 12]

Preoperative measurement of desired correction

Clinical measurement of loss of abduction, flexion and medial rotation gives a very crude estimate of the degree of correction required. The different components of the deformity are best determined radiologically.

Varus

21

Southwick recommends an anteroposterior film of the pelvis taken with both legs in a neutral position. The axis of the epiphysis (*a–a*) and a line at right angles to this down the neck of the femur (*A–B*) are drawn. The long axis of the shaft is drawn (*B–C*) and the angle *A–B–C* measured. The difference between the normal and abnormal sides represents the amount of correction needed on the anterior aspect of the femur.

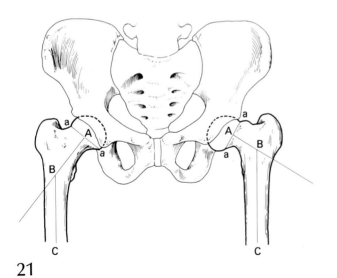

21

Posterior angulation

22

Comparable frog lateral radiographs are taken of both hips. If positioning is difficult the pelvis may be tilted to give an accurate lateral film of the proximal end of each femur. Southwick draws the axis of the head (*x–x*) and the vertical to it (*X–Y*) and measures the angle between *X–Y* and the long axis of the shaft (*X–Z*). The difference between the normal and abnormal sides represents the amount of correction needed on the lateral aspect of the femur.

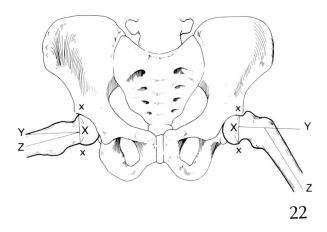

22

Lateral rotation

Correction of the varus and posterior tilt restores normal rotation. If the posterior tilt exceeds 60° Southwick prefers to undercorrect the deformity lest excessive shortening occurs, and to compensate for this by medial rotation of the shaft of the femur according to the range of movement achieved at the time of operation.

23

A piece of metal foil is cut as a template, the anterior part corresponding to the measured angle of valgus required and the lateral part to the flexion required. The hypotenuse of the lateral triangle should be 2 cm long to ensure good bony contact when the wedge is closed.

Surgical technique

The patient lies supine with the leg draped free. The anterolateral aspect of the upper femoral shaft is exposed through a lateral incision in line with the posterior edge of the greater trochanter, the lesser trochanter identified round the front of the shaft, and the psoas tendon detached.

At the junction of the relatively flat anterior surface and the rounded lateral surface of the upper femur, an orientation mark is made with an osteotome, and at the level of the lesser trochanter a second mark made at right angles to the first, representing the vertical and horizontal lines on the template. The template is bent and applied and the edges of the intended osteotomy marked.

Anterior | Lateral

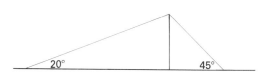

15° | 30°

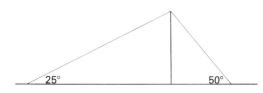

20° | 45°

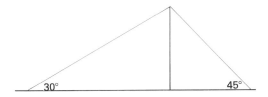

25° | 50°

30° | 45°

23

24

A threaded Steinmann pin is drilled from the base of the greater trochanter distally and medially towards the lesser trochanter in line with the anterior edge of the intended osteotomy. Keeping to the guide lines, the wedge of bone is removed. The wedge should not be larger than necessary for good bony apposition. The greater the wedge the more shortening is produced.

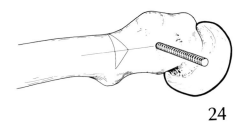

24

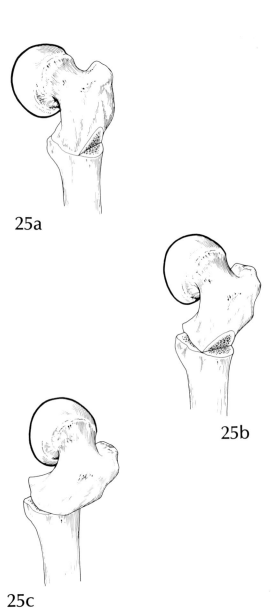

25a

25b

25c

25 a, b & c

The transverse part of the osteotomy is continued through the shaft of the femur.

The proximal fragment is controlled by a pin and the osteotomy closed anterolaterally by flexion and abduction of the limb. This opens a gap posteromedially.

The position is stabilized either by two pins in each fragment brought out through the wound and fixed to an external bar, or a plate and screws with or without compression. The range of hip movement is checked and should show at least 90° of flexion in neutral rotation and 30° of abduction. The skeletal fixation is supplemented by a plaster of Paris hip spica.

The spica is removed after about 8 weeks. Union of the osteotomy occurs in 8–12 weeks, by which time the affected growth-plate has become closed. Weight-bearing is then allowed.

Unacceptable deformity with growth-plate closed

Operations on the femoral neck are contraindicated and correction of the deformity has to be undertaken in the intertrochanteric region. Southwick's biplane trochanteric osteotomy is the established operation of choice. The author has used an alternative geometric flexion osteotomy on 14 patients. In one patient there was failure of fixation due to placement of two screws in the trochanteric growth-plate, and this required further surgery; another patient developed chondrolysis. The remaining patients regained an almost full range of pain-free movement, although one has radiological evidence but no symptoms of early osteoarthritis 13 years later. The operation has only been used after closure of the growth-plate for fear of subsequent slipping.

GEOMETRIC FLEXION OSTEOTOMY[1]

Theoretical considerations

The metaphyseal surface of the proximal femoral growth-plate may be represented by one-quarter of a cylinder. The epiphysis slips round the curved surface of this cylinder. The centre of rotation lies in the middle of the intertrochanteric region, as seen on the lateral radiograph, and in a plane parallel to the slope of the original growth-plate as seen on the anteroposterior view (this can be best measured on the normal hip).

The aim of the operation is to remove a wedge of bone with its apex at the geometric axis of rotation of the epiphysis and thus rotate the epiphysis back to its normal relationship to the acetabulum and femur.

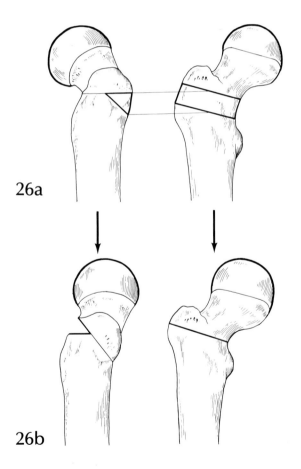

26a

26b

Surgical technique

26a & b

The anterior surface of the proximal end of the femur is exposed. A wedge of bone is removed from the intertrochanteric region, the apex of the wedge lying along the axis of rotation of the epiphysis. The proximal surface of the wedge is cut first. The line of division is in the intertrochanteric region and usually inclines medially and distally at 70° to the long axis of the shaft of the femur. The oscillating saw should be held at right angles to the anterior surface of the femur and should pass only half-way through the shaft at this stage.

The distal surface of the wedge is then cut so that the wedge is equal to the angle of rotation of the epiphysis. The apex of the wedge should be half-way through the shaft of the femur and should lie in the anteversion plane – that is, it should be a little more posterior on the lateral than on the medial side of the shaft. The cortex on the medial side of the shaft is then divided completely, leaving the posterolateral cortex intact. This facilitates application of the osteotomy plate. The osteotomy plates are made to provide angles of correction of 45°, 50°, 60° and 70°.

27

If the osteotomy is made distal to the axis of rotation of the epiphysis, either inadvertently or because the patient has an excessively long valgoid femoral neck, a secondary deformity of the femur will occur.

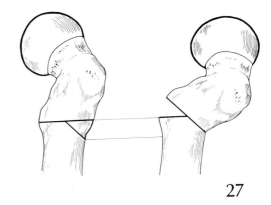

27

28

The appropriate plate is screwed to the proximal fragment so that the long axis of the plate lies at right angles to the osteotomy surface. The posterolateral cortex is then divided. Once the femur is completely divided, the proximal fragments tend to move into abduction. The shaft of the femur is abducted a similar amount and flexed to align it to the osteotomy plate, to which it is fixed with three screws. Care should be taken to avoid rotation of the shaft of the femur.

Postoperative management

After operation the hip is held in a flexed position by light Hamilton Russell traction and early gentle movement of the hip is encouraged. At 6–8 weeks the patient is allowed to walk with crutches, but weight-bearing is prohibited until the osteotomy is united.

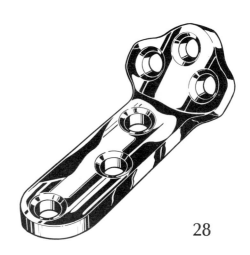

28

References

1. Griffith MJ. Slipping of the capital femoral epiphysis. *Ann R Coll Surg Engl* 1976; 58: 34–42.

2. Billing L, Severin E. Slipping epiphysis of the hip: a roentgenological and clinical study based on a new roentgen technique. *Acta Radiol* 1959; Suppl 174.

3. Oram V. Epiphysiolysis of the head of the femur: follow-up examination with special reference to end results and social prognosis. *Acta Orthop Scand* 1953; 23: 100.

4. Boyer DW, Mickelson MR, Ponseti IV. Slipped capital femoral epiphysis: long-term follow-up study of one hundred and twenty-one patients. *J Bone Joint Surg [Am]* 1981; 63-A: 85–95.

5. Heyman CH, Herndon CH. Epiphysiodesis for early slipping of the upper femoral epiphysis. *J Bone Joint Surg [Am]* 1954; 36-A: 539–55.

6. Melby A, Hoyt WA Jr, Weiner DS. Treatment of chronic slipped capital femoral epiphysis by bone-graft epiphyseodesis. *J Bone Joint Surgery [Am]* 1980; 62-A: 119–125.

7. Heyman CH, Herndon CH, Strong JM. Slipping femoral epiphysis with severe displacement – a conservative operative treatment. *J Bone Joint Surg [Am]* 1957; 39-A: 293.

8. Dunn DM, Angel JC. Replacement of the femoral head by open operation in severe adolescent slipping of the upper femoral epiphysis. *J Bone Joint Surg [Br]* 1978; 60-B: 394–403.

9. Colton CL. Slipped upper femoral epiphysis. In: Catterall A, ed. *Recent advances in orthopaedics* No. 5. Edinburgh: Churchill Livingstone, 1987: 61–77.

10. Crock HV. A revision of the anatomy of the arteries supplying the upper end of the human femur. *J Anat* 1965; 99: 77–88.

11. Southwick WO. Osteotomy through the lesser trochanter for slipped capital femoral epiphysis. *J Bone Joint Surg [Am]* 1967; 49-A: 807–35.

12. Southwick WO. Compression fixation after biplane intertrochanteric osteotomy for slipped upper femoral epiphysis. *J Bone Joint Surg [Am]* 1973; 55-A: 1218–24.

13. Ireland J, Newman PH. Triplane osteotomy for severely slipped upper femoral epiphysis. *J Bone Joint Surg [Br]* 1978; 60-B: 390–3.

Illustrations by Gillian Oliver

Correction of flexion contracture of the hip

B. Helal MChOrth, FRCS
Honorary Consultant Orthopaedic Surgeon, The Royal London Hospital and The Royal National Orthopaedic Hospital, London, and Enfield Group of Hospitals, UK

S. C. Chen FRCS
Consultant Orthopaedic Surgeon, Enfield Group of Hospitals, UK

Introduction

In cerebral palsy the hip joint may become flexed due to contractures of the iliotibial tract, rectus femoris muscle, iliopsoas and gluteal muscles. Usually the flexion contracture is associated with either an adduction deformity due to contractures of the adductor muscles or with a medial rotation deformity due to overactivity of the medial rotator muscles of the hip. It is important to establish clearly the type of deformity present in the hip, for the typical spastic scissor gait of a child suffering from cerebral palsy can be due to a simple flexion contracture, or to a contracture producing both flexion and medial rotation, or flexion and adduction of the hip. Severe cases can secondarily affect the lumbar spine producing, in longstanding cases, a fixed scoliosis due to pelvic tilt. Mild cases can be treated by regular stretching and exercises in the physiotherapy department.

Operations

RELEASE OF A TIGHT ILIOTIBIAL TRACT
(Yount procedure[1])

The tensor fasciae latae muscle flexes and abducts the hip while at the same time it flexes the knee and laterally rotates the tibia. When this muscle becomes contracted, deformities will occur in the direction of its actions.

Incision

1

The skin is incised along the lateral aspect of the knee, extending from the joint line to just above the femoral condyle.

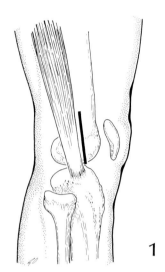

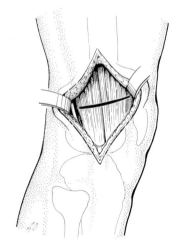

Procedure

2

The iliotibial tract and fascia lata are exposed and both these structures divided transversely backwards to the lateral head of the biceps femoris and forwards to just above the upper pole of the patella. Care should be taken not to damage the quadriceps tendon and muscles and the lateral popliteal nerve.

Postoperative management

A plaster cast is applied from the foot to the upper thigh with the knee in full extension. The patient can walk with the plaster cast on for 2 weeks. Then the plaster is removed and physiotherapy to mobilize the knee can commence. A removable backslab is applied for 3 more weeks during the day for walking, and this is used as a night splint for 6 months before discarding it completely.

ILIOPSOAS TENOTOMY

An iliopsoas tenotomy is necessary when the hip is flexed more than 15° but less than 45°, and passive stretching cannot correct the deformity. An adductor tenotomy may have to be done at the same time, for an associated adductor deformity.

Incision

3

The attachment of the iliopsoas to the lesser trochanter of the femur is found through a medial approach. A vertical incision is made on the medial aspect of the thigh, 2 cm distal to the pubic tubercle.

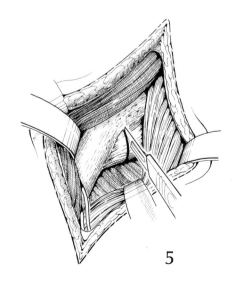

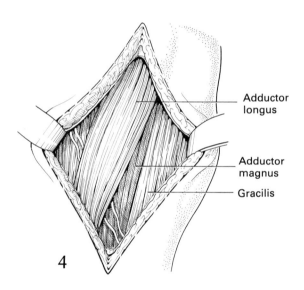

Adductor longus

Adductor magnus

Gracilis

Procedure

4

The adductor longus and gracilis muscles are identified. The tissue plane between the adductor longus and brevis anteriorly and the gracilis and adductor magnus posteriorly is identified and the muscles separated, taking care to protect the branches of the obturator nerve and blood vessels in this area.

The lesser trochanter is identified, and the iliopsoas is detached. The tendons of the adductor longus, brevis and magnus can be cut at the same time if necessary.

Postoperative management

Hip abduction and extension exercises are commenced early. Full weight-bearing is permitted after a few days. The patient is encouraged to sleep prone at night.

SOUTTER OPERATION FOR HIP FLEXION CONTRACTURE[2]

In severe flexion contracture of the hip there is extensive involvement of the sartorius, rectus femoris, tensor fasciae latae and glutei. These have to be released if full correction is to be achieved. An iliopsoas tenotomy is almost always necessary.

Incision

6

The incision runs from the anterior part of the iliac crest to the anterior superior iliac spine and downwards for about 12 cm towards the lateral side of the patella.

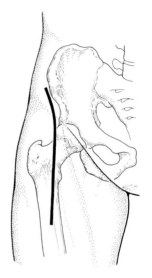

6

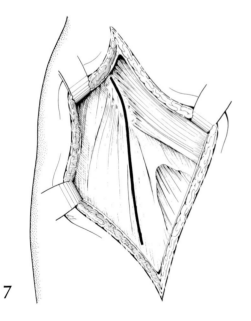

7

7

The skin and subcutaneous tissue are reflected distally and backwards to expose the crest of the ilium and deep fascia. The deep fascia is incised from the anterior superior iliac spine downwards and backwards to the greater trochanter.

Release

8

The sartorius, tensor fasciae latae and glutei are released from their attachments to the ilium, with a combination of sharp and blunt dissection deep to the deep fascia on the lateral side of the ilium. The hip is extended and the released structures allowed to retract. The subcutaneous tissue and skin only are sutured.

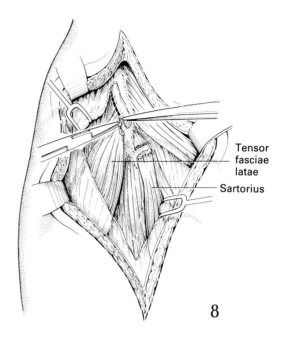

Tensor fasciae latae

Sartorius

8

Postoperative management

Skin traction is applied to the affected leg for 3 weeks. Hip abduction and extension exercises are commenced and full weight-bearing is permitted after this period. The patient should be encouraged to sleep prone at night.

References

1. Yount CC. The role of the tensor fasciae femoris in certain deformities of the lower extremities. *J Bone Joint Surg* 1926; 8: 171–93.

2. Soutter R. A new operation for hip contractures in poliomyelitis. *Boston Med Surg J* 1914; 170: 380–1.

Adductor release (with or without partial anterior obturator neurectomy)

W. J. W. Sharrard MD, ChM, FRCS
Emeritus Consultant Orthopaedic Surgeon, Royal Hallamshire and Children's Hospital, Sheffield;
Professor of Orthopaedic Surgery, University of Sheffield, UK

Preoperative

Indications and assessment

Before adductor release the range of abduction must be assessed with the hips and knees extended to ensure that any contracture of the gracilis, which is frequently affected, is recognized. Abduction of the hip is limited to 40° or less owing to strong and probably spastic adductor muscle in the presence of weaker hip abductors in cerebral palsy, myelomeningocele, poliomyelitis or other paralytic conditions and is the main indication for the operation. If abductor power is greater than MRC Grade 3 (antigravity) and there is minimal radiological subluxation of the hip, adductor release only is needed, often only of adductor longus and gracilis. If abductor power is less than Grade 3 and/or there is more than one-third subluxation of the femoral head, adductor release should be combined with neurectomy of the anterior branch of the obturator nerve. Adductor longus, gracilis, adductor brevis and, in severe contracture, adductor magnus, may need to be released until a full range, or as full a range of abduction as possible, is achieved. If the hip has been completely dislocated before operation, it may reduce. The operation may be combined with iliopsoas tendon lengthening or recession by the medial approach (see the chapter on pp. 936–939).

The operation can be performed at any age in a child or an adult and is often needed bilaterally.

A radiograph of the hips should be taken before operation.

Anaesthesia and position of patient

General anaesthesia is normally needed. In children thought to be unfit for general anaesthesia because of severe respiratory dysfunction, local anaesthesia can be used. The degree of limitation of abduction is confirmed under anaesthesia. The patient is placed supine with a small sandbag under the buttocks. After skin preparation the limbs are enclosed in stockinette to just above the level of the knee. A vertical narrow drape is used to cover the genitalia and other towels are applied to leave the upper medial aspects of the thigh exposed. The operative area may be covered by transparent adhesive. The lower limbs should be free to allow the hips to be manipulated in all directions.

A diathermy plate should be placed to give adequate skin contact, usually under the back or upper part of the buttock.

Operation[1]

Incision

1

A 3–4 cm incision, depending on the size of the patient, is made parallel to the groin crease and 2.5–3 cm below it, centred over the adductor longus tendon. The subcutaneous tissue is divided down to, but not through, the deep fascia and is mobilized proximally for about 2 cm and distally for 1 cm to expose the fascia over the proximal end of the adductor muscle.

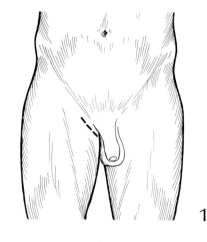

1

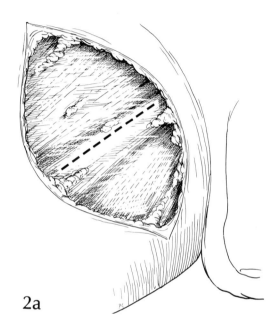

2a

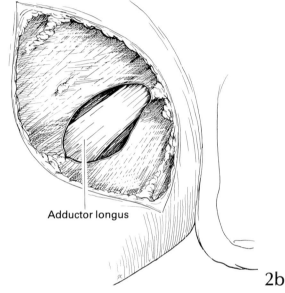

Adductor longus

2b

Exposure

2a, b & 3

A vertical incision is made along the line of the adductor longus, which is usually identifiable by the prominence of its tendon. The fascia is undermined medially and laterally to expose the gracilis medial to and the pectineus and adductor brevis lateral to the adductor longus. The muscles and tendons can be identified by their shape. The adductor longus arises by a thick oval tendon attached to the pubis and rapidly expanding into a broad fleshy belly. The gracilis arises by a thin flattened aponeurosis, vertically disposed and taking origin from the medial margins of the lower half of the body of the pubis and the ischium. The flat muscle lies immediately below the surface of the skin with a thin covering layer of fascia, and can easily be obscured beneath a medially placed retractor. The pectineus arises by a muscular origin anteriorly. It does not normally require division and is separated and retracted forward to expose the adductor brevis beneath it.

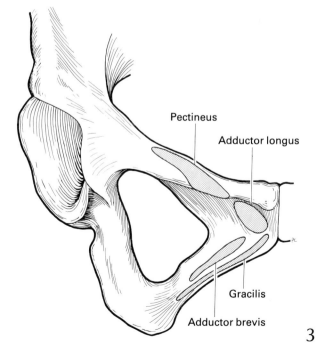

Pectineus

Adductor longus

Gracilis

Adductor brevis

3

Musculotendinous division

4a, b & c

The uppermost part of the adductor longus is defined by passing a MacDonald blunt dissector behind its tendon and uppermost muscular fibres. It is divided transversely 1 cm from its origin by cutting through the tendon onto the blunt dissector. The distal muscle should retract distally when it has been completely divided; only occasionally a small vessel may require coagulation by diathermy.

The aponeurosis of the gracilis is defined by blunt dissection on its medial and lateral sides. The aponeurosis is wide, extending well posteriorly. It is divided by a slightly oblique cut parallel and 1 cm distal to its origin. At its most posterior attachment, a small vessel is always encountered which needs to be coagulated by diathermy. The distal muscle should retract distally. Complete division of the adductor longus and gracilis is confirmed by abduction of the hip with the knee extended. The range of abduction should now be considerably improved. If the abduction range is more than 65°–70°, no further adductor release is required. If it is still limited, the adductor brevis and possibly the adductor magnus muscle, exposed beneath the divided adductor longus and gracilis, are palpated.

Some lengthening of the adductor brevis can be made without incision by teasing its fibres with a blunt dissector whilst slowly stretching them by abducting the hip further. The adductor magnus rarely requires division except in very severe adduction deformity. If the hip was dislocated or severely subluxated before operation, a radiograph may be taken to check whether reduction has been achieved.

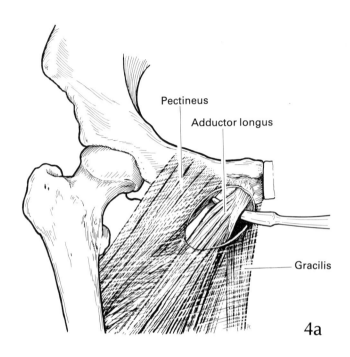

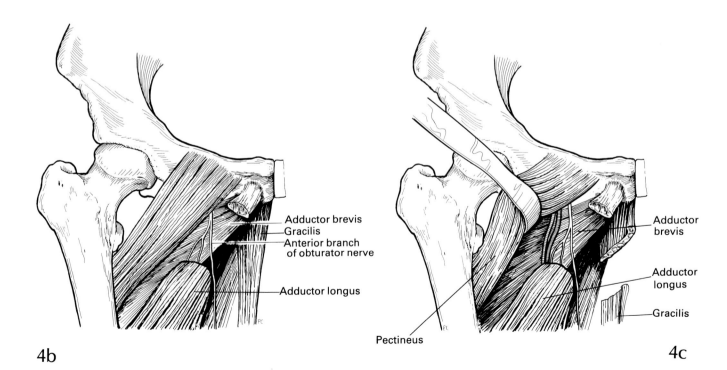

Additional procedure – posterior adductor transfer

If adduction deformity is associated with hip flexion deformity, owing to weakness of hip extension and abduction, adductor release and iliopsoas lengthening or recession may be combined with posterior transfer of the adductors. The approach is similar, except that the skin incision is extended posteriorly by an additional 2 cm. The origins of the adductor longus and gracilis and, if desired,

adductor brevis are detached close to the pubic ramus[2]. The upper 5 cm of the muscles are mobilized, retaining their nerve supply. The tendons of origin are moved posteriorly and attached to the ischial tuberosity or to the common tendon of origin of the hamstrings with strong unabsorbable sutures using a Mayo's cutting needle. Care must be taken to ensure that adductor tightness is not reproduced in the attempt to attach the tendons of origin to the bone; if there is a tendency for this to occur, it is better to attach the tendons to the common tendon of origin of the hamstrings.

Partial neurectomy of the obturator nerve

5

The anterior branch of the obturator nerve passes obliquely across the surface of the adductor brevis accompanied by branches of the obturator artery and vein. It may present as a single nerve dividing into two branches or as two separate branches. If necessary, it can be identified by gently pinching it with non-toothed dissecting forceps and noting twitching of the adductor muscles. If there are two nerve branches, the posterior branch of the obturator nerve should be identified on the posterior aspect of the adductor brevis to confirm that one of the anterior branches is not a posterior branch taking an anomalous course on the anterior surface of the muscle.

The nerve is separated from its accompanying vessels and retracted by blunt hooks. Artery forceps are applied proximally and distally and the nerve divided with removal of 1–1.5 cm of nerve. If the artery or vein are accidentally divided, brisk bleeding may occur, but the vessel can be coagulated by diathermy without important after-effects.

The posterior branch of the obturator nerve should not be divided, but it may be crushed in cases of severe adductor spasticity.

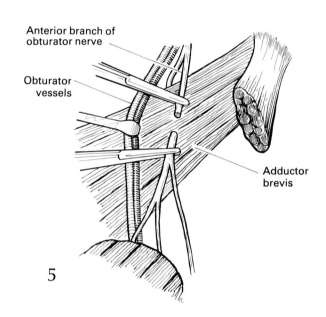

Anterior branch of obturator nerve

Obturator vessels

Adductor brevis

5

Wound closure

6

After diathermy of any outstanding smaller vessels, the wound is closed in three layers. The deep fascia is closed by vertical interrupted sutures and serves to limit haematoma formation. The subcutaneous fat is closed transversely by a continuous or interrupted suture and the skin is closed by interrupted sutures or a continuous subcuticular suture. A suction drain is not normally needed in children but is advisable in adolescents or adults for 48 hours.

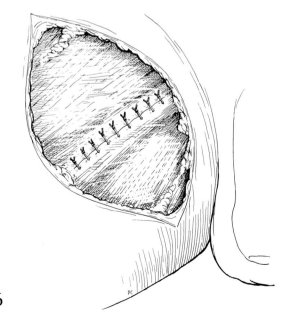

6

Immobilization

7

If the hip joint was not dislocated or markedly subluxated before operation and spasticity is not severe, no plaster immobilization is necessary in a child below the age of 10 years. The limbs can be maintained in abduction by a pillow between the thighs.

If the hip joint has been unstable, the lower limbs are immobilized in a groin-to-ankle or groin-to-toe plaster cast with the knees extended and both hips abducted as far as possible. The plaster casts are connected by two metal, wood or plaster bars.

Spasm can be limited by oral diazepam or baclofen for 2–3 days or longer if necessary.

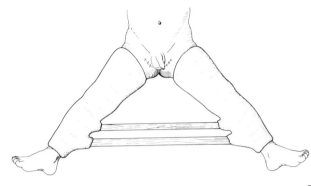

7

Postoperative management

The patient, if a child, can usually return home after 2 or 3 days. Sutures, if not absorbable, are removed after 10–12 days. If plaster casts have been needed, they are retained for 2–3 weeks in children below the age of 5 years, 3–4 weeks in children between the ages of 5 and 10 years and 4–5 weeks in patients over this age. Physiotherapy is given to encourage active and passive movements, including hip flexion, in joints not immobilized by plaster. After removal of plaster casts physiotherapy to encourage passive and active abduction should be instituted immediately.

References

1. Banks HH, Green WT. Adductor myotomy and obturator neurectomy for the correction of adduction contractures of the hip in cerebral palsy. *J Bone Joint Surg [Am]* 1960; 42-A, 111–26.

2. Root L, Spero CR. Hip adductor transfer compared with adduction tenotomy in cerebral palsy. *J Bone Joint Surg [Am]* 1981; 63-A, 767–72.

Hip flexor release: iliofemoral approach

W. J. W. Sharrard MD, ChM, FRCS.
Emeritus Consultant Orthopaedic Surgeon, Royal Hallamshire Hospital and Children's Hospital, Sheffield;
Professor of Orthopaedic Surgery, University of Sheffield, UK

Preoperative

Indications and assessment

The main indication for hip flexor release is flexion deformity of the hip of between 20° and 80°, arising from the activity of strong hip flexors in the presence of weak hip extensors in cerebral palsy, myelomeningocele, poliomyelitis and other paralytic conditions in which the deformity is due to musculotendinous contracture rather than bony deformity.

Before operation an assessment should be made of the part contributed to the flexion deformity by the iliopsoas, tensor fasciae latae, sartorius and rectus femoris. An increase of flexion on medial rotation of the hip suggests tightness of the iliopsoas or sartorius or both. An increase of hip flexion when the knee is flexed indicates tightness of the rectus femoris. An increase of hip flexion when the hip is adducted suggests tightness of the tensor fasciae latae. In most cases, the iliopsoas is likely to be the predominantly short tendon.

When there is more than 45° of fixed flexion, the hip tends to fall into abduction and lateral rotation. When the hip is adducted, the true degree of flexion deformity becomes apparent. Inability to adduct to neutral even when the hip is allowed to flex indicates that there is an abduction or a combined flexion and abduction deformity, often owing to contracture in the tensor fasciae latae.

Anaesthesia and position of patient

General anaesthesia is needed. An intravenous infusion should be begun. One or two units of blood may be needed during the operation. The patient is placed supine with a small sandbag under the buttock of the affected side. The skin is prepared. The limb is enclosed in stockinette to above the knee. Drapes are placed to expose the upper third of the thigh, the anterior superior iliac spine and the anterior half of the iliac crest. The operative area is covered either by stockinette or a transparent adhesive drape. When there is a marked flexion deformity, the limb may need to be held in semi-flexion until some correction has been obtained. Stockinette is applied to the opposite limb so that it can be flexed fully to perform a Thomas' test during the operation.

A diathermy plate is placed to give adequate skin contact, usually under the back or upper part of the buttock.

Operation

Incision

1

The incision is made along the outer side of the anterior third of the iliac crest, immediately lateral to the anterior superior iliac spine and obliquely along the line of the sartorius in the upper third of the thigh. The subcutaneous tissue is divided in the same line down too deep fascia. A vein running transversely just distal to the anterior superior iliac spine may need to be coagulated. The incision must not be made too deeply just distal to the anterior superior iliac spine to avoid dividing the lateral cutaneous nerve of the thigh as it emerges from beneath the inguinal ligament.

To avoid postoperative breakdown of the skin over a prominence, the incision should not cross directly over the anterior superior iliac spine.

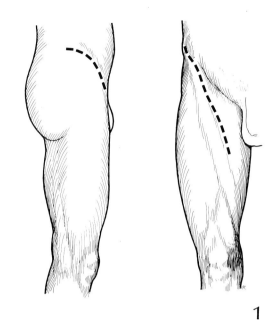

1

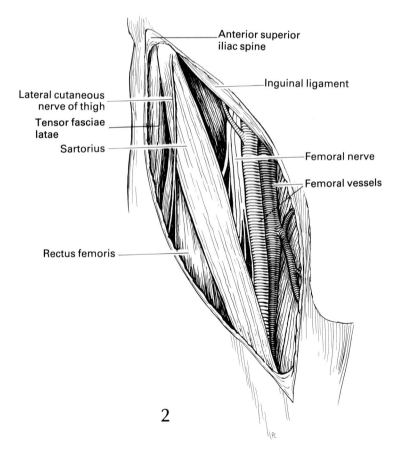

2

Anterior superior iliac spine

Inguinal ligament

Lateral cutaneous nerve of thigh

Tensor fasciae latae

Sartorius

Femoral nerve

Femoral vessels

Rectus femoris

Exposure

2

The deep fascia is incised from the anterior superior iliac spine distally along the proximal half of the sartorius, which can often be seen through the fascia. The lateral cutaneous nerve of the thigh lies immediately beneath the fascia just distal and medial to the anterior superior iliac spine, running obliquely distally and laterally, and should be preserved. In the incision of the thigh, small cutaneous branches of the femoral nerve may be encountered and their division should, if possible, be avoided. The aponeurosis on the inner and outer side of the tensor fasciae latae is defined up to its origin from the iliac crest from which it is detached in its anterior two-thirds, and sometimes completely, if it is found to be contributing significantly to the flexion deformity.

Division of sartorius

3

The origin of the sartorius from the anterior iliac spine and an adjoining 1 cm of the inguinal ligament medial to it is defined over a distance of 2 cm. The sartorius tendon is divided obliquely to allow for the possibility of suture with elongation at the end of the operation. A number of vessels require coagulation with diathermy. The conjoint tendon of rectus femoris at the junction of its straight and reflected heads is found beneath the sartorius. If it is tight, the tendon is defined by blunt dissection and also divided obliquely. If, with the knee extended, the rectus femoris is not tight, it should be left untouched, but, as release of hip flexors continues, especially after release of the iliopsoas tendon, its tension should be reviewed and division made if necessary.

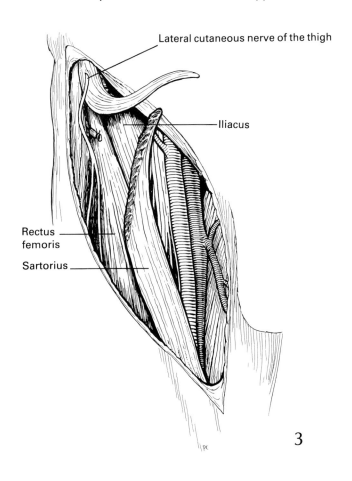

3

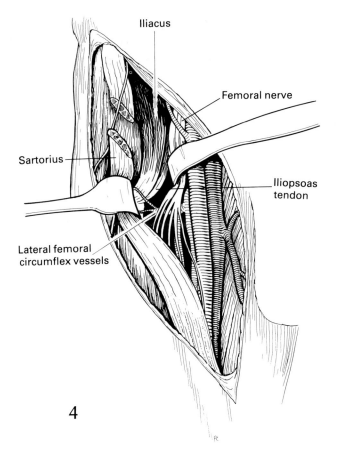

4

Anterolateral approach to the iliopsoas tendon

4

A thin layer of fascia immediately medial to the origin of the sartorius, attached to and just distal to the inguinal ligament, is incised and opened up with a haemostat to expose the femoral nerve as it emerges from beneath the inguinal ligament lying on the medial part of the iliacus muscle. The same fascial plane is extended distally to expose the branches of the femoral nerve. The hip is allowed to flex a little so that the nerve and its branches may be freed and retracted forwards and medially. In the distal third of the incision, the lateral femoral circumflex vessels cross the wound from the medial to the lateral side and must be divided and ligatured to allow further retraction of the femoral nerve and vessels to expose the iliopsoas tendon.

Division of iliopsoas tendon

5

The lesser trochanter should be palpated deeply on the medial side of the femur with the hip laterally rotated to facilitate this.

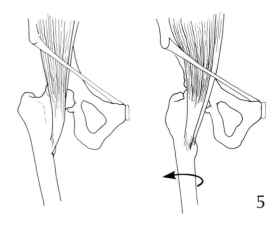

5

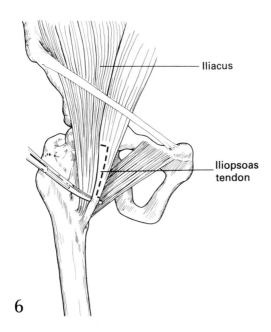

Iliacus

Iliopsoas tendon

6

6

If the lesser trochanter is not too posteriorly situated and lateral rotation and flexion of the hip allows it to be brought into view with the aid of deep retractors, elongation of the iliopsoas tendon or recession of it can be done as described on pp. 936–939.

If the lesser trochanter lies posteriorly, as it often does in paralytic conditions of the hip, adequate exposure by this approach is difficult or impossible. In that event, it is better to expose the iliopsoas tendon between the femoral nerve and the femoral vessels.

Alternative approach to the iliopsoas tendon

The femoral nerve and its proximal branches are exposed as in the preceding section. The most medial branch, the saphenous nerve, is traced distally by blunt dissection until it crosses the femoral artery. The femoral vessels are then exposed by opening the femoral sheath from this level proximally up to the level of the inguinal ligament.

7

The proximal part of the femoral nerve is retracted gently to the lateral side and the femoral vessels are retracted medially. The superficial circumflex iliac vessels arising from the lateral side of the femoral vessels are identified, divided between haemostats and either ligated or coagulated with diathermy. About 1 cm more distally, the profunda artery, and slightly more distally still, the profunda vein are exposed; the lateral femoral circumflex vessels passing laterally are identified with extreme gentleness and divided between haemostats and double ligated. The femoral and profunda vessels can then be easily retracted medially to expose the iliopsoas tendon deeply, passing down to the lesser trochanter. The tendon is defined, freed and lengthened or recessed as described on pages 936–939.

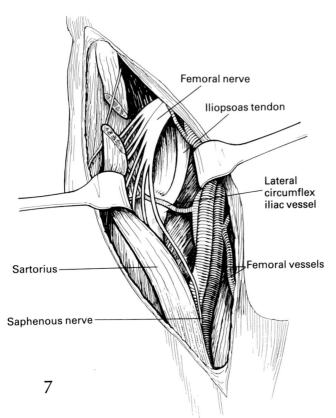

Femoral nerve

Iliopsoas tendon

Lateral circumflex iliac vessel

Sartorius

Femoral vessels

Saphenous nerve

7

Additional release

After division of the tensor fasciae latae, sartorius, rectus femoris and iliopsoas, an assessment is made of the degree of correction of the flexion deformity by flexing the opposite hip fully. If further correction is prevented by tightness of the femoral vessels and nerve, no further release of soft tissue is indicated and any additional correction can only be achieved by division and shortening of the femur. If the vessels and nerve are not unduly tight, the remaining flexion deformity may be due to tightness of the iliofemoral ligament which can be divided to provide a further, but limited amount of correction. Excessive division of the anterior capsule of the hip should be avoided lest it should result in anterior dislocation of the hip.

8

Wound closure

The tensor fascia latae is left unsutured. The sartorius is sutured with lengthening, either by attaching its obliquely cut ends to each other by two or three sutures or by suturing the distal end of the tendon to any available deep fascia. The rectus femoris tendon is similarly treated. It may be possible to close a layer of deep fascia, but, more usually in marked flexion deformity, it is only possible to suture the deep layer of superficial fascia and to close the skin with interrupted sutures or a continuous subcuticular suture. In children over the age of 6 years, one or two suction drains are inserted.

Immobilization

The hip is immobilized in maximum extension, neutral abduction and neutral rotation in a hip spica plaster cast extending to the toes on the operated side and to the knee on the opposite side.

Sartorius
Femoral nerve
Femoral vessels
Rectus femoris

8

Postoperative management

Intravenous dextrose saline infusion is continued for 24 hours, or, if necessary, additional blood is given if there was substantial loss during the operation. The circulation to the toes is kept under observation as is the upper thigh for any evidence of haematoma. Paralytic ileus is a rare but possible complication. Plaster immobilization is continued for 3½ to 4 weeks; it is not normally necessary to remove the sutures, even if they are non-absorbable, until the plaster cast is removed. Mobilization and physiotherapy treatment is started immediately after removal of the plaster spica.

Iliopsoas tendon lengthening or recession: medial (Ludloff) approach

W. J. W. Sharrard MD, ChM, FRCS
Emeritus Consultant Orthopaedic Surgeon, Royal Hallamshire Hospital and Children's Hospital, Sheffield; Professor of Orthopaedic Surgery, University of Sheffield, UK

Preoperative

Indications and assessment

The main indication for operation on the iliopsoas tendon is flexion deformity of the hip of 20°–40° owing to strong and possibly spastic iliopsoas and hip flexor muscles in the presence of weaker hip extensors in cerebral palsy, myelomeningocele, poliomyelitis or other paralytic conditions. Flexion and adduction deformity are often combined together so that adductor and flexor release are both needed, possibly combined with posterior transfer of the adductors to the ischium. If so, this approach is the recommended one. Assessment is made as described in the chapter on 'Hip flexor release: the iliofemoral approach' (pp. 931–935) and should confirm that there is no excessive tightness of the tensor fasciae latae or sartorius.

Anaesthesia and position of patient

General anaesthesia is needed. The degree of fixed flexion and adduction should be confirmed under anaesthesia. The patient is placed supine with a small sandbag under the affected hip. The approach to the iliopsoas tendon is made easier if the hip is flexed and laterally rotated during the operation. Skin preparation and the application of drapes is as for adductor release (see chapter on 'Adductor release' pp. 926–930).

Operation

Incision

1

The incision is the same as for adductor release with a distal extension of the medial end of the incision to allow sufficient distal mobilization of the lower flap.

Exposure

The deep fascia is incised and the muscles exposed as for adductor release (see p. 927). If adductor release is required, this is done first. If only iliopsoas lengthening or recession is needed, it can be performed through this approach if the adductors are relaxed and the knee semiflexed to allow their retraction.

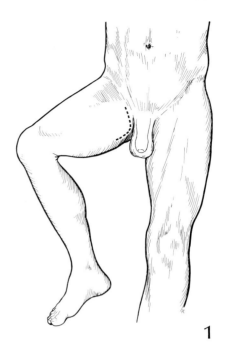

1

Approach to the iliopsoas tendon

2

The approach, originally attributed to Ludloff[1], was described for iliopsoas release by Keats and Morgese[2]. The plane between the adductor longus and pectineus anteriorly and the gracilis and adductor brevis posteriorly is opened up by blunt dissection. The iliopsoas tendon and the lesser trochanter are obscured by a layer of fat. The lesser trochanter is palpated beneath this fat layer on the posteromedial aspect of the femur and its position confirmed by rotation of the thigh.

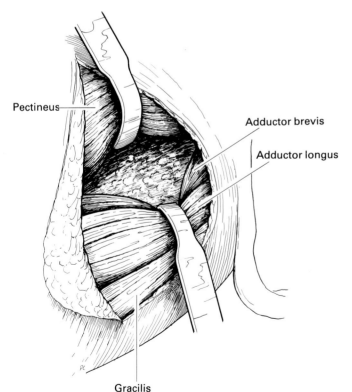

Pectineus

Adductor brevis

Adductor longus

Gracilis

2

3

Deep retractors are placed to expose the lesser trochanter, which is covered by a layer of fascia and fat which needs to be lightly incised: one or two small vessels need to be coagulated. The direction of the iliopsoas tendon as it passes from the pelvis to the lesser trochanter needs to be appreciated: the tendon runs almost vertically from above downwards and backwards. Once the plane of the tendon has been defined, it can be cleared proximally to visualize 5–7 cm of its length. Branches of the medial femoral circumflex vessels cross the tendon about 1 cm above the lesser trochanter and may need to be divided and coagulated by diathermy.

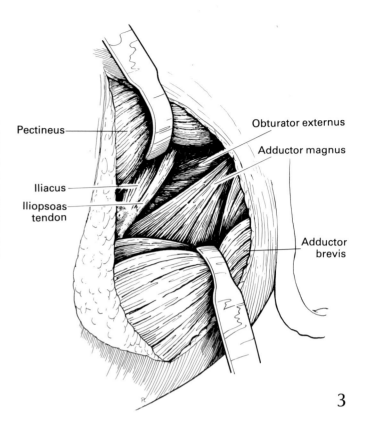

3

Procedure

4

The tendinous part of the iliopsoas tendon needs to be defined from the muscular fibres of the iliacus which lie lateral to the tendon and are inserted into it and to the femur just above the lesser trochanter. The iliopsoas tendon is often present as two bands: a more superficial one attached to the lesser trochanter and a deeper one which passes more posteriorly to be attached to the shaft of the femur. A pair of long-handled curved artery forceps is insinuated between the tendon and the femoral shaft just above the lesser trochanter to lift it up and to allow the precise definition of its deep surface.

4

5

If sufficient tendon is available, it can be divided by a Z-incision over a distance of 4–5 cm. If there are two well-defined bands they can be used as the two portions of tendon for lengthening, dividing the anterior band from the lesser trochanter and the deep band as far proximally as possible. Before the two portions of the tendon are divided, the ends should be secured by Kocher's forceps. The proximal portion is likely to retract into the depths of the wound proximally. Confirmation of correction of the flexion deformity is made by flexing the opposite hip fully (Thomas' test). The ends of the tendon are approximated and sutured to each other by two or three stout non-absorbable sutures using a small curved needle.

If the iliopsoas tendon is too short or exposure of a sufficient length is not possible, the iliacus fibres are not separated from the tendon. The iliopsoas tendon is divided just above the lesser trochanter and allowed to stretch. If the iliacus fibres prove to be too tight, they can be sectioned as well but it is usually better to leave the iliacus to prevent too much proximal displacement of the iliopsoas tendon. Alternatively, the proximal end of the tendon can be sutured more proximally to the anterior aspect of the hip capsule near the base of the femoral neck as an iliopsoas recession[3].

Because the dissection takes place between muscle planes, blood loss is minimal and blood transfusion is not normally required.

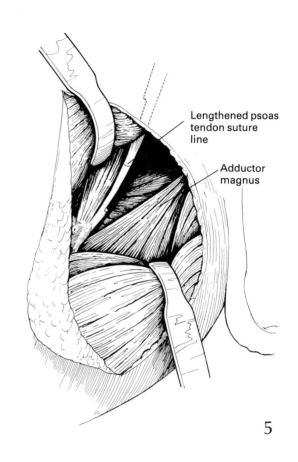

Lengthened psoas tendon suture line

Adductor magnus

5

Wound closure

The wound is closed in the same way as for adductor release (*see* p. 929). If the preoperative flexion deformity was 30° or less and the hip is not significantly unstable, no plaster fixation is required. A crêpe hip spica bandage is applied. If there is more severe deformity or hip instability a plaster hip spica may be needed (*see* chapter on 'Hip flexor release: iliofemoral approach', pp. 931–935).

Postoperative management

Rest in bed either prone or supine is needed for 3 weeks, with pillows between the thighs if plaster is not used. If there is considerable spasm in spastic patients, diazepam is a useful drug for its control after operation. Gentle passive hip movements and active hip extension exercises can be started on the second or third day. The skin sutures are removed after 10–12 days. Active mobilization and return to preoperative activities can start after the third week.

References

1. Ludloff K. Zur blutigen Einrenkung der angeborenen Hüftluxation. *Z Orthop Chir* 1908; 22: 272–6.

2. Keats S, Morgese AN. A simple anteromedial approach to the lesser trochanter of the femur for the release of the iliopsoas tendon. *J Bone Joint Surg [Am]* 1967; 49-A: 632–6.

3. Bleck EE. Postural and gait abnormalities caused by hip-flexion deformity in spastic cerebral palsy: treatment by iliopsoas recession. *J Bone Joint Surg [Am]* 1971; 53-A: 1468–88.

Illustrations by Peter Cox after F. Price

Proximal hamstring release

W. J. W. Sharrard   MD, ChM, FRCS
Emeritus Consultant Orthopaedic Surgeon, Royal Hallamshire Hospital and Children's Hospital, Sheffield;
Professor of Orthopaedic Surgery, University of Sheffield, UK

Preoperative

Indications and assessment

The indication for this operation is limited to shortness of the hamstring muscle in the absence of significant flexion deformity of the knee in cerebral palsy or other paralytic conditions. The effect is to cause limitation of hip flexion, so that the patient's length of stride is much reduced and he has to walk with flexed knees or with rotation of the pelvis or both. He cannot sit with the knees extended. The degree of shortness is assessed either by determining the range of straight-leg raising, that is flexion of the hip with the knee extended, or the limitation of extension of the knee when the hip is flexed to a right angle. Straight-leg raising of less than 35° or limitation of extension of the knee by 35° or more when the hip is flexed is an indication for operation. If there is more than 20° of limitation of knee extension when the hip is extended, distal hamstring release is preferable (*see* pp. 981–984). Proximal hamstring release is also contraindicated when there is marked lumbar lordosis, which may be increased by proximal hamstring release.

Anaesthesia and position of patient

General anaesthesia is needed. The shortness of the hamstring is confirmed under anaesthesia. The patient is placed prone with the pelvis elevated on sandbags and the hip flexed 30°–40° by breaking the operating table. A diathermy pad is applied. The skin is prepared. The lower limbs up to the level of the mid-thigh are covered by sterile stockinette and drapes are placed to expose the distal part of the buttock and the upper half of the posterior aspect of the thigh. The operative area may be covered by a transparent adhesive drape.

Operation

Incision

1

A transverse incision is made in the natal fold 2.5 cm distal to the ischial tuberosity over medial two-thirds of the posterior aspect of the thigh. The incision is deepened through subcutaneous fat, which is often thick, down to the deep fascia from which it is mobilized proximally and distally for 6 or 7 cm in each direction.

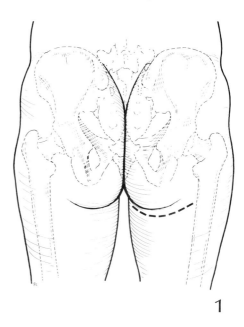

1

Gluteus maximus

Quadratus
femoris

Sciatic nerve

Biceps and semitendinosus

Semimembranosus

2

Exposure of the hamstring tendons

2

The lower border of the gluteus maximus is defined, separated from the deep fascia and mobilized upwards and laterally. Care must be taken to avoid damage to the sciatic nerve which lies deep to the gluteus maximus. The ischial tuberosity is palpated and the site of the hamstring tendons arising from it and running distally is established. A vertical incision is made through the deep fascia overlying the tendons which are cleared over a distance of 6 or 7 cm and their origin from the ischial tuberosity is defined. The long head of biceps arises in common with the semitendinosus from the inferomedial facet of the ischial tuberosity, and the semimembranosus arises from the superolateral facet expanding into an aponeurosis closely associated with the other two tendons. The sciatic nerve should be identified and a tape passed beneath it with which to retract it laterally. Occasionally the nerve may present in its two main branches at this level.

Musculotendinous division

3

The more superficial tendon arising from the ischial tuberosity is the common tendon of the long head of biceps and semitendinosus. It is divided by a long incision as oblique as possible, the proximal end of the distal fragment being held by Kocher's forceps to prevent its excessive distal retraction. The tendon and upper aponeurosis of the semimembranosus is similarly exposed and divided. If the adductor magnus tendon is tight, it, too, can be divided at its attachment to the ischial tuberosity and allowed to retract. The tips of the elongated hamstring tendons are sutured by thick non-absorbable sutures. The tendons should not be allowed to retract or there is a danger of excessive lengthening and the production of pelvic lordosis. Bleeding is not usually significant and any small vessels can be coagulated by diathermy.

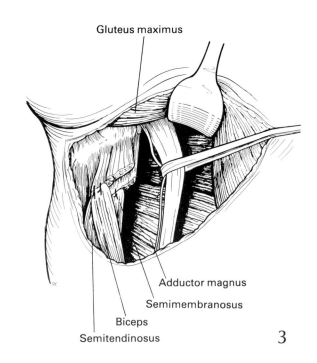

3

Wound closure

The deep fascia is closed vertically by interrupted or continuous non-absorbable sutures and the subcutaneous tissue is closed by absorbable interrupted sutures in a transverse line. The skin is closed by interrupted sutures or continuous subcuticular sutures. A simple adhesive dressing is applied.

Postoperative management

For the first 24 hours, the patient is nursed supine. After this the patient is encouraged to sit in bed with the hips progressively flexed by 20° more per day whilst the knees are kept straight by means of a draw sheet. He is allowed to lie in a straight supine posture at night. In younger children, in whom it may be difficult to keep the knees extended, or in patients with considerable spasm, a plaster backslab or a plastic splint may be needed to keep the knees extended, and diazepam may help to limit muscle spasm.

The sutures are removed on the tenth to twelfth day. By the end of the second week, straight-leg raising should reach 90° and walking can be resumed, using, if necessary, a simple brace to maintain knee extension for 2 or 3 weeks.

Further reading

Reimers J. Contracture of the hamstrings in cerebral palsy: a study of the three methods of operative correction. *J Bone Joint Surg [Br]* 1974; 56-B: 102–9.

Seymour N, Sharrard WJW. Bilateral proximal hamstring release of the hamstrings in cerebral palsy. *J Bone Joint Surg [Br]* 1968; 50-B: 274–7.

Illustrations by Robert Lane and Gillian Lee

Total hip replacement arthroplasty

Kevin Hardinge   MChOrth, FRCS
Hunterian Professor, Royal College of Surgeons of England; Honorary Lecturer, Victoria University of Manchester;
Consultant Orthopaedic Surgeon, Centre for Hip Surgery, Wrightington Hospital, Wigan, UK

Introduction

Cemented total hip replacement is firmly established as a highly successful procedure giving total relief of pain and good movement in painful osteoarthritis from a variety of causes for periods up to 15 years. Infection rate is low and the chief problem is component loosening. Longer-lasting prostheses wear more, producing particles which cause inflammation and bone resorption leading to loosening. New, low-wear materials will be required in future. The early promise of uncemented prostheses, which should be easy to revise in the absence of cement, has been marred by slow recovery from operation and persistent thigh pain.

Indications

Total hip replacement aims to eradicate pain and stiffness in the operated hip and restore a physiological gait. To obtain this goal there must be optimum conditions for joint visualization, cementation, implant orientation and correction of leg length inequality.

The total hip arthroplasty, using a stemmed femoral component and an ultra-high molecular weight polyethylene (UHMWPE) acetabular cup, has the longest record of proven benefit in the treatment of degenerative arthrosis of the hip. The components are bonded to the bone by methylmethacrylate cement and this bond depends upon an intimate interdigitation of the cement with cancellous bone, producing sound mechanical interlocking – the bond responding well to compression but poorly to tension and shear.

A femoral component with a head of small diameter is an essential feature of the Charnley low-friction arthroplasty as the low frictional torque reduces shear at the cement–bone interface of both the acetabular component and the femoral stem. The small-diameter component needs precise orientation to minimize postoperative dislocation.

Primary osteoarthrosis

1a & b

The total hip arthroplasty was originally indicated for 'idiopathic' osteoarthrosis in old patients because of the limited lifespan of the procedure: these patients may have loss of joint space, sclerosis of bone and marginal osteophytes, leading to pain and stiffness. However, the success of the operation in this group of patients has led to the application of the technique to a greater variety of pathological abnormalities.

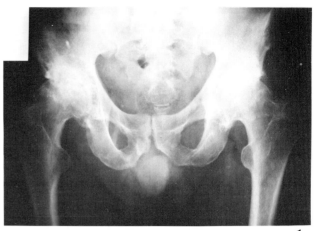

1a

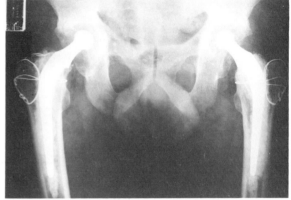

1b

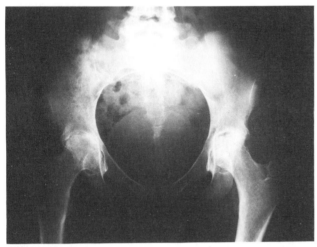

2a

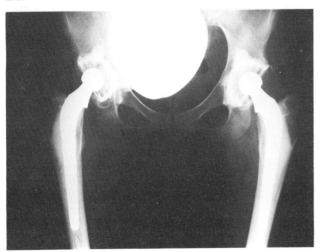

2b

Rheumatoid arthritis

2a & b

The earliest alternative application was for rheumatoid arthritis where the hip degeneration can be severe. Many of these patients are young but the alternative to operation can be a wheelchair existence. The lady depicted in the illustration was 27 years old, having suffered with rheumatoid arthritis since the age of 11 years. The arthroplasties have been performed using the direct lateral approach. It is noteworthy that the pre-operative film shows that Shenton's line is almost intact, thus leg length discrepancy is not marked. The post-operative film shows complete restoration of Shenton's line; good walking ability was restored.

Ankylosing spondylitis

3a & b

Ankylosing spondylitis affects young adults presenting usually with pain and stiffness in the spine. Spontaneous fusion of the hip was frequently seen formerly and was possibly due to prolonged immobilization. The preoperative illustration shows fusion of the sacroiliac joints, which is diagnostic of ankylosing spondylitis; the hips have also fused, in addition to the symphysis pubis. Note how Shenton's line is intact, indicating that the hips have fused in the anatomical position[1]. The mobilization of this fusion and conversion to total hip arthroplasty can be a difficult technical procedure, but it is certainly made easier by the wide exposure gained from trochanteric osteotomy. The postoperative radiograph shows the appearance after bilateral total hip arthroplasty where trochanteric osteotomy has been employed to facilitate the exposure and femoral neck section.

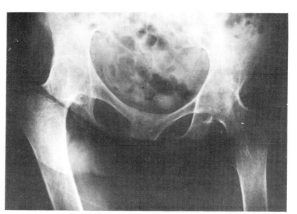

3a

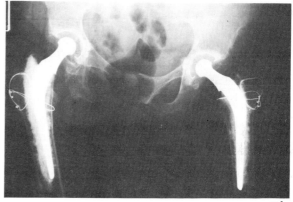

3b

Protrusio acetabuli

4, 5a & b

Stress fracture of the medial wall of the acetabulum with subsequent healing can occur idiopathically or in rheumatoid arthritis, Paget's disease, ankylosing spondylitis or osteoarthritis. It is typified radiologically by the medial wall of the acetabulum being shown to have protruded past the ilio-ischial line (Y–Y). The medial acetabular wall may become fragmented and total hip replacement may be technically difficult because of the lack of constraint on the fixation of the prosthetic cup. Grafting the medial wall with slices taken from the femoral head constitutes a useful method of containing the cement.

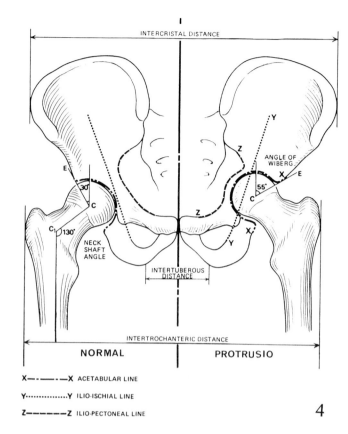

X—·—·—X ACETABULAR LINE

Y·············Y ILIO-ISCHIAL LINE

Z— — — — —Z ILIO-PECTONEAL LINE

4

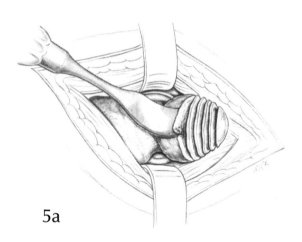

5a

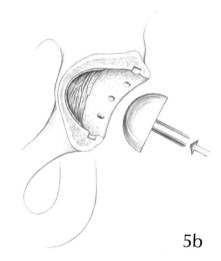

5b

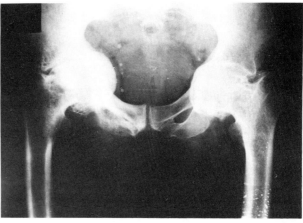

6a

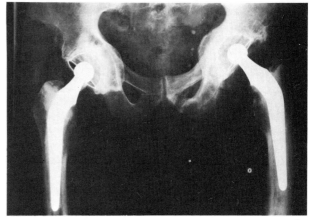

6b

6a & b

This method was used in a 67-year-old man who had suffered gradually increasing pain and stiffness in the hips for 10 years, having enjoyed an exceptional level of physical activity until the age of 50 years[2]: he had medial migration of the acetabular walls, with thick sclerotic bases to the acetabula. As a result of the bone graft allowing the cup to be lateralized to the face of the pelvis, Shenton's line was restored, and the patient has become much more mobile.

The bone graft has become incorporated with the fragmented medial acetabular wall and remodelled so the the pelvic brim (ilio-pectineal line)is restored to normal.

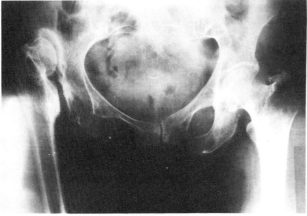

7a

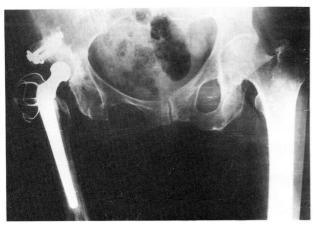

7b

Congenital dislocation of the hip

7a & b

Congenital dislocation of the hip occurs when there is variable disproportion between the head of the femur and the acetabulum. In many cases the head has never been in the true acetabulum, and indeed moulds a false acetabulum on the side of the ilium. Secondary degenerative arthrosis can supervene in the third and fourth decade and impose a severe restriction on walking as a result of pain and stiffness. The acetabulum in these cases is abnormally small and a bone graft, taken from the head of the femur and bolted to the side of the ilium, can provide an improved bone cover for the prosthetic acetabular cup. Clearly, in these cases a wide exposure is mandatory and can be obtained using a trochanteric osteotomy.

Degenerative hip conditions due to old sepsis

8a & b

Septic arthritis and tuberculous hip disease lead to a variable damage of the articular surfaces. This joint damage can lead, after full healing of the primary infection, to a secondary degenerative arthrosis or to a spontaneous fusion in the healing process. In this case, after a tuberculous infection of both hips in childhood, there has been spontaneous fusion of the right hip in marked abduction with ossification of the sacrospinous ligament, and a severe degenerative arthrosis of the left hip in marked adduction. The right hip was not painful because it was fused. The left hip was very painful and was the primary reason for the patient's referral. There was flexion contracture of both hips and lumbar lordosis. It is important to note that the symptoms in the left hip are due to the position of marked adduction producing a subluxation that is *secondary* to the deformity of the right hip. It could be incorrect to offer a total hip arthroplasty for the left hip alone as it would still function in marked adduction and would be in danger of dislocating.

It was necessary to correct the primary deformity; in this case, converting the right hip to a total arthroplasty with correction of the abduction deformity, so that the subsequent arthroplasty of the left hip could function in a more neutral position. The pelvic tilt and lordosis were thus reduced and mobility increased.

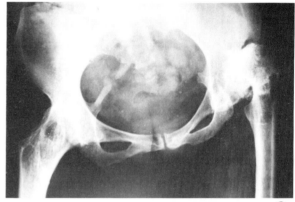

8a

Criteria for arthroplasty after infection

Clearly it is important to avoid reactivation of a pre-existing septic or tuberculous infection as the total hip arthroplasty would fail. It is vital to ensure that the previous infection is cured and this can be achieved with a high level of certainty using clinical, radiological and haematological criteria[3].

Clinically, the patient must have a clear-cut history of the infective condition and have recovered from it. This course of events may have entailed from 1 to several years in hospital or under treatment, but been followed by complete subsidence of the infection and the restoration of walking with useful function. The history must also reveal that the period of recovery and improvement in function has lasted several years. If the patient's symptoms are due to the supervention of secondary arthritis there will also typically be a gradual decline in overall function over a period of years. The onset of pain and stiffness will have been in the remote past and both will have gradually increased in severity. Physical examination shows stiffness of the joint without local signs of inflammation and an absence of spasm.

The radiographs show sound bony ankylosis in these cases with spontaneous fusion of the joint or, if the joint is mobile, loss of joint space, sclerosis of joint surfaces and marginal osteophytosis. The haematological tests should show a normal erythrocyte sedimentation rate and white cell count. It is important to repeat the radiographs and blood tests after a 6-month period when it should be possible to establish that the patient's symptoms are due to secondary degenerative arthrosis, and that total hip arthroplasty is a safe procedure.

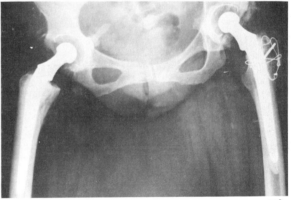

8b

9a & b

Where septic arthritis before skeletal maturity has led to severe bone destruction and limb shortening, it is not always possible to restore the leg length fully, because of tension in the pelvifemoral intermuscular septa. In a similar way, active movement will not be full and a limp will persist as a result of the overall limb-length discrepancy. It must be emphasized to the patient that total hip arthroplasty in the presence of severe bone destruction cannot fully restore movement and limb length, and must be considered 'a limited goal' procedure. There can, however, occasionally be quite gratifying results after septic arthritis of the hip in infancy has caused loss of the head of the femur. The illustration shows a hip that had always been mobile, and it was possible to restore leg length by total hip arthroplasty.

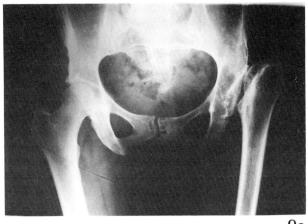

9a

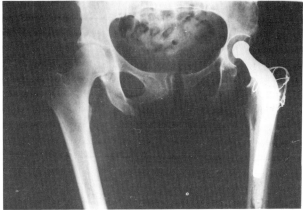

9b

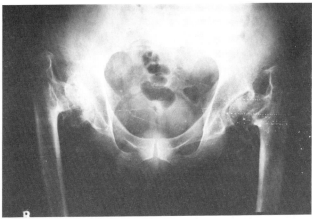

10a

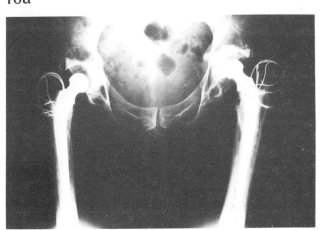

10b

Congenital hip dysplasia other than dislocation

10a & b

Infantile coxa vara can present as an idiopathic condition or may be present in association with craniocleidodysostosis. Both these conditions, and also multiple epiphyseal dysplasia, can lead to a severe secondary degenerative arthrosis in the fourth and fifth decade: the patient illustrated could not abduct the hip, so that ankle separation was limited to 12 cm. Considerable improvement in function can be bestowed by total hip arthroplasty, but it is necessary to improve exposure by performing trochanteric osteotomy in these cases of distorted anatomy.

The secondary degenerative arthrosis that follows Perthes' disease and slipped upper femoral epiphysis does not require variation in surgical technique, and will not be considered separately.

Failed previous surgery

11a & b

The success and dependability of the total hip arthroplasty in primary and secondary arthrosis has led to wide application in cases where surgery has failed.

In the decade before successful total hip arthroplasty, a variety of surgical methods were employed to treat osteoarthrosis. The illustration shows the result of attempted fusion of the hip in osteoarthrosis by the use of a transarticular pin (which broke) and an ischiofemoral graft (which also fractured). Movement of the joint still occurred, and caused severe local pain. Impressive relief of pain resulted from conversion of the unsound fusion to a total hip arthroplasty, when, to improve exposure, a trochanteric osteotomy was performed[4,5].

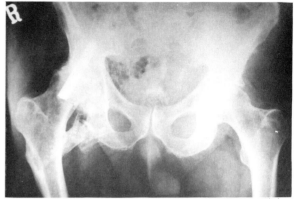

11a

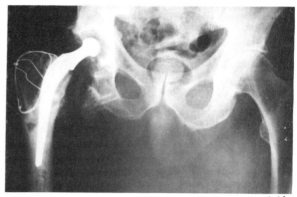

11b

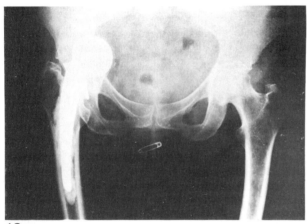

12a

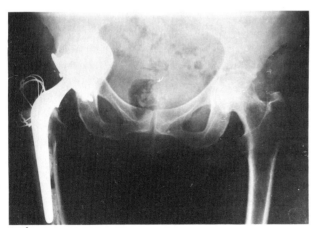

12b

12a & b

Femoral head replacement after fracture of the neck of the femur has been the method of choice where wide separation of the capital fragment has occurred and reduction is poor. On occasion the femoral replacement can loosen, migrate upwards, erode the acetabulum and penetrate the pelvis. In one patient there was a large defect of the base of the acetabulum and the femoral head was not available to use for grafting. When the total hip arthroplasty was performed, a metallic reinforcement ring was used to support the prosthetic acetabular cup, and when placed into the acetabulum prevented migration of the cement used for fixation. Before the total hip arthroplasty, this patient had had severe leg length discrepancy due to migration of the prosthetic head which had occurred within 12–18 months of operation. After this relatively short history and previous normal leg length, it was possible to restore equality.

The original indication for total hip arthroplasty was severe degenerative osteoarthrosis of the hip in the elderly. Yet a large group of patients in their seventh decade had pain in the hip, stiffness and a limp due to shortening of the limb as a result of destruction of the joint surfaces. Initially, the procedure was confined to the elderly because it was felt that the lifespan of the implant was limited to at most 10 years, but the success of the early results led to a cautious extension of the time period, and use in the younger patient.

Surgical approaches

General principles

Surgical exposure of the hip joint must take account of muscle innervation and blood supply and must avoid, if possible, detachment of muscle insertions, since detachment prolongs recovery time and increases morbidity. Thus, the advantage of any approach that minimizes muscle detachment must be contrasted with the disadvantage that may arise from limited exposure which may necessitate heavy soft tissue retraction. Poor visibility of the joint cavity may similarly lead to poor orientation of the implants so that movement may be compromised or instability and dislocation occur.

Orientation of the implant to the bony pelvis is certainly facilitated if the patient is placed in the supine position. In this way the anterior superior iliac spine and the greater trochanter can be palpated through the surgical drapes and thus implant orientation can be facilitated by alignment to the horizontal plane, and leg length equalization promoted by direct comparison to the contralateral limb. The supine position is used in the original technique of McKee, Müller and Charnley while the lateral decubitus position is employed for the posterior approaches to the hip joint.

An appreciation of the development of the various surgical approaches to the hip joint in an historical sense serves to emphasize their original indication and can illustrate potential shortcomings. For example, Moore's southern exposure[6] was originally described for insertion of the self-locking femoral head prosthesis, and while it is adequate for this purpose it does not give a sufficient view of the acetabulum for total hip arthroplasty. In addition, the acetabulum is anteverted or anteriorly disposed to a varying extent, and necessitating as it does the lateral decubitus position, the posterior approach of Moore does not facilitate accurate orientation of the implant.

The anterolateral approach of Watson-Jones[7] was originally described for open reduction of fractures of the neck of the femur; although it gives good exposure of the neck of the femur, exposure of the acetabulum depends upon heavy retraction of the soft tissue and can be associated with damage to the femoral vein, artery and nerve, particularly in obese patients or those with well-developed musculature. Similarly access to the femur is possible only with the femur held in strong lateral rotation, adduction and flexion, so that orientation of the femoral component may be difficult.

The lateral approach with trochanteric osteotomy, the patient lying in the supine position, has always been associated with Charnley[8]. Trochanteric osteotomy has been the traditional approach used in hip surgery in Manchester, having been brought from Boston, Massachusetts, by Platt where he had worked with Brackett and also visited Whitman in New York. It has the advantage of a wide exposure of the hip for correction of deformity, implant orientation, and leg length equalization.

Trochanteric osteosynthesis remains a difficult problem, particularly with scarred tissue and osteoporotic bone. In Charnley's hand the level of complication was accepted, but trochanteric osteotomy has not been widely practised, except by a few devotees[9].

The direct lateral approach[10] developed from that described by McFarland and Osborne[11], offers the advantages of the supine position, without trochanteric osteotomy, and adequate exposure of the acetabulum and femur for implant orientation and leg length equalization, but is suitable only for the patient without severe deformity or marked leg length inequality (the 'anatomical' hip). These patients account for 85 per cent of primary arthritic hips. It has distinct advantages in this respect over the anterolateral and posterior approaches.

Anterior approaches to the hip were described by Smith-Petersen[12] and others. They were used exclusively for the original cup arthroplasty and by Wagner[13] for his double-cup arthroplasty. The approach has not gained popularity with other surgeons because of the need for extensive detachment of tendinous insertions and retraction of muscle, with potential damage to vital structures such as femoral artery and nerve, and because of traction exerted on the lateral cutaneous nerve of the thigh, causing numbness or meralgia paraesthetica. Whereas the Smith-Petersen approach can be recommended for operation on the innominate bones (Chiari and Salter osteotomy), it is not recommended for total hip arthroplasty as better exposures exist.

POSTERIOR APPROACH

Anatomical considerations

13

The muscles covering the posterior aspect of the hip joint form two layers. The outer layer, the 'pelvic deltoid of Henry'[14], is the gluteus maximus, the largest muscle in the body; the fascia lata covers the gluteus medius and the tensor fasciae latae forms a continuous muscle sheath. This outer layer can be incised at different points, each of which changes the surgical approach.

The Moore or southern exposure splits the gluteus maximus at the junction of the anterior and intermediate thirds, and because of poor access to the acetabulum is not advised for total hip arthroplasty.

The Gibson approach[15] is in the inter-nervous plane between gluteus maximus (inferior gluteal nerve) and gluteus medius (superior gluteal nerve). Whereas the Gibson approach detaches gluteus medius and minimus from the greater trochanter, the further refinement of Marcy and Fletcher[16] leaves the gluteus medius and minimus insertions intact and effects dislocation by strong flexion and medial rotation.

The deep layer of muscle consists of the short lateral rotators of the hip, the piriformis, the superior gamellus, the obturator internus, the inferior gamellus and the quadratus femoris. The sciatic nerve runs down through the operative field between the layers closely applied to the posterior capsule of the hip joint.

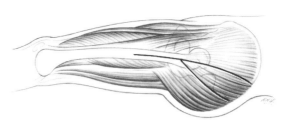

13

Position of patient

14

The patient is placed in the true mid-lateral position with the affected limb uppermost. The limb is draped free to allow for movement and manipulation during the procedure.

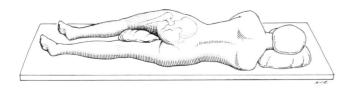

14

Incision

15

The greater trochanter forms the landmark for the incision and the posterior edge can be palpated through the drapes.

The incision is 12–15 cm long, curved and centres on the greater trochanter. Its starts 6–8 cm above and posterior to the greater trochanter, in line with the posterior superior iliac spine, and passes towards the trochanter in the same direction as the fibres of the gluteus maximus. The incision curves over the posterior aspect of the greater trochanter and continues down along the shaft of the femur for 6–8 cm.

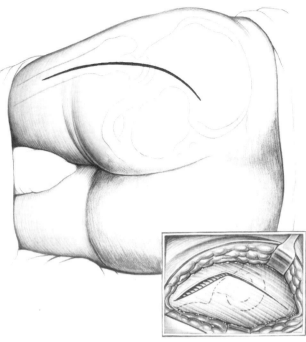

15

Superficial dissection

16

The fascia lata on the lateral aspect of the femur is incised and this fascial incision is developed proximally and enters the plane between gluteus maximus and gluteus medius. The fibres of the gluteus maximus are coarser than gluteus medius and the plane is developed between them to split the fascia and open it up. In this way the blades of the retractors are placed on the gluteus maximus and gluteus medius to avoid traction on the sciatic nerve which will not be exposed in this procedure, although it can be palpated in the fat lying in the posterior aspect of the deeper space.

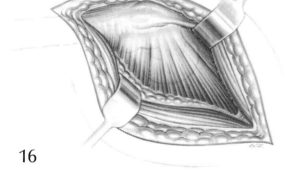

16

Deep dissection

17

The space between the gluteus medius and gluteus maximus is floored by the short lateral rotators which cover the posterior aspect of the hip joint. The thigh is medially rotated to stretch the short lateral rotators and to distance the deep incision from the sciatic nerve.

Stay sutures are inserted into the piriformis and obturator internus tendons before their insertion to leave a skirt of tendon inserted into the femur for later suture. The tendons are divided to expose the neck of the femur and laid over the sciatic nerve to protect it. Part of quadratus femoris may need to be divided, at which point troublesome bleeding from the lateral circumflex femoral artery can be encountered.

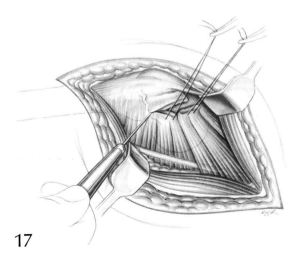

17

18

The capsule of the hip joint is now exposed and is longitudinally incised; if the hip is stiff part of the posterior capsule is excised to permit dislocation by medial rotation of the femur. With excision of the capsule and placement of the Hohmann's retractors, the acetabulum is exposed.

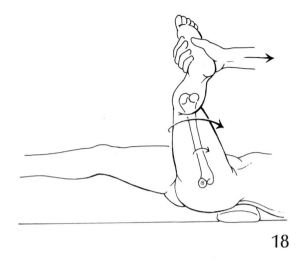

18

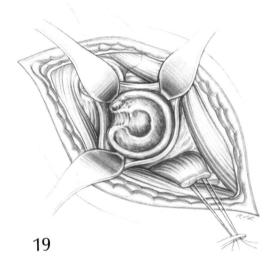

19

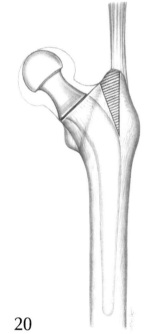

20

19 & 20

The femoral head is excised by Gigli saw or oscillating saw and the femur is prepared for insertion of the prosthesis by removal of bone at the trochanteric fossa.

21

Clearly alignment of the acetabular component depends upon the patient being firmly secured in the true lateral decubitus position, whilst the femoral prosthesis is inserted with the femur held in full medial rotation.

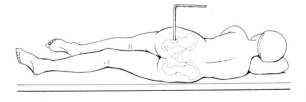

21

THE ANTEROLATERAL APPROACH

Anatomical considerations

The fascia lata covers all the thigh and hamstring muscles; it covers the sartorius and then splits into a deep and superficial layer to enclose the tensor fasciae latae and the gluteus maximus. The gluteus medius is covered by the fascia lata on its superficial surface only and is not enveloped by it.

The anterolateral approach develops the intermuscular plane between the tensor fasciae latae and the gluteus medius. The origins of the two muscles are almost continuous but they diverge towards their insertions.

The tensor fasciae latae arises superficially from the anterior portion of the outer lip of the iliac crest and inserts into the iliotibial band; whereas the gluteus medius, arising from the outer surface of the ilium between the anterior and posterior gluteal lines, inserts deeply into the anterior and lateral aspects of the greater trochanter. They share a common nerve supply from the superior gluteal nerve.

To exploit this intermuscular plane, the overlying fascia is incised below the posterior margin of the tensor fasciae latae, so that, because the fascia lata envelops the tensor muscle, retracting the fascia takes the muscle up with it. The nerve supply lies in the interval and can be damaged inadvertently as the capsule is exposed.

Position of patient

The patient is placed in the supine position, although some proponents place a small pillow beneath the buttocks on the operative side[17] or slightly tilt the table to raise the buttocks[18].

Incision

22

The incision begins 2 cm distal and 2 cm posterior to the anterior superior iliac spine, curves distally and laterally to the apex of the greater trochanter, and extends down over the greater trochanter to end 6 cm distal to the vastus lateralis ridge.

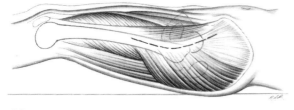

22

Superficial dissection

23

The deep fascia is incised over the femur distally to the greater trochanter, and the incision continued proximally keeping to the palpable posterior lower border of the tensor fasciae latae. As the cut edge of the fascia lata, with its contained tensor fasciae latae, is brought forwards, the anterior border of the gluteus medius is exposed. The plane between the two muscles is now developed by blunt dissection using the fingers. There are blood vessels in this plane that need to be coagulated.

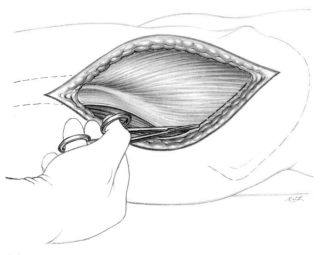

23

24

A retractor placed on the anterior border of the gluteus medius muscle border retracts the muscle posteriorly to expose the fat lying on the hip capsule.

The femur should now be fully rotated laterally to stretch the capsule. The upper border of the vastus lateralis is thus exposed at the anterior surface of the femoral neck and reflected for 1 cm, extending down to the vastus lateralis ridge laterally.

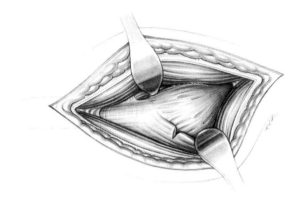

24

Deep dissection

25

The capsule is visible at this stage and further exposure is only possible with full lateral rotation of the femur and release of the neck of the femur to allow the neck to fall backwards. This is necessary to facilitate exposure of the acetabulum and femoral reaming.

A stay suture is placed into the anterior border of gluteus medius tendon, leaving a skirt of tendon attached to the trochanter for later reattachment. The exact amount of gluteus medius that needs to be detached in this way will vary with the stiffness of the hip and anatomical distortion, but this clearly represents a limitation of the surgical exposure.

A complete capsulectomy is then performed, including the fibres of the reflected head of rectus femoris and vastus lateralis apex inferiorly. Anterior dislocation can now be facilitated by removal of the osteophytes with nibblers followed by traction, lateral rotation and adduction; the neck is sectioned at the desired level with a Gigli saw.

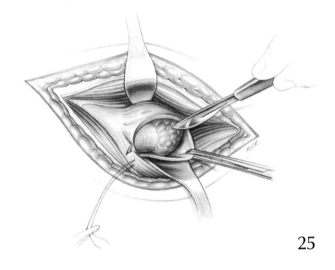

25

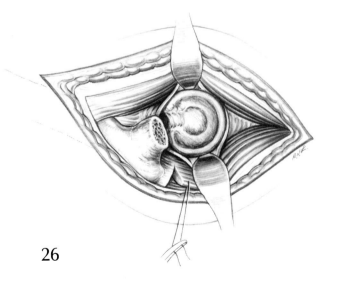

26

The exposure of the acetabulum is then completed by Hohmann retractors placed anteriorly, posteriorly and inferiorly, whilst access to the femur is promoted by full lateral rotation after partial detachment of the gluteus medius insertion.

26

THE DIRECT LATERAL APPROACH

Anatomical considerations

The direct lateral approach, with or without trochanteric osteotomy, and with the patient lying in the supine position, offers the optimum conditions for joint visualization, adequate cementation, implant orientation and correction of leg length discrepancy.

If there has been a previous arthroplasty, previous surgery such as an intertrochanteric osteotomy, arthrodesis or if there is severe anatomical deformity such as occurs in osteoarthrosis secondary to congenital hip dysplasia or coxa vara, then trochanteric osteotomy gives the preferred wide exposure to the hip joint and ilium to deal with the distorted anatomy. Trochanteric osteosynthesis remains a difficult procedure and problems can occur postoperatively with trochanteric detachment, wire breakage and trochanteric bursitis. If the degenerative arthrosis has occurred in a hip that has an 'anatomical' appearance, then trochanteric osteotomy is not necessary.

A strong physiological gait should be possible in this group of patients if an attempt is made to restore Shenton's line, thus ensuring that all of the pelvifemoral muscles are able to act in a normal fashion. There has been a tendency in the past to concentrate on abductor power only; it must be realized, however, that strong hip function is dependent upon all of the muscle groups that act around the hip joint. If the centre of the axis of rotation of the total hip replacement (the locus) is sited at the centre of the head of the femur, and thus Shenton's line is restored, then excellent function can be expected to return as a result of rehabilitation.

Optimum joint visualization with the patient in the supine position ensures the following.

1. Accurate implant orientation – which permits a maximum range of movement without instability leading to dislocation
2. Adequate cementation – with pressurization in an attempt to ensure a long-term bond that will reduce implant loosening
3. Leg length equalization – the use of bony landmarks enables direct comparison to aid accurate correction of leg length which, combined with correct lateralization, helps to produce a physiological gait.

The gluteus medius tendon blends into the greater trochanter by a crescentic insertion. Taking a pair of blunt forceps it is possible to demonstrate the mobile tendon of the gluteus medius insertion as it merges with the periosteum of the greater trochanter.

Position of patient

The patient is placed in the supine position, with the greater trochanter lying at the edge of the table, thus freeing the buttock muscles from the table. In this way if there are 10 cm or so of subcutaneous fat this is made to hang over the edge of the table so that the actual bony edge of the trochanter is lying at the table edge.

Incision

27

A curved longitudinal incision is made which has the greater trochanter at the midpoint. From the midpoint it proceeds distally along the lateral midline of the shaft of the femur. Proximally it curves posteriorly and ends at a vertical line dropped through the anterior superior iliac spine. If the patient is heavily muscled, it may be necessary to extend this incision slightly more proximally in the posterior direction. The incision will usually be 24 cm in length.

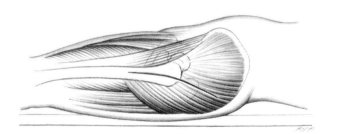

27

Superficial dissection

28

The gluteal fascia and iliotibial band are exposed in line with the skin incision. It is useful to go straight down to the greater trochanter and palpate the bony landmark before exposing the deep fascia.

The incision of the deep fascia begins over the middle of the trochanter and passes distally, the tissue layer being recognized by bulging of the vastus lateralis, with the fascia here being incised, once again, in the lateral midline of the femur. The deep fascial incision is completed by passing proximally and posteriorly in the direction of the fibres of the gluteus maximus, thus splitting them[19].

The trochanter is then exposed and any soft tissue adhesions on the front of the gluteus medius or the gluteus maximus are freed by blunt dissection.

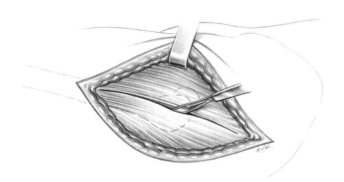

28

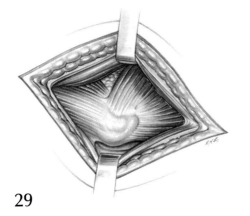

29

29

There may be a bursa over the trochanter and this must be incised and partially excised to expose the gluteus medius insertion into the greater trochanter. The initial-incision retractor is now inserted, the anterior blade beneath the deep fascia anteriorly at the level of the anterior border of the gluteus medius, and the posterior blade at the level of the gluteus maximus insertion into the posterior aspect of the femur. Tension on the bow of the initial-incision retractor enables the deep fascia to be distracted and the greater trochanter exposed.

Deep dissection

30

In the average subject the incision of the gluteus medius tendon is approximately 1 cm from the musculotendinous junction anteriorly. The incision extends distally to leave the anterior border of the gluteus medius where it borders the vastus lateralis intact, and it divides the vastus lateralis at the junction of the anterior quarter and intermediate half (thus preserving its innervation) for a distance of approximately 6 cm. Posteriorly, the incision of the gluteus medius tendon is extended to the apex of the trochanter and then passes horizontally in a proximal direction so that it splits the fibres of gluteus medius for a distance of 3 cm from the apex of the trochanter. This avoids the innervation of the muscle, that is, the superior gluteal nerve, which is some distance away.

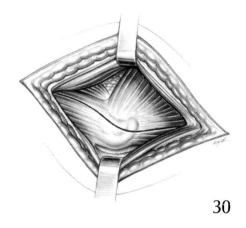

30

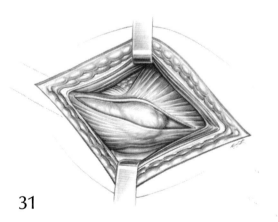

31

31

Using a cutting diathermy the tendinous insertions of the gluteus medius and minimus are then lifted from the greater trochanter; mild adduction of the thigh causes the neck of the femur to come into view as the gluteus medius muscle opens up anteriorly, while the thick tendinous posterior portion is undisturbed. Using the cutting diathermy the neck of the femur is exposed and the ligament of Bigelow is separated from the prominent ridge on the front of the neck of the femur. Further adduction allows the capsule of the hip joint to come into view. The capsule is incised circumferentially until the posterior aspect of the head of the femur is reached (in the left hip at the 4 o'clock position and in the right hip at the 8 o'clock position), where a radial incision is made into the capsule of the joint down to the edge of the acetabulum.

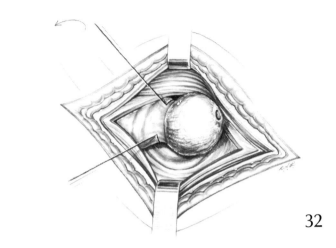

32

32 & 33

Further adduction of the thigh then brings the head of the femur into view, and gentle further adduction combined with some lateral rotation usually allows dislocation to occur. It will occasionally be necessary to put a curved cholecystectomy-type forceps underneath the neck of the femur to produce gentle traction on the neck to aid dislocation. Dislocation occurs when full adduction of the thigh takes place so that the femur is hanging over the contralateral extended leg. With the tibia in the vertical position neutral section of the neck of the femur is accomplished using the Gigli saw. This takes advantage of the anatomical observation that the trochanter is a posterior structure and the undisturbed part of the gluteus medius is isolated from the femoral neck section.

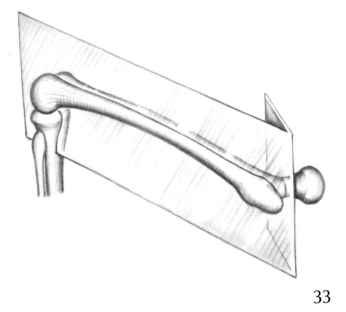

33

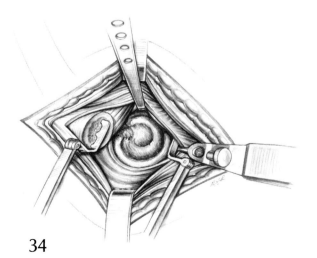

34

34

The capsule on the superior aspect of the acetabulum is then retracted using a pin retractor (superior capsular retractor) which is hammered firmly home into the innominate bone (in the left hip at the 3 o'clock position, in the right hip at the 9 o'clock position). The blades of the horizontal retractor engage distally with the stump of the cut end of the neck of the femur and proximally with the pin of the superior capsular retractor. Distraction of the horizontal retractor exposes the acetabulum. The anterior capsular retractor is then placed underneath the anterior capsule at the 12 o'clock position in both hips and, by means of the chain, attached to the upper or anterior blade of the initial-incision retractor.

35

The remains of the ligamentum teres is dissected and excised using cutting diathermy. A Hohmann's retractor may be placed into the obturator foramen if prominent synovium obscures the lower lip of the acetabulum. Correlation of the radiographs and the anatomical findings at operation will give an indication of the thickness of the medial wall of the pelvis. A large curette can be used to remove bone from the fovea or insertion of ligamentum teres so that the glistening medial wall of the pelvis is exposed. Preparation of the acetabulum, removing the fibrocartilage and sclerotic bone, is carried out using the deepening and expanding reamers as in the original Charnley technique, or 'potato-grater' reamers. The Charnley technique necessitates a pilot hole to be drilled into the fovea whereas a 'potato-grater' reamer does not. The acetabulum is prepared, removing all fibrous tissue and sclerotic bone, so that raw, bleeding corticocancellous bone is obtained. A series of 5 mm holes is drilled through the cortico-cancellous bone to a depth of 8 mm to augment the keying of the cement into the acetabulum. Lavage is used to remove all fat, blood and debris.

The orientation of the pelvis is then ascertained using the bony landmarks of the anterior superior iliac spines for orientation in the coronal plane, and also the degree of rotation. The acetabular gauge is then placed in the acetabulum to ascertain the cup size required. Familiarization takes place for the correct orientation of the cup and to ensure that full bony cover occurs. The trimming of the cement injection flange is performed at this stage. Mixing of the cement is then permissible and this is pressurized into the acetabulum using either a dome-shaped pressurizer or the inflatable pressurizer of Ling. The cup is then inserted and pressed until full bony cover takes place in its favoured orientation. Excess cement is removed. The cup holder remains on the cup until the cement is set fully, firm pressure being applied continuously.

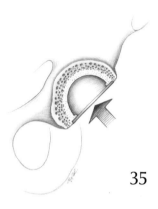

35

Preparation of the femur and insertion of the prosthesis

36

The bone on the lateral aspect of the neck of the femur, from the cut end of the femoral neck into the trochanteric fossa, is removed using Trotter's forceps to obtain neutral entry into the shaft of the femur (that is, no valgus or varus). Rotatory taper reamers are passed down the shaft of the femur until they bite into the corticocancellous bone. A blunt curette is used to remove the loose swarf and weak cancellous bony trabeculae. A trial prosthesis is inserted that will fit easily into the shaft of the femur. It is mandatory to have this trial prosthesis lying with the neck in the neutral plane with no anteversion or retroversion. A trial reduction takes place and the range of movement of the trial prosthesis is decided. It is important to ensure that the prosthesis is stable in adduction. This can only be performed with the patient in the supine position. Flexion, rotation and abduction are also assessed. At this stage the equalization of leg length can be determined to a high degree of accuracy using the bony landmarks of the anterior superior iliac spines, the patellae and the medial malleoli, comparison being made with the normal side. Having determined that the range of movement and leg lengths are satisfactory, the trial prosthesis is removed and the femoral cement restrictor is inserted to a distance of 13.5 cm from the calcar to prevent excessive migration of the femoral cement.

The first stage of the soft tissue repair of the anterior aspect of the hip joint now takes place. A braided Mersilene suture (Ethicon, Edinburgh, UK) is passed anteriorly through the neck of the femur to reattach the ligament of Bigelow and the tendon of gluteus minimus.

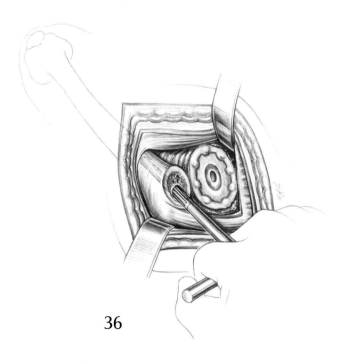

36

37

The ligament of Bigelow is attached to a horizontal ridge on the front of the neck of the femur at its midpoint. The gluteus minimus is attached to the outer aspect of this ridge. When these sutures have been passed through the neck of the femur the cement is mixed and is then pressurized into the shaft of the femur. The cement can either be inserted using a cement piston gun, preferably, or less favourably by finger packing, a femoral vent being necessary with the latter technique. The stem of the prosthesis is then inserted into the pressurized cement in the neutral axis *vis-à-vis* valgus/varus, with the neck of the prosthesis being maintained in the neutral plane *vis-à-vis* anteversion/retroversion. The hip joint socket and surrounding soft tissues are then irrigated with isotonic saline or chlorhexidine solution to clear debris, and when the cement is set the hip is reduced.

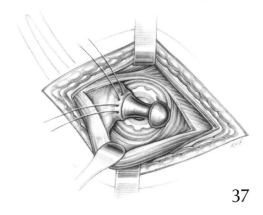

37

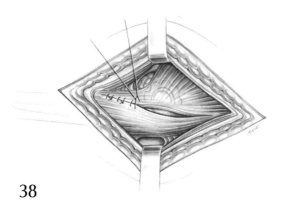

38

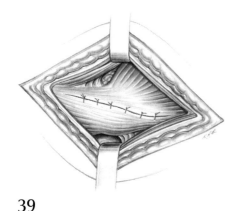

39

Closure

38 & 39

The ligament of Bigelow and gluteus minimus are reattached to their insertions. Closure of the gluteus medius is performed with a series of interrupted non-absorbable sutures. This is a tendinous closure and allows early mobilization. The deep fascia is similarly closed with non-absorbable interrupted sutures. Two drains are inserted beneath the deep fascia and one subcutaneously. These are removed at 48 hours.

Postoperative management

The patient begins active movement of the legs in flexion and extension as soon as consciousness returns. Adduction of the hip is avoided for 4 weeks postoperatively.

Standing is allowed at 48 hours when the drains have been removed, and usually the intravenous infusion is terminated. Standing and walking are accomplished using two elbow crutches. These elbow crutches are usually retained for 6 weeks after operation, some two of which are spent in hospital. Patients are allowed to go home when they can get out of bed, arise from a chair and climb stairs using two elbow crutches, which varies from 10 to 14 days postoperatively depending on age, general fitness and recovery from surgery.

TROCHANTERIC OSTEOTOMY

The patient position, skin incision and superficial dissection is the same as for the lateral approach.

Deep dissection

40 & 41

The trochanter is elevated using a Gigli saw passed through the trochanteric fossa to leave the gluteus medius and minimus insertions undisturbed; it is secured in position with a superior capsular retractor. Dislocation is achieved by adduction and slight lateral rotation, as previously described (see *Illustration 32*), and the insertion of the implants follows the same pattern.

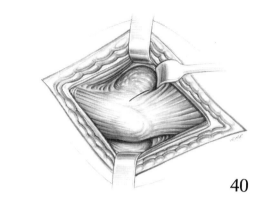

40

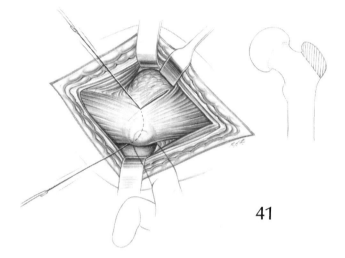

41

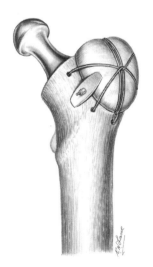

42

42

Trochanteric osteosynthesis is achieved by securing the trochanter back onto the trochanteric bed by wires and staples. It is important to locate the trochanter accurately and to hold it securely during the healing phase. During this time, approximately 6 weeks, the patient needs to have protected weight-bearing using elbow crutches.

Acknowledgement

Illustrations 4, 5a and 5b are reproduced from the Journal of Bone and Joint Surgery, 1987; 69-B: 229–33, by kind permission of the Edito

References

1. Hardinge K. Reconstructive su, ry of the hip in ankylosing spondylitis. In: Kelly WN, Harris ᴅ, Ruddy S, Sledge CB, eds. *Textbook of rheumatology*. Philadelphia: Saunders, 1981: 1973–9.

2. Hirst P, Esser M, Murphy JCM. Hardinge K. Bone grafting for protrusio acetabuli during total hip replacement: a review of the Wrightington method in 61 hips. *J Bone Joint Surg [Br]* 1987; 69-B: 229–33.

3. Hardinge K, Cleary J, Charnley J. Low friction arthroplasty for healed septic and tuberculous arthritis. *J Bone Joint Surg [Br]* 1979; 61-B: 144–7.

4. Hardinge K, Williams D, Etienne A, McKenzie D, Charnley J. Conversion of fused hips to low friction arthroplasty. *J Bone Joint Surg [Br]* 1977; 59-B: 385–92.

5. Hardinge K, Murphy JCM, Frenyo S. Conversion of hip fusion to Charnley low friction arthroplasty. *Clin Orthop* 1986; 211: 173–9.

6. Moore AT. The Moore self-locking vitallium prosthesis in fresh femoral neck fractures: a new low posterior approach (the southern exposure). *Am Acad Orthop Surg Instr Course Lect*. 1959; 16: 309.

7. Watson-Jones R. Fractures of the neck of the femur. *Br J Surg* 1936; 23: 787–808.

8. Charnley, J. *Low friction arthroplasty of the hip: theory and practice*. Berlin: Springer-Verlag, 1979.

9. Eftekhar N. Charnley "low friction torque" arthroplasty: a study of long-term results. *Clin Orthop* 1971; 81: 93–104.

10. Hardinge K. The direct lateral approach to the hip. *J Bone Joint Surg [Br]* 1982; 64-B: 17–9.

11. McFarland Osborne G. Approach to the hip. *J Bone Joint Surg [Br]* 1954; 36-B: 364–7.

12. Smith-Petersen MN. Approach to and exposure of the hip joint for mold arthroplasty. *J Bone Joint Surg [Am]* 1949; 31-A: 40–6.

13. Wagner H. Surface replacement arthroplasty of the hip. *Clin Orthop* 1978; 134: 102–30.

14. Henry AK. *Extensile exposure*. 2nd ed. Edinburgh: Churchill Livingstone, 1973.

15. Gibson A. Posterior exposure of the hip joint. *J Bone Joint Surg [Br]* 1950; 32-B: 183–6.

16. Marcy GH, Fletcher RS. Modification of the postero-lateral approach to the hip for the insertion of femoral head prosthesis. *J Bone Joint Surg [Am]* 1954; 36: 142–3.

17. McKee, GK, Watson-Farrar J. Replacement of arthritic hips by the McKee–Farrar prosthesis. *J Bone Joint Surg [Br]* 1966; 48-B: 245–59.

18. Müller ME. Total hip prostheses. *Clin Orthop* 1970; 72: 46–68.

19. Brady LP. Lateral oblique incision for the Charnley low friction arthroplasty. *Clin Orthop* 1976; 118: 7–9.

Girdlestone's pseudarthrosis of the hip

E. W. Somerville FRCS (Ed), FRCS
Emeritus Consultant Orthopaedic Surgeon, Nuffield Orthopaedic Centre, Oxford, UK

Introduction

During the past 30 years the treatment of arthritis of the hip has become more precise. High femoral osteotomy with internal fixation is an operation of value in the younger patient when degenerative changes are not advanced. When gross changes have developed in rheumatoid arthritis or osteoarthritis, total hip replacement is the procedure of choice. In such circumstances it is easy to forget the value of other well-tried procedures, such as arthrodesis and pseudarthrosis.

Girdlestone developed the use of the pseudarthrosis operation in the treatment of osteoarthritis from its previous use in tuberculosis of the hip joint. In this condition a complete joint clearance combined with excision of the head and neck of the femur was found to lead to healing of the disease and still allow a mobile and painless joint. A similar operation in osteoarthritis was found to provide a mobile and painless joint although this joint was subsequently unstable. Nevertheless, it allowed walking with a stick and sitting in comfort which, in the elderly patient for whom the operation was advocated, provided an excellent result.

Indications

There are certain indications for this operation.

It is particularly useful as a salvage operation following failure of an arthroplasty. The scarring which will have resulted from the previous operation greatly improves the stability of the joint, and in these patients a very satisfactory result is often obtained.

In ankylosing spondylitis the problem of restoring mobility to the hip joint is great. In such a case Girdlestone's pseudarthrosis gives comparatively good results, and after the operation a range of movement sufficient to allow sitting in comfort and for the legs to be separated adequately for nursing purposes is usually obtained. There is also a sufficient range of movement to allow walking, but it is probable that the patient will need to use either two sticks or crutches. Nevertheless, in such cases the patient is usually well satisfied with the result.

Contraindications

Generally speaking the operation is contraindicated in young patients where other procedures will probably be of greater value, but occasionally, as the result of very severe trauma, the results of pseudarthrosis in these patients have been good.

Pseudarthrosis performed bilaterally, except in the case of ankylosing spondylitis, as already mentioned, produces a degree of bilateral instability which is extremely disabling, so that the operation is contraindicated when arthritis is bilateral, unless it is combined with some other procedure to provide stability in the other hip.

Limitations

Pseudarthrosis is an operation which, although successful when carried out in the right patient, has strict limitations. It is an operation which relieves pain and preserves mobility, but at the same time produces an unstable hip. The degree of instability will usually condemn patients to using one stick, sometimes two, for the rest of their lives, although they usually manage to walk indoors without support. The pain which has been relieved by the operation is often rapidly forgotten, but the instability continues to be a source of great annoyance. Before this operation is carried out it is of the greatest importance that the nature of these limitations should be made perfectly clear to the patient and, because patients so easily forget, it is wise to explain this to the relatives as well.

Results

In 1950, Taylor[1] reported the results obtained in 93 patients. In 83 the results were considered to be satisfactory, in seven they were poor and three patients died as a result of the operation.

Operation

Approach

1

The operation may be carried out through any of the standard approaches to the hip joint. Girdlestone used the anterior Smith-Petersen approach, but the Gibson lateral approach is often preferable to this, particularly if a severe flexion contracture is present.

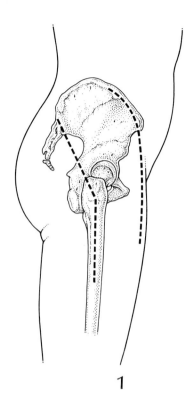

1

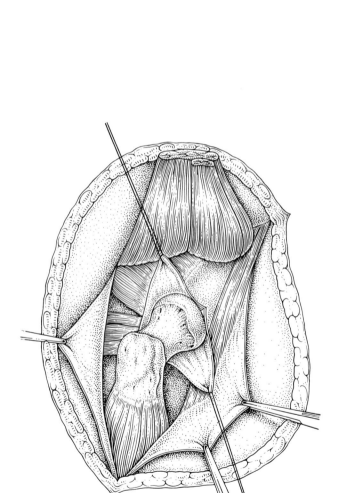

2

Exposure of joint capsule

2

Whatever approach is used the capsule of the joint is exposed and the anterior and superior portions are widely excised, allowing the hip to be dislocated arteriorly.

Division of neck of femur

3 & 4

The neck of the femur is divided along the inter-trochanteric line, care being taken to see that none is left protruding. This division may be carried out either with a Gigli saw or an osteotome, provided that care is taken to avoid splintering. The lip of the acetabulum is examined, and if it is found to be prominent, it must be excised flush with the side of the pelvis so that no protruding spur is left which might make contact with the upper end of the femur, since this invariably causes pain and stiffness. It is not necessary to interpose soft tissue between the pelvis and the upper end of the femur deliberately.

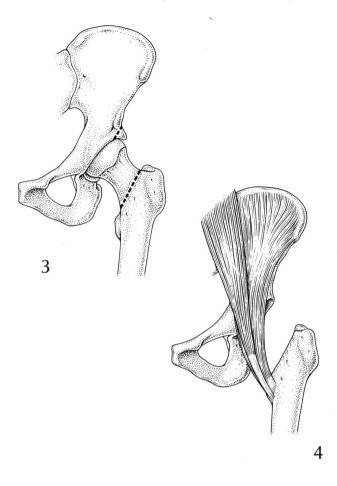

3

4

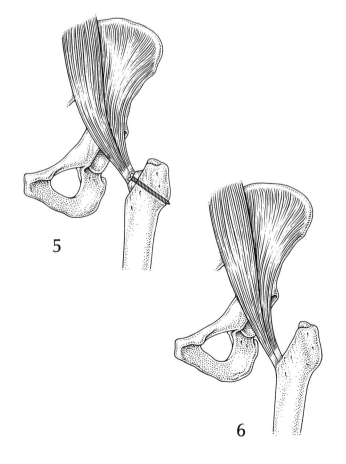

5

6

Useful modifications

5 & 6

There are two modifications to this operation which can be often usefully employed at this stage. There is a tendency for the leg to lie in lateral rotation because the fulcrum of the head of the femur has been removed, and the psoas muscle acts as a powerful lateral rotator. To reduce this tendency to lateral rotation the lesser trochanter can be removed with the psoas attached to it, and this can be displaced upwards and reattached to the raw surface at the base of the neck of the femur; or what is simpler still, the lesser trochanter can simply be excised and the iliopsoas will reattach itself in a more suitable position. After this the leg will lie more easily in neutral rotation.

Traction

7

Postoperatively, the leg is suspended in traction which is usually obtained by adhesive strapping to the skin with a 19 kg weight, although fixed traction can often be used provided it is carefully attended. If an anterior incision has been used, the leg is most satisfactorily suspended on a Thomas' splint with the knee flexion piece, but if the lateral incision has been employed it is better to use simple modified Russell traction and thereby avoid pressure from the ring of the splint on the wound. If there is a tendency for the leg to lie in lateral rotation this must be controlled, or the deformity will become fixed and make walking more difficult later. Usually a medial rotation bandage will be adequate, although of course this has the disadvantage of producing some circulatory constriction, which should be avoided in view of the risk of thrombophlebitis after such hip operations; traction by means of a Steinmann pin, which can also control rotation, may be better.

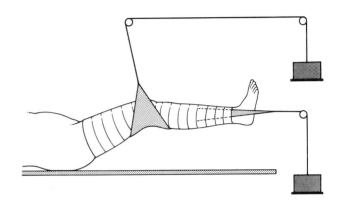

7

Batchelor's modification

8

The operation has been modified by Batchelor[2]. In this operation, after excision of the head and neck of the femur, an osteotomy is carried out at the level of the lesser trochanter, and the fragments are joined together with a plate in valgus position. This is said to improve stability when walking.

8

Postoperative management

Balanced traction, as descibed, is maintained for 3 weeks, after which time it is replaced by a simple form of traction with the leg lying on the bed over a pillow. From the beginning, quadriceps, foot and calf exercises will have been regularly carried out. Now with simple traction, hip and gluteal exercises are started. At 6 weeks from the time of the operation, the fixed traction is removed and removable extensions are applied, so that the patient can start getting up and can have hydrotherapy and sling exercises in the gymnasium and start walking between the bars. Classically a bucket-top caliper with knee flexion hinge is used when walking is started, a plaster of Paris cast being taken for this at the time the stitches are removed, so that the caliper will be ready by the time the patient is able to get up. Such a caliper is helpful to many patients, but to some a caliper is quite intolerable however well it may have been fitted, and in these patients there is no point in insisting on the caliper being used – they will get on very much better without it. A certain degree of shortening always occurs after this operation, usually amounting to 25–38 mm, which is compensated for by a 19 mm raise on the heel of the shoe, tapering to 6 mm at the toe. About 1 week after getting up, the patient will be allowed to start standing and walking between bars, and as soon as it is possible he should start with elbow crutches, which he will have to use for approximately 3 months. By this time the patient should be able to graduate to the use of two sticks. At 6 months the patient is encouraged to walk with the knee hinge unlocked and gradually during the next 2 or 3 months progressively to give up the caliper altogether and practise walking with one stick only in the opposite hand.

References

1. Taylor RG. Pseudoarthrosis of the hip joint. *J Bone Joint Surg [Br]* 1950; 32-B: 161–5.

2. Batchelor JS. Pseudoarthrosis for ankylosis and arthritis of the hip. *J Bone Joint Surg [Br]* 1949; 31-B: 135.

Arthrodesis of the hip

J. Crawford Adams   MD, MS, FRCS
Consulting Orthopaedic Surgeon, St Mary's Hospital, London, UK

Introduction

Arthrodesis of the hip is carried out much less often now than it was two or three decades ago. The main reason for this is the successful development of total replacement arthroplasty, which has revolutionized the treatment of osteoarthritis and rheumatoid arthritis of the hip, for which arthrodesis was formerly often advocated. A secondary reason is the dramatic decrease in the incidence of tuberculous arthritis in the western world – a benefit of the general improvement of living standards and the large-scale elimination of tuberculosis by antibacterial drugs. Arthrodesis is nevertheless still a useful method of treatment in certain special situations.

Indications

The present indications for arthrodesis of the hip may be summarized as follows.

1. For certain cases of destructive arthritis of the hip in which conditions are unsuitable or difficult for replacement arthroplasty – particularly in cases of tuberculous arthritis or pyogenic arthritis with much destruction of bone.
2. For certain cases of major disintegration of the hip from trauma – as for instance in central dislocation of the hip, especially in a young person.
3. For certain cases of slipped upper femoral epiphysis complicated by avascular necrosis of the femoral head and consequent disorganisation of the joint.
4. For certain cases of untreated or relapsed congenital dislocation of the hip in which the femoral head is displaced high up on the ilium – especially when an ill-developed lateral wall of the pelvis offers poor support for the socket of a replacement hip.
5. Very occasionally, for a hip that lacks muscle control from selective paralysis, in order to provide stability.

None of the above conditions is an absolute indication for arthrodesis, and much will always depend upon other factors – especially upon the age of the patient, upon the requirements of his or her occupation and leisure activities, and upon the patient's religious or cultural habits.

So far as age is concerned, arthrodesis of the hip is much more acceptable to a young adult patient than to the elderly. In general, it is more suitable for an active patient than for one with a sedentary occupation. Arthrodesis is always much more readily acceptable to a patient whose hip is already partly stiff – as for instance in a case of fibrous ankylosis – than to one who has retained a good range of movement.

The advantages of arthrodesis are that it abolishes pain completely; that the result is permanent; and that it provides good stability for the limb. Disadvantages – accentuated if the position of the fused hip is imperfect – are that it throws a strain upon the corresponding knee and upon the lumbar region of the spine. Sitting has to be modified, and squatting is precluded. Sexual function is not seriously prejudiced, provided that the other hip is fully mobile.

Contraindications

Arthrodesis of the hip should be avoided if the opposite hip shows significant impairment of mobility; or if the knee on the same side is disordered. It should usually be avoided in those whose national or religious habits demand the adoption of a squatting position.

A cautious attitude should be adopted towards hip arthrodesis in children. While the epiphyseal plate at the upper end of the femur is still open there is a strong tendency for progressive adduction to occur after hip fusion, to the extent that corrective osteotomy may be required. When practicable, therefore, arthrodesis should be deferred until growth is complete.

Position for arthrodesis

It is fundamentally important that the hip be fused in the optimal position: fusion in an incorrect position may badly mar the patient's functional ability for the remainder of his or her life. The optimal position for hip fusion is: 15°–20° of flexion; no adduction or abduction; and no medial or lateral rotation. If the limb on the affected side is short, it is a mistake to try to gain length by fusing the hip in abduction. An abducted position severely prejudices the integrity of the opposite hip and of the lumbar spine.

Technique

Of the many techniques of hip arthrodesis that have been described, there are two that have stood the test of time rather more successfully than the others. These are: (1) intra-articular arthrodesis with nail fixation and iliofemoral graft[1,2]; and (2) ischiofemoral arthrodesis by nail and graft[3]. These two methods will be described.

INTRA-ARTICULAR ARTHRODESIS WITH ILIOFEMORAL GRAFT

In this technique the hip joint is opened, the remains of articular cartilage are removed to expose vascular subchondral bone, the parts are reassembled in the required position, the hip is locked by a long nail transfixing the joint, and a bridge of bone is constructed by grafts between the wing of the ilium and the greater trochanter of the femur.

Preoperative

It is important to establish that the arterial circulation in the limb is adequate. Extensive atheroma in the proximal limb arteries presents a hazard. In elderly men, any prostatic obstruction should be dealt with before the hip operation is undertaken: otherwise acute obstruction may be precipitated.

Anaesthetic

General anaesthesia is usually to be preferred, but the operation may be done under spinal or epidural anaesthesia.

Position of patient

The patient is placed supine upon the raised platform of the orthopaedic table, the footpieces being in position to accept the feet at the appropriate stage of the operation: that is, while the hip is fixed with a transfixion nail.

The whole length of the affected limb should be draped in a sterile occlusive tube (e.g. stockinette) to facilitate handling of the limb during the operation.

Operation

Incision

1

The anterior (Smith-Petersen) approach to the hip is used. The skin incision follows the anterior half of the iliac crest to the anterior superior spine, whence it extends vertically downwards into the thigh for about 12.5 cm.

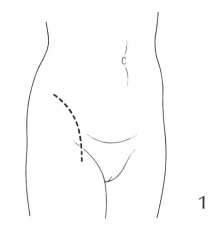

1

Deep dissection

2

The deep fascia is incised in the line of the incision, revealing in the proximal part of the thigh the line of separation between the sartorius medially and the tensor fasciae latae laterally. These muscles are separated and retracted apart. The sartorius may be divided. More proximally, the tensor fasciae latae muscle is stripped from the outer aspect of the wing of the ilium, and a large gauze pack is inserted to hold it away. Deep to this layer, the gap between the iliopsoas muscle medially and the rectus femoris laterally is developed, with care to avoid damage to laterally directed branches of the femoral nerve. A leash of vessels crossing laterally to the rectus muscle needs to be divided. The rectus muscle is detached and retracted downwards and medially to expose the capsule of the hip joint, the front of which is excised.

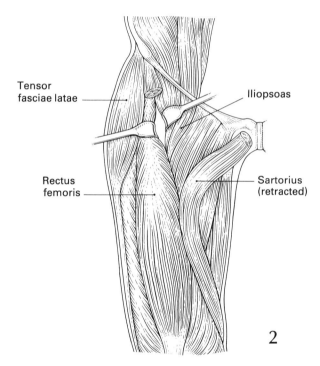

2

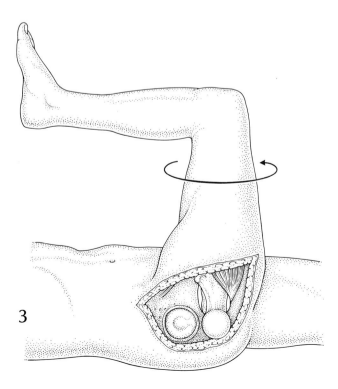

3

Dislocation of hip

3

The hip is dislocated by first flexing the thigh and then rotating the limb laterally. If dislocation is impeded by large osteophytes these may be chiselled away, and dislocation may be further aided by a stout skid or gouge inserted between the femoral head and the acetabulum to serve as a lever, or by a large hook around the femoral neck. Strong rotational force must not be used for fear of breaking the shaft of the femur.

Rawing of articular surface

4

The limb is laid on its outer side in order to direct the femoral head towards the operator. With chisels and gouges, or, if preferred, by a powered burr, all the articular cartilage is removed from the femoral head and from the acetabulum. The subchondral bone is lightly imbricated to leave a rough, oozing surface.

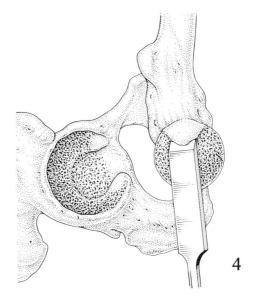

4

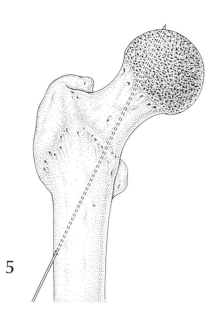

5

Introduction of guide wire

5

A guide wire is introduced into the lateral aspect of the femoral shaft 2–3 cm distal to the commencing flare of the greater trochanter, and is so directed within the femoral neck that its point emerges through the femoral head at its superior (weight-bearing) surface. The point is left almost flush with the surface of the bone at this stage.

Reduction of dislocation and adjustment of position of hip

6

The dislocation is reduced by guiding the femoral head towards the acetabulum and then rotating the limb medially and extending it. The feet are then strapped to the footpieces of the orthopaedic table, and by adjustment of the push-pull attachments both hips are brought to the neutral position so far as abduction/adduction is concerned. (If the limbs are of equal length the feet will now be level.) The footpieces may now be raised as far as is necessary to ensure that the hip rests in a position of flexion of 15°–20°.

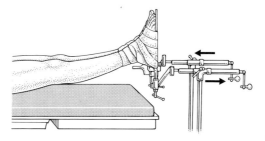

6

Locking of hip by transfixion nail

7

The length of the trifin nail required is calculated by determining the length of guide wire contained within the femur (by measuring the length protruding) and adding 3 cm for penetration of the acetabular roof. The guide wire is advanced across the joint to emerge, ideally, from the brim of the pelvis at the iliopectineal line, where its tip may be felt by a finger directed along the inner aspect of the ilium. The chosen three-flanged hip nail is driven in over the guide wire, with care to ensure that the wire is not inadvertently driven on with the nail. An impactor is used to correct any 'rebound' of the femoral head that might have left a space between the femoral head and the acetabulum. Alternatively, two AO cancellous screws may be used to secure the femur and acetabulum under compression.

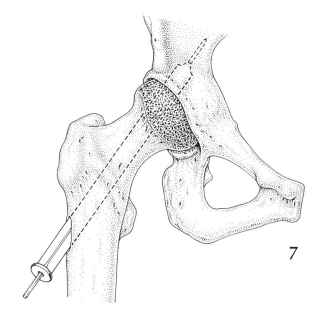

7

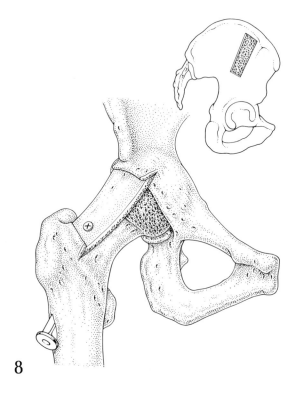

8

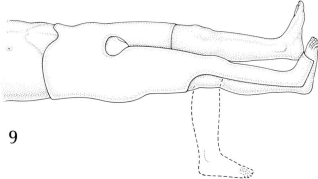

9

Iliofemoral grafting

8

A graft cut from the outer aspect of the ilium just below the crest is trimmed appropriately and inserted in a precise fit between the ilium and the greater trochanter of the femur, being engaged in slots cut in the ilium just above the hip joint, and in the medial aspect of the greater trochanter. Additional sliver or chip grafts are laid about the main graft to fill up any crevices. The graft may be secured by a screw transfixing it to the base of the femoral neck.

Closure and plaster

9

The wound is closed in layers, with provision for suction drainage. A double plaster hip spica is applied: this extends to include the foot of the limb operated upon, and to just above the knee on the opposite side. The plaster may be bivalved posteriorly below the lower thigh, to permit knee flexion exercises.

Postoperative management

After a week the patient may be got out of bed and encouraged to walk with crutches, minimal weight being taken on the affected side. A closer-fitting plaster may be applied after 2 or 3 weeks, when the sutures are removed. The spica should remain for 12 weeks when a radiograph out of the spica will show if fusion has occurred. If this is not certain, a short hip spica extending to above the knee may be used with full weight-bearing until fusion is solid.

ISCHIOFEMORAL ARTHRODESIS

In this technique the hip is first transfixed by a long three-flanged nail. Without exposure of the hip joint itself, the interval between the femur and the ischium is then bridged by a rigid tibial graft inserted through a drill hole in the femur and driven on to enter a hole drilled in the ischium.

Special contraindications

Since in this operation the hip joint itself is not opened, the technique is inappropriate if the hip shows a fixed deformity that cannot be overcome in the way now to be described.

Preoperative

Correction of fixed deformity

10

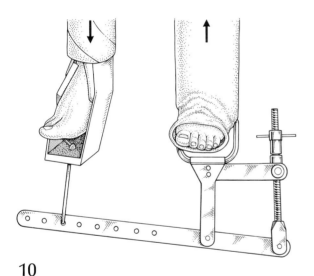

10

Moderate adduction or abduction deformity, and a flexion deformity not exceeding 30°, may usually be corrected by the push-pull method described by Roger Anderson[4] in 1932 and known as 'well-leg traction' because traction is exerted against, or sometimes upon, the well leg.

In the correction of fixed adduction deformity – the usual pattern – a full-length plaster of Paris splint is applied to the well leg, with the knee almost fully extended. The plaster includes the foot, and the Roger Anderson well-leg traction apparatus is incorporated in it. Through the lever arm of the apparatus sustained traction is then applied to the disordered limb, usually through the medium of skin strapping, though a lower tibial Steinmann pin may be used if desired. The correcting force acts on the hip by a parallelogram of forces. If the fixed deformity is severe and of long duration, correction may be aided by tenotomy of the taut adductor tendons.

If abduction deformity is to be corrected the system is reversed, the plaster splint and the apparatus being applied to the disordered leg and traction to the well leg. Again, tenotomy of contracted tendons or muscles may be carried out if necessary.

If correction of fixed deformity is to be achieved by this method it will usually be gained within a week. If the deformity resists correction beyond this time, either the hip must be opened to correct the deformity before ischiofemoral arthrodesis is undertaken, or this method of arthrodesis must be abandoned in favour of intra-articular arthrodesis.

Operation

Position of patient

11

Because of the fundamental requirement that the hip be fused in precisely the optimal position, the first stage of the operation should be carried out with the patient supine upon the orthopaedic table and the feet strapped to the push-pull footpieces. By appropriate adjustment of the footpieces, the correct position of the hip can be assured before the joint is transfixed with a long nail. For the second stage of the operation the patient must be turned to the prone position. (It is impracticable to adjust the position of the hip with the patient prone.)

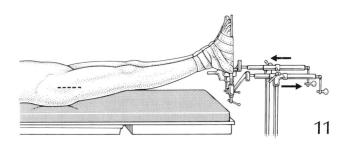

FIRST-STAGE OPERATION: TRANSFIXION OF HIP BY THREE-FLANGED NAIL

Incision

12

In this first stage a lateral incision is made immediately below the prominence of the greater trochanter to expose the lateral aspect of the upper part of the shaft of the femur. A second incision is made over the anterior part of the crest of the ilium, through which the iliacus muscle is stripped away from the inner aspect of the pelvis by a blunt periosteal elevator. The purpose of this incision is to allow a finger to reach the brim of the pelvis to palpate an emerging guide wire, inserted in the manner now to be described.

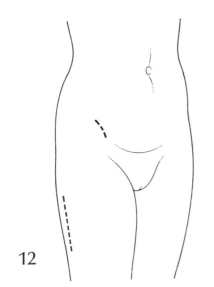

Insertion of guide wire

13

Through the lateral incision a small hole is made with a gouge or drill in the cortex of the femur 2.5 cm below the outward flare of the greater trochanter, and slightly behind the mid-lateral line of the bone. This allows the insertion of a long (30 cm) guide wire, which is directed obliquely upwards, medially and slightly forwards towards a doubly-gloved finger inserted deeply in the iliac wound. The wire is best introduced in the chuck of a powered drill. Edged forwards by degrees, its point should be felt as it emerges through the bone of the pelvic brim. If necessary the position of the guide wire may be checked radiographically, but this is not essential if the tip of the wire is palpated as described.

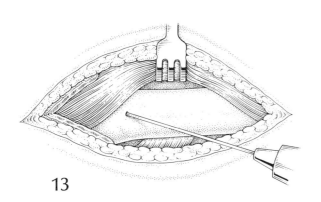

Driving of nail

14

By measurement of the length of guide wire still protruding from the femur the length that is within the bone is calculated, and hence the length of nail required to transfix the hip joint and to enter strong iliac bone is determined. The chosen three-flanged nail, held in a Smith-Petersen punch, is then driven in over the guide wire, with special care to ensure that the guide wire is not inadvertently driven forward with the nail. To prevent this, the wire should be rotated after every few hammer blows, and the length of wire protruding remeasured.

The incision over the crest of the ilium is now closed. The lateral incision is closed temporarily with towel clips.

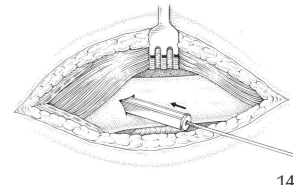

14

Cutting and preparation of bone graft

15

The bone graft is cut from the subcutaneous surface of the tibia. Twin parallel or tandem grafts exactly 12.5 mm wide and 10 cm long are required. The anterior and postero-medial corners of the tibia must be preserved to minimize the risk of fracture. After extraction, the two grafts are wired together cortex to cortex, and one end is finely tapered to a blunt point over a length of 1.5 cm. Finally the composite graft is rounded with a chisel or with a powered burr so that it forms a cylindrical peg exactly 12.5 mm in diameter.

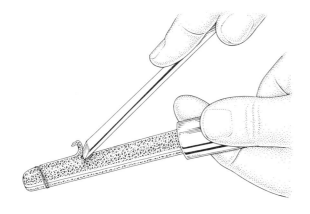

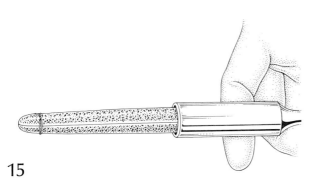

15

SECOND-STAGE OPERATION: INSERTION OF BONE GRAFT

For the second stage of the operation the patient is turned and placed prone upon the operation table, with care not to apply any undue force to the hip, the position of which has been locked with the nail. Fresh drapes are placed in position.

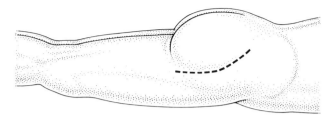

16

Incision

16

The existing lateral incision is prolonged upwards and medially across the buttock, towards the posterior superior spine of the ilium.

The deep exposure

17

The gluteus maximus is split in the direction of its fibres and its femoral insertion is detached. The two sides are retracted apart to expose, more deeply, the short posterior muscles of the hip – namely the obturator internus and gemelli above, and the quadratus femoris below. The sciatic nerve is identified lying on these muscles before disappearing proximally beneath the piriformis muscle. The nerve must be carefully protected. The interval between the inferior gemellus above and the quadratus femoris below is opened up. In the gap thus created the tuberosity of the ischium is first palpated and then exposed by blunt dissection.

Drilling of channel for bone graft

18

The drill enters the lateral aspect of the femur 2 cm below the head of the transfixion nail (already inserted) and in a plane slightly anterior to the mid-lateral axis. The pilot hole, 9.5 mm (⅜ inch) in diameter, is directed towards the tuberosity of the ischium under direct vision: it passes almost horizontally, with a slight posterior inclination. When the drill has penetrated the femur it is carefully advanced to strike the outer aspect of the ischium (usually 5 cm distant from the femur), which is then penetrated by the drill. (If desired, a guide wire may first be introduced into the ischium and the hole then made by a cannulated drill passed over the guide wire.) When the pilot hole has been made it is enlarged to 11 mm (⁷⁄₁₆ inch). The femoral hole is further enlarged to 12.5 mm (½ inch) in diameter but the ischial hole is left undersize to ensure a jam-fit of the graft.

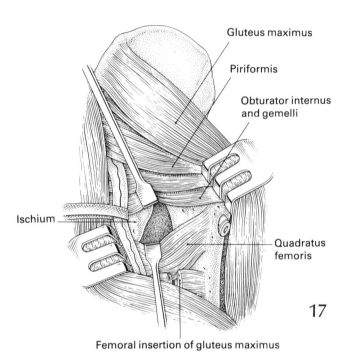

Gluteus maximus

Piriformis

Obturator internus and gemelli

Ischium

Quadratus femoris

17

Femoral insertion of gluteus maximus

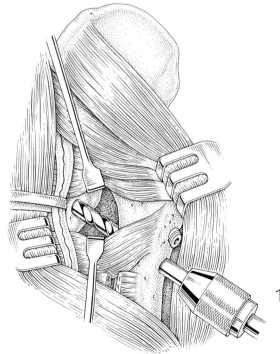

18

Insertion of graft

19

The prepared graft, with the point carefully tapered, is held in the hollow end of a Smith-Petersen punch and driven through the hole in the femur and on into the ischial tunnel. It should preferably penetrate right through the ischium, which has a depth of about 2.5 cm. The graft is impacted so that its outer end is flush with the lateral cortex of the femur. The wound is closed in layers.

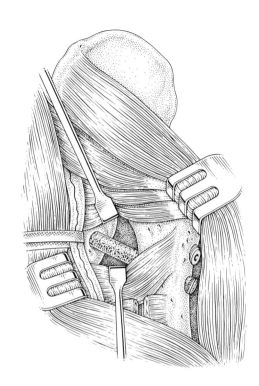

19

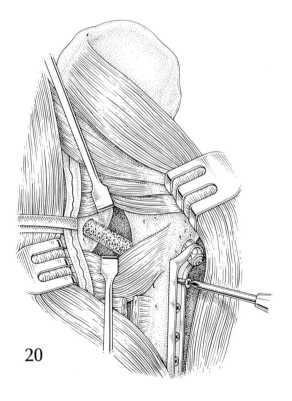

20

Alternative fixation

20

Some surgeons recommend the use of a two-piece nail–plate in preference to a plain three-flanged nail, in order to forestall the risk of fracture of the femoral shaft through the drill hole. If this is the case the plate component of the nail–plate is screwed in place after the graft has been driven home.

Postoperative management

21

The patient is turned back to the supine position on the orthopaedic table; the feet are strapped to the adjustable footpieces of the table, or the feet may be held by an assistant while the pelvis rests upon a portable support. A close-fitting plaster spica is applied, extending high up on the thoracic cage and including the thigh on the affected side to just above the knee. (Since the graft as well as the nail provides stability this minimal spica is adequate.) Walking with crutches is encouraged after 3 or 4 days, with some weight being taken upon the affected limb. Knee movements are practised with the patient prone. The plaster spica is changed as necessary to maintain a snug fit: it is retained for a total of 8 weeks.

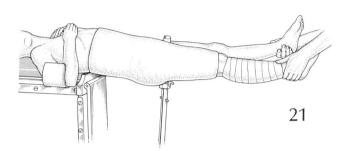

21

Special complications

The most frequent complication has been fracture of the graft near the point where it enters the ischium. This has occurred usually about 2 months after the operation. It may be in the nature of a stress fracture. If the nail remains firm, and the hip immobile, the fracture will often heal spontaneously, often with the formation of abundant callus. Exceptionally, if the nail loosens and the fracture fails to heal, regrafting and fresh nailing may be required. The incidence of primary incorporation of the graft has been about 90 per cent. It is followed many months later by obliteration of the acetabulofemoral joint space. Fracture of the femur through the drill hole has been a rare complication. In the author's experience it has occurred only in frail women.

References

1. Watson-Jones R, Robinson WC. Arthrodesis of the osteoarthritic hip joint. *J Bone Joint Surg [Br]* 1956; 38-B: 353–77.

2. Wiles P. The surgery of the osteoarthritic hip. *Br J Surg* 1958; 45: 488–97.

3. Adams JC. *Ischio-femoral arthrodesis*. Edinburgh: Livingstone, 1966.

4. Anderson R. New method for treating fractures utilising the well leg for counter-traction. *Surg Gynecol Obstet* 1932; 54: 207–19.

Illustrations by Peter Cox

Distal hamstring release

W. J. W. Sharrard MD, ChM, FRCS
Emeritus Consultant Orthopaedic Surgeon, Royal Hallamshire Hospital and Children's Hospital, Sheffield;
Professor of Orthopaedic Surgery, University of Sheffield, UK

Preoperative

Indications and assessment

A flexion deformity of the knee of 20°–50° due to moderate imbalance of muscle activity at the knee in paralytic conditions such as cerebral palsy, poliomyelitis and spina bifida is the main indication for distal hamstring release, though it may be used in other non-paralytic lesions associated with knee flexion contracture.

Distal hamstring release is ideally performed when there are strong knee flexor muscles associated with an active but weak quadriceps muscle with a power of MRC Grade 3 or 4. The assessment of the degree of knee flexion contracture is best made with the patient prone. Sometimes, one or more of the hamstring tendons or gracilis tendon may be more severely affected, but it is more usual to find that all the hamstring tendons require release.

Before performing a hamstring release, a check should be made on the presence of any contractures at the hip or foot. Knee flexion may arise as a secondary consequence of hip flexion deformity, which puts the hamstring muscles under tension and which should be corrected first.

Anaesthesia and position of patient

General anaesthesia is needed. The limb is normally exsanguinated by an Esmarch bandage, and a pneumatic tourniquet cuff is applied as proximally as possible and inflated with the knee extended. The operation is performed with the patient prone. A diathermy plate is applied.

The skin is prepared. A sterile stockinette is applied to the level of the upper calf. Drapes are applied to leave the knee and lower third of the thigh exposed. The operation area can be covered by a transparent adhesive drape, though is does not mould well to the contours of a knee with a flexion deformity and it may be easier to leave the skin undraped, or to cover it with stockinette stuck to the skin with adhesive solution and to incise the stockinette.

Operation

Incisions

1

The operation is done through two vertical incisions, posteromedial and posterolateral. The posteromedial incision is made along the line of the semitendinosus tendon, which is usually the most prominent medial hamstring tendon, extending for a distance of 12–15 cm in the lower third of the thigh and across the back of the knee to end by curving slightly forwards. The postero-lateral incision is made for a similar distance over the biceps tendon, extending distally to the level of the head of the fibula.

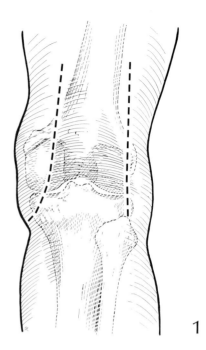

1

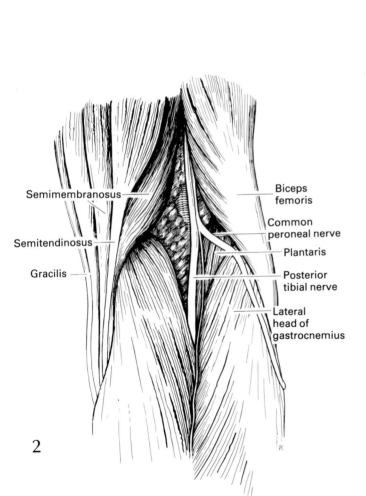

Semimembranosus

Semitendinosus

Gracilis

Biceps femoris

Common peroneal nerve

Plantaris

Posterior tibial nerve

Lateral head of gastrocnemius

2

Exposure of the medial tendons

2

The incision is deepened through the subcutaneous tissue; a few subcutaneous veins need to be identified and coagulated. The tendons to be exposed are the semitendinosus, gracilis and semimembranosus. The semitendinosus and gracilis tendons are enclosed in sheaths of paratenon, often associated with a consider-able amount of fat which may make the tendons difficult to find, isolate and uncover. Both tendons are fairly superficial and can become hidden under a retractor.

The semitendinosus is usually the most prominent tendon and is exposed by a vertical incision along its sheath for as much of its extent as the incision allows. Additional length can be exposed by allowing the knee to flex and retracting the distal end of the incision. It is differentiated from the gracilis tendon in that it is more substantial, oval and does not have muscle fibres along most of its length.

The gracilis tendon lies medial to the semitendinosus. It is finer and muscle fibres extend on one side of the tendon along the upper half of its extent.

The semimembranosus muscle and tendon lies deep to the semitendinosus. It is in the form of a flat aponeurosis on the superficial surface of a substantial bulk of muscle fibres which extend well distally. It narrows to about half its width from above downwards.

The tibial (medial popliteal) nerve, which lies between and deep to the semimembranosus and biceps muscles proximally and becomes more superficial distally, should be identified by careful blunt dissection to avoid injury to it.

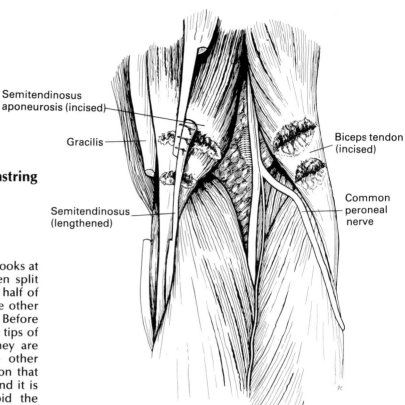

Semitendinosus
aponeurosis (incised)

Gracilis

Biceps tendon
(incised)

Semitendinosus
(lengthened)

Common
peroneal
nerve

3a

Musculotendinous release of the medial hamstring tendons

3a, b & c

The semitendinosus tendon is lifted up by single hooks at each end to put it under some tension. It is then split longitudinally by incising it along its length. One half of the tendon is divided transversely distally and the other half of the tendon proximally to form a Z-incision. Before the tendon is divided, a stay suture is put into the tips of each tendon slip to avoid losing them when they are released. They are not resutured until all the other tendons have been released. The length of tendon that will need to be divided is sometimes deceptive and it is wise to lengthen as much as possible to avoid the embarrassment of being unable to approximate the tendon ends when the deformity has been corrected.

The gracilis tendon can either be split longitudinally in the same way as the semitendinosus or simply divided and allowed to retract without suturing it.

The aponeurosis of the semimembranosus is lengthened by several transverse incisions into it, without cutting the muscle fibres beneath. The muscle and tendon will stretch easily when the knee is extended. There is no need to suture it.

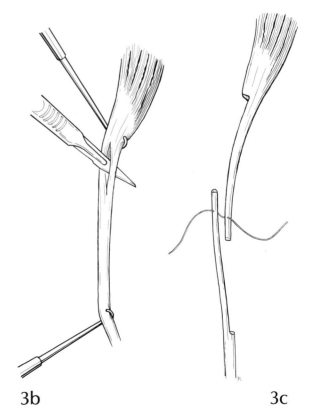

3b   3c

Exposure and release of the biceps femoris

The biceps tendon is exposed through the posterolateral incision over a length of 7–10 cm by a vertical incision through the thin fascia overlying it. It is formed of a substantial bulk of muscle fibres extending well distally on the surface of which a thick but flattened tendon arises, which is exposed down to the point at which it divides to enclose the lateral ligament of the knee. Immediately medial and posterior to the biceps tendon, the common peroneal nerve should be identified by careful blunt dissection. Distally it approaches close to the tendon and must be seen and retracted out of harm's way before the biceps tendon is incised. The biceps tendon can be lengthened by multiple transverse incisions into it in its proximal part leaving the muscle fibres to stretch in the same way as the semimembranosus, or the tendon can be separated from its attached muscle fibres and lengthened by a Z-incision, dependent on the amount of lengthening that is required.

Correction of knee flexion deformity and tendon suture

The knee is now extended as far as possible, watch being kept on the tension on the tibial and common peroneal nerves. There may be need to divide the deep fascia of the posterior aspect of the thigh lying beneath the subcutaneous tissue if it has not already been released sufficiently. If there is still incomplete extension of the knee, a small amount of further correction may be obtained by posterior capsulotomy of the knee. The posterior capsule is exposed by dissecting carefully beneath the tibial nerve and the popliteal vessels, with care being taken not to damage the medial or lateral geniculate vessels. The capsule is divided transversely at the joint line. It is doubtful whether this manoeuvre, by itself, is justified, since, if the capsule and ligaments of the knee are short, only division of the medial, lateral, and possibly the cruciate ligaments is likely to provide significant further improvement in knee extension.

The slips of the divided semitendinosus tendon are approximated under moderate physiological tension and sutured side-to-side to each other with 3 or 4 non-absorbable sutures. The gracilis and biceps tendons are similarly sutured only if they have been lengthened by Z-incisions. If not, no other tendon sutures are required.

Wound closure

The subcutaneous layer of each incision is closed with interrupted non-absorbable sutures after putting in suction drains to the deep layers. The skin is sutured with non-absorbable intermittent sutures or absorbable subcuticular sutures. Dressings are applied and mutual pressure applied to the posterior aspect of the thigh and popliteal fossa whilst the tourniquet is released and removed. The toes need to be observed for the adequacy of circulation in them before the plaster is applied. If the circulation is not adequate the knee should be allowed to flex until the blood supply is restored. The corrected position is held by a plaster cast applied from the top of the thigh, as near to the groin as possible, down to the toes, over an adequate layer of plaster wool, particularly over the front of the knee and the back of the heel which are likely to be subject to pressure. The suction drain tubes are brought out of the top of the plaster cast and are not sutured to the skin, so that they may be removed after 48 or 72 hours by directly pulling on them without the need to remove the plaster.

Postoperative management

The circulation in the toes is kept under observation. If the toes become swollen and the circulation in them diminishes, the plaster should be split immediately and the knee allowed to flex if necessary to restore circulatory flow. The plaster cast is changed on the tenth day and any non-absorbable sutures removed. This is best performed under sedation or general anaesthesia in young children. If some flexion deformity remains, further correction may be possible. The plaster cast is retained for 4–5 weeks, after which active mobilization and physiotherapy is begun to encourage the return of active knee extension and the maximum range of knee movement.

Illustrations by Philip Wilson after P. Henry

Transfer of the hamstrings to the quadriceps in the adult

J. A. Fixsen MChir, FRCS
Consultant Orthopaedic Surgeon, The Hospital for Sick Children, Great Ormond Street, London, and St Bartholomew's Hospital, London, UK

Introduction

Indications

Transfer of the hamstring muscles to the quadriceps can be used to reinforce a weak or paralysed quadriceps muscle. However, several criteria must be fulfilled if the operation is to be a success.

1. Both biceps femoris and semitendinosus muscles must be of power 4 or more on the Medical Research Council scale.
2. The biceps femoris muscle should not be transferred on its own as this can lead to lateral instability and dislocation of the patella[1].
3. Transfer of the biceps femoris and semitendinosus should not be performed unless one other knee flexor is active and the gastrocnemius is also functioning to flex the knee and prevent genu recurvatum.
4. The patient should have active hip flexors and extensors. If the hip flexors are weak the patient will have difficulty in clearing the floor with the foot. This is a serious contraindication to the operation.
5. Any flexion deformity at the hip or the knee must be corrected before performing the transfer. Valgus or varus at the knee and equinus at the foot should also be corrected.

Operation

The operation is performed under general anaesthesia with the patient supine. A tourniquet placed high as possible on the thigh is used to provide a bloodless field.

Incisions

1

The first incision is made over the anteromedial aspect of the knee centred on the patella and long enough to expose the patella, quadriceps tendon and patellar tendon when retracted laterally.

2

The second incision is made longitudinally over the lateral side of the lower third of the thigh extending distally to the head of the fibula. The deep fascia is divided.

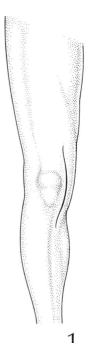

1

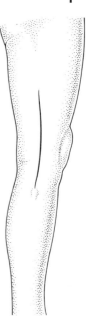

2

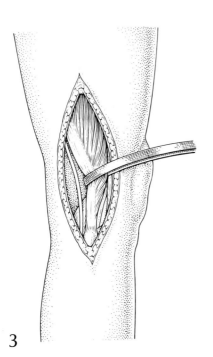

3

3

The biceps femoris tendon is dissected out, taking particular care not to damage the lateral popliteal nerve which lies immediately behind the tendon and winds round the neck of the fibula.

4

The biceps tendon is divided distally at its insertion on the lateral aspect of the head of the fibula, taking care not to damage the lateral ligament of the knee joint which it surrounds. A slip of the tendon inserts onto the lateral tibial condyle and must also be divided.

The tendon and muscle belly are mobilized proximally, detaching the short head from the femur as far proximally as the entry of its nerve and blood supply on the medial side will permit. A wide subcutaneous tunnel is made as obliquely as possible from the first to the second incision so the pull of the tendon after transfer is as straight as possible.

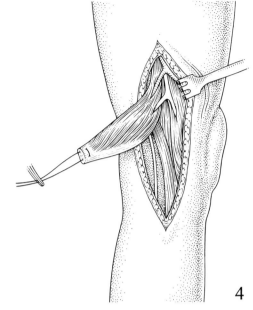

4

5

A third incision is now made on the medial side of the lower third of the thigh extending as far distally as the medial tibial condyle. The semitendinosus tendon, which is round with no muscle belly, is found lying behind the sartorius and gracilis muscles. It is divided at its insertion on the tibia and mobilized proximally to the mid-thigh. Blunt finger dissection is very useful for this. A second oblique subcutaneous tunnel is made from the first to the third incision so that the semitendinosus tendon can be transferred to the patella. Both tendons are passed through their respective tunnels. It is most important to make sure that they can move quite freely in the tunnels and their line is as straight as possible.

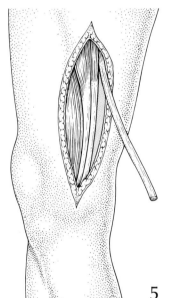

5

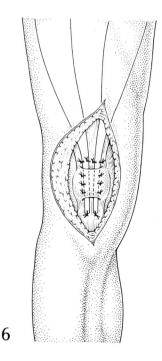

6

6

A subperiosteal tunnel is made on the anterior surface of the patella and the two tendons passed through it. Alternatively, the periosteum may be raised as two longitudinal flaps and the tendons placed beneath them. With the knee in extension the tendons are then firmly sutured with non-absorbable sutures to the patella and its periosteum, to the quadriceps tendon proximally and the patellar tendon distally. The tourniquet is removed and haemostasis obtained. The wound is closed in layers, usually without drainage.

Postoperative management

A long-leg plaster is applied for 3 weeks with the knee in extension but not hyperextended. Care must be taken during this period not to stretch the transferred muscles by flexing the hip.

At 3 weeks the plaster is removed and physiotherapy started to mobilize the knee and re-educate the transferred muscles. Protective splintage is retained until adequate muscle control of the knee has been achieved. Some surgeons prefer to retain a protective orthosis and night splintage for up to 6–12 months postoperatively.

Complications

Provided the initial criteria described have been adhered to, good control of the knee without an orthosis should be obtained. Lateral instability of the patella should not occur if both tendons are transferred. Serious genu recurvatum should not develop if the gastrocnemius and semimembranosus are working adequately.

Reference

1. Schwartzmann JR, Crego CH Jr. Hamstring-tendon transplantation for the relief of quadriceps femoris paralysis in residual poliomyelitis: follow-up study of 134 cases. *J Bone Joint Surg [Am]* 1948; 30-A: 541–9.

Proximal gastrocnemius release

W. J. W. Sharrard MD, ChM, FRCS.
Emeritus Consultant Orthopaedic Surgeon, Royal Hallamshire Hospital and Children's Hospital, Sheffield;
Professor of Orthopaedic Surgery, University of Sheffield, UK

Preoperative

Indications and assessment

This operation may be used for equinus deformity due to gastrocnemius tightness, for which the indications are the same as in distal gastrocnemius release (*see* p. 1169). It may also form part of an operation for the release of knee flexion deformity, in association with distal hamstring release (*see* pp. 981–984). It is particularly indicated in combined equinus and knee flexion deformity in neglected cases of cerebral palsy or for equinus deformity when there is weakness of ankle dorsiflexion to less than MRC Grade 3, indicating the need for gastrocnemius release combined with partial gastrocnemius neurectomy.

Anaesthesia and position of patient

This is the same as for distal gastrocnemius release (*see* p. 1169). A pneumatic tourniquet is applied to the upper thigh.

Operation

Incision

1

A transverse incision is made in the popliteal fossa parallel with the skin creases from a point 1 cm lateral to the biceps tendon to 1 cm medial to the semitendinosus tendon. If the operation is combined with lengthening of the hamstring tendons, the gastrocnemii may be exposed through the incisions used for that operation. The incision is deepened through the deep fascia and a small flap retracted proximally.

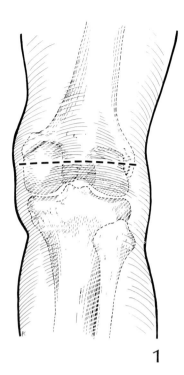

1

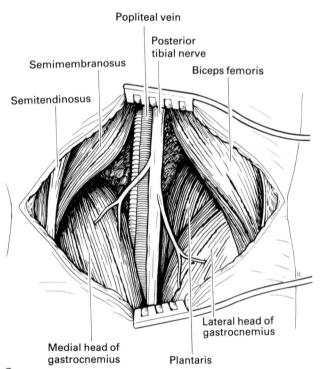

Popliteal vein

Posterior
tibial nerve

Semimembranosus

Biceps femoris

Semitendinosus

Medial head of
gastrocnemius

Plantaris

Lateral head of
gastrocnemius

2

Exposure of gastrocnemius origins

2

The posterior tibial nerve is identified by blunt dissection in the fat of the popliteal fossa and its motor branches to the heads of the gastrocnemii traced to the point where they enter the muscle. One or two of the branches to each head are divided with removal of a small amount of nerve to effect a partial denervation.

By blunt dissection, the medial and lateral heads of the gastrocnemius are exposed with care to avoid injury to the popliteal vein which lies immediately deep to the posterior tibial nerve. On the lateral side of the incision, the common peroneal nerve should be exposed and retracted.

Musculotendinous division

3

The origins of the medial and lateral heads of the gastrocnemius from the lower end of the femur are defined. The medial head arises from the femoral shaft above the medial femoral condyle, whilst the lateral head arises from the lateral side of the lateral femoral condyle more distally. A curved clamp is passed beneath each origin which is divided transversely near its attachment to the bone and mobilized distally. The plantaris origin arising immediately proximal to the lateral head is also divided. The medial and lateral genicular vessels pass medially and laterally, respectively, proximal to the gastrocnemius heads and care is needed to avoid damage to them or to the posterior tibial nerve.

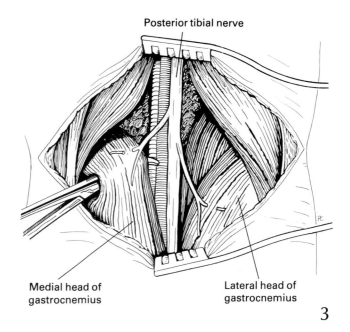

Posterior tibial nerve

Medial head of gastrocnemius

Lateral head of gastrocnemius

3

4

The two gastrocnemius heads are freed so that they move freely distally when the ankle is dorsiflexed with the knee extended and the equinus deformity corrected.

Wound closure

It is advisable to release the tourniquet at this point to identify and coagulate by diathermy or ligate any bleeding vessels. The wound is closed by interrupted or continuous non-absorbable sutures to the deep fascia and interrupted absorbable sutures to the subcutaneous fat. The skin is closed by a subcuticular suture or interrupted non-absorbable sutures and a plaster cast is applied from the groin to the toes with the knee fully extended and the ankle dorsiflexed as fully as possible.

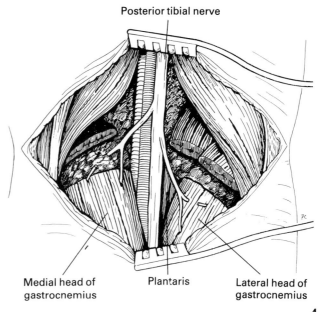

Posterior tibial nerve

Medial head of gastrocnemius   Plantaris   Lateral head of gastrocnemius

4

Postoperative management

The postoperative management is the same as for distal gastrocnemius release (*see* p. 1171).

Further reading

Silfverskiold N. Reduction of the uncrossed two-joint muscle of the leg to one-joint muscle in spastic conditions. *Acta Chir Scand* 1924; 56: 315–30.

Illustrations by Philip Wilson after P. Henry

Supracondylar osteotomy of the femur

J. A. Fixsen MChir, FRCS
Consultant Orthopaedic Surgeon, The Hospital for Sick Children, Great Ormond Street, London, and St Bartholomew's Hospital, London, UK

Introduction

Osteotomy of the lower end of the femur in the supracondylar region can be used to correct valgus or varus, flexion or extension deformities mainly in children but also in adults. Rotational deformities can be corrected at this level but the author prefers to correct pure rotational deformity in the subtrochanteric region. In children, fixation by staples is sufficient but in adults a plate and screws can be used. When the femur is very small or delicate the two-stage osteotomy–osteoclasis described by Moore[1] can be used. This method avoids the problems of inadequate fixation in a small or soft bone and the danger of losing control of a small bony fragment close to the joint. At the first stage the required wedge of bone is removed leaving the cortex at the apex intact. The bone wedge is cut into chips and replaced in the gap left by the wedge. Two to three weeks later closed osteoclasis is performed, bending or cracking the intact cortex to close the gap and correct the deformity while retaining stability without internal fixation.

Varus and valgus deformities can be corrected at any age. It is tempting to correct severe soft tissue flexion deformity at the knee in conditions such as arthrogryposis, spina bifida and lumbar agenesis by supracondylar osteotomy. Unfortunately this produces a forward angulation of the epiphyseal plate which with growth results in a very ugly and functionally awkward deformity of the femur. Osteotomy should be avoided until near maturity in these patients.

In the adult, extension supracondylar osteotomy may be indicated rarely for old poliomyelitis. The main indication in the adult is for valgus deformities resulting from osteoarthritis or trauma. Although rigid fixation and early movement can be achieved by use of an angled blade–plate and screws placed on the lateral aspect of the femur, as described for supracondylar fractures (see pp. 242–251), fixation with one or two staples and a high cylinder plaster of Paris cast for 6 weeks postoperatively will give good results and the exposure is much less extensive.

Preoperatively the deformity must be carefully assessed and measured clinically and radiologically in the weight-bearing position. This is vital to achieve the right amount of correction.

Operation

The correction of a valgus deformity by medially based wedge will be described.

To correct other types of deformity the position of the base of the wedge is altered accordingly. To correct a varus deformity by removal of a laterally based wedge a lateral approach is used.

1

The patient lies supine under general anaesthesia. A high thigh tourniquet may be used. A medial longitudinal incision, approximately one quarter the total length of the thigh, is made, extending proximally from the apex of the medial femoral condyle.

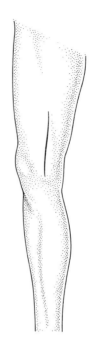

1

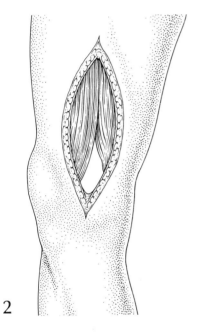

2

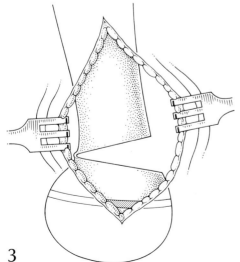

3

2

The deep fascia is divided and the vastus medialis exposed. To avoid damaging the muscle it is lifted forwards developing the plane between it and the adductor magnus. The femur is exposed and a longitudinal incision made in the periosteum on the medial side. The periosteum is raised and the supracondylar region is exposed widely by retracting the periosteum with bone levers. The epiphyseal plate can be clearly seen and care taken not to damage it either when removing the wedge of bone or inserting the fixation device.

3

A medially based wedge of bone is then removed proximal to the epiphyseal line making sure there is sufficient room to insert the fixation device, staple or plate, without damaging the epiphyseal plate. The wedge can be removed with a power saw or an osteotome and multiple drill holes. It is most important to leave the periosteum and the apex of the wedge intact to retain control of the bony fragments when the wedge is closed. The exact size of the wedge required must be measured from a weight-bearing radiograph and accurately marked out on the bone to ensure that the right amount of bone is removed. To avoid undesirable rotational deformity the bone can be marked above and below the wedge so that the surgeon can check rotational alignment at the end of the operation.

4

In children two or three staples are inserted to hold the wedge closed. It is advisable to start the points of the staples in small drill holes. This avoids displacing the osteotomy when the staples are hammered in. It also ensures that they are inserted evenly as the cortical bone of the proximal fragment is usually harder than that of the distal.

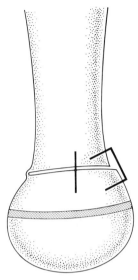

4

Postoperative management

The wound is closed in layers. Suction drainage is not usually necessary. A long leg plaster is applied with the knee in a few degrees of flexion. The foot may or may not be included in the plaster depending on the surgeon's preference. It is normally not necessary to immobilize the hip in a single spica unless the femur is very short. The plaster is retained until union occurs, usually 6 weeks in children and 8–10 weeks in adults. Weight-bearing in the plaster is allowed as soon as the surgeon feels it is safe, usually after 1 week.

Complications

The commonest error is failure to obtain the right amount of correction. Care in the clinical and radiological measurement of the correction required when the limb is weight-bearing should avoid this. Some surgeons use a sterile template to measure the angle for the wedge. In young children and patients with soft porotic bone adequate fixation can be difficult and the two-stage osteotomy–osteoclasis method is very useful.

Damage to the epiphyseal plate while it is still open must be avoided.

Reference

1. Moore JR. Osteotomy-osteoclasis: method for correcting long-bone deformities. *J Bone Joint Surg* 1947; 29: 119–29.

Illustrations by Gillian Oliver after B. Hyams

Rupture of the quadriceps mechanism

B. Helal   MChOrth, FRCS
Honorary Consultant Orthopaedic Surgeon, The Royal London Hospital and The Royal National Orthopaedic Hospital, London, and Enfield Group of Hospitals, UK

S. C. Chen   FRCS
Consultant Orthopaedic Surgeon, Enfield Group of Hospitals, UK

Introduction

The quadriceps mechanism can be disrupted at one of three levels depending on the age of the patient.

1. Rupture of the ligamentum patellae in children and young adults.
2. Fracture of the patella in young adults.
3. Rupture of the quadriceps tendon in the middle and older age groups.

RECENT RUPTURE

RUPTURE OF LIGAMENTUM PATELLAE

This occurs usually at the attachment of the ligamentum patellae to the inferior border of the patella as a result of a severe flexion injury against resistance. A haemarthrosis is present but the gap in the tendon may only be palpable after administration of a general anaesthetic. The treatment is always surgical.

Incision

1

A slightly curved anterior midline vertical incision is made over the knee from above the patella to below the tibial tuberosity.

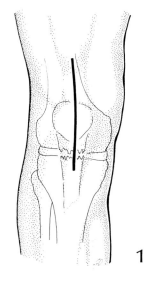

1

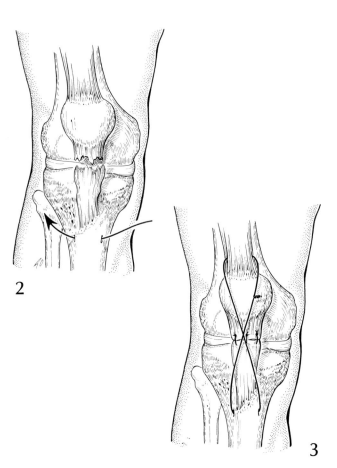

2

3

Procedure

2 & 3

A horizontal drill hole is made in the tibia at the level of the tibial tuberosity. A steel wire, 1.2 mm diameter, is threaded through the drill hole and passed across into the quadriceps tendon just above the patella, forming a figure-of-eight stitch. This stitch is tightened so that the ruptured ligamentum patellae is brought together. The tendon is stitched back using thick synthetic slowly absorbable sutures (polydioxanone-PDS). The subcutaneous tissue and skin are then closed.

Postoperative management

A well-padded crêpe bandage is applied over the knee and static quadriceps exercises including straight-leg raising exercises are commenced immediately. At 1 week, gentle knee flexion exercises can begin. The patient should walk on crutches at the end of 2 weeks but weight-bearing on the affected leg should not begin until 3 weeks have elapsed. Once the quadriceps muscles can lift the leg against gravity and some resistance, and the knee will flex to 90°, the crutches can be discarded for a walking-stick, which in its turn is discarded with the return of power and mobility.

RUPTURE OF QUADRICEPS TENDON

Incision

4

A midline vertical incision is made over the knee.

The surgeon must identify and ascertain the extent of the rupture of the quadriceps tendon. The rupture is usually across the musculotendinous junction of the quadriceps and the edges are ragged.

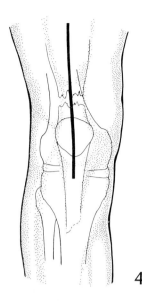

4

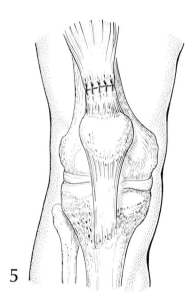

5

Repair

5

The ruptured muscle is stitched with interrupted thick synthetic, slowly absorbable sutures (polydioxanone-PDS). The wound is closed in layers.

Postoperative management

A plaster cylinder is applied from the ankle to the upper thigh and static quadriceps exercises are started the following day. At the end of 1 week straight-leg raising exercises are started and at the end of 2 weeks partial weight-bearing with the leg in plaster is allowed, using crutches. At the end of 4 weeks the plaster cylinder is removed and knee flexion exercises commenced. Unprotected weight-bearing is allowed when the knee can flex to 90° and the quadriceps muscles are strong.

OLD RUPTURE

OLD RUPTURE OF LIGAMENTUM PATELLAE
(modified Kelikian, Riashi and Gleason technique[1])

In old rupture, the quadriceps muscle becomes contracted. This has to be overcome and the patella brought down to its normal position before the ligamentum patellae can be replaced. The operation is carried out in two stages.

Stage 1

6 & 7

A vertical midline incision is made over the knee. The incision is deepened and the knee joint entered. The patella and the quadriceps muscle are freed so that any adhesions are broken down, enabling the patella to move freely.

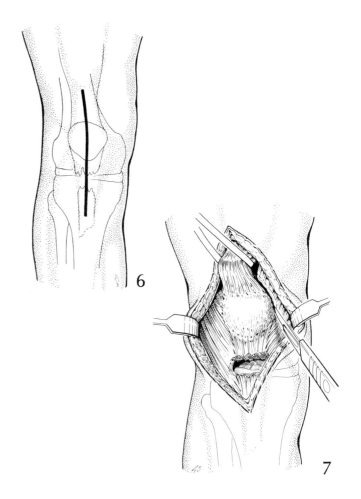

6

7

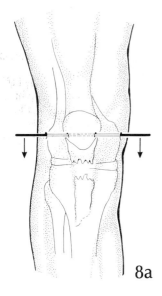

8a

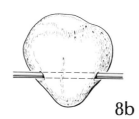

8b

8a & b

A skeletal pin (Steinmann or Denham pin) is passed transversely across the lower third of the patella. It is important to position the pin accurately as the pin track is later enlarged in Stage 2 to accommodate the semitendinosus tendon.

The skin incision is closed and traction applied to the skeletal pin in order to stretch the quadriceps muscle. Traction is continued until the patella is brought down to its normal level, the position being checked by radiography. This usually takes up to 2 weeks. In the meantime, the patient is encouraged to perform static quadriceps exercises.

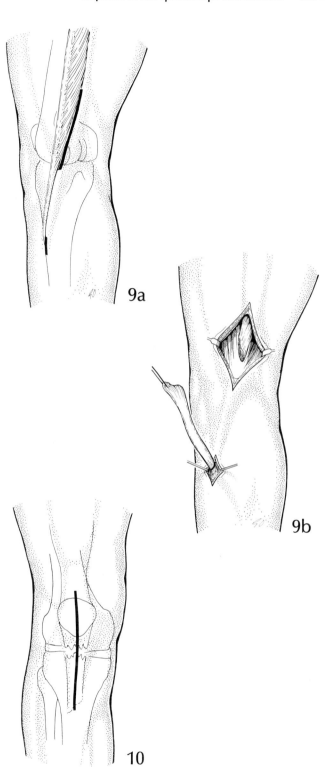

Stage 2

9a, b & 10

The skeletal pin is removed.

A longitudinal incision is made on the posteromedial aspect of the thigh. The semitendinosus tendon is identified and cut at the musculotendinous junction. Another small incision is made at the insertion of the semitendinosus tendon and the severed tendon withdrawn through this incision.

A third incision, a vertical midline incision, is made along the line of the initial incision in Stage 1.

11

A transverse hole is drilled across the tibia at the level of the tibial tuberosity. This hole must be of adequate size to accommodate the semitendinosus tendon. The pin track in the patella is enlarged in a similar manner.

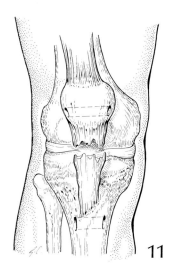

11

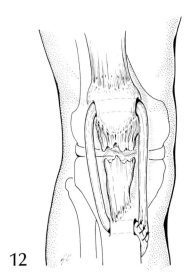

12

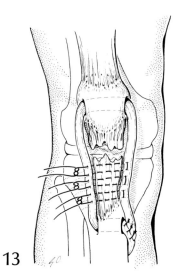

13

12 & 13

The semitendinosus tendon is passed subcutaneously from its insertion into the front of the tibia. It is threaded through the holes in the tibia and patella. The tendon is tightened and stitched back to itself as shown. The crumpled ligamentum patellae is pulled up and stitched to the two parts of the semitendinosus tendon with thick synthetic, slowly absorbable, sutures (polydioxanone-PDS).

Postoperative management

A plaster cast is applied from the toes to the upper thigh with the knee in extension. At the end of 6 weeks, the plaster cast is removed and passive and active knee exercises started.

OLD RUPTURE OF QUADRICEPS TENDON

Here again, the quadriceps muscle may be contracted.

Incision

14

A curved incision is made along the front of the knee extending from the lower thigh to the lower pole of the patella and the ruptured quadriceps tendons exposed.

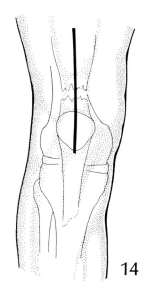

14

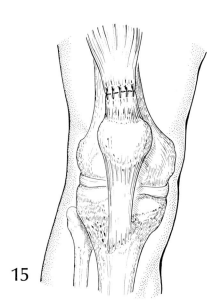

15

Repair

15

If the ruptured ends can be approximated with the knee fully extended, the ends are sutured together with interrupted thick chromic catgut sutures.

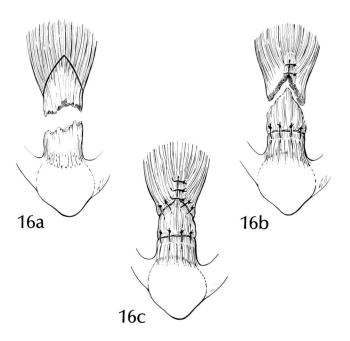

16a

16b

16c

Lengthening and repair

16a, b & c

If, however, the ruptured ends cannot be approximated, the quadriceps tendon can be lengthened by an inverted V-Y-plasty. An inverted V-inc'sion is made completely through the proximal segment of the quadriceps tendon 1 cm proximal to the ruptured end.

The ruptured ends are sutured with interrupted thick chromic catgut sutures.

The inverted V-incision is closed converting it into an inverted Y.

Postoperative management

A plaster cast is applied from the toes to the upper thigh with the knee in extension. At the end of 6 weeks, the plaster cast is removed and passive and active knee exercises started.

CONTRACTURE IN INFANCY

Repeated injections into the quadriceps, e.g., of antibiotics in the neonatal period, can lead to the muscle becoming fibrosed and contracted. This results in an inability to flex the knee. The fibrosis may occur in the deep fascia and in the quadriceps muscle.

Incision

17

The fibrosed part of the quadriceps should be sought. A longitudinal incision is made over the anterior part of the lower thigh to include the fibrosed area of the quadriceps.

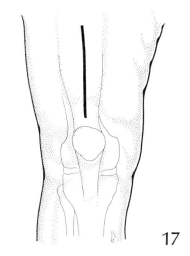

17

Release

18 & 19

The deep fascia is incised transversely across the front and sides of the thigh. Knee flexion should be assessed. If it is still restricted, the fibrosed parts of the quadriceps muscle are excised. This is rarely necessary. Usually the vastus intermedius is involved, but the rectus femoris and vastus lateralis may also be involved. The wound is then closed.

Postoperative management

A plaster cast is applied from the toes to the upper thigh with the knee flexed to 90°. The plaster cast is removed at the end of 3 weeks and passive and active exercises started.

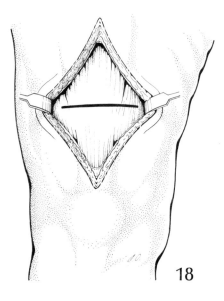

18

Reference

1. Kelikian H, Riashi E, Gleason J. Restoration of quadriceps function in neglected tear of the patellar tendon. *Surg Gynecol Obstet* 1957; 104: 200–4.

Further reading

Thompson TC. Quadricepsplasty to improve knee function. *J Bone Joint Surg* 1944; 26: 366–79.

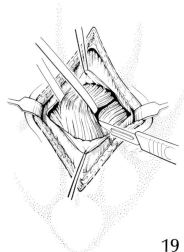

19

Quadricepsplasty in the adult

J. A. Fixsen MChir, FRCS
Consultant Orthopaedic Surgeon, The Hospital for Sick Children, Great Ormond Street, London, and St Bartholomew's Hospital, London, UK

Introduction

Indications

This operation can be used to correct limitation of flexion of the knee due to soft tissue scarring in the anterior aspect of the thigh involving the quadriceps muscle and its expansion. The commonest cause of such scarring and fibrosis are fractures of the femoral shaft, extensive soft tissue wounds of the thigh and immobilization following trauma. At operation limitation of flexion is usually found to be due to one or more of the following factors, all of which block the distal movement of the patella[1].

1. Fibrosis of the intermedius.
2. Adhesion of the patella to the femoral condyles.
3. Fibrosis and shortening of the lateral expansions of the vasti with adherence to the femoral condyles.
4. Actual shortening of the rectus femoris muscle, but this is rare.

Thompson, when describing the operation in 1944, commented that success depends on[2]:

1. whether the rectus femoris has escaped injury;
2. how well the rectus femoris can be isolated from the scarred parts of the quadriceps mechanism; and
3. how well the muscle can be developed by active use postoperatively.

Patients should have had a thorough course of active conservative treatment, including manipulation under anaesthesia to mobilize the knee, before considering this operation. The procedure is rarely indicated if the patient can flex his knee to 70° or more, and in the majority of patients considered for operation flexion is less than 30°.

Operation

The operation is usually performed under general anaesthesia. The patient lies in the supine position. A tourniquet can be used to facilitate the dissection in the early part of the operation if it is possible to place it high enough on the thigh to avoid the operation site. It must be removed before completing the operation to allow careful haemostasis and remove any tethering effect it may have on the quadriceps mechanism. Careful haemostasis using diathermy is essential throughout the operation.

1

A straight or slightly curving S-shaped anterior longitudinal incision is made through the skin, subcutaneous tissue and superficial fascia from the distal pole of the patella to the mid-thigh. The precise position and length of the incision are determined by the site of the scarring.

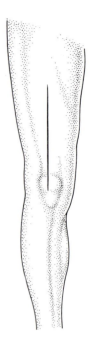

1

2

The rectus is then separated out by dividing the deep fascia on each side of the muscle to separate it from the vastus medialis and lateralis. The incisions are continued distally into the medial and lateral expansion of the capsule of the knee as far as is necessary to overcome any contracture. If the tendon of the rectus femoris has been obliterated by scarring it is necessary to fashion a new one by making a longitudinal strip out of scar tissue to replace it.

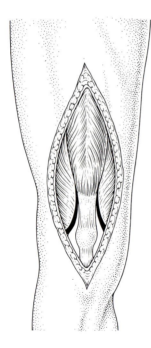

2

3

The scarred vastus intermedius which commonly binds down the rectus femoris and patella to the femur is excised completely, preserving the integrity of the rectus femoris and, if possible, a fibrous or periosteal covering over the anterior aspect of the femur. Following each step in the release of the quadriceps mechanism, the knee can be flexed to gauge how much flexion has been achieved. After removal of the scarred vastus intermedius the knee should be flexed to at least 110° to break down any intra-articular adhesion. If the rectus femoris is the sole remaining tight structure preventing flexion it can be lengthened but this will result in some permanent loss of active extension. If the patella itself is severely damaged on its articular surface, Nicoll[1] advises that it should be removed, but Hesketh[3] warns that this will weaken the quadriceps tendon and adversely affect postoperative mobilization.

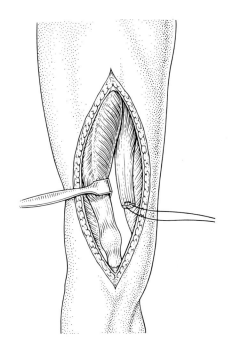

3

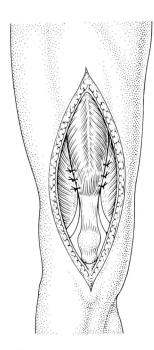

4

4

If the vastus medialis and lateralis are severely scarred, subcutaneous tissue and fat should be interposed between them and the rectus femoris. If they are reasonably normal, they may be sutured back to the sides of the rectus as far as the distal third of the thigh. The incisions in the capsule of the knee and lateral expansions are left open. If a tourniquet has been used this should be removed and careful haemostasis obtained. The wound is then closed with suction drainage.

Postoperative management

There is a variety of regimens for treatment of the limb postoperatively. Thompson immobilizes the leg in a Thomas' splint with a Pearson kneepiece. Balanced traction is applied and continued for 3 weeks. Active and passive stretchings are started as soon as possible after surgery. This is a slow and painful process and considerable determination on behalf of the patient and the physiotherapist are necessary to mobilize the knee at this stage. The author prefer Nicoll's method of immobilizing the knee in plaster in flexion of about 20°–30° less than that obtained at operation for the first 48–72 hours. The plaster and drain are then removed and the knee exercised during the day. At night it is immobilized in extension provided the range of flexion is being maintained during the day. Once the wound is healed, a gentle manipulation under anaesthesia may be necessary if flexion is being lost. The constant passive motion (CPM) machine can also be very useful in the postoperative management.

Complications

All authors writing on the subject of quadricepsplasty stress that the postoperative mobilization of the knee is usually slow and painful and requires determination and fortitude on the part of the patient. Hesketh[3] recommends that the operation should not be offered to patients over 55 years, unless they are unusually determined. The variety of postoperative regimens for mobilizing the knee also points to the difficulty of regaining the range of movement obtained at the time of operation by this extensive soft tissue procedure. Pool therapy is often helpful in regaining movement. An initial extension lag is almost invariable but usually disappears gradually over a period of up to a year, except in those patients where the rectus femoris has been lengthened, when some permanent loss of active extension is the rule.

References

1. Nicoll EA. Quadricepsplasty. *J Bone Joint Surg [Br]* 1963; 45-B: 483–90.

2. Thompson TC. Quadricepsplasty to improve knee function. *J Bone Joint Surg* 1944; 26: 366–79.

3. Hesketh KT. Experiences with the Thompson quadricepsplasty. *J Bone Joint Surg [Br]* 1963; 45-B: 491–5.

Illustrations by Gillian Oliver

Diagnostic arthroscopy of the knee

George Bentley ChM, FRCS
Professor of Orthopaedic Surgery, The Institute of Orthopaedics, University of London; Honorary Consultant
Orthopaedic Surgeon, Royal National Orthopaedic Hospital, Stanmore and the Middlesex Hospital, London, UK

Anthony J. B. Fogg FRCS
Consultant Orthopaedic Surgeon, Princess Margaret Hospital, Swindon, UK

Introduction

Endoscopic examination of the knee joint was first performed by Professor K. Tagaki in 1918, primarily for the assessment of tuberculosis. Eugen Bircher[1] of Switzerland reported the first European series in 1921 and the procedure was popularized by Watanabe in the 1950s[2,3] and by Jackson in the 1970s[4,5] and 1980s[6].

Arthroscopy is now routinely used in the diagnosis of knee joint injuries and disorders and as a prelude to endoscopic procedures, providing the surgeon with a method of accurate intra-articular assessment without the attendant risks of open arthrotomy.

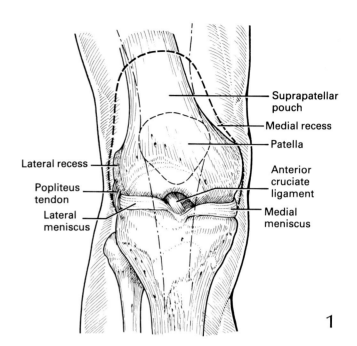

1

Anatomy

1, 2 & 3

With practice, a more extensive view of the interior of the joint can be achieved than is possible by arthrotomy. The structures visible through the routine anterolateral approach are as follows:

1. Articular surfaces of patella, patellar groove, femoral condyles and tibial condyles.
2. Anterior two-thirds of the medial meniscus and its posterior horn.
3. Entire lateral meniscus.
4. Anterior cruciate ligament.
5. Retropatellar fat pad and synovial folds.
6. Popliteus tendon.
7. Suprapatellar pouch.
8. Medial patellar plica.
9. Lateral and most of the medial femoral recess.

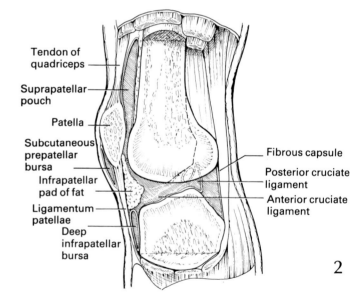

2

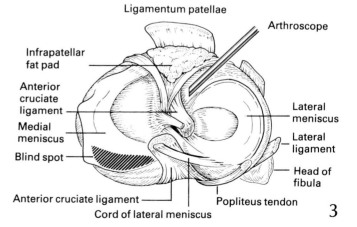

3

Preoperative

Indications

Arthroscopy should always be used in conjunction with a thorough history and clinical examination of the patient and is not an adequate substitute for either. Plain radiographs of the knee are an essential prerequisite: anteroposterior, weight-bearing and lateral views of the knee with views of both patellae at 30° of flexion are ideal. The procedure is used for the following purposes:

1. Confirmation of suspected meniscal lesions prior to arthroscopic or open surgery.
2. Assessment of anterior cruciate ligament integrity.
3. Diagnosis of acute injuries associated with haemarthrosis.
4. Investigation of anterior knee pain.
5. Evaluation of chondromalacia patellae and estimation of patellar 'tracking'.
6. Localization of loose bodies.
7. Assessment of osteochondritis dissecans.
8. Diagnosis and assessment of osteoarthritis.
9. Diagnosis of inflammatory joint disease and synovial biopsy.
10. Assessment of articular cartilage and synovium before and after treatment (e.g. tibial osteotomy, synovectomy, osteochondral grafting).
11. Examination of knee joint prostheses.

Equipment

4a

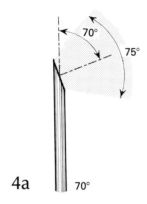

The rod lens system designed by Professor Hopkins of Reading University can provide the modern surgeon with a 4 mm, wide-angle (75°) viewing lens giving sharp bright images.

4b

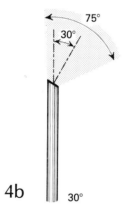

The preferred instrument for general use is the 30° fore-oblique arthroscope.

4c

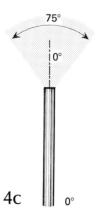

0° telescopes are available for the novice and give a straight-ahead view which allows for easier orientation. Visualization of certain areas is, however, impossible with the 0° telescope.

A 70° telescope provides greater access to the posteromedial and posterolateral joint compartments and is a useful addition to the experienced arthroscopist.

Modern arthroscope design has incorporated the bridge of the old cystoscope-based instrument into a stainless steel sheath down which sharp and blunt trocars are passed prior to insertion of the telescope. The risk of breakage of the telescope has consequently been reduced. Narrow diameter (2.7 mm) telescopes are available for paediatric use. A fibre-optic cold light source with a 150 watt lamp provides adequate illumination for routine examination. More powerful 250 watt sources are essential for television and video documentation.

Still slide photographs are obtainable using camera and flash attachments.

All diagnostic arthroscopy sets are equipped with at least one blunt hook with which to manipulate the menisci and cruciate ligaments and assess the articular cartilage for fissuring and softening.

Sterilization

The arthroscope is sterilized according to the manufacturers' instructions. The telescope may be subjected to flash autoclaving with great care, or gas sterilization using carboxide (88 per cent) and ethylene oxide (12 per cent) can be used (4 hour cycle at 71°C) in a gas autoclave. All parts of the instrument can be sterilized by immersion in an activated glutaraldehyde solution for 20 minutes provided that they are thoroughly washed in sterile water before use, and this is the commonly used method.

Anaesthesia

General anaesthesia

This is the preferred method in the majority of cases, and has advantages for both the surgeon and the patient. It allows for the comfortable use of a tourniquet, avoids the need for multiple injections of local anaesthetic, and presents the surgeon with a totally relaxed patient. Under a general anaesthetic, the joint is readily unlocked or manipulated for the purpose of improving the surgeon's view and arthrotomy can be performed if necessary.

Local anaesthesia

This method should be employed only by the experienced surgeon with confidence in his technique. It precludes the use of a tourniquet and, where multiple incisions are contemplated, is best conducted with the smaller diameter telescope. Each entry site is infiltrated with 0.5 per cent bupivacaine containing 1/100 000 adrenaline. A similar concentration of anaesthetic can be added to the irrigation fluid and the joint left for 5 minutes before proceeding. Femoral nerve block will facilitate this procedure and reduce postoperative pain.

Examination under anaesthesia

In an anaesthetized, fully relaxed patient, no diagnostic arthroscopy is complete without a thorough clinical examination of the knee. The examination should preferably be carried out prior to application of tourniquet and drapes and should include an assessment of the range of movement, collateral ligament stability, Lachman's test, pivot shift or 'jerk' test, anterior and posterior drawer signs, and patellar stability.

Tourniquet

A high thigh pneumatic tourniquet is applied to the leg prior to draping. Unless it is essential to assess the vascularity of the synovium arthroscopically, the leg is exsanguinated by elevation and/or application of a 'roll-on exsanguinator' and the tourniquet inflated to approximately twice systolic blood pressure.

It is considered useful to flex the knee as much as possible before inflation. This minimizes 'tightness' in the quadriceps muscles and allows greater freedom of movement of instruments within the joint.

Preparation and position

The leg should be shaved preoperatively and the skin prepared as for an arthrotomy. Although gaining in popularity as a day case procedure, the operation should be carried out in a fully equipped operating theatre under routine aseptic conditions. Because of the inevitable contact of the surgeon's mask, eyelash or hood with the eyepiece of the arthroscope, and the unavoidable spillage of irrigating fluid, it is impossible to keep the procedure completely sterile. Careful handling of the instruments by the eyepiece or handles and avoidance of contact with the barrel will help to minimize the introduction of potentially infective agents into the joint. The use of a video camera also reduces the risk, but the operator must be aware of potential contamination of the instruments, especially if the procedure proves difficult.

With the patient supine on the operating table, the limb is cleaned with an appropriate antiseptic solution such as 0.5 per cent chlorhexidine in 70 per cent alcohol and draped in such a manner that the hip and knee can both be flexed towards 90° and the perineum can remain completely isolated. Single-handed operators can use table-mounted thigh rests to assist control of the limb if necessary.

5

To avoid entanglement of the operatives with essential lengths of cable and tubing used during the procedure, it is wise to spend a short time in planning the positioning of personnel and equipment before embarking on diagnostic arthroscopy. Special attention should be paid to the positioning of the light source to avoid undue tension on the cable, and also to the provision of irrigation control which should be sterile and within easy reach of the surgeon.

The investigation is most comfortably performed sitting on a mobile stool with the table elevated to an appropriate height and the leg supported by the foot in the operator's lap. Where video photography is available, the operator stands or sits facing the television screen.

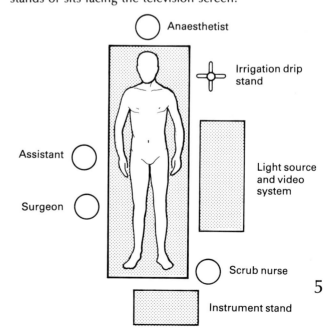

Anaesthetist

Irrigation drip stand

Assistant

Surgeon

Light source and video system

Scrub nurse

Instrument stand

5

Operation

Aspiration and irrigation

Prior to insertion of the arthroscope, any effusion or haemarthrosis in the joint is aspirated using a large bore irrigation or hypodermic needle and syringe, introduced via a lateral suprapatellar approach. Wide-bore, disposable trocars and cannulae are commercially available and serve equally well as fluid entry or exhaust portals.

Approach and assembly

6a & b

The anterolateral approach is the most useful for routine initial arthroscopic examination of the knee. With the knee flexed to 90°, it is easy to locate the small depression in the joint line to the lateral side of the patellar tendon with a fingertip. With a size 10 blade, a 5 mm transverse stab incision, 5 mm above the lateral tibial condyle (to avoid the lateral meniscus) and 5 mm lateral to the patellar tendon, is made in the skin and extended down through the joint capsule. The arthroscope sheath with the sharp trocar is then introduced and directed medially, upwards and backwards towards the intercondylar notch, using gentle pressure and a rotational force. Once the capsule is penetrated, the tip lies just above the anterior horn of the lateral meniscus. The blunt trocar is now substituted for the sharp trocar.

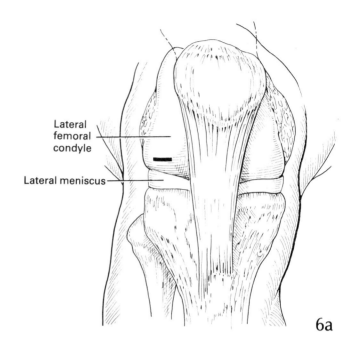

Lateral femoral condyle

Lateral meniscus

6a

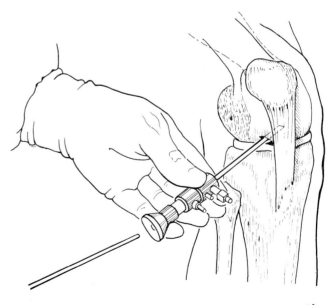

6b

6c

The knee is extended and, with a sudden controlled push, the tip is introduced beneath the patella into the suprapatellar pouch. The trocar is removed and replaced by the telescope, which is locked into the sheath. The light cable, VDU and video systems are attached and the distension and irrigation system assembled. Distension of the joint is achieved by a sterile 'giving-set' connected from a 1 litre bag of normal saline (suspended 1 metre above the knee) to the inlet tap on the arthroscope sheath. A drainage tube is connected to the outlet tap of the arthroscope and led to a bowl beneath the table. For diagnostic procedures it is often not necessary to use continuous irrigation but the joint can be irrigated at intervals by alternate use of inlet and outlet taps. The joint may be filled prior to insertion of the arthroscope by a wide-bore needle if preferred. Continuous irrigation may be performed by this method also. Examination of the joint commences. With practice it is easier to view the TV monitor directly than to use the eye-to-telescope method.

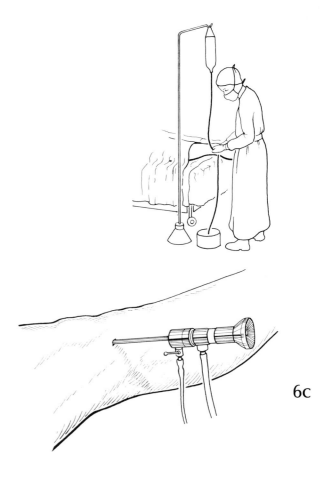

6c

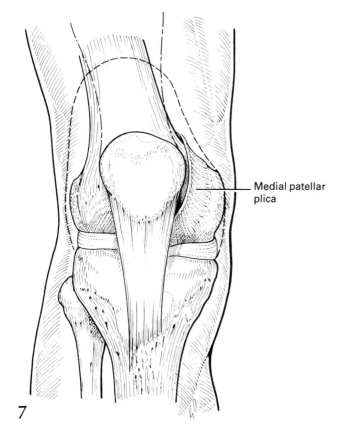

Medial patellar plica

7

7

With the knee extended the arthroscope is pushed gently towards the apex of the pouch and gradually withdrawn, inspecting the synovium en route (*Plate 11**). At the superior medial pole of the patella and running upwards and backwards to the femur is the medial suprapatellar plica which very occasionally divides the pouch into two distinct cavities and may obscure the presence of loose bodies. This structure is not to be confused with the more common medial patellar plica (medial synovial shelf or Aoki's band) (*see Illustration 7*), which runs in the coronal plane from the medial side of the joint to insert distally below the inferior pole of the patella into the infrapatellar fat pad (*Plate 12*). This latter structure, although infamous, rarely causes symptoms. When pathological, it is visible as a thickened, fibrous crescentic band which can be seen to impinge between the patella and femur as the knee is flexed and may cause a groove in the medial femoral condyle. These structures can be further assessed by probing them with an irrigation needle or arthroscopy hook. Biopsy of the synovium, especially in the absence of a tourniquet, is deferred until completion of the examination to avoid bleeding and interference with the visual field.

*Colour plates 11–30 are on pages 1033–1036.

Patellofemoral joint

By withdrawing the instrument and rotating it to direct the line of vision upwards, the undersurface of the patella can be inspected. The lateral half of the patella can be examined easily by carefully running the arthroscope along its length and, by pushing the patella laterally and tilting it towards the examiner, the median ridge, the medial articular cartilage and the most medial (odd) facet can be visualized.

Aoki's band is best seen by directing the arthroscope medially and upwards at this juncture. Further assessment of the patellar articular cartilage can be gained by probing with a blunt hook introduced through an anteromedial stab incision, special note being taken of any areas of softening, 'blistering' or fissuring on the medial or odd facets suggestive of chondromalacia patellae.

The relationship of the median patellar ridge to the intercondylar groove of the femur is now inspected during an arc of flexion of 0–60°. In normal subjects, the ridge strikes just lateral to the floor of the groove and gradually comes to lie centrally by approximately 60° flexion (*Plate 13*).

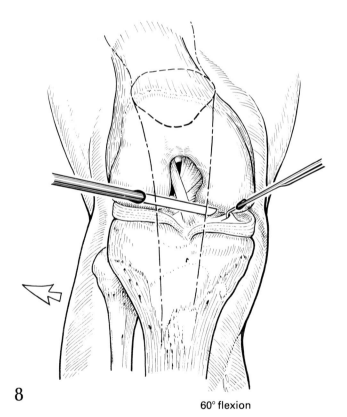

8

60° flexion

Infrapatellar fat pad

The infrapatellar fat pad is occasionally traumatized (Hoffa's syndrome) or caught between the patella and femoral condyles during violent extension (hurdler's knee). The normal pad can be seen easily as a fatty globular structure immediately below the patella with a covering of synovium containing a fine plexus of blood vessels (*Plate 14*). The alar fold can also be seen. Occasionally, if introduced too medially, the arthroscope penetrates the suspensory ligament of the patella, impeding visualization. This is remedied by reinsertion of the instrument in a more posterior direction.

Medial compartment

8

By turning the arthroscope downwards after examination of the patellofemoral joint, the rolled edge of the medial femoral condyle can be identified and followed downwards to gain entry to the medial compartment. The knee is now placed in 60° of flexion and a valgus/lateral rotation strain applied. The meniscosynovial attachment is readily identifiable and, as the telescope is very slightly withdrawn, the sharp free edge of the medial meniscus and the anterior horn are seen (*Plate 15*). Further inspection of the femoral and tibial condyles is also possible and particular note should be made of irregularities in the articular cartilage of the femoral condyle where it abuts on the anterior horn in full extension. 'Abrasions' of the cartilage are frequently associated with meniscal tears. The anterior two-thirds of the medial meniscus are easily inspected but the posterior third is not so readily visualized, although its free edge may be seen beneath the femoral condyle if a considerable valgus strain is applied to the knee in 30° flexion. At the junction of the two parts, a 'flounce' or 'kink' is regularly noted (*Plate 16*). This is a normal finding, unless excessive, in which case a detachment of the posteromedial portion may be present. The inspection is assisted by introducing a blunt probe through the anteromedial portal and lifting the free edge to explore for inferior cleavage tears (*Plate 17*). The hook can also be used to try to displace the meniscus into the joint, as may occur with a peripheral detachment (*Plate 18*). By placing the hook into the meniscosynovial junction and rotating the knee laterally, large flap tears previously hidden beneath the femoral condyle may emerge. Further information about the posterior horn is gained by accessing the posteromedial compartment.

Intercondylar notch and anterior cruciate ligament

9 & 10

By gently withdrawing the tip of the arthroscope from the anteromedial compartment, the anterior cruciate ligament will present itself as a silver striated bundle, covered with synovium. Blood vessels are arranged longitudinally along the length of the ligament which travels posteriorly and laterally, tapering towards its attachment on the medial surface of the lateral femoral condyle (*Plate 19*). The ligament is occasionally bifurcate but is still distinguishable from a partial tear by the presence of an intact synovial membrane. The integrity of the ligament can be assessed under direct vision while the assistant performs the anterior drawer test. The ligament may also be probed with the hook.

To gain access to the posteromedial compartment, the knee is flexed 10° and, under direct vision, the telescope is passed over the anterior cruciate ligament and between it and the posterolateral edge of the medial femoral condyle (*see Illustration 10*). This manoeuvre is occasionally hampered by the presence of excessive synovial folds or osteophytes but, in the majority of cases, gives the surgeon a rewarding view of the posterior horn of the medial meniscus and an area behind the medial tibial condyle where a loose body may be concealed. The back of the meniscus can be examined in greater detail by substituting the 70° lens at this stage. The instrument is now withdrawn and, if rotated medially and slightly upwards, may identify a raised area on the lateral aspect of the medial femoral condyle corresponding to the attachment of the posterior cruciate ligament. This structure is otherwise not seen through the anterolateral approach unless there is a complete rupture of the anterior cruciate ligament. In a proportion of such cases where diagnosis has been delayed, the anterior cruciate ligament may be identified running posteriorly and medially to become adherent to the posterior cruciate ligament.

The arthroscope is rotated downwards so that the anterior cruciate ligament again enters the field. The ligamentum mucosum (infrapatellar synovial fold) sometimes impedes passage of the instrument across the notch and may be confused with the ligament itself. By keeping the anterior cruciate in constant view, orientation is not lost and the telescope can gradually be withdrawn and moved laterally into the lateral compartment of the joint.

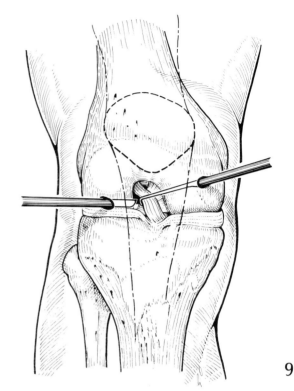

9

10° flexion

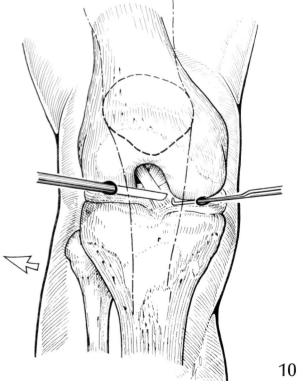

10

10° flexion

Lateral compartment

11

With the knee flexed to 30° and the foot placed across the table onto the opposite leg, a varus strain can be applied to the knee joint, thereby opening up the lateral compartment for inspection. An alternative method is to place the foot over the edge of the operating table with the knee in 30° flexion and apply a varus strain with the surgeon's thigh against the patient's foot, using the table edge as a fulcrum.

The first structure visible is the free edge of the posterior horn of the lateral meniscus lying under the lateral femoral condyle (*Plate 20*). This is easily visualized on its inferior surface by passing the arthroscope directly beneath it into a small recess where loose bodies may lodge. It may also be inspected by elevating the meniscal margin with a hook introduced through the anteromedial portal.

By advancing the instrument under direct vision between the anterior cruciate ligament and the medial edge of the lateral femoral condyle, the posterolateral compartment is entered. The superior and posterior surfaces of the posterior horn of the lateral meniscus and the back of the lateral femoral condyle are now easily seen. Use of the 70° telescope will again provide a more detailed inspection. The instrument is now withdrawn back into the joint and the sharp edge of the lateral meniscus followed laterally and anteriorly. During this manoeuvre the popliteus tendon is usually seen running obliquely downwards and medially behind the posterior third of the meniscus towards its insertion on the posteromedial aspect of the tibia (*Plate 21*).

Occasionally it is difficult to see the attachment of the anterior horn of the lateral meniscus and, if serious doubt exists, then an entry from the anteromedial portal should be made.

Lateral gutter

If difficulty is encountered in traversing the intercondylar notch, then a bucket-handle tear of either meniscus should be suspected. In this instance, the lateral compartment is best reached by returning the telescope to the suprapatellar pouch with the knee in extension and passing the tip down into the lateral gutter, adjacent to the lateral surface of the lateral femoral condyle. While here, the gutter can be inspected for loose bodies (*see Plate 22*) and, by guiding the instrument backwards through the synovial folds, a different perspective of the popliteus tendon may be obtained. In cases of suspected lateral patellar instability, one should assess the degree of 'overhang' between the lateral margin of the patella and the lateral femoral condyle by turning the tip of the instrument upwards and observing the relationship during flexion. The lateral joint compartment can then be entered by withdrawing the tip of the arthroscope and directing it medially.

After inspection of the lateral compartment, including visualization of the articular surfaces, the procedure is at an end.

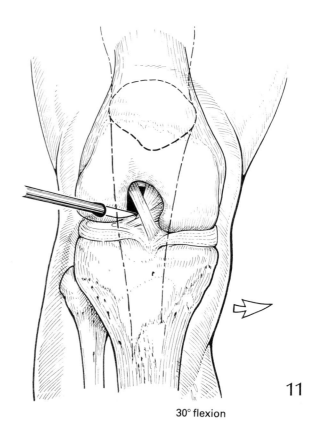

30° flexion

11

Wound closure

Fluid is expressed from the joint at the end of the procedure down the empty sheath which is then withdrawn completely. The skin is closed using sterile skin 'closure strips' or fine microfilament nylon sutures through skin and subcutaneous tissues and the wound dressed with non-adhesive material. The knee is supported with a compression bandage of wool and crêpe extending from the tibial tuberosity to the lower thigh.

If the surgeon wishes to proceed to arthrotomy at the end of the arthroscopy, the leg should be prepared anew and draped in the usual manner and the surgeon and assistant should change gloves and gowns.

Postoperative management

Straight-leg raising should commence immediately postoperatively and flexion and weight-bearing should begin within 24 hours, following reduction of the compression dressing. The patient may be discharged when recovered from the anaesthetic. Sutures, if used, are removed 10 days postoperatively, at which time full activity may be able to recommence, depending on the findings.

Alternative approaches

Anteromedial approach

12

As a visual portal, this approach (labelled 2 in illustration) is not recommended unless there is considerable suspicion of an anterior horn lesion of the lateral meniscus. If the arthroscope is to be introduced through this approach, then a stab incision approximately 1 cm above the tibial plateau and 1.5 cm medial to the edge of the patellar tendon will allow an acceptable view of the anterior horn of the lateral meniscus, the posterior attachment of the medial meniscus and the intercondylar notch. The anteromedial approach is, however, the routine portal of entry for arthroscopic surgical instruments including the blunt hook or probe. To facilitate the choice of site of entry, a hypodermic needle can first be inserted under direct vision until the ideal position is obtained and a stab incision then made at this point.

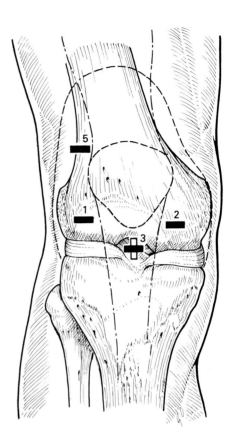

12

Central approach

This route (3), popularized by Gillquist[7], allows more detailed inspection of the posterior compartments of the knee. A transverse skin crease stab incision is made in the midline, 1 cm below the inferior pole of the patella through skin and subcutaneous fat. The patellar tendon is then incised along the length of its fibres and the trocar and sheath directed upwards and backwards through it.

The suprapatellar pouch can be examined with the knee in extension and the rest of the joint inspected with the knee flexed and appropriate strains applied. The postero-medial compartment is accessed by guiding the instrument between the anterior cruciate ligament and the medial femoral condyle. With a 70° lens, the posterior cruciate ligament can be seen if the tip is rotated laterally and downwards. Tension can be introduced into the ligament by applying medial tibial rotation. The authors of this approach claim to reduce significantly the numbers of unseen tears of the posterior horn of the medial meniscus, this being the most common diagnostic error when using the standard anterolateral approach.

Posteromedial approach

13

This approach (4), described by Dashefsky[8], allows optimal examination of the 'blind area' of the medial meniscus. Entry is gained under direct vision by inserting the telescope through a stab wound in the posteromedial angle of the joint, with the knee in 90° of flexion. Initial passage of a hypodermic needle into a fluid-filled joint will reassure the surgeon that the extracapsular structures remain undamaged. The posterior aspect of the meniscus, posterior cruciate ligament and the inferior recess are best visualized with the knee flexed to 90°.

Lateral suprapatellar[9] (approach 5), *posterolateral* and *medial suprapatellar* approaches are all described but have no place in routine diagnostic arthroscopy.

Note. It is very unwise for the novice to embark on any but the routine anterolateral approach until total familiarity with intra-articular landmarks and common abnormalities has been achieved. Proficiency at 'visual triangulation' is also essential before proceeding to any arthroscopic surgical procedure, and this is most rapidly achieved by regular use of the blunt hook introduced via the anteromedial portal.

Biopsy

This can be achieved under direct vision using either a specially adapted 2.7 mm telescope with attached biopsy forceps or by directing, under vision, a second instrument through the anteromedial or lateral suprapatellar portals.

Photography

Normal and pathological features can be documented on both still photographs and video tape. The former method requires a modified single lens reflex camera and a flash attachment, operated by a non-sterile member of the team. Three shots at different exposures are recommended. Video tape recording not only allows the surgeon a greater freedom of movement, but is extremely valuable as a teaching aid and provides a more dynamic record of intra-articular pathology. Sterilizable video cameras have now achieved a high level of sophistication and compactness.

Pathological findings

Tears of the meniscus (semilunar cartilage)

The edge of the meniscus is a sharp, clearly defined border although the edge, especially of the lateral meniscus, may be slightly fibrillated over the age of 25 years. Degenerated menisci are more fibrillated and have a rough edge with fibrils floating into the joint. These may conceal a horizontal tear and should be carefully examined with a blunt hook (*Plate 23*). Bucket-handle tears can be confusing, especially if one end is free or the

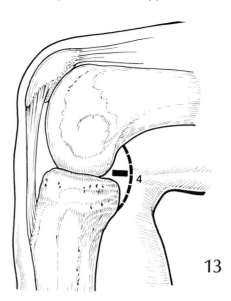

13

handle is displaced into the centre of the joint. Peripheral detachment can be recognized if care is taken to ensure that the arthroscopic view extends out to the junction of the synovium and the meniscus and the junction is probed with the blunt hook. The stability of the meniscus can then be checked. The doubtful area of the posterior one-third of the meniscus can be viewed partially from the intercondylar notch, but generally speaking a small cleft, fibrillation or irregularity of the meniscus can be seen when there is a posterior tear. A normal-looking meniscus which is stable on probing usually is normal and not a cause of symptoms.

A discoid lateral meniscus (*Plate 24*) may be difficult to recognize but can be defined by exerting pressure on the lateral joint line, thus moving the meniscus edge further towards the centre of the joint.

Synovial membrane

This is visible throughout most of the joint and covers the intra-articular structures such as the infrapatellar fat pad and cruciate ligaments. Normally a thin vascularized film, it is hypertrophied when the joint is inflamed from any cause (*Plate 25*) and can be biopsied under vision by a forceps passed through the anteromedial portal.

Articular cartilage

Chondromalacia patellae is easily recognized at all stages and careful probing of the cartilage surface will indicate softening (*Plates 26, 27* and *28*). In osteoarthritis pitting of the femoral condyle (*Plate 29*) is an early change, whilst in the later stages erosion of the tibial articular surface is seen with multiple tears of the meniscus (*Plate 30*).

Osteochondritis dissecans

Sometimes it is difficult to see any change in the articular cartilage arthroscopically, even with a clearly defined bony defect on the radiographs. Probing the affected area will indicate any soft or unstable cartilage.

References

1. Bircher E. Die Arthroendoskopie. *Zentralbl Chir* 1921; 48: 1460.

2. Watanabe M, Takeda S. The number 21 arthroscope. *J Jap Orthop Assoc* 1960; 34: 1041.

3. Watanabe M, Takeda S, Ikeuchi H. *Atlas of arthroscopy*. 2nd ed. Tokyo, Igaku: Shoin Ltd, 1969.

4. Jackson RW, Abe I. The role of arthroscopy in the management of disorders of the knee; analysis of 200 consecutive examinations. *J Bone Joint Surg [Br]* 1972; 54-B: 310–22.

5. Jackson RW, Dandy DJ. *Arthroscopy of the knee*. New York: Grune and Stratton, 1976.

6. Jackson RW. The scope of arthroscopy. *Clin Orthop* 1986; 208: 69–71.

7. Gillquist J, Hagberg G, Oretop N. Arthroscopic examination of the posteromedial compartment of the knee joint. *Int Orthop* 1979; 3: 13–8.

8. Dashefsky JH. Arthroscopic visualization of the 'blind area' in the posteromedial compartment of the knee. *Orthop Rev* 1976; 5: 51.

9. Dandy DJ. *Arthroscopic surgery of the knee*. Edinburgh: Churchill Livingstone, 1981.

Illustrations by Peter Cox

Arthroscopic surgical procedures

Ian Stother MA, FRCS(Ed), FRCS(Glas)
Consultant Orthopaedic Surgeon, Glasgow Royal Infirmary and The Glasgow Nuffield Hospital, Glasgow, UK

Introduction

The range of surgery performed on the knee joint is very large. Arthroscopic surgery is by definition intra-articular surgery. In theory it should be possible to carry out any intra-articular procedure through the arthroscope; indeed, the range of arthroscopic surgical procedures is continually increasing, and includes not only procedures such as meniscectomy but also such diverse procedures as the insertion of prosthetic ligaments and abrasion arthroplasty for degenerative arthritis.

Arthroscopic surgery offers a number of advantages. Firstly, the surgical incisions and subsequent scars are small. Secondly, the postoperative recovery is usually rapid when compared with the equivalent open operation. Thirdly, arthroscopy allows access to all areas of the joint without extensive scarring.

Triangulation

1 & 2

The basic technique used in arthroscopic surgery is triangulation. The arthroscope is inserted through one incision or portal. The operating instrument is usually inserted through a separate incision and manipulated into the field of view of the arthroscope. Most surgeons use a 25° or 30° telescope for arthroscopic surgery. Sometimes two instruments are used simultaneously (*see* chapter on 'Arthroscopic meniscectomy', pp. 1043–1055). Before the actual operating instruments are inserted it is recommended that a hypodermic needle or probe be inserted along the proposed route to check that access to the site of operation is possible.

Distension of the joint

It is essential that all the surgical manoeuvres are carried out under direct vision (either via the telescope itself or via a television monitor attached to the arthroscope). To achieve this the knee joint must be distended with either gas or liquid (*see* chapter on 'Diagnostic arthroscopy of the knee', pp. 1007–1018).

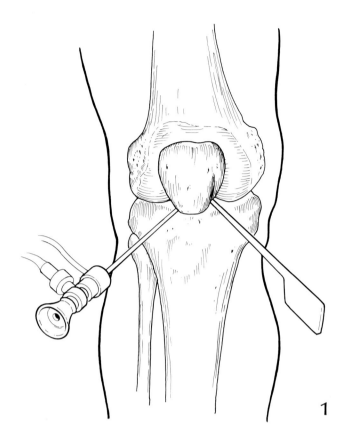

1

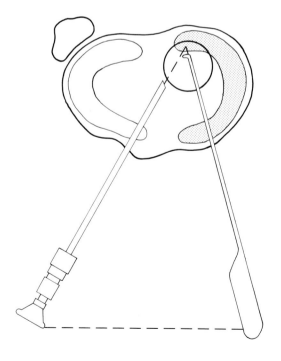

2

Arthroscopic surgical instruments

The equipment needed for diagnostic arthroscopy is required (*see* chapter on 'Diagnostic arthroscopy of the knee', pp. 1007–1018). In addition many special instruments are also available. There are two major types of instrument; hand instruments and power instruments.

In general both groups of instruments serve the same functions. Power instruments are potentially more dangerous than hand instruments and should probably only be used by experienced arthroscopic surgeons.

It is useful to have instruments of different diameters. Small (2.7 mm) diameter instruments are useful to reach the posterior parts of the medial meniscus. Curved instruments also make access easier on occasion. All the instruments serve a number of basic functions:

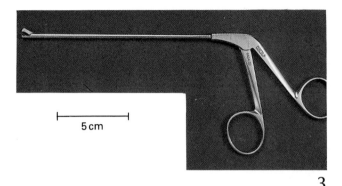

5 cm

3

Cutting instruments

3, 4 & 5

Small scissors (*Illustrations 3* and *4*). Small knife (preferably with retractable blade) (*Illustration 5*). 'Draw knives' which cut towards the operator as the knife is withdrawn are useful for short bucket-handle tears.

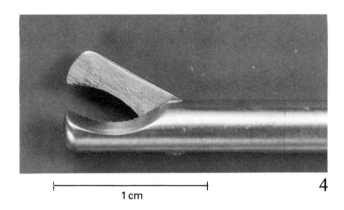

1 cm

4

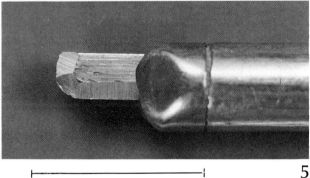

1 cm

5

Grasping instruments

6 & 7

Various grasping forceps are available. It is helpful if they have teeth in the jaws and ratchet handles.

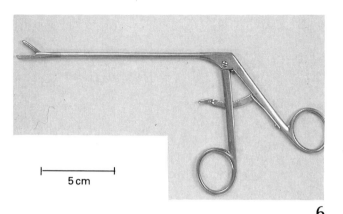

5 cm

6

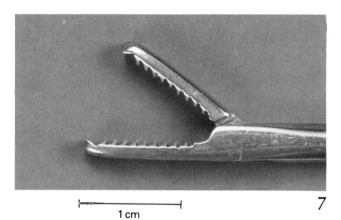

1 cm

7

Nibbling instruments

8 & 9

Pituitary rongeurs of small size and with different head angles are useful for degenerate meniscus and articular cartilage flaps.

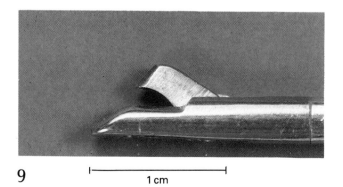

5 cm

8

9

Punch forceps in several sizes are useful for trimming and cutting. Side-cutting punch forceps may be easier to manipulate into the desired position near the back of the joint, and at the front of the joint.

During arthroscopic surgery it may be necessary to insert the telescope and instruments through several different portals, and to exchange the position of the telescope and instruments.

9

1 cm

Operative procedures

Surgery of the synovium

SYNOVIAL BIOPSY

Indications

A diagnostic procedure for chronic effusion or synovitis of the knee joint.

Serology for the various causes of chronic synovitis should be performed preoperatively. These include tests for rheumatoid arthritis, *Salmonella* and *Shigella* antibody titres, and on occasion the antituberculin titre and tests for syphilis.

Preparation of the patient

The operation may be performed under local or general anaesthesia. The patient is placed supine on the operating table. A mid-thigh tourniquet placed well clear of the suprapatellar pouch reduces bleeding and aids viewing in the presence of synovitis. Some surgeons prefer not to inflate the tourniquet as this allows a better appreciation of the synovial colour and vascularity.

The skin is cleaned and drapes applied to give a sterile operating field.

Insertion of irrigation cannula

This is inserted laterally above the patella. Usually there will be an effusion and a sample of this should be sent for culture.

As much effusion as possible should be drained. The joint should then be distended with normal saline. A sample should then be drained and if it is turbid the joint should be drained and re-filled until clear fluid emerges.

Insertion of the arthroscope

The arthroscope is inserted in the anterolateral portal. A stab skin incision is made with the knee flexed and then the arthroscope inserted and the knee extended so the scope enters the suprapatellar pouch. The view here may be very limited in the presence of florid synovitis.

Assessment of the synovitis

Continuous irrigation with clear saline entering via the arthroscope is usually required. All compartments of the joint should be inspected. An area of florid synovitis should be chosen for biopsy. Any invasion of the joint surfaces and their state should be carefully documented.

Insertion of the biopsy forceps

10

It is usually convenient to biopsy synovium in the suprapatellar pouch. Pituitary rongeurs make suitable biopsy forceps. It is easiest to insert the forceps through a stab incision made directly through skin and joint capsule some distance from the proposed biopsy site. This makes it easier to manipulate the forceps into the field of view by triangulation.

The telescope passes from an anterolateral portal across the patellofemoral joint in the extended knee. The rongeurs are inserted in a midpatellar medial position. *Plate 31** shows the biopsy being taken; two or three bites of abnormal synovium should be sent for histology.

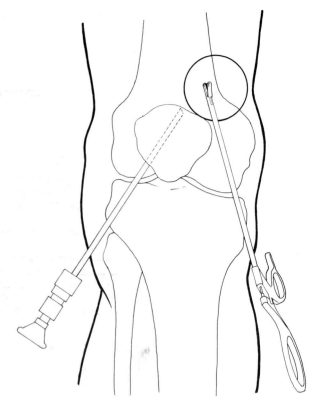

10

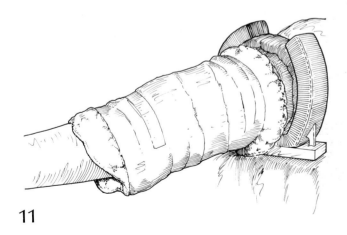

11

Closure of wounds

11

The fluid is drained from the knee joint. The skin incisions are closed with single sutures. A padded crêpe compression bandage is applied.

Postoperative management

The patient starts quadriceps exercises on recovery from the anaesthetic and mobilizes weight-bearing as comfort allows as soon as straight-leg raising can be performed with minimal lag. Knee flexion can be started at the same time. The speed of recovery depends upon the extent of the synovitis. If the recovery is very slow this may be because of a haemarthrosis. If this is suspected the dressings should be removed and the haemarthrosis aspirated after 48 hours. The sutures can be removed after 7 days.

*Colour plates 31–43 are on pages 1037–1039.

DIVISION OF A SYNOVIAL FOLD OR SHELF

Indications

Pathological synovial folds usually catch against the femoral condyle, often at the junction of the patellar and tibial surfaces where the articular cartilage heaps up. The folds can usually be detected clinically as a fibrous band which suddenly snaps over the femoral condyle during flexion or extension.

There may be a history of direct trauma to this area of the knee. The folds may be asymptomatic, but removal is indicated if the abnormal movement of the fold causes pain or a feeling of instability.

Preparation of the patient

The approximate position of the fold should be marked on the skin preoperatively. The patient is placed supine on the operating table. General or spinal anaesthesia should be used. A mid-thigh tourniquet should be in position and inflated to control bleeding. The skin is cleaned and drapes are applied to give a sterile operating field. The knee is distended with normal saline inserted via the suprapatellar pouch.

Insertion of the arthroscope

The arthroscope should be inserted on the side opposite the fold visualized, anteromedially for lateral folds and anterolaterally for medial folds.

Definition of the fold

The fold must be palpated, both through the skin and also with a probe inserted into the joint. Abnormal folds are firm or hard and do not stretch out of the way of a probe (see *Plate 32*). The probe may be inserted anteriorly or from the suprapatellar pouch. The presence of an erosion of the femoral condyle should be sought (see *Plate 33*).

Division of the fold

12

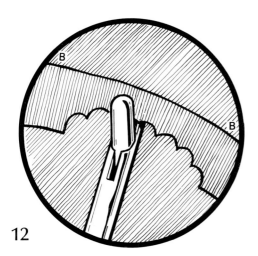

A length of 1 cm or more of the abnormal fold is removed. The base of the fold (marked B–B) must be excised so that no tight band remains.

The excision is often most easily achieved using punch forceps – either end-cutting or side-cutting. A power meniscotome with a rotating side-cutting blade and suction is also very suitable. Scissors may also be used to divide the fold, but once the initial cut has been made the tension in the fold is relaxed and subsequent excision is more difficult.

The joint is irrigated and drained. The instruments are removed. The joint is palpated through the skin to check that the fold no longer catches. If it still catches, then a further length of fold must be removed. A check should be made that a length of the base of the fold has been excised. If these measures fail to stop the fold catching, a lateral release may be helpful if the fold is on the lateral side.

Closure of wounds

As for Synovial biopsy (p. 1024).

Postoperative management

As for Synovial biopsy (p. 1024).

EXCISION OF SYNOVIAL TAGS

Indications

Pedunculated synovial tags, often of abnormal synovium, e.g. localized villonodular synovitis, may interpose between the joint surfaces and cause episodes of locking or giving way. They may mimic a loose body or a tag of torn meniscus.

Preparation of the patient

The patient is placed supine on the operating table. General or spinal anaesthesia is required. A mid-thigh tourniquet may be useful to control bleeding. The skin is cleaned and the leg draped to provide a sterile operating field. The joint is distended with isotonic saline.

Insertion of the telescope

The arthroscope is inserted anterolaterally. Synovial tags are commonly associated with the fat pads and interfere with the front of the joint (see Plates 34a, 34b). If they cannot easily be defined from an anterolateral insertion of the telescope then it should be reinserted in the mid-patellar lateral position. Tags may also jam between the patella and its groove (see Plate 35a, 35b).

Definition of the synovial tag

The size of the tag and the position of its base should be defined with a probe (see Plate 36). If the telescope is in the anterolateral portal the probe may be inserted through a high anteromedial portal. If the telescope is in the midpatellar lateral portal the probe can be inserted anteromedially or anterolaterally.

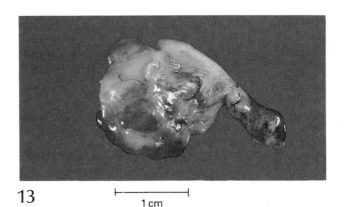

13

| 1 cm |

13

Tags which cause symptoms are probably at least 1 cm in diameter, and if they have been catching between the articular surfaces they are often oedematous and bruised.

Removal of the synovial tag

Pedunculated tags can often be removed by putting scissors in place of the probe and subtotally dividing the base. The scissors are then removed and a pair of grasping forceps or rongeurs are inserted to grasp the tag across its base.

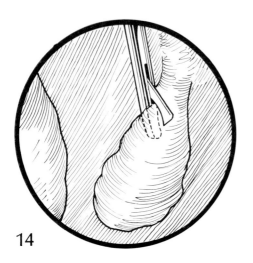

14

14

The telescope views from anterolaterally and scissors have been inserted from a high anteromedial portal for a medial tag. Large tags may be removed piecemeal with rongeurs. Care must be taken to remove the whole of any abnormal tag (see Illustration 13). A check must be made for the presence of two or more tags. The excised tissue should be sent for histology.

Closure of wounds

As for Synovial biopsy (p. 1024).

Postoperative management

As for Synovial biopsy (p. 1024).

SYNOVECTOMY

Indications

As for open synovectomy (see chapter on 'Synovectomy of the knee', pp. 1109–1112).

The range of movement and stability of the joint as well as the state of the joint surfaces shown on the radiograph and the presence of synovial thickening and an effusion should be noted. Marked instability or stiffness are contraindications.

Equipment

Some form of power instrumentation with a rotary cutting head and suction is required. Large volumes of irrigation fluid are also needed.

Preparation of the patient

As for Excision of synovial tags (pp. 1026).

The operation

A tourniquet should be applied. A telescope is inserted in the anterolateral portal. A power shaver may be inserted supermedially to shave the suprapatellar pouch. All hypertrophic synovium should be excised, although some areas will inevitably be inaccessible. Some tissue may be more easily removed with pituitary rongeurs. The medial gutter should be accessible with the superomedial insertion of the shaver. The lateral gutter may require a superolateral insertion. The area around the anterior cruciate ligament may be accessible via an anteromedial portal. All shaving must be done under direct vision. The operation is a long one.

Closure of wound

As for Synovial biopsy (p. 1024).

Postoperative management

A compression bandage is applied for 48 hours, and then the leg is gradually mobilized. A continuous passive motion machine may be useful in the postoperative period.

Surgery of the articular cartilage

SURGERY OF OSTEOCHONDRITIS DISSECANS

Diagnosis of the condition is primarily radiological. Diagnostic arthroscopy is useful to determine whether or not the articular cartilage is breached and to see if there is an unstable area of joint surface.

In young patients with open epiphyses the initial treatment is conservative. In older patients and in young patients who do not respond to conservative measures diagnostic arthroscopy is indicated. Further treatment depends upon the findings:

1. Where the osteochondritic areas have separated and formed loose bodies they should be removed unless they are very large, when an attempt may be made to fix them back in place (see chapter on 'Loose bodies in the knee', pp. 1073–1078).
2. Where the osteochondritic area is unstable and the articular cartilage is breached the abnormal area should be fixed rigidly after freshening the base (see Fixation of osteochondritic fragments, below).
3. Where the osteochondritic area is covered by intact articular cartilage, treatment may consist of immobilization alone, or immobilization after drilling – the latter especially if the base of the abnormal area is very sclerotic on the radiograph (see Removal of fixation devices used to treat osteochondritis dissecans, p. 1028).

Fixation of osteochondritic fragments

Indications

See previous section. It should be noted that even after arthroscopic surgery a period of immobilization is required. The main advantage of the arthroscopic technique is therefore reduced scarring.

Preparation of the patient

As for Excision of synovial tags (p. 1026).

Insertion of the telescope

A 25° or 30° telescope should be inserted anterolaterally.

Definition of the abnormal area

The area to be inspected can be identified from radiographs. If the articular surface is not breached then the abnormal area is often slightly dulled and shows some loss of normal contour (*see Plate 37*).

The suspect area should then be probed via the anteromedial portal. Instability can often be demonstrated by abnormal movement of an area of the articular surface. If there is a breach in the articular surface a probe can be inserted into this and the breach extended to allow the osteochondritic fragment to be elevated on a hinge of articular cartilage (*see Plate 38*). It is important not to detach the fragment completely.

Fixation of the fragment

15

Using a small curette, the base of the deficit is freshened via the same portal as the probe.

The fragment is replaced in its bed. It may be fixed there with Smillie pins or small screws. Two or preferably three should be inserted. The position for inserting the pin holder or screwdriver should be piloted with a hypodermic needle. The skin and capsular incision should allow the instruments easy access so that the pin or screw is not displaced. The Smillie pin holder is a good instrument to use as the pins can be withdrawn almost completely into the instrument until the latter is positioned. With flexion and extension of the knee it is often possible to insert all the pins or screws through the same skin incision. After insertion of the pins or screws the head of the fixation device should be slightly below the articular surface. The stability of the fixed fragment should be checked with a probe.

Closure of wound

As for Synovial biopsy (p. 1024).

Postoperative management

The knee should be immobilized in a plaster cylinder for 6 weeks during which time the patient remains non-weight-bearing. After removal of the plaster the knee is mobilized gradually but the patient should remain non-weight-bearing for a further 6 weeks. The fixation device should be removed after 3 months.

Removal of fixation devices used to treat osteochondritis dissecans

Indications

Fixation devices should be removed when healing has occurred. It is the author's practice to remove pins or screws about 3 months after insertion and before full weight-bearing is allowed.

Radiographs should be taken immediately prior to operation to check the position of the pins or screws.

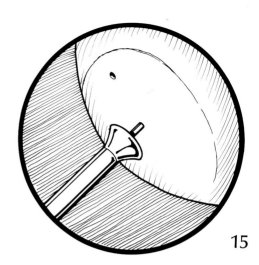

15

Preparation of patient

See Excision of synovial tags (p. 1026).

Location of the pins or screws

The arthroscope should be inserted anterolaterally if the area of osteochondritis is in the usual place on the medial femoral condyle. The knee should be flexed and extended to bring the pins or screws into view. They may have become covered with articular cartilage.

A large diameter hypodermic needle should be inserted anteromedially to gain access to the pins. If they are covered with articular cartilage they may be visible as dark areas beneath the joint surface.

The overlying cartilage may need to be moved away with the edge of the needle to expose the pins. The needle may also be used to tease articular cartilage out of the grooves in the pins or the slots in the screws (*see Plate 39*).

Removal of the pins or screws

The needle should be removed. Smillie pins can usually be removed using pituitary rongeurs. Small bone nibblers are sometimes useful. Screws should be removed with an appropriate screwdriver with screw-retaining clip.

The stability of the osteochondritic area should be checked after removal of the fixation. If it is loose it also should be removed. If the fragment is stable the state of its articular cartilage should be noted.

The joint should be irrigated.

Closure of wound

As for Synovial biopsy (p. 1024).

Postoperative management

The patient mobilizes fully weight-bearing as soon as he has adequate muscle control. A radiograph of the knee should be taken to check the union of the osteochondritic fragment after a further 6 weeks.

Drilling of osteochondritis dissecans

Indications

See Surgery of osteochondritis dissecans (p. 1027).

Preoperative preparation

See Excision of synovial tags (p. 1026).

Insertion of telescope

A standard anterolateral insertion of a 30° telescope should be suitable for osteochondritis in the common sites.

Definition of the abnormal area

The suspect area can be approximately located from radiographs. If the articular surface is not breached (which it must not be for this procedure) the abnormal area is slightly dulled. There is a slight loss of normal contour. The affected area often lies slightly below the normal surrounding area.

On probing (via an anteromedial portal), the articular surface is slightly soft and there may be a jog of movement between the normal and abnormal areas if the abnormal area is pressed with the probe.

16

Drilling of the abnormal area

Usually access via an anteromedial portal is suitable. Access may be piloted using a hypodermic needle. The actual drilling is most easily performed using a short Kirschner wire or toe pin with a shaped end, inserted into a small power drill. Only a puncture wound needs to be made in the skin. The drilling must be done under direct vision and no undue pressure applied.

The pin can usually be felt to penetrate the sclerotic base of the lesion. Multiple drill holes are made 3–4 mm apart. It may be necessary to insert the drill through more than one puncture.

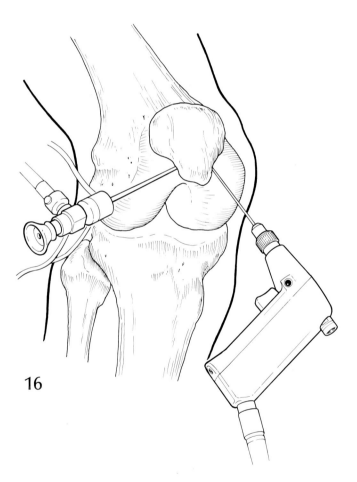

16

Closure of wound

As for Synovial biopsy (p. 1024).

Postoperative management

The knee should be immobilized in a plaster cylinder for 6 weeks and the patient should remain non-weight-bearing during this time.

After 6 weeks the plaster is removed and the knee mobilized. The state of the articular surface should be checked radiographically after 6 weeks and 3 months.

SURGERY OF CHONDROMALACIA PATELLAE

Shaving of chondromalacia patellae

Indication

Shaving is indicated when chondromalacia patellae involves less than one-third of the articular surface. It should be noted that the results of this operation are not consistently good. Surgery is only indicated if conservative measures have failed and the patient has moderate or severe symptoms.

At diagnostic arthroscopy the patellar groove should not be involved. The aetiology of the chrondromalacia should be determined whenever possible. If there is a patellar tracking problem this should be identified and corrected to prevent recurrence.

Preparation of patient

See Excision of synovial tags (p. 1026).

Insertion of telescope

Anterolateral insertion of the telescope is usually satisfactory. A 70° telescope may be useful to assess extent of the condition. Probing of the articular surface to assess softening is important. The probe may be inserted via the suprapatellar pouch or anteromedially. Where there are areas of fibrillation the probe can be inserted down to the subchondral bone.

Assessment of the abnormal area

The severity and extent of the condition must be assessed.

Removal of the fibrillated articular cartilage

This may be carried out using pituitary rongeurs. Instruments which are straight and instruments angled upwards at the tip are useful. They should be inserted in place of the probe. Fibrillated cartilage should be removed as completely as possible leaving a sharp edge to the deficit. Alternatively a power shaver may be used. The joint should be extensively irrigated to remove the articular cartilage debris.

Closure of wound

Wounds should be closed with single sutures and a compression bandage applied. The sutures are removed at 7–10 days.

Postoperative management

Static quadriceps exercises should commence at once. Crutches should be used for 3–4 weeks. The flexed knee should not be loaded for this period. (In theory this should allow fibrous tissue to fill the defect in the patella.)

Removal of loose and foreign bodies

Removal of loose and (rarely) foreign bodies from the knee joint utilizes one of the main advantages of arthroscopic surgery. Through one or two portals the whole of the knee joint is accessible. This is important for the removal of loose and foreign bodies which by definition may move within the joint.

Foreign bodies are much less common than loose bodies. Small pieces of needle may puncture the skin and break off in the joint. If they cannot be located they should be sought in the articular cartilage (especially in children) and in the sheath of the popliteus tendon (*see Plate 40*). Rust staining may be a useful guide to the location.

There are three stages to the removal of a loose or foreign body. It must be (a) located, (b) trapped and (c) removed. A search must then be made to seek for additional loose bodies and also their origin.

Indications

Loose bodies almost always cause locking and giving way – not pain, which is usually from the origin of the loose body and may not be helped by its removal.

Many, but not all, loose bodies are radio-opaque. Preoperative radiographs are important to determine the number, size and position of any loose bodies. Serial radiographs will show whether or not radio-opaque bodies are truly loose, i.e. they are seen in different positions on different occasions. If a body is in a fixed position it may well be stuck to the synovium and may not be causing any symptoms.

Preparation of the patient

As for Excision of synovial tags (p. 1026).

Insertion of the telescope

A routine anterolateral insertion of a 30° telescope is used first. It is best to have a 70° telescope available.

Locating the loose body

Loose bodies may be found in many sites. If a loose body is not easily seen the following sites should be inspected:

17

1. Lateral gutter.
2. Medial gutter (via an anteromedial insertion).
3. Intercondylar notch.
4. Posterior compartments (via a 70° telescope inserted anteromedially or anterolaterally). *Illustration 17* and *Plate 41* show a 70° telescope across the notch and a needle being used to triangulate the loose body in the posterolateral compartment.
5. Under the lateral meniscus and around the popliteus sheath.
6. Any folds within the suprapatellar pouch.

Trapping the loose body

Once the loose body has been seen it is important to try not to lose it again. The surgeon should therefore stop irrigation via the telescope.

Loose bodies in the medial and lateral gutters and in the suprapatellar pouch can usually be impaled with a needle inserted transcutaneously (*see Plate 42*). If the loose body is too hard to impale, then one or more needles may be inserted behind the loose body to prevent its escape.

Removal of the loose body

Some form of grasping instrument needs to be used. The author routinely uses pituitary rongeurs, but other instruments such as artery forceps and Kochers forceps may also be used.

The grasping instrument should be inserted some distance from the loose body, so that it is not disturbed by the insertion of the graspers. Access to the suprapatellar pouch, medial recess and lateral recess is easily achieved. If the proposed portal of entry is dubious it can be piloted with a hypodermic needle inserted first.

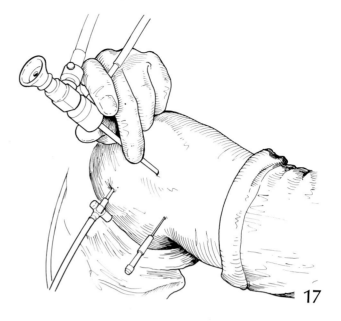

17

Access to loose bodies in the posterior compartment

Loose bodies in the posterior compartments can usually be located using a 70° telescope inserted across the intercondylar notch.

18

The loose body can often then be removed with rongeurs inserted posteromedially or posterolaterally (*see also Plate 43*). (see chapter on 'Diagnostic arthroscopy of the knee', pp. 1007–1018). These portals should be piloted with a hypodermic needle viewed into the joint. It is important to angle the needle and then the grasping forceps forwards, towards the patella and away from the popliteal fossa.

If access across the intercondylar notch is difficult, e.g. in an arthritic knee, it may be necessary to insert the telescope posteromedially or posterolaterally. In this case the grasping instrument can be inserted through an extension of the same incision. Angled rongeurs are useful in this situation.

Checks

After removing the loose body always check for (a) further loose bodies and (b) the origin of the loose bodies.

Closure of wound

As for Synovial biopsy (p. 1024).

Postoperative management

Quadriceps exercises are started on recovery from the anaesthetic and the patient is mobilized when he has muscle control.

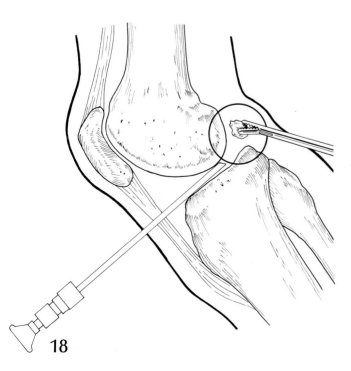

18

Lateral release

Indications

These are not well defined, but as an isolated procedure lateral release may be indicated in recurrent subluxation of the patella, excessive lateral pressure syndrome and perhaps chondromalacia patellae. *See also* the section on Division of a synovial fold or shelf (p. 1025).

Preoperative preparation

As for Excision of synovial tags (p. 1026).

Insertion of telescope

The arthroscope may be inserted anterolaterally or (perhaps better) anteromedially.

The release

19

The lateral release must extend from the joint line up to the vastus lateralis muscle. The release should be a little away from the patella. A skin incision about 2 cm long is made at about the level of the middle of the patella and is deepened through the subcutaneous fat. The capsular release is started with a scalpel. Branches of the lateral geniculate vessels are tied. The capsular release is extended up and down with scissors or a Smillie knife. The inner edge of the blade is inserted deep to the capsule. The synovium may be left intact.

The incision is extended up to the muscle and then down to the joint line. As the incision is extended the irrigation fluid escapes and it is usually necessary to complete the incision by feel rather than under direct vision.

Before closure the joint should be flexed and extended. In flexion the cut capsular edges should separate. Any tethers should be divided.

Closure of wound

Skin closure only is performed, using monofilament polyamide sutures. A compression bandage is applied.

Postoperative management

A haemarthrosis is said to be relatively common after this procedure, so bandaging should be retained for 5 days. A large haemarthrosis should be aspirated. Knee flexion should commence as soon as comfort allows or at any rate after 1 week.

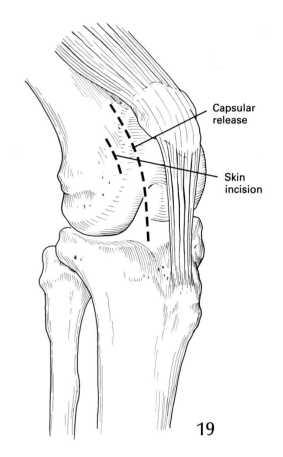

Capsular release

Skin incision

19

Further reading

Dandy DJ. *Arthroscopic surgery of the knee.* Edinburgh: Churchill Livingstone, 1981.

Jackson RW. Current concepts review – arthroscopic surgery. *J Bone Joint Surg [Am]* 1983; 65-A: 416–9.

Sherman OH, Fox JM, Snyder SJ, Del Pizzo W, Friedman MJ, Ferkel RD, Lawley MJ. Arthroscopy – 'no problem surgery' – an analysis of complications in 2640 cases. *J Bone Joint Surg [Am]* 1986; 68-A: 256–65.

Stother IG, Illingworth G, Ayoub M. Arthroscopic removal of loose bodies from the knee. *J R Coll Surg Edinb* 1984; 29(4): 246–8.

Vaughan-Lane T, Dandy DJ. The synovial shelf syndrome. *J Bone Joint Surg [Br]* 1982; 64-B: 475–6.

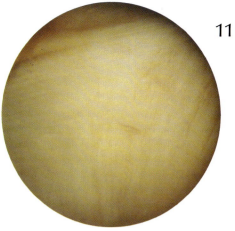

Plate 11. Synovial membrane of suprapatellar pouch, characterized by small ridges produced by the underlying capsular fibres and by the fine arterioles running just beneath the surface.

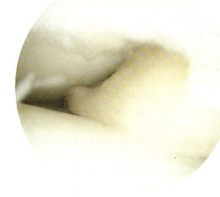

Plate 12. Arthroscopic view of the patellofemoral joint with the patella uppermost. A medial synovial shelf or plica can be seen which lies between the edges of the two articular surfaces and usually slips medially out of the articulation as flexion proceeds.

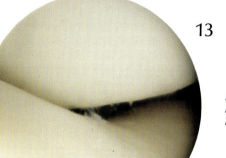

Plate 13. View of the patellofemoral joint showing the patella lying in the femoral groove, slightly laterally placed, with the knee flexed to 30°.

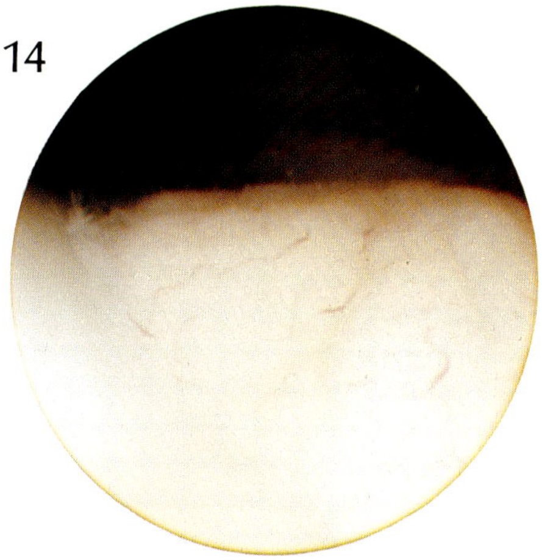

Plate 14. Normal infrapatellar fat pad covered with thin synovial membrane containing fine blood vessels on the fatty base.

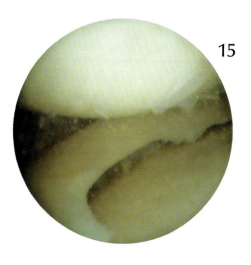

Plate 15. Free edge of the medial meniscus with slight fibrillation of the femoral condyle. The normal kinking of the junction of the anterior two-thirds and the posterior one-third is seen.

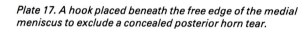

16

Plate 16. Normal kinking of the inner edge of the medial meniscus.

17

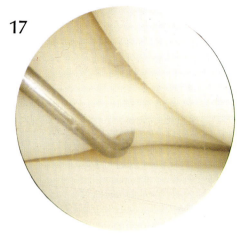

Plate 17. A hook placed beneath the free edge of the medial meniscus to exclude a concealed posterior horn tear.

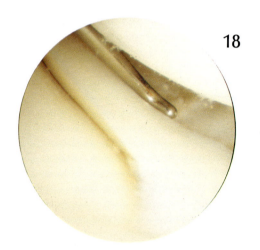

18

Plate 18. The hook is placed over the top of the meniscus and pulled towards the centre of the joint to assess its stability.

19

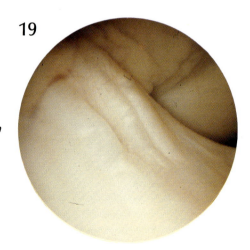

Plate 19. Normal anterior cruciate ligament with fine arteries in the synovial membrane which covers the surface.

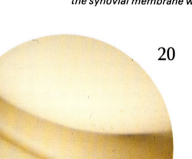

20

Plate 20. Normal free edge of the posterior horn of the lateral meniscus.

21

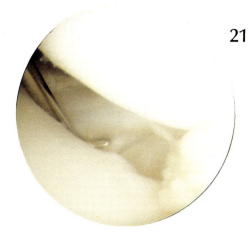

Plate 21. The posterolateral compartment of the knee with the hook placed over the posterior edge of the lateral meniscus, in the gap between it and the popliteus tendon which can be seen running obliquely downwards and medially.

22

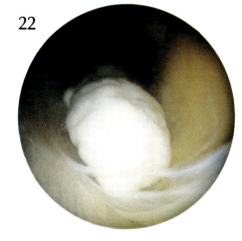

Plate 22. Osteocartilaginous loose body in the lateral parafemoral gutter.

23

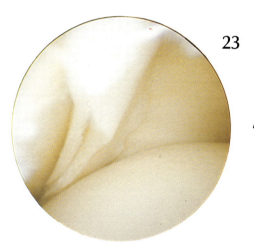

Plate 23. Horizontal tear of the medial meniscus.

24

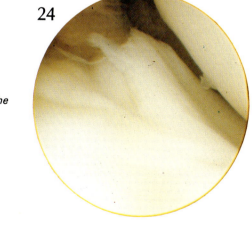

Plate 24. Discoid lateral meniscus showing the edge near the intercondylar area.

25

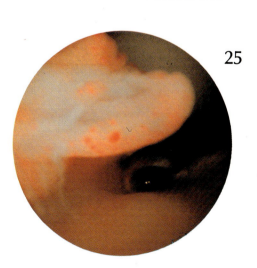

Plate 25. Typical hypervascular synovial villus in rheumatoid arthritis.

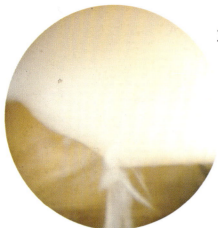

26

Plate 26. Grade I chondromalacia patellae.

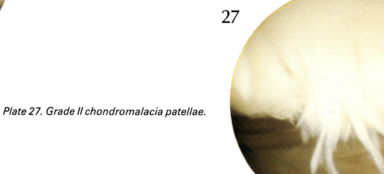

27

Plate 27. Grade II chondromalacia patellae.

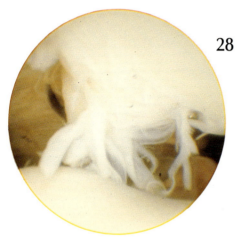

28

Plate 28. Grade III chondromalacia patellae.

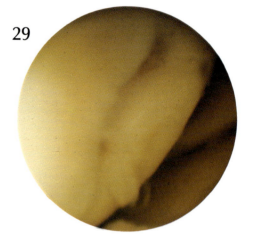

29

Plate 29. Osteoarthritic, pitted femoral condyle.

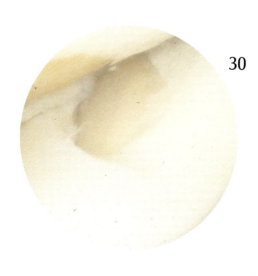

30

Plate 30. Advanced osteoarthritis with erosion of the medial femoral and tibial articular surfaces and multiple tears of the medial semilunar cartilage.

31

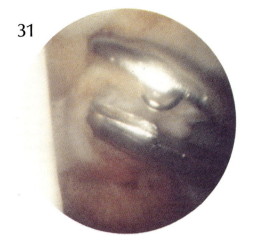

Plate 31. Synovial biopsy.

32

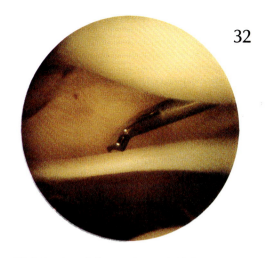

Plate 32. Palpation of abnormal synovial fold using a probe.

33

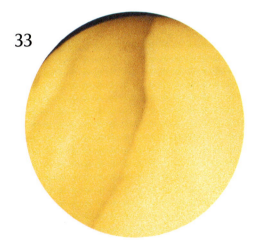

Plate 33. Erosion of the femoral condyle.

34a

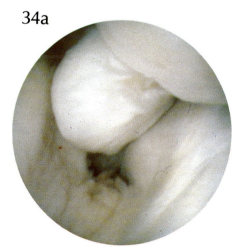

34b

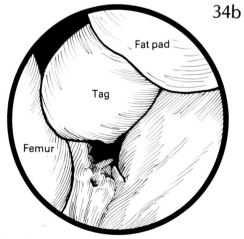

Plates 34a, b. Synovial tag and associated fat pad.

35a

35b

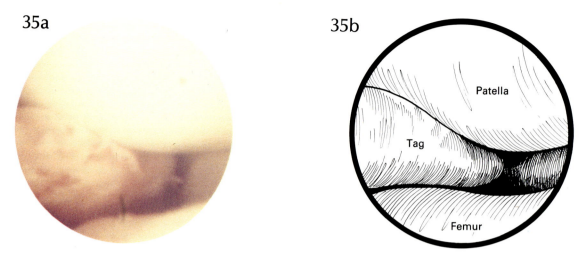

Plate 35a, b. Synovial tag jammed between the patella and its groove.

36

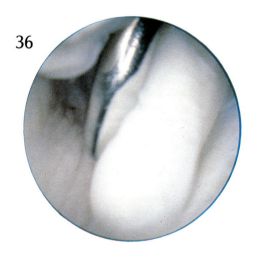

Plate 36. Defining the synovial tag by means of a probe.

37

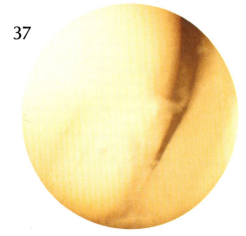

Plate 37. Appearance of the abnormal articular cartilage in osteochondritis dissecans.

38

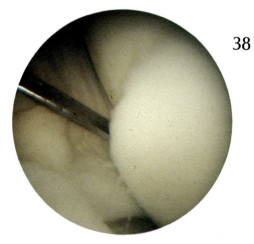

Plate 38. Probing a breach in the articular cartilage to elevate, and therefore define, the osteochondritic fragment.

39

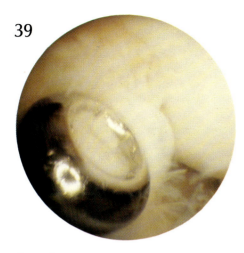

Plate 39. Screw head exposed after the removal of articular cartilage.

40

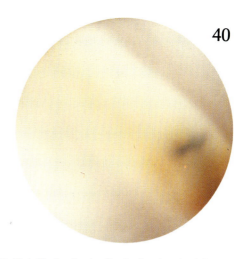

Plate 40. Metallic foreign bodies in the sheath of the popliteus tendon.

41

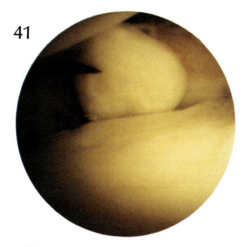

Plate 41. Triangulation of a loose body in the posterolateral compartment using a needle.

42

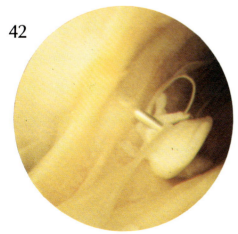

Plate 42. A loose body impaled with a needle inserted transcutaneously.

43

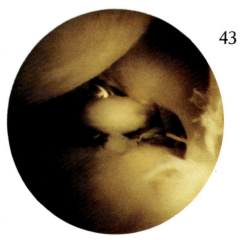

Plate 43. Removal of the loose body using rongeurs.

Arthroscopic meniscectomy

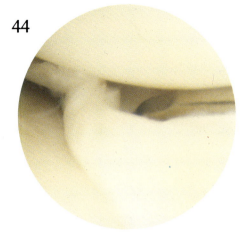

Plate 44. Defining the junction of a full bucket-handle tear and the rim using a probe.

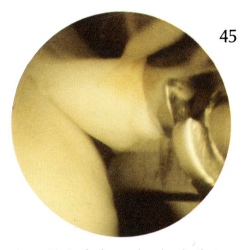

Plate 45. Lower blade of scissors placed under the tear.

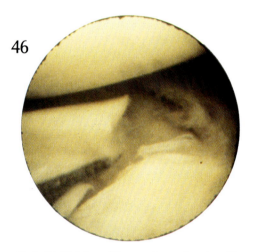

Plate 46. Division of the meniscus—tear junction.

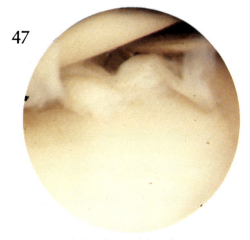

Plate 47. Tags remaining after excision of the tear.

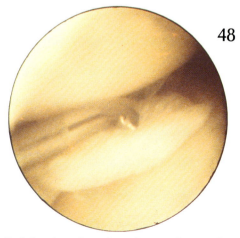

Plate 48. Defining the points of attachment of a tag using a probe.

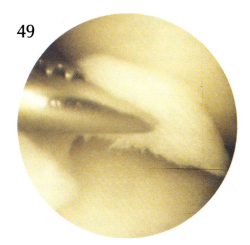

49

Plate 49. Avulsion of a tag using rongeurs.

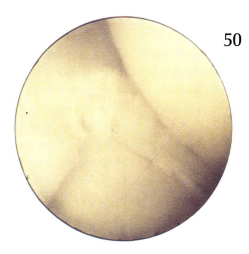

50

Plate 50. Appearance after avulsion of a tag.

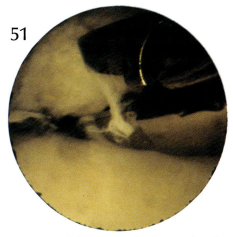

51

Plate 51. Using punch forceps to trim the remains of an excised tear.

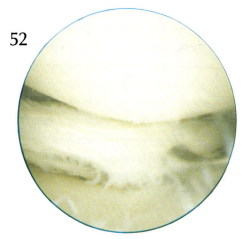

52

Plate 52. Using a hook to define a posterior third bucket-handle tear.

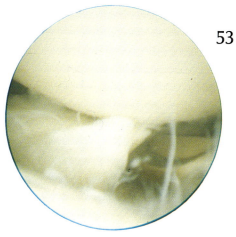

53

Plate 53. Dividing a tear with scissors passed across the intercondylar notch.

54

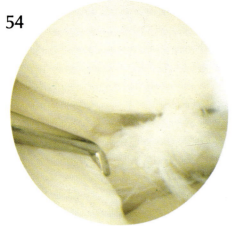

Plate 54. Hingeing a divided tear forwards with a hook to lie in front of the femoral condyle.

55

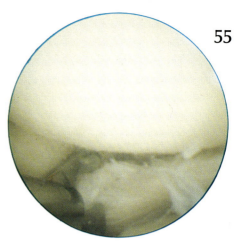

Plate 55. Dividing the anterior attachment of the tear using scissors.

56

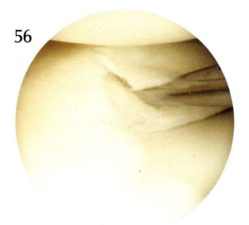

Plate 56. Defining a posterior horn cleavage tear using a probe.

57

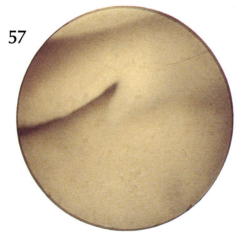

Plate 57. A radial tear of the lateral meniscus.

58

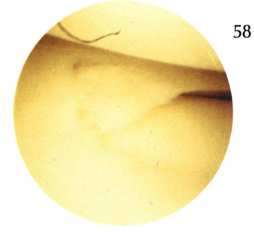

Plate 58. A parrot-beak tear of the lateral meniscus.

Illustrations by Peter Cox

Arthroscopic meniscectomy

Ian Stother   MA, FRCS(Ed), FRCS(Glas)
Consultant Orthopaedic Surgeon, Glasgow Royal Infirmary, Glasgow, UK

Introduction

Meniscus pathology is a common cause of knee morbidity. Initial diagnostic arthroscopy allows precise assessment of the site and extent of meniscus damage. It therefore allows logical treatment of meniscus tears. The main treatment options to be considered are:

1. No procedure.

2. Meniscal suture (*see* chapter on 'Arthroscopic meniscal repair', pp. 1056–1061).
3. Partial meniscectomy.
4. Total meniscectomy (*see* chapter on 'Open meniscectomy of the knee', p 1062–1072).

Arthroscopic partial meniscectomy is considered in this chapter. The long-term results of partial meniscectomy are better than those of total meniscectomy[1] and closed partial meniscectomy allows a more rapid early recovery[2].

Basic technique

Arthroscopic meniscectomy has three essential stages:

1. Definition of the abnormal area
2. Excision of the abnormal area
3. Trimming of the remaining rim.

These stages are carried out by the 'double puncture' or 'triple puncture' technique.

1

In the double puncture technique the arthroscope is inserted through one skin puncture or portal, usually the anterolateral, and one or more instruments are inserted through a second portal, often the anteromedial.

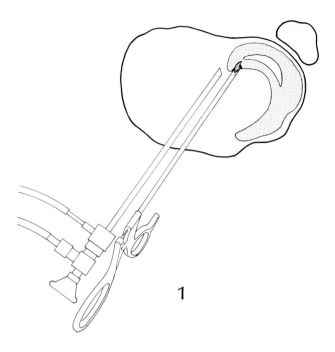

1

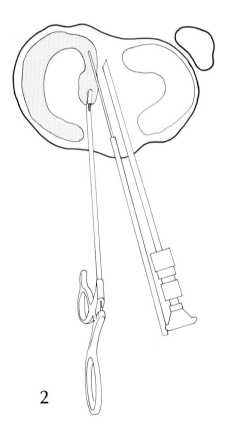

2

2

In the triple puncture technique, three portals are used, one for the telescope and two for instruments – most commonly one grasping and one cutting instrument.

Hand instruments

The equipment needed for diagnostic arthroscopy is required (see chapter on 'Diagnostic arthroscopy of the knee', pp. 1007–1018).

In addition special hand instruments are required for performing three basic functions – cutting, grasping and nibbling. Curved instruments are useful for access to the horns of the menisci.

Power instruments

Various power instruments are available. Most have a rotating cutting blade or burr and an attached suction mechanism for removing debris. On the whole these instruments are an alternative to hand instruments. With the possible exceptions of synovectomy and patellar shaving, power instruments do not increase the range of surgery.

Special diathermy cutting instruments are also available.

EXCISION OF A FULL BUCKET-HANDLE TEAR OF THE MENISCUS

Medial bucket-handle tears

Indications

The procedure is indicated for locked knee or recurrent giving way.

Preparation of the patient

A general or spinal anaesthetic is administered. The patient lies supine on the operating table and the knee ligaments are examined under anaesthesia. A mid-thigh tourniquet is applied (optional). The skin is cleaned and drapes are applied to give a sterile operating field.

Insertion of the telescope

3

The knee is distended with irrigation fluid inserted via the suprapatellar pouch. A 30° telescope is inserted via an anterolateral portal. Irrigation is continued via the telescope.

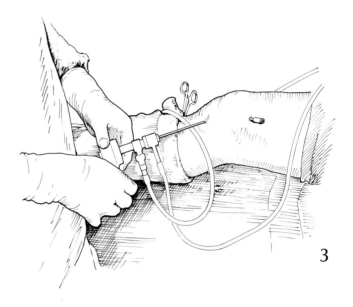

3

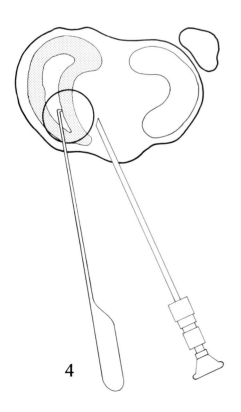

4

Defining the tear

4

The bucket-handle tear will be either displaced or undisplaced. The junctions of the tear and the rim are defined with a probe inserted via an anteromedial portal. *Plate 44** shows the hook between the bucket-handle tear and the rim, and *Illustration 4* is a plan view of this.

*Colour plates 44–48 are on pages 1040–1042.

5

If the tear is displaced it may be reduced with the probe whilst a valgus force is applied. To do this the leg may be dropped over the side of the table onto the operator's knee.

Excising the tear

Ideally each end of the bucket-handle tear should be divided as close as possible to the rim so that one large fragment is removed, leaving no tags to trim. If at all possible the tear should be reduced with the probe.

If the tear can be reduced, its posterior attachment should be divided first. The telescope remains in the anterolateral portal. A probe is manipulated across the intercondylar notch from the anteromedial portal to the posterior horn of the meniscus. The probe is then replaced with a small pair of hook scissors and the posterior attachment of the tear is divided. The completeness of the division is then checked with the probe.

The anterior attachment of the tear is then approached. Initially the telescope should remain in the anterolateral portal and the probe should be manipulated through the anteromedial portal. If access to the anterior attachment of the tear is difficult, the insertions of the telescope and probe should be reversed.

Occasionally a third portal further anteromedially may be required. The site for such a portal can be piloted with a hypodermic needle. Such an approach may enable the meniscus to be divided from the angle between the rim and the tear.

Once access to the anterior attachment of the tear has been achieved with the probe then the probe should be replaced with a pair of scissors or a small knife and the attachment subtotally divided. The cutting instrument is then removed and a pair of grasping forceps gently inserted and the torn fragment of meniscus seized. With a twisting action the tear is completely detached from the rim and removed.

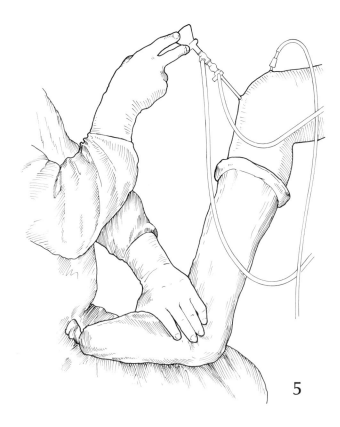

5

6

If the tear cannot be reduced or if the fat pad is becoming oedematous and tending to obscure the anterior attachment of the tear then the anterior attachment should be divided first.

The probe is manipulated through an anteromedial portal into the position where it is desired to divide the meniscus. The probe is then replaced with scissors or a knife. *Plate 45* and *Illustration 6* show a pair of scissors with the lower blade under the tear. The meniscus–tear junction is divided (*Plate 46*). The completeness of division is checked with the probe.

The cut anterior end of the bucket handle is seized with grasping forceps inserted in the anteromedial portal. The tear is then gently displaced into the intercondylar notch.

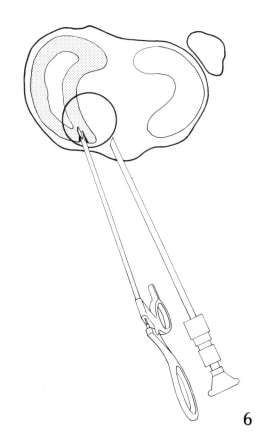

6

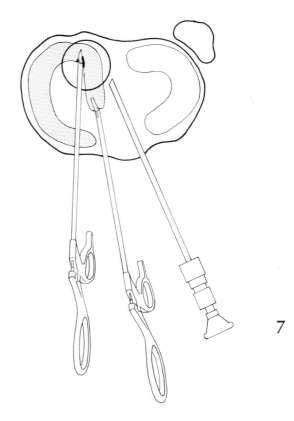

7

7

The telescope is moved across the intercondylar notch to view the posterior end of the tear. Scissors or a retractable bladed knife are inserted via a third portal, usually placed medial to the graspers.

The cutting instrument is manoeuvred posteriorly to divide the posterior end of the tear under direct vision. The bucket-handle tear can be kept under tension with the graspers. Care must be taken not to damage the anterior cruciate ligament. The torn fragment is then withdrawn from the joint in the graspers.

Checking the remaining rim

8

The size of the excised fragment is a good guide as to the likelihood of any remaining tags to be trimmed. Ideally the excised bucket-handle tear should measure about 2 cm in length. Any tags such as those seen in *Plate 47* may be excised as described below.

Closure of the wound

The joint should be irrigated. Skin wounds are closed with single sutures or sterile wound closure strips.

Postoperative management

A wool and crêpe bandage is applied. When the patient can achieve straight-leg raising he is mobilized with a walking stick and discharged home, usually within 24 hours.

Sutures are removed at 1 week. Most sedentary workers can return to work at or before this time. If the quadriceps are poor at this time a course of physiotherapy should be given. Final review is usually 6 weeks after operation, when the patient's knee should be clinically normal.

Lateral bucket-handle tears

The procedure for excision of a bucket-handle tear from the lateral meniscus is similar, except that the knee should be opened into varus.

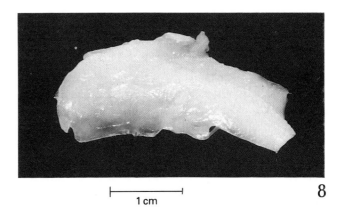

├── 1 cm ──┤   8

EXCISION OF TAG TEARS

Indications

The tags must be large enough to cause mechanical symptoms of pain and tenderness medially. Minor fraying of the meniscus edge is not an indication for surgery.

Preparation of the patient

As for Excision of a full bucket-handle tear, p. 1045.

Insertion of the telescope

A routine anterolateral insertion is used.

Defining the tear

9

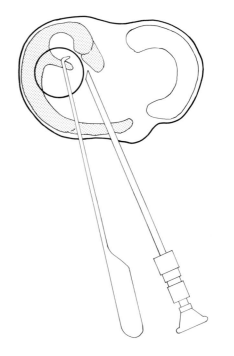

The free and attached ends of the tag must be defined using an anteromedially inserted probe, as shown in *Illustration 9* and *Plate 48*. Sometimes tags are the ends of a transected bucket-handle tear. If a tag is seen antero medially it is important to check for a second tag at the posterior horn.

Occasionally a tag of meniscus from the lower surface of the meniscus will fold underneath the meniscus and cause a palpable joint line swelling mimicking a cystic meniscus. Such tags can be retrieved by careful probing under the meniscus.

9

Excising the tear

If the tag has a broad base this should be divided subtotally with scissors, which can usually be inserted in place of the probe. Once the width of the base of the tag has been reduced the tag can be avulsed or excised using rongeurs or grasping forceps inserted in place of the probe, as shown in *Plates 49* and *50*.

Tags at the posterior horn can be pulled forwards with a probe and excised using angled rongeurs or grasping forceps, inserted either anteromedially across the inter-condylar notch or occasionally posteromedially with the telescope across the notch.

Checking the remaining rim

The surgeon should always check for a second tag. Any sharp angles should be trimmed using punch forceps (*Plate 51*).

Closure of the wound

As for Excision of a full bucket-handle tear, p. 1047.

Postoperative management

As for Excision of a full bucket-handle tear, p. 1047.

EXCISION OF POSTERIOR THIRD BUCKET-HANDLE TEARS

Indications

10

Tears such as those shown in *Illustration 10* are often associated with ligament injuries and cause intermittent giving way when they sublux in front of the femoral condyle. In young patients with recent short tears, consideration should be given to suturing the tear (*see* chapter on 'Arthroscopic meniscal repair', pp. 1056–1061).

The longer the tear, the longer the duration of symptoms and the older the patient, the greater the indication for excision. These tears are among the most difficult to gain access to, especially on the medial side.

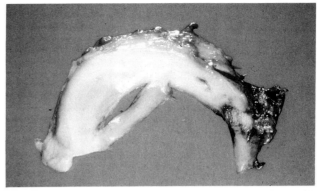

10

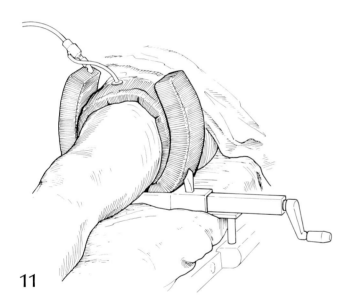

11

Preparation of the patient

11

As for Excision of a full bucket-handle tear, p. 1045. It is always useful to have a leg holder to immobilize the thigh in order to gain access to the posterior third of the meniscus.

Insertion of the telescope

As for Excision of a full bucket-handle tear, p. 1045.

Defining the tear

12

Using a hook, the tear can often be subluxated forward in front of the femoral condyle (*Plate 52*) but usually slips back immediately. It is important to try and define the ends of the tear and to check the ease of access to each end.

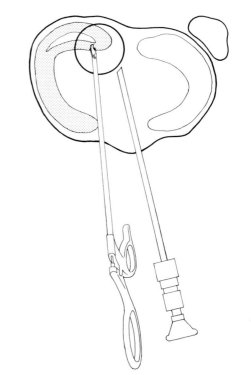

12

Excising the tear

It is often easiest to divide the posterior end first, provided the knee is not arthritic and there is access to the posterior horn across the intercondylar notch. If a small pair of scissors can be passed across the notch, the tear can be divided right to its edge (*Plate 53*). Once divided, the tear can be hinged forwards with a hook to lie in front of the femoral condyle (*Plate 54*). Grasping forceps can then be inserted anteromedially to put traction on the cut end of the tear.

13

Using a third incision medial to the graspers, small scissors or a sheathed knife can be used to cut the anterior attachment of the tear while gentle traction is applied with graspers (*Plate 55*).

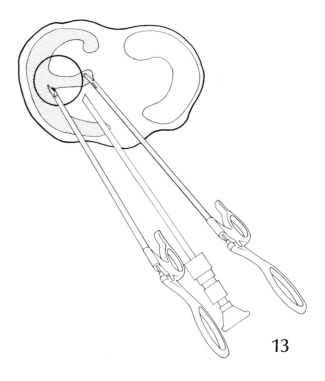

Checking the remaining rim

The rim should be checked with a hook. Small posterior horn tags can be ignored. The anterior edge of the excision should be as smooth as possible and should be trimmed with punch forceps, or perhaps with powered instruments. On the lateral side care should be taken to leave a popliteus bridge.

Closure of the wound

As for Excision of a full bucket-handle tear, p. 1047.

Postoperative management

As for Excision of a full bucket-handle tear, p. 1047.

13

EXCISION OF POSTERIOR HORN CLEAVAGE TEARS

Indications

So-called cleavage or degenerative tears of the posterior horn of the medial meniscus have been associated with both pain and mechanical symptoms. Mechanical symptoms are usually due to tag tears which can be excised as outlined previously. Where the meniscus is degenerate but there are no major tags, there may be a place for removing the abnormal tissue for relief of pain.

Preparation of the patient

As for Excision of a full bucket-handle tear, p. 1045.

Defining the tear

14

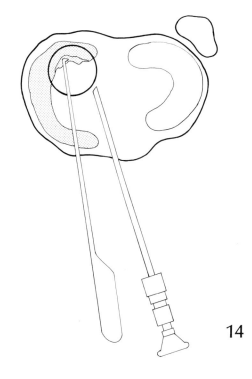

14

Visualization of the tear requires the knee to be opened into valgus. The abnormal area should be defined with the probe as shown in *Illustration 14* and *Plate 56*. Occasionally a posteromedial insertion of the arthroscope may be useful.

Excising the tear

15

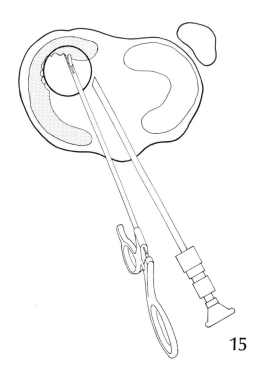

15

The degenerate meniscus is soft and fragmented. It therefore needs to be removed piecemeal. Access to the posterior third from the anteromedial portal can be limited and it can be difficult to open instruments such as punch forceps and rongeurs. Side-cutting punches and powered rotating instruments may make the operation easier. Care must be taken not to damage the articular surface.

Bites of abnormal meniscus should be removed until a stable peripheral rim remains. The ends of the area should be contoured back to the normal meniscus edge. The loose bites of meniscus should be flushed out down the arthroscopic sheath or removed with a suction probe.

Checking the remaining rim

A small rim of meniscus should be left *in situ*, even if it is somewhat degenerate. There should, however, be no remaining tags.

Closure of the wound

As for Excision of a full bucket-handle tear, p. 1047.

Postoperative management

As for Excision of a full bucket-handle tear, p. 1047.

RADIAL TEARS OF THE LATERAL MENISCUS

Indications

These tears, as shown in *Plate 57* indicate instability of the posterior third of the lateral meniscus. The tears themselves should be 'saucerized' and the posterior third of the lateral meniscus should either be stabilized with a suture or excised. Stabilization is preferable, as excision usually requires removal of the popliteus bridge which is functionally undesirable.

Preparation of the patient

As for Excision of a full bucket-handle tear, p. 1045.

Defining the tear

16

The edges of the tear should be defined using a hook, placing the hook into the popliteus groove. Usually the posterior third of the meniscus can be subluxated forwards in front of the femoral condyle.

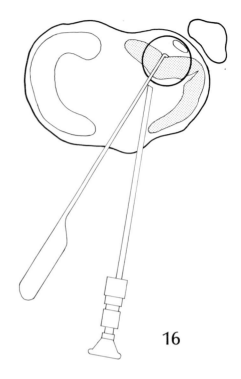

16

Excising the tear

The margins of the tear should be 'saucerized'. Lateral cutting punches are useful for this. Next either the posterior third should be sutured to the capsule (*see* chapter on 'Arthroscopic meniscal repair', pp. 1056–1061) or alternatively the posterior third should be removed using large punch forceps.

Checking the remaining rim

The surgeon should ensure that no large tags can cause symptoms by interposition.

Closure of the wound

As for Excision of a full bucket-handle tear, p. 1047.

Postoperative management

As for Excision of a full bucket-handle tear, p. 1047.

SURGERY OF TORN CYSTIC LATERAL MENISCUS

In such cases there is both intra-articular and extra-articular pathology. The tear can be excised arthroscopically, but the area of cystic change extends outside the periphery of the meniscus and often involves a considerable length of the meniscus itself. To excise the abnormal tissue therefore often involves both breaching the continuity of the meniscus edge and removing a large part of the meniscus itself. Where extensive cystic changes are found at diagnostic arthroscopy, and where the tear itself is complex and involves a considerable length of the meniscus, an open complete lateral meniscectomy is often the easiest operation to perform. Alternatively, resection with a powered meniscotome may be performed.

Care must be taken not to mistake a flap tear of the inferior surface of the lateral meniscus, which has come to be extruded peripherally, for a small meniscus cyst.

If a partial arthroscopic meniscectomy is performed for a cystic lateral meniscus the procedure is as described in the next section. In the author's experience, recurrence of symptoms after partial meniscectomy for cystic degeneration is quite common.

EXCISION OF PARROT-BEAK TEARS OF THE LATERAL MENISCUS

Indications

17

Tears such as those shown in *Plate 58* and *Illustration 17* may cause lateral pain and also recurrent instability, in which case the abnormal area of lateral meniscus should be removed.

Parrot-beak tears are complex tears of the posterior half of the lateral meniscus. They extend obliquely through the substance of the meniscus. They are sometimes associated with cystic changes in the affected area. The tears can be excised arthroscopically but care needs to be taken to remove the whole of the abnormal area.

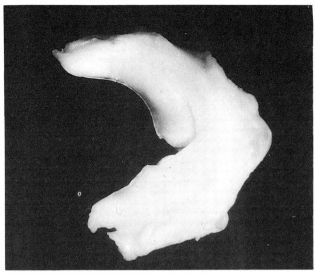

17

Preparation of the patient

As for Excision of a full bucket-handle tear, p. 1045.

Insertion of the telescope

The 30° telescope should be inserted anterolaterally through a portal as close to the patellar tendon as possible. The probe should be inserted anteromedially. Where the lateral femoral condyle is very convex, care should be taken not to insert the probe too low. It is often helpful to reverse the positions of telescope and probe.

Defining the tear

The upper surface of the tear usually does not indicate the extent of the meniscal involvement. The tear itself and the inferior surface of the meniscus should be probed to assess the posterior extent of the tear.

Excising the tear

Care must be taken to excise the whole of the abnormal area of meniscus. Usually the posterior and inferior part of the tear has a very broad base, so the tear cannot be treated like a tag tear. Instead the posterior component of the tear needs to be excised piecemeal with punch forceps or power instruments (*see Illustration 15*). It may also be necessary to trim the anterior or superior part of the tear with punch forceps. The base of the tear needs to be carefully probed. Some of these tears extend to the capsular margins of the meniscus. In this case, or if cystic changes in the meniscus are encountered as bites of meniscus are being removed, consideration can be given

to performing a subtotal meniscectomy, removing the posterior half of the meniscus (behind the tear) piecemeal with punch forceps. The remaining rim of the anterior part of the meniscus is often gently sloping towards its capsular attachment and requires little trimming.

After removing the meniscus piecemeal, the portions of the meniscus should be flushed out of the joint, either down the telescope sheath or through a sucker.

Checking the remaining rim

If possible, a rim of the posterior part of the meniscus should be left *in situ* to preserve meniscal function. If such a rim is left, a hook should be placed over it into the popliteal groove and traction applied. If the rim can be subluxated forwards in front of the femoral condyle the rim should be removed or sutured, otherwise it may interpose between the joint surfaces and cause instability.

Closure of the wound

As for Excision of a full bucket-handle tear, p. 1047.

Postoperative management

As for Excision of a full bucket-handle tear, p. 1047.

SURGERY OF THE DISCOID LATERAL MENISCUS

Indications

The only definite indication for surgery is the presence of mechanical symptoms together with the finding of a torn discoid meniscus.

Such tears commonly involve the central area of the meniscus. If the discoid meniscus is a complete one, the tear may involve only the upper surface or the lower surface, one surface of the meniscus remaining intact.

Preparation of the patient

As for Excision of a full bucket-handle tear, p. 1045. If the patient is a child, the normal arthroscope and instruments are quite suitable.

Insertion of the telescope

As for Excision of a full bucket-handle tear, p. 1045.

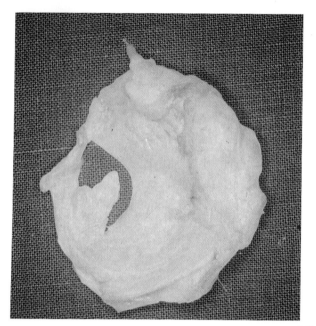

18

Defining the tear

It is very important to determine exactly the size of the meniscus and the location of any tears. In complete discoid menisci the inferior surface of the meniscus must be viewed. The telescope may be easier to manoeuvre under a discoid meniscus from the anteromedial portal.

Two main types of tear occur:

18, 19 & 20

1. There is separation of the thickened medial margin of the meniscus (a 'perforated' discoid meniscus).
2. There is a 'flap' tear of one surface of an imperforate meniscus. *Illustrations 19* and *20* show the intact upper and torn lower surface of such a meniscus.

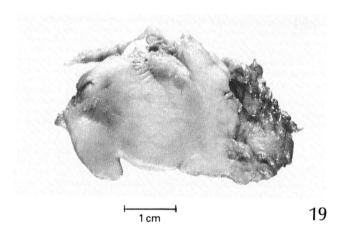

1 cm   **19**

Excision of the medial part of a perforated discoid meniscus

The operation is similar to excising a displaced bucket-handle tear, except that the 'bucket handle' is bulky and its attachments more extensive than usual.

The space occupied by the inner edge of the meniscus is large and access to it is tight. The anterior end of the inner edge of the meniscus should be divided first. Because of the difficult access the cutting instrument may be best introduced from the anteromedial portal.

The procedure is essentially that described for Excision of a full bucket-handle tear, p. 1046.

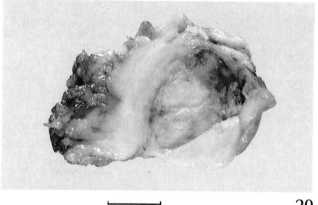

1 cm   **20**

Closure of the wound

As for Excision of a full bucket-handle tear, p. 1047.

Postoperative management

As for Excision of a full bucket-handle tear, p. 1047.

Excision of a superior surface flap tear

Such a tear usually has a broad base. The base can be divided with scissors or a knife inserted on the same side of the patellar tendon as the tear. The tear can then be grasped and removed.

The remainder of the discoid meniscus may be left *in situ*. Alternatively it may be trimmed creating a bucket-handle type of tear, which is then excised to leave a relatively normal rim.

If such a procedure is undertaken and becomes difficult it should be abandoned and an open total meniscectomy carried out rather than damage the joint surfaces. The large volume of tissue which needs to be removed may be dealt with more quickly by power instruments, provided the anatomy is carefully defined first.

Excision of an inferior surface flap tear

If there is a flap tear of the inferior surface then the options are:

1. Arthroscopic partial meniscectomy, fashioning a 'normal' meniscus by excising the central area (as for Excision of a superior surface flap tear, above).
2. Open total meniscectomy.

References

1. Tapper EM, Hoover NW. Late results after meniscectomy. *J Bone Joint Surg [Am]* 1959; 51-A: 517–26.

2. Dandy DJ. Early results of closed partial meniscectomy. *Br Med J* 1978; i: 1099–100.

Arthroscopic meniscal repair

Robert W. Jackson   MD, MS (Tor), FRCS(C)
Chief of Staff/Surgery, Orthopaedic and Arthritic Hospital, Toronto; Professor of Surgery, University of Toronto, Canada

Sanford S. Kunkel   MD
Orthopaedic Surgeon, Methodist Hospital, Indiana, USA

Introduction

Since Thomas Annandale published his description of the surgical repair of a torn semilunar meniscus one century ago, the pendulum of opinion has swung back and forth in regard to the ideal method of treatment of a meniscal disruption. In the early part of this century the trend was towards removal of the entire meniscus, based on the theory that this would allow nature to produce a fibrous replica of the original. In spite of the trend towards total meniscectomy, some voices of moderation pointed out that partial removal of the mobile or damaged portion of the meniscus was probably the better method of treatment[1,2]. Eventually, the thought evolved that total removal of the meniscus might actually be the precipitating cause of the degenerative changes that were seen so frequently after total meniscectomy[2-4], a theory that was soon supported by numerous clinical studies[5-7]. Further support came from biomechanical studies which demonstrated the importance of the meniscus in several ways, including load distribution, lubrication and stability[8-10]. The trend then quickly moved towards partial meniscectomy, usually under arthroscopic control, as the 'gold standard' of treatment[7,11,12].

It was then logical, that if retention of the peripheral portion of the meniscus produced better results than total meniscectomy, preservation of the entire meniscus, through successful repair of the torn structure, might result in a virtually normal knee. This concept was supported by the good clinical evidence obtained in follow-up after primary suturing of both torn collateral ligaments and torn menisci[13,14]. Several studies of a clinical nature and some of an experimental nature endorsed the fact that a torn meniscus could indeed heal itself given the right conditions[15,16].

The first arthroscopic repair of a torn meniscus was carried out by Ikeuchi in 1969[17]. Since that time there has been considerable interest in this minimally-invasive arthroscopic technique for two important reasons. First, the morbidity with an arthroscopic procedure is generally less than with an open procedure. Secondly, the selection, preparation, and stabilization of many meniscal tears is easier. Arthroscopy not only allows the surgeon to see further back in the joint, but also to see better (due to the fibre-light illumination and the magnification) than with open techniques[18]. Moreover, tears that are situated towards the centre of the knee are accessible to arthroscopy, whereas only those that are at the periphery of the meniscus can be repaired by open procedures. Coincident with the clinical interest in closed meniscal repair, came scientific evidence in dogs and humans to support the concept[19,20]. Now, with favourable medium term results, meniscal repair is becoming a standard method of treatment for suitable cases.

Indications

The ideal indication for meniscal repair would appear to be a vertical tear in the vascular outer third of the meniscus, longer than 1.5 cm in length and inherently unstable, in a young athletically-orientated individual, with no other pathology in his knee. A further strong indication for repair would be the meniscal lesion that exists in association with ligamentous instability, such as that following torn anterior cruciate or medial collateral ligament. Various studies have shown that lesions suitable for repair are present in only 20 to 30 per cent of all knees with torn menisci, with 70 per cent of those lesions existing in the medial compartment and 30 per cent in the lateral compartment.

Contraindications

1

Contraindications to repair are somewhat relative. A surgeon might not wish to repair a knee in an older individual (35 years plus) if the tear was relatively short (less the 1.5 cm) and stable, or where there was associated ligamentous instability and no attempt was going to be made (for whatever reasons) to stabilize the joint. Further contraindications include the various types of meniscal tears other than vertical – such as horizontal cleavage tears, radial tears, flap tears, or degenerative tears of the posterior horn. Also, most surgeons would agree that a tear in the inner two-thirds of the meniscus (Zone B), in the avascular or white zone, would best be treated by partial meniscectomy, as the chance of successful healing is greatly reduced in this area. By contrast, a tear in the vascular zone (Zone A) can be successfully treated by suture.

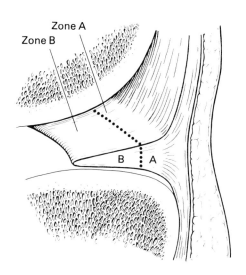

1

Special investigations

The role of arthrography remains to be established. Some surgeons feel that an arthrogram can give useful information regarding the integrity of the inner portion of the meniscus and demonstrate better than arthroscopy the position of the tear in terms of its relative vascularity. Most competent arthroscopists, however, feel that this information can easily be obtained at arthroscopy and that the arthrogram is no longer of any significant value in assessing the lesion preoperatively. Arthrography might be of some value in the postoperative evaluation of healing; however, the overall usefulness of this technique is doubtful.

Magnetic resonance imaging promises to clarify the location and extent of tears preoperatively.

Experimental studies using fluorescent dyes injected intravenously, and viewed with ultraviolet light under arthroscopic control, are being carried out in an effort to visualize the vascularity of the meniscus, and thus select the most suitable cases for repair. Such studies have not as yet been successful.

Technique

The important stages involved in successful arthroscopic meniscal repair can be described as follows.

1. Selection of the case for treatment.
2. Preparation of the tissues to obtain the maximum biological healing response.
3. Fixation or stabilization of the meniscal fragments to allow healing to occur. Stabilization techniques involve either inside-out techniques or outside-in techniques relating to the placement of sutures.

Selection

Selection of appropriate cases is by arthroscopy. The lesion should be in the vascular periphery of the meniscus, of more than 1.5 cm in length, unstable and vertical.

Preparation

2

The peripheral rim should be debrided of scar tissue and the synovial area should be abraded or otherwise stimulated, to promote a maximum vascular response during the healing phase. This may be carried out using rotating burrs, rasps, or punch forceps, either from the anterior approach under direct vision or through additional posterior portals. The vascular peripheral side of the defect obviously deserves the most attention in order to promote vascularity to the area. Some recent evidence suggests that vascular access channels can be made from the peripheral vascular area to lesions that are more central in the meniscus. However, clinical experience in this area is still meagre and these techniques are not commonly practised, for fear of weakening the inner meniscal tissue by creating stress-risers. Recent evidence also suggests that an autogenous fibrin clot placed in the healing area can enhance the repair process. Again however, long-term studies to prove or disprove the effectiveness of clot placement are not available.

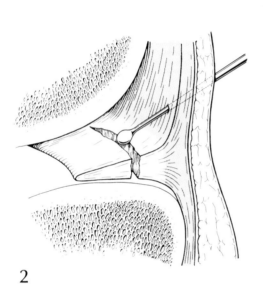

2

Stabilization

3

Whether the technique is from inside out, or outside in, most surgeons feel that sutures should be placed approximately 2 to 3 mm apart, either on the inferior or superior border of the meniscus, and in such a way that stability and firm apposition of the internal fragment to the peripheral rim is obtained at the conclusion of the procedure. Some controversy exists as to whether the suture material should be placed horizontally or vertically to the plane of the meniscus. Those advocating vertical placement suggest that the circular orientation of the peripheral fibres of the meniscus can best withstand the tension of a suture if it is placed vertically. Most sutures placed by arthroscopy are horizontal, because it is easier to do. The suture material that is most commonly used is an absorbable material, either polyglactin 910 or PDS (polydioxanone) of either 0 gauge or 2/0 gauge strength.

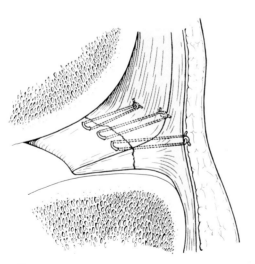

3

'Inside-out' technique

4

In this technique the sutures are placed from anterior portals through cannulae. The suture material is usually attached to a long, thin, and relatively malleable needle which can be passed through the inner fragment, across the defect, through the peripheral rim, and out through capsule and other soft tissues surrounding the knee. This can be done through a single-channel cannula or double-channel cannula, forming a loop of tissue on the inner fragment which is then pulled tight and tied outside the capsule, thus holding the meniscal fragment against the peripheral rim. Sufficient sutures are placed to obtain good stability, usually 2 to 3 mm apart.

One of the major problems associated with passing sutures from inside out is the risk of damage to extra-articular structures such as the sartorial branch of the saphenous nerve on the medial side, the peroneal nerve on the lateral side, and the popliteal vessels posteriorly. Most arthroscopists now prefer to dissect down to the capsule in the posterior regions of the joint so that these vital structures will not be compromised by inadvertent passage of the suture through the structures or by tying the suture around them.

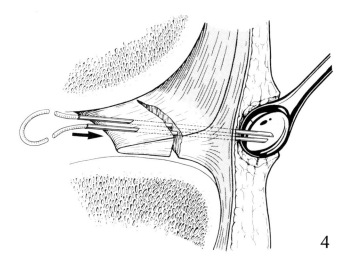

4

Once appropriate sutures have been placed, they should be tied extracapsularly, and therefore buried subcutaneously. Early attempts at bringing sutures out through the skin, and tying them over a bolster, was complicated by infection in several instances.

A retractor is commonly inserted through a posterior incision which dissects down to the capsular layer. The tip of the malleable needle strikes the retractor and is deflected outwards to an area where there is no danger. A common tablespoon is of good shape to provide such deflection and act as a retractor posteriorly.

'Outside-in' technique

5a, b, c & d

In this technique needles are passed from the exterior through the peripheral rim and then through the mobile inner fragment. This is usually carried out with a number 18 spinal needle through which suture material can be threaded. The advantage of this technique is that with the knee appropriately flexed and a knowledge of surface anatomy, one can choose the appropriate sites for penetration of the skin and thus avoid the neurovascular structures that are at risk with blind placement from the inside-out technique.

Once the spinal needles have been placed under arthroscopic control, two stabilization techniques are possible. One method involves suture material passed through the needle and threaded through a second needle and withdrawn so that it becomes a loop inside the joint. The second method involves passing a suture into the joint where it is retrieved, and pulled out through an anterior portal. Then a knot is tied in the end of the suture material, and it is then pulled back into the joint so that the knot abuts against the mobile fragment and pulls it firmly against the peripheral rim. Again, with the outside-in technique, dissection is carried out so that the sutures are tied over the capsule and not left exterior on the skin surface.

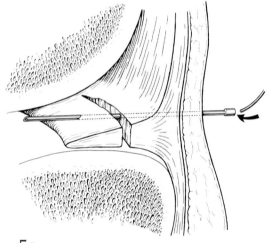

5a

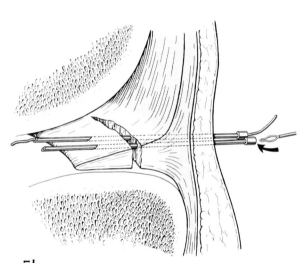

5b

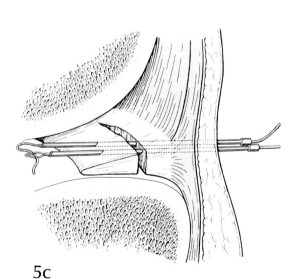

5c

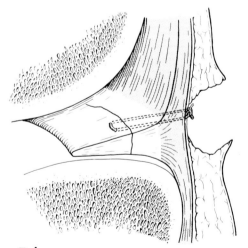

5d

Postoperative management

Most authors recommend immobilization of the knee at 30° to 40° to avoid weight-bearing strains during the initial healing phase. Immobilization is maintained from 4 to 6 weeks. Other authors have advocated tying the sutures with the knee in full extension and immobilizing the limb in this position with immediate full weight-bearing. They argue that in this position there is little stress on the periphery of the meniscus, and if there is no pivoting or weight-bearing in flexion, the repaired area is not stressed and the patient is able to maintain function during the immobilization phase. It now appears that primary healing does occur within 4 to 6 weeks; however, consolidation of the repair probably does not occur for many months. Consequently, it is recommended that the individual be restricted from running and impact-loading for at least 4 months, and from squatting, pivoting, or other sporting activities for at least 6 months after the repair has been done.

Complications

Major complications include damage to neurovascular structures, sepsis and postoperative stiffness. On the medial side, the sartorial branch of the saphenous nerve has been damaged, through the formation of scar tissue, through the actual perforation by needles, or by tying a suture over the nerve structure. On the lateral side, similar problems have been encountered with the peroneal nerve. The disastrous effect on the lateral side is one of peroneal nerve palsy which has a far greater significance than mere sensory loss.

The most serious complications to date have been damage to the popliteal artery and vein, either through perforation by the passage of sutures or through sutures encircling the vessels and obstructing the circulation to the lower leg. Cases of amputation have been reported following this complication.

Knee infections can occur at any time but deep joint infection or pyarthrosis has been reported largely in association with sutures that were tied externally over bolsters, for a long enough period of time which allowed the ingress of bacteria to the joint. A septic knee should be treated in the usual fashion with arthroscopic lavage, appropriate distension-irrigation of the joint, and antibiotics.

Flexion contractures have been reported, presumably due to an inadvertent suture imbrication of the posterior capsule which prevents the knee from coming into full extension. For this reason, some authors advocate tying sutures with the knee in full extension. The use of absorbable sutures might minimize this complication, as any loss of extension might be regained once the suture material has been absorbed.

References

1. Cargill AO'R, Jackson JP. Bucket handle tear of the medial meniscus: a case for conservative surgery. *J Bone Joint Surg [Am]* 1976; 58-A: 248–51.

2. Dandy DJ, Jackson RW. Meniscectomy and chondromalacia of the femoral condyle. *J Bone Joint Surg [Am]* 1975; 57-A: 1116–9.

3. Fairbank TJ. Knee joint changes after meniscectomy. *J Bone Joint Surg [Br]* 1948; 30-B: 664–70.

4. Tapper EM, Hoover NW. Late results after meniscectomy. *J Bone Joint Surg [Am]* 1969; 51-A: 517–26.

5. Dandy DJ, Jackson RW. The diagnosis of problems after meniscectomy. *J Bone Joint Surg [Br]* 1975; 57-B; 349–52.

6. Gillquist J, Oretorp N. Arthroscopic partial meniscectomy: technique and long term results. *Clin Orthop* 1982; 167: 29–33.

7. McGinty JB, Geuss LF, Marvin RA. Partial or total meniscectomy: a comparative analysis. *J Bone Joint Surg [Am]* 1977; 59-A: 763–6.

8. Frankel VH, Burstein AH, Brooks DB. Biomechanics of internal derangement of the knee: pathomechanics as determined by analysis of the instant centers of motion. *J Bone Joint Surg [Am]* 1971; 53-A: 945–62.

9. Kurosawa H, Fukubayashi T, Nakajima H. Load-bearing mode of the knee joint: physical behaviour of the knee joint with or without menisci. *Clin Orthop* 1980; 149: 283–90.

10. Seedhom BB, Dowson D, Wright V. Functions of the menisci: a preliminary study. *J Bone Joint Surg [Br]* 1974; 56-B: 381–2.

11. Dandy DJ. Early results of closed partial meniscectomy. *Br Med J* 1978; 1: 1099–1100.

12. Jackson RW, Rouse, DW. The results of partial arthroscopic meniscectomy in patients over 40 years of age. *J Bone Joint Surg [Br]* 1982; 64-B: 481–5.

13. Hughston JC, Barrett GR. Acute anteromedial rotatory instability: long term results of surgical repair. *J Bone Joint Surg [Am]* 1983; 65-A: 145–53.

14. Price CT, Allen WC. Ligament repair in the knee with preservation of the meniscus. *J Bone Joint Surg [Am]* 1978; 60-A: 61–5.

15. DeHaven KE. Peripheral meniscus repair: an alternative to meniscectomy. *J Bone Joint Surg [Br]* 1981; 63-B: 463.

16. King D. The healing of semilunar cartilages. *J Bone Joint Surg* 1936; 18: 333–42.

17. Ikeuchi H. Meniscus surgery using the Watanabe arthroscope. *Orthop Clin North Am* 1979; 10: 629–42.

18. Johnson LL. *Arthroscopic surgery, principles and practice*, 3rd ed. St Louis: Mosby, 1986.

19. DeHaven KE. Meniscus repair in the athlete. *Clin Orthop* 1985; 198: 31–5.

20. Rosenberg TD, Scott SM, Coward DB, Dunbar WH, Ewing JW, Johnson CL, Paulos LE. Arthroscopic meniscal repair evaluated with repeat arthroscopy. *Arthroscopy* 1986; 2(1): 14–20.

Illustrations by Peter Cox after P. Archer

Open meniscectomy of the knee

Adrian N. Henry MCh, FRCS, FRCSI
Formerly Senior Consultant Orthopaedic Surgeon, Guy's Hospital, London, UK

Introduction

Indication

Lesions of the menisci are but one cause of symptoms of mechanical derangement of the knee joint. It is essential that an accurate preoperative diagnosis be made concerning the state of the menisci since adequate visualization of the menisci at arthrotomy is not possible and removal of a normal meniscus is undesirable. Confirmation of the clinical diagnosis should be obtained by arthroscopy or magnetic resonance imaging. The descriptions of the operations which follow relate to total meniscectomy. Current practice places much more emphasis on conservative operations on the menisci, such as removal of torn fragments or repair of peripheral detachments, under arthroscopic control.

Preoperative preparation

It is unnecessary and undesirable to shave the part prior to operation. An exsanguinating tourniquet is used, the skin prepared and the part towelled off as for other operations on the knee joint.

Operations

MEDIAL MENISCECTOMY

Incision

1

With the end of the table lowered and the knee flexed 90° with a pad beneath it, a slightly oblique, vertical, medial, parapatellar incision of approximately 5 cm in length is made one thumb's-breadth medial to the border of the patella and patellar tendon and just crossing the upper margin of the tibial plateau distally.

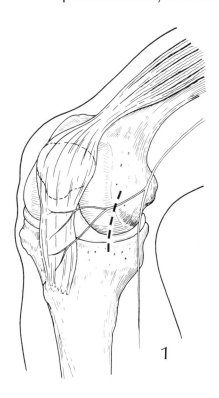

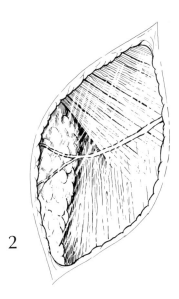

Exposure

2

The infrapatellar branch of the saphenous nerve is sought in the subcutaneous fat immediately superficial to the fibrous capsule. This nerve crosses the operative field at an inconstant level and if identified should be resected wide of the incision by sharp division.

3

Next, the two layers of the fibrous capsule are divided in the same direction and length as the skin incision. The synovial membrane is also opened in a similar manner at the upper end of the incision to avoid damage to the meniscus. A medium-sized Langenbeck retractor is placed in the lateral edge of the incision, retracting the infrapatellar fat pad laterally.

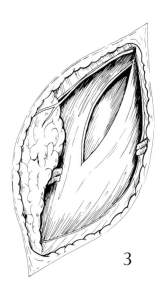

4

A Stamm or similar retractor is inserted into the medial aspect of the incision, retracting the fibrous and synovial capsules medially. This retraction exposes the anterior horn of the medial meniscus together with the distal insertion of the anterior cruciate ligament and part of the articular cartilage of the medial femoral condyle on its lateral aspect.

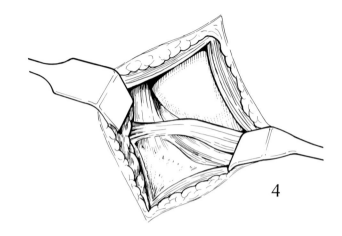

4

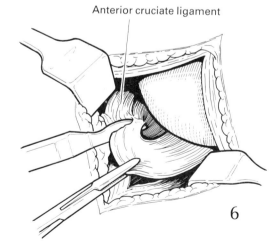

5

Mobilization of anterior horn of the medial meniscus

5

A blunt hook is inserted under the free margin of the anterior horn to emerge through the coronary ligament on the inferior aspect of the meniscus.

6

Using the plane of the hook as a guide, a scapel with rounded tip incises the coronary ligament at the tip of the hook and is directed in a horizontal plane laterally and then vertically to detach the anterior horn of the meniscus. Care must be taken to avoid damage to the anterior cruciate ligament.

Anterior cruciate ligament

6

Excision of medial meniscus

7

The detached anterior horn is now gripped by Kocher's forceps and, with the scalpel, the meniscus is divided along its periphery just inside its attachment to the synovial membrane.

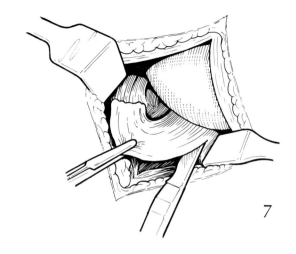

8

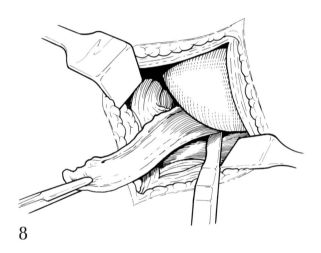

This division continues along the periphery of the meniscus at the same time as the Kocher's forceps are exerting a laterally directed pull on the meniscus. Mobilization of the periphery of the meniscus is continued posteromedially until the structure displaces into the centre of the joint.

9

Finally, the attachment of the posterior horn is divided and the meniscus removed.

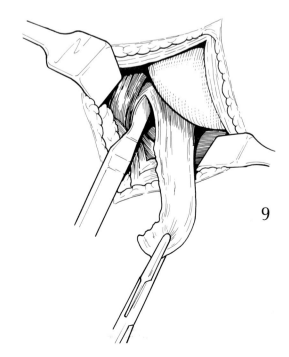

Closure

10

The synovial membrane is closed by a continuous haemostatic plain catgut or polyglactin 910 suture.

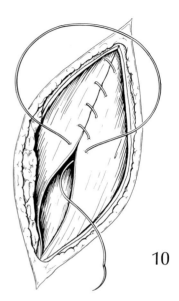

10

11

The two layers of the fibrous capsule are closed together with interrupted chromic catgut polyglactin sutures. Skin may be closed by interrupted sutures or a continuous subcuticular stitch of nylon or polypropylene.

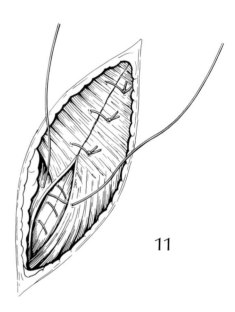

11

Postoperative management

A two-layer wool and crêpe bandage is applied from ankle to groin before removal of the tourniquet. On regaining consciousness the patient is immediately instructed to start quadriceps exercises and these are continued with bedrest until 48 hours postoperatively, when the patient may begin partial weight-bearing on crutches. The compression bandage is maintained for 10–14 days when the sutures are removed and flexion exercises may then be commenced in addition to continuing the quadriceps drill. At this stage crutches may be discarded and the patient may gradually resume normal activity, which should be possible at approximately 4–6 weeks after operation depending on his occupation.

LATERAL MENISCECTOMY

Incision

12

Without lowering the end of the table, the knee is flexed 120°. A horizontal incision is made in the skin from the lateral edge of the patellar tendon to the fibular collateral ligament and approximately 0.5 cm above the level of the lateral tibial plateau.

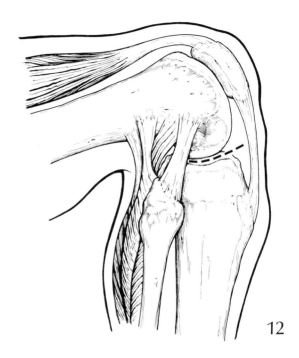

12

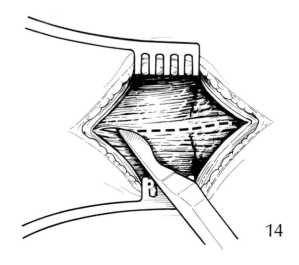

13

Exposure

13

After retraction of the skin edges the fibres of the iliotibial tract are divided in the direction in which they run, which is approximately similar to that of the skin incision. The tract is divided throughout the same length as the skin incision.

14

The edges of the iliotibial tract are retracted by a self-retaining retractor. This exposes the extrasynovial lateral infrapatellar fat pad in the anterior half of the wound and the synovial membrane in the posterior half. An incision is made in the latter and carried forward through the fat pad almost to the patellar tendon.

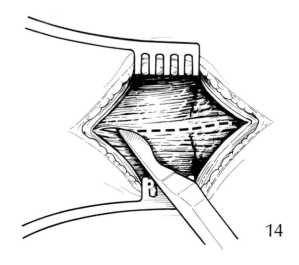

14

15

A medium-sized Langenbeck retractor is then inserted into the anterior end of the wound, retracting the fat pad. This exposes the anterior aspect of the lateral meniscus.

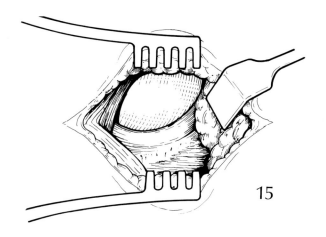

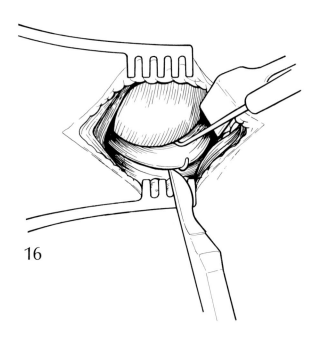

Mobilization of the meniscus

16

A blunt hook is inserted under the anterior horn of the lateral meniscus, as in medial meniscectomy, and the anterior horn mobilized in a similar manner.

17

After the anterior horn has been gripped by Kocher's forceps, the meniscus is detached from the synovial membrane by a scalpel and a small Langenbeck retractor is inserted into the posterior end of the wound to retract the popliteal tendon and the leash of lateral inferior geniculate vessels running just anterior to it.

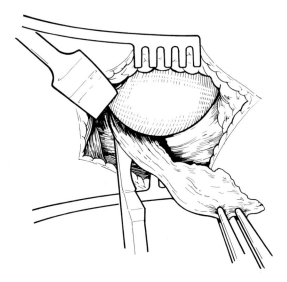

18

The peripheral attachment of the meniscus is deficient surrounding the popliteal tendon and is continued posteriorly by a loose tenuous attachment to the posterior horn. The peripheral attachment is divided posteriorly beyond the popliteal tendon, at the same time exerting an anterior strain by the Kocher's forceps on the meniscus. The extreme attachment of the posterior horn from the tibia is divided with removal of the whole meniscus.

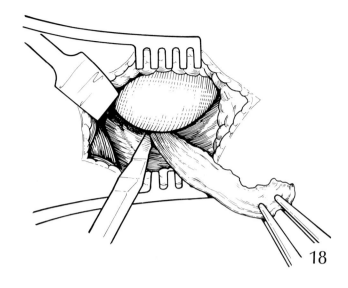

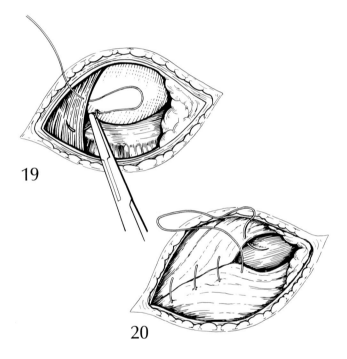

Closure

19 & 20

The synovial membrane is closed with a continuous haemostatic plain catgut or polyglactin suture, particular attention being paid to inclusion of the lateral inferior geniculate vessels in the initial stitch.

21

The iliotibial tract is closed with interrupted chromic catgut or polyglactin and the skin is closed according to the surgeon's choice.

Postoperative management

The postoperative programme for lateral meniscectomy is similar to that for the medial side. However, the incidence of postoperative haemarthrosis is greater following lateral meniscectomy owing to haemorrhage from the lateral inferior geniculate vessels. This complication must be watched for and dealt with at an early date by aspiration or evacuation of the haematoma or haemarthrosis, otherwise the patient's postoperative recovery is delayed.

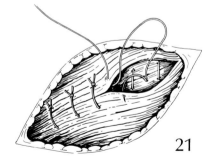

EXCISION OF RETAINED POSTERIOR HORN OF MEDIAL MENISCUS

Occasionally the posterior horn of the meniscus may become detached during the procedure of medial meniscectomy. If the retained fragment is large and mobile it should be removed through a separate postero-medial incision. The patient should be placed supine on the table with a sandbag under the opposite buttock and the knee flexed 90° to expose the posteromedial corner of the knee joint.

Incision

22

An oblique incision is made in the skin approximately 2.5 cm in length on the posteromedial aspect of the knee joint.

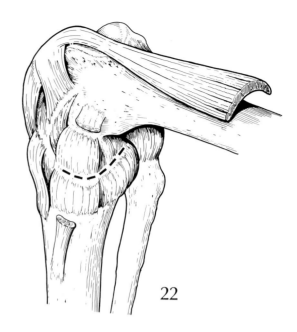

22

Exposure

After retraction of the skin edges the important postero-medial component of the medial capsule is exposed and an incision made through this structure in the direction of its fibres. Deep to the fibrous capsule the synovial membrane is exposed and divided in a similar manner. Small Langenbeck retractors are inserted to expose the posterior horn of the medial meniscus and this is removed by peripheral division as during medial meniscectomy.

Closure

Closure is carried out in a similar manner to that for the anterior incision during medial meniscectomy, particular care being taken to repair the posteromedial capsular ligament.

EXCISION OF POSTERIOR HORN OF LATERAL MENISCUS

Position of patient

The patient is positioned on his side with the affected knee uppermost and flexed 70°.

Incision

23

The skin is incised along the posterior border of the iliotibial tract for approximately 5 cm distal to the styloid process of the fibula.

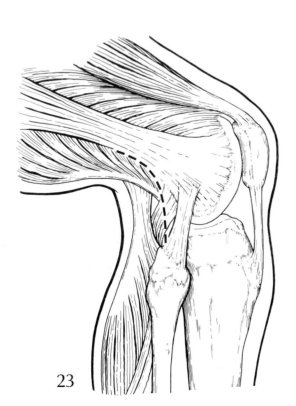

23

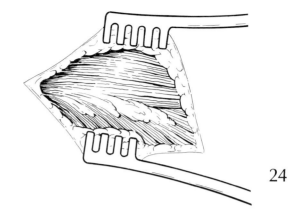

Exposure

24

The posterior margin of the iliotibial tract is freed from the fascia overlying the biceps muscle.

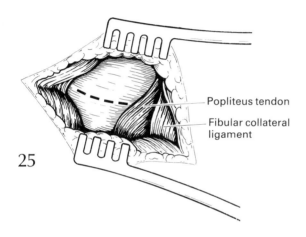

Popliteus tendon

Fibular collateral ligament

25

The iliotibial tract is retracted superiorly and the biceps muscle inferiorly. After separation of these structures the fibular collateral ligament is seen running vertically in the distal part of the incision, and just deep to the ligament the popliteal tendon runs obliquely upwards and forwards.

26

Both these structures are retracted to reveal the underlying synovial membrane which is divided horizontally just above the posterior horn of the lateral meniscus.

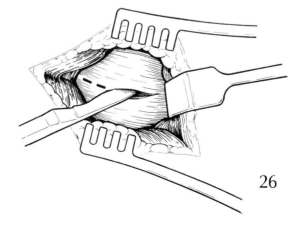

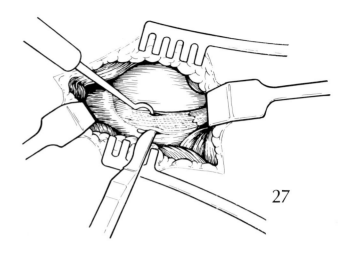

27

Langenbeck retractors are inserted to show the posterior horn of the meniscus. This is then detached peripherally and at its insertion to the tibial intercondylar area.

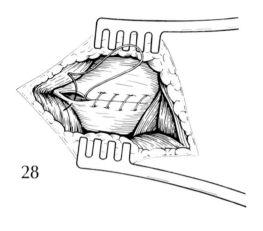

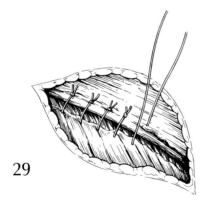

Closure

28 & 29

Closure is effected in layers in similar fashion to closure of other meniscectomy incisions.

Loose bodies in the knee

Paul Aichroth MS, FRCS
Consultant Orthopaedic Surgeon, Westminster Hospital and Westminster Children's Hospital, London; Queen Mary's Hospital, Roehampton, UK

Introduction

Loose bodies form in the knee joint in a variety of different conditions. The majority are due to the following conditions.

Osteochondritis dissecans

A fragment of articular cartilage and subchondral bone separates from a joint surface. This condition may be considered an ununited osteochondral fracture of the femoral condyle. Rarely is the patellar surface involved.

Acute osteochondral fractures

A fragment is avulsed from the femoral condyle in a severe knee injury. Also, fragments separate by shearing stresses from the lateral margin of the femoral groove of the femur and the patella in twisting injuries.

Osteoarthritis

Rarely, an osteophyte separates from the articular margin and becomes free in the joint. The cartilage component may increase in size as the articular cartilage proliferates.

Synovial osteochondromatosis

Metaplasia of the synovial membrane results in the formation of a multitude of small chondromatous bodies. The cartilaginous material then ossifies and the bodies become radio-opaque. These may float free in the synovial cavity. The posterior synovial pouch is frequently involved.

Avascular necrosis of bone

Loose fragments of necrotic bone together with hyaline cartilage separate in steroid arthropathies, caisson disease and other conditions where massive necrosis of the femoral condylar bone occurs. Loose fragments shed from a necrotic femoral condyle are an increasing problem in the post-renal transplantation arthropathies.

Symptoms and signs of a loose body

The loose body may sometimes be palpated in the parapatellar or suprapatellar region. The knee joint becomes internally deranged only when the fragment becomes jammed between the joint surfaces. It produces the following.

1. Pain
2. Locking of the joint during movement
3. Synovial effusion.

Indications for removal

Loose bodies may be present in the knee joint singly or in large numbers. They may remain asymptomatic but if the above symptoms of an internal derangement occur they should be removed. A patient may present with pain and disability in an osteoarthritic knee and on X-ray examination loose bodies are found. Episodes of locking will necessitate an arthrotomy or arthroscopy to remove the loose fragments; but, in the absence of locking, the joint may be treated by conservative means.

Arthroscopic removal of loose bodies

The removal of loose bodies may be undertaken arthroscopically as described in the chapter on 'Arthroscopic surgical procedures' (see pp. 1019–1032). It may be very simple to remove the loose body in the anterior compartment after appropriate visualization, localization and then extraction using the pituitary rongeur or spiked grasping forceps. However, the loose body may move to a difficult position or to the posterior recesses. It will then become much more difficult and before embarking on such an arthroscopic procedure the operator must be conversant with all arthroscopic approaches to the knee.

Arthrotomy may be indicated if there are multiple or very large loose bodies.

OPEN REMOVAL

Preoperative

The position of the loose body should be determined by palpation. The fragment in the suprapatellar pouch is best approached with the knee extended. Fragments seen radiologically to be lying on the tibial plateau are usually not palpable, and these, together with loose bodies posteromedially and posterolaterally, are best approached with the knee flexed over the end of the table. An Esmarch bandage is applied to exsanguinate the limb and a pneumatic cuff is inflated around the upper thigh. The knee should be palpated again and the joint position arranged as indicated above. A radiograph must be taken in the anteroposterior and lateral planes – with the knee in the position in which it will be opened – if the fragment cannot be felt with certainty.

These careful preoperative precautions must be undertaken to avoid the situation where the joint is opened with one incision and the fragment has moved to another area, where a second incision is required.

Operations

LOOSE BODY REMOVAL FROM THE SUPRAPATELLAR POUCH AND ANTERIOR CAVITY

The skin of the knee, the thigh and the leg is prepared and towelled in such a way that the knee may be flexed. An incise drape may be used. If the loose body can be palpated it should be transfixed with a sterile needle through the skin.

Incision

A vertical parapatellar incision is recommended. Ideally, this should be over the loose body if it can be palpated or in the appropriate position if the site of the fragment has been identified radiologically. When the fragment is due to osteochondritis dissecans, or osteochondral fracture, the parapatellar incision may be extended inferiorly to allow inspection of the condylar crater from which the loose body came. After skin incision, the parapatellar aponeurosis is opened in the same line. The synovium is then exposed and should be incised in the same line, with the incision entering the joint cavity. The loose fragment sometimes pops through, with a rush of synovial fluid, but more commonly it is obscured from view by a synovial fold.

Technique

1 & 2

As soon as the fragment is sighted a large curette should be positioned behind it so that there is little chance of the body being squeezed by the approaching broad forceps and moved to another part of the joint. If this technique fails, and the loose body moves, then it may be retrieved by palpating the area through the skin and pushing it back into view. Flexing and extending the joint may be helpful but, if this fails, syringing the joint cavity with a large quantity of normal saline may be successful.

The above manoeuvres are usually successful, but if they are not a second glove may be donned, and the joint cavity explored with the finger. A further radiograph may be helpful, or the arthroscope inserted through the wound may reveal the site of the loose fragment.

Closure

The synovium is closed with a fine chromic catgut or polyglactin 910 (Vicryl, Ethicon, Edinburgh, UK) continuous suture. Interrupted 1/0 or 2/0 chromic catgut or Vicryl sutures will approximate the patellar expansion and the subcutaneous tissues. The skin is closed with intradermal nylon or Prolene (Ethicon, Edinburgh, UK) reinforced by surgical tapes.

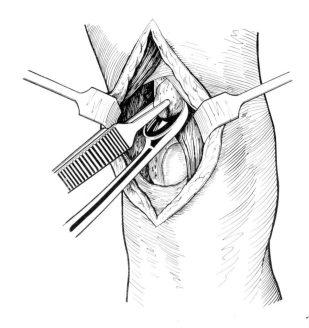

1

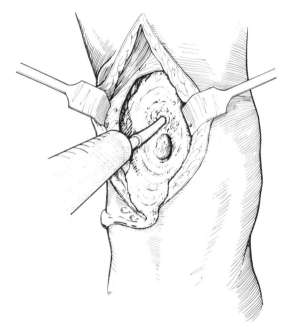

2

Dressing

3

The limb is wrapped in cotton wool from the thigh to above the ankle and compression bandages applied. Side slabs of plaster of Paris within the layers of bandage will give extra support and strength. The patient can walk, weight-bearing, after 48 hours and begin knee flexion after 5 days. Sutures should be removed after 14 days if the wound is satisfactory.

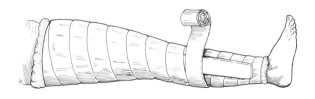

3

REMOVAL FROM THE POSTERIOR COMPARTMENT

The posterior cruciate ligament and its synovial reflection separates the posterior aspect of the knee into two compartments. It is therefore essential to identify the particular compartment containing the posterior loose body.

Posteromedial approach

4

The knee is flexed and a vertical incision is made, centred on the joint line posteromedially. The oblique fibres of the posteromedial capsule behind the medial collateral ligament are exposed. This layer is incised vertically, and after entering the synovium the posterior horn of the medial meniscus and the posterior compartment is exposed.

Posterolateral approach

5

The knee is flexed and a posterolateral curved incision is made anterior to the fibular head and the biceps femoris tendon. The lateral popliteal nerve is behind these two structures. The popliteus tendon is seen between the biceps tendon and the lateral collateral ligament. This is retracted posteriorly, the capsule and synovium are incised and the posterior compartment opened.

TREATMENT OF OSTEOCHONDRITIS DISSECANS

6

Osteochondritis dissecans may be considered a subchondral or osteochondral surface fracture. Some lesions will heal and others will remain ununited in a crater and will later separate as a loose body. Eighty-five per cent affect the medial femoral condyle and 70 per cent are situated in the classic site on the intercondylar region of the medial femoral condyle. Fifty per cent of patients with such a lesion give a history of substantial trauma, and as a group they are excellent athletes.

Arthroscopic procedures

The fragment may be removed and the crater curetted using arthroscopic techniques. Alternatively, the fragment may be drilled under direct arthroscopic inspection using powered instruments.

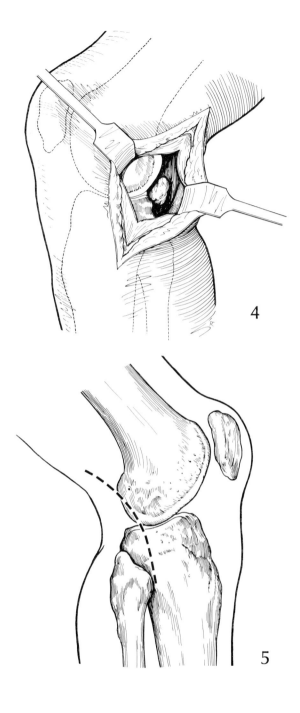

4

5

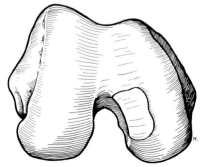

6

Osteochondritis dissecans with the fragment *in situ*

7 & 8

If the fragment remains in its crater, and the symptoms are slight, then it should be left alone. Arthroscopy is useful to confirm the fixity of the fragment and to exclude any other internal derangement. Regular clinical and radiological follow-up will be required to confirm the healing or separation of the fragment. If the knee locks or regularly gives way, it is likely that the fragment is hinging or moving in its crater. Arthrotomy is then required with approaches similar to those used in meniscectomy. If the fragment is loose in its crater, it should be excised and the crater curetted. All fibrous tissue should be removed and drilling performed to expose bleeding bone. This allows the proliferation of fibrocartilaginous material in the crater and produces a remarkably smooth surface.

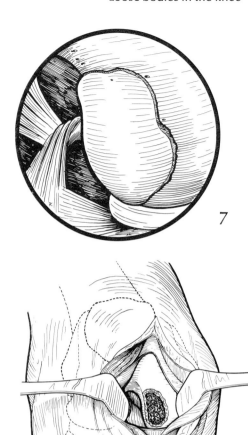

7

8

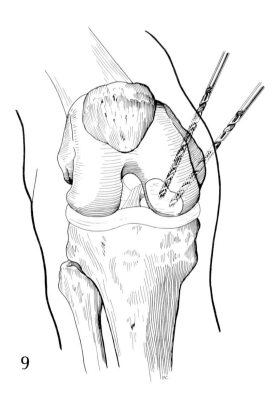

9

9

If at arthrotomy the fragment is found very tightly *in situ* or the fragment is not visible from the intact cartilaginous surface (the fracture being entirely subchondral), then the bony fragment may be drilled from the condylar side. The twist-drills traverse the pseudarthrosis but do not pierce the condylar surface cartilage and so stimulate healing and revascularization from the subchondral bone. Alternatively, the fragment may be drilled at arthroscopy with a fine bone wire on a power drill.

Osteochondritis dissecans with a loose body

The loose body should be removed as described above and the crater from which it came should be inspected and curetted. There is no definite indication for replacement of the loose fragment using internal fixation for it is only rarely possible to produce enough stability of the fragment with a good fit of the articular surfaces and bony apposition to allow union to occur.

TREATMENT OF THE ACUTE OSTEOCHONDRAL FRACTURE

Osteochondral fractures are sustained in severe injuries to the knee joint. Avulsion or shearing off of a fragment is associated with a rapid large haemarthrosis, and oblique, tunnel and sky-line radiographs may be required for its detection. Small fragments should be removed at arthrotomy but larger fragments (2 × 2 cm or more) may be repositioned accurately and internally fixed.

Technique

10

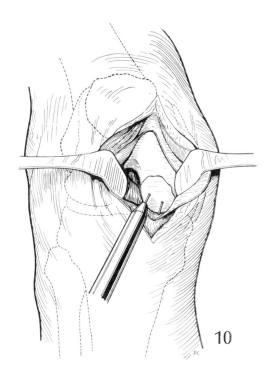

10

The crater is approached as above (p. 1074) and is debrided. The fragment is similarly prepared and is repositioned with the correct orientation. Two or more Smillie pins are inserted to transfix the fragment with their heads punched just beneath the cartilage surface. The wound is closed and dressed as above (p. 1075). Alternatively, small Herbert screws with reverse threads are ideal and produce good fixation with compression.

Postoperative management

A compression bandage of wool and crépe is applied from ankle to groin and the leg is elevated for 24 hours. Quadriceps exercises begin as soon as pain allows and weight-bearing in the bandages with crutches at 48 hours.

The knee is mobilized when the wound is healed at 2 weeks after operation. Minimal weight-bearing on crutches is recommended until the fragment unites. A further arthrotomy may then be required after 1 year to remove the pins or screws.

SYNOVIAL OSTEOCHONDROMATOSIS

This is a poorly understood condition in which the whole synovial lining is involved. Symptoms are frequently severe and on opening the joint vast numbers of loose bodies gush out. A synovectomy will be required (see pp. 1109–1112) and a posterior synovial mass may require excision through the popliteal fossa via a formal posterior approach.

Repair and reconstruction of knee ligament injury

Paul Aichroth MS, FRCS
Consultant Orthopaedic Surgeon, Westminster Hospital and Westminster Children's Hospital, London; Queen Mary's Hospital, Roehampton, UK

Introduction

Injury to a knee ligament may be partial or complete. A sprain or partial tear of the medial collateral ligament may occur in isolation and is very painful. The stability of the ligament, however, remains intact and treatment is that of pain relief and then full rehabilitation. Temporary splintage may be required in the most painful stage.

The complete tear of a knee ligament is rarely in isolation. O'Donoghue described his 'unhappy triad' of medial collateral ligament tear, anterior cruciate avulsion and an injury to the medial meniscus.

The assessment of a knee ligament injury must include a full history and a detailed clinical examination. The type of injury sustained often indicates the structures damaged. For example, a dashboard injury to the knee is frequently associated with a tell-tale anterior bruise and abrasion on the tibial tubercle, and a posterior cruciate ligament tear is detected when undertaking posterior drawer and Lachman tests.

Clinical examination of the knee must be undertaken carefully to assess the medial and lateral collateral stability by means of a valgus and varus strain in a few degrees of flexion. Cruciate ligaments are assessed by anterior and posterior drawer signs with the knee at right angles, and, more importantly, by the Lachman test, in which the tibia is brought forwards and backwards on the femur in 20° flexion. Rotary instability of the knee joint must also be assessed, and anterolateral rotary instability with a 'pivot shift' and a jerk is present in an anterior cruciate ligament tear with associated capsular laxity.

Posterior cruciate ligament laxity is best assessed with the knee at right angles when a posterior sag of the tibia on the femur is noted. The posterior drawer sign is positive at this angle, and a posterior drawer or posterior Lachman manoeuvre may also be positive with the knee at 20° flexion. Rotary instability may also be detected with a posterior cruciate ligament injury if the posteromedial and posterolateral structures are damaged in association. There may be a reverse pivot shift or, alternatively, a hyperextension lateral rotation sign if the great toe is lifted high. Immediately following a knee injury, swelling, tenderness and general irritability may prevent movement and adequate examination. The sight of a strong athlete walking into the examination room with a complete rupture of the medial and cruciate ligaments must not fool the surgeon. In these circumstances it is vital to assess the knee ligament structures and their integrity by examination under anaesthesia. At the same time an arthroscopy is undertaken to elucidate any problem of internal derangement fully. There is an associated haemarthrosis in most patients with an acute injury of this type, and at arthroscopy patient and copious irrigation is required to obtain a good view of all internal structures. A hook is always necessary to assess the stability of the menisci and anterior cruciate ligament. The meniscal damage may be treated arthroscopically at this stage.

The presence of clinical physical signs together with the results of examination under anaesthesia and arthroscopy will allow a plan of surgical action to be made. Early and accurate diagnosis is necessary so that appropriate treatment may avoid the need for reconstruction later.

Operations

MEDIAL COLLATERAL LIGAMENT REPAIR

Examination under anaesthesia is undertaken to assess knee ligamentous damage fully. Arthroscopy is also performed to elucidate any internal derangement. A plan of repair and reconstruction is then made and any meniscal damage may be treated arthroscopically.

After exsanguination, a high thigh tourniquet is applied. The knee is flexed over the end of the table or is maintained in this position with a knee rest.

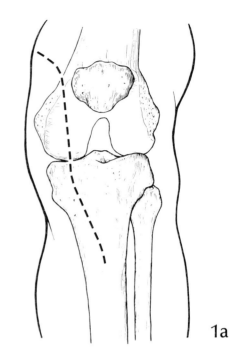

1a

Incision

1a & b

A long, curved, medial parapatellar incision is made. The middle portion of the incision is situated in the appropriate place for formal medial arthrotomy. The superior part of the incision is curved posteriorly to allow access to the more posterior portions of the joint and its posteromedial capsule.

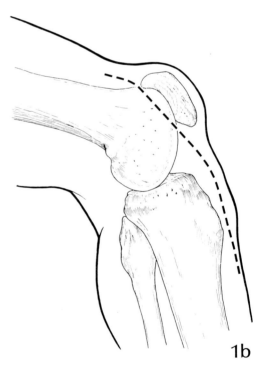

1b

Exploration

2

The whole of the medial capsule and medial collateral ligament is exposed. A swab is used to wipe away the superficial areolar tissue which is frequently infiltrated by blood or oedema. It is important to explore as far as the posterior aspect of the capsule as this structure is frequently ruptured behind the medial collateral ligament. It may be obvious that the superficial part of the medial collateral ligament is ruptured from the femur above or the tibia below.

The superficial collateral ligament is then incised in the line of its fibres to expose the deep layer of the medial collateral ligament beneath. The deep ligament may be ruptured at the midpoint of its attachment to the medial meniscus or it may be shredded and stretched at this site.

The medial meniscus may be torn peripherally and an assessment must be made to determine whether it is to be repaired or removed. If removal is indicated, a formal anteromedial arthrotomy is made through the capsule and a routine meniscectomy undertaken unless prior arthroscopic treatment has been performed. If the anterior cruciate is to be repaired or reconstructed, this must be planned before the medial collateral ligament and medial capsule repair sutures are finally tightened.

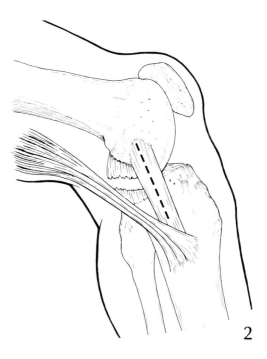

2

Technique of repair

3a & b

The exact reposition site for the superior attachment of the medial collateral ligament must be identified. However, it is ideal to repair the posterior capsule and also the posterior oblique fibres of the medial collateral ligament initially. Sutures of 1/0 Dexon (Davis and Geck, Gosport, UK) or Vicryl (Ethicon, Edinburgh, UK) are recommended. The sutures should be placed obliquely to bring the superior fibres in this repair more anterior.

Superior or inferior reattachment of the medial collateral ligament must be accurately undertaken with sutures which pass through the bone. The bone is drilled with an awl or fine drill entering the bone surface at 45°. A stout trocar/small-radius needle is used to pass the sutures through interconnecting holes in the bone to reattach the collateral ligament tightly. If, however, a main portion of the medial collateral ligament has been avulsed from the bone, it may be reattached using a barbed staple of the Richards type.

Tears of the midpoint of the deep medial collateral ligament may require attachment to the medial meniscus, and the peripheral edge can be used to receive the suture material. Shreds in this position are again brought into a more anterior position with appropriate placement of the sutures. It should be noted that the tibia is rotated medially whilst the sutures are tightened and the layers are advanced anteriorly.

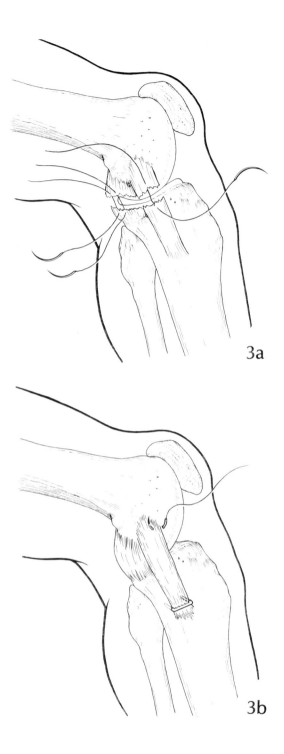

3a

3b

Postoperative management

The wound is closed with suction drainage and the limb is placed in a cast in some 30°–40° flexion with the tibia rotated medially. At 5–6 weeks the cast is removed and physiotherapy is continued, followed by progressive rehabilitation. However, if the repair is thought to be strong and tight, the surgeon may decide that gentle early restricted movement is possible followed by a brace. In this situation, a constant passive motion machine may be used with the movement setting between 30° and 80° of flexion. When the wound is quiescent and movement may be maintained, a brace is applied with a setting at approximately 20°–80° of flexion. This must be maintained for 6 weeks after operation and during this period the patient does not bear weight and remains on crutches.

POSTERIOR CRUCIATE LIGAMENT REPAIR

This is a large structure which may be torn in isolation or in combination with any other knee ligament. The posterior capsule is frequently injured and the combination may constitute a posteromedial or posterolateral instability. The tibia is posteriorly displaced on the femur, the ligament is either pulled off the bone or, frequently, a bone fragment is avulsed from its inferior tibial attachment.

After exsanguination of the limb, a high thigh tourniquet is applied and the patient is positioned prone.

Incision

4

An S-shaped incision is made across the popliteal fossa with the inferior limb on the medial side. The deep fascia is divided in the same line and the posterior cutaneous nerve of the calf is preserved.

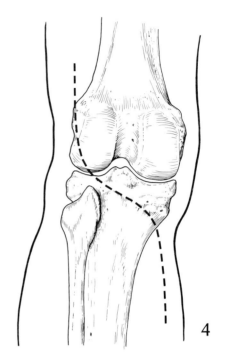

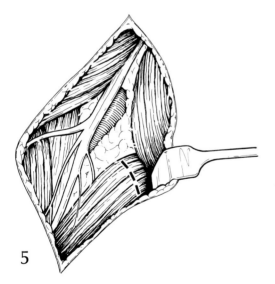

Dissection

5

The medial head of gastrocnemius is isolated and dissected superiorly to its attachment on the back of the femoral condyle. It is divided transversely near its attachment to the bone. The medial edge of the muscle is then dissected free and the whole structure retracted to the lateral side.

Repair

6

The medial superior genicular vessel may be over the site
of the capsule incision and require division after ligation.
The middle genicular vessel must be similarly ligated. A
vertical incision is made through the capsule and posterior
oblique ligament near the midline, and the posterior
cruciate and its bone fragment detachment can be seen.
The bone fragment may then be screwed back into the
bed from which it has been avulsed using a cancellous
screw. If the ligament has been torn above the bone it may
be sutured back and multifilament Dacron (du Pont de
Nemours and Company, UK) sutures may be used,
passing through bony tunnels. However, midsubstance
posterior cruciate tears are best reconstructed using a
tendon transfer of semitendinosus and gracilis as discussed below.

Postoperative management

The capsular incision is repaired and the medial head of
the gastrocnemius resutured. The wound is closed with
drainage and the knee is placed in a cast in a few degrees
of flexion for 5–6 weeks. Vigorous rehabilitation em-
phasizing active movement follows. Sporting activity is
forbidden for 6 months.

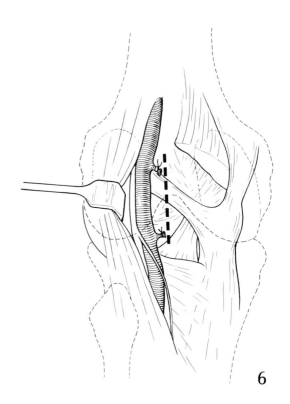

6

ANTERIOR CRUCIATE LIGAMENT REPAIR

Rupture of the anterior cruciate ligament may occur in isolation or with medial collateral ligament and medial meniscus injuries. If an anterior cruciate ligament injury occurs in isolation, full counselling of the patient is necessary to determine his or her future physical and sporting aims. Many patients may wish to avoid a major repair or reconstruction at this stage and simply concentrate on muscle rehabilitation.

With midsubstance tears the ligament is frequently so torn and shredded that repair is not possible, and reconstruction using a tendon transfer of semitendinosus and gracilis is necessary.

If the cruciate is avulsed with a bone fragment, a good repair may be effected by fixation of this bone portion with a screw or other fixation device. From time to time the cruciate is avulsed from either the superior or inferior attachments with a small fragment of bone removed. If the bone avulsion fragment is small, then a screw cannot be used and the fragment, together with the ligament, is reattached with sutures.

When the anterior cruciate is ruptured from its upper attachment it is best repaired by an 'over the top technique' taking the sutures through the intercondylar region and over the top of the lateral femoral condyle. The most appropriate repair suture consists of a heavy 2/8 circle, round-bodied, taper-cut needle swaged to a loop of multifilament polyester.

Technique of repair

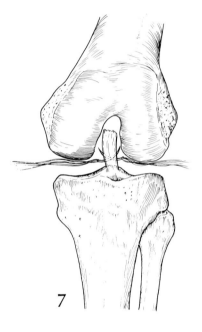

7

A routine medial arthrotomy incision is made, and two sutures and needles are positioned in the upper attachment of the anterior cruciate as shown.

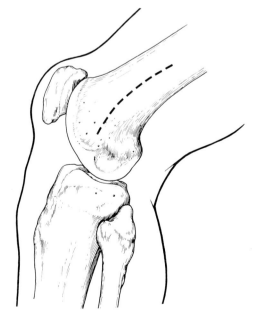

8

An incision is made over the lateral femoral condyle and the supracondylar region. The iliotibial tract is incised in the same line, and, using a self-retaining retractor, the posterior aspect of the femoral condyle is palpated and the lateral gastrocnemius muscle identified. The lateral gastrocnemius is then separated from the posterior capsule.

9

A director is then passed through the posterior capsule and through the intercondylar region. A tape may be taken along the same path by attaching it to the notch in the director. The four ends of the Dacron sutures are attached to this tape and brought through the posterior capsule and over the top of the condyle.

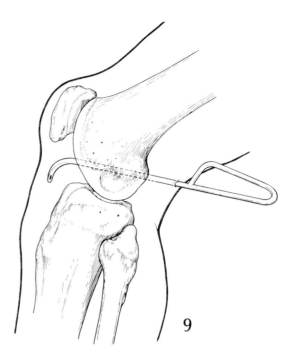

9

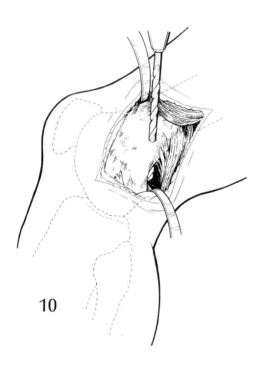

10

10

An oblique hole is then drilled in the supracondylar bone just above the attachment of the lateral gastrocnemius. Sutures are tied tightly through this bone tunnel with the knee in flexion and lateral rotation.

11

The inferior attachment of the anterior cruciate ligament may also be repaired using the same two sutures. The Dacron fibres are then brought through two bone tunnels drilled in the tibia. A hook is used to pull the Dacron suture through these holes and they are then tied tightly on the surface of the medial upper tibia.

Postoperative management

A cast is applied for 5–6 weeks in 40° flexion with the tibia in lateral rotation.

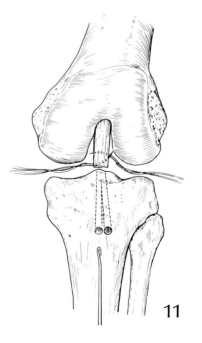

11

ANTERIOR CRUCIATE REPAIR/RECONSTRUCTION USING TENDON TRANSFER FOR ACUTE INJURY

The large majority of anterior cruciate injuries occur in the midsubstance or at the upper end without bone avulsion. The diagnosis will be made by examination under anaesthesia and confirmed arthroscopically. Sometimes the arthroscope will show a bruised but essentially intact synovium over the anterior cruciate ligament. When the ligament is apparently partially torn or is very lax, dissection with a hook reveals the extent of the cruciate ligament damage. The anterior cruciate ligament is in two portions, anteromedial and posterolateral. One or other, or both, portions may be ruptured. If one portion is intact it may still be considered necessary to reconstruct the ligament using tendon transfers, as the laxity may be substantial.

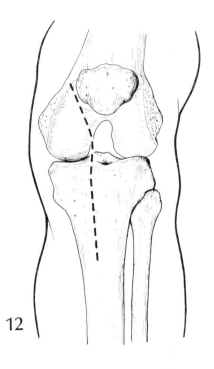

12

Incision

12 & 13

A medial parapatellar incision with inferior extension to allow access to the pes anserinus is made. A routine medial parapatellar arthrotomy is also undertaken through the upper end of this incision. A lateral incision is made to allow access to the lateral supracondylar region.

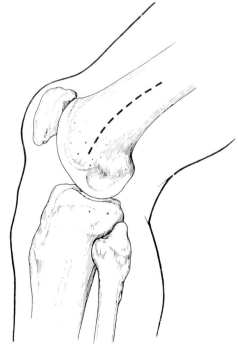

13

Dissection of pes anserinus

14, 15 & 16

The semitendinosus and gracilis tendons are identified by careful dissection of the whole pes structure. They are traced back into the posteromedial thigh and the maximal length is achieved by means of a special rotary tenotome or by open dissection superiorly. A small incision is made in the posteromedial thigh. The tendons are dissected free and isolated; they are then separated from surrounding muscle and cut off as high as possible.

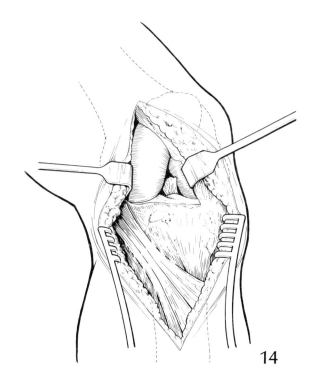

14

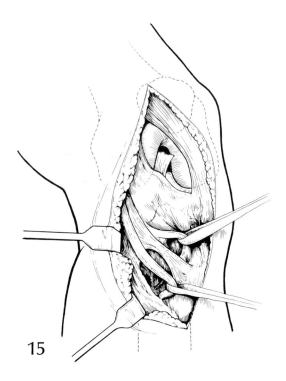

15

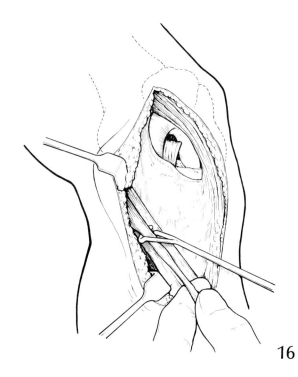

16

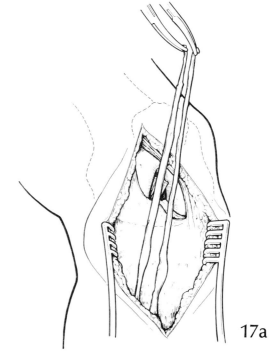

17a

17a & b

The gracilis and semitendinosus tendons are sutured together. A Bunnell-type suture is then inserted superiorly.

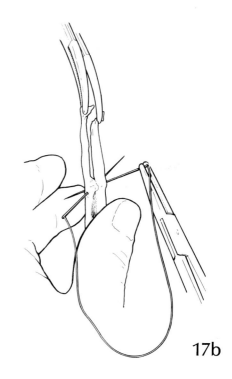

17b

18

A jig is used to drill a tibial tunnel. The drill enters the tibia just above the insertion of the two tendons and emerges from the tibial plateau at the normal inferior attachment of the anterior cruciate ligament – just at, and slightly posterior to, the bifid anterior tibial spine. This point is often better felt than observed.

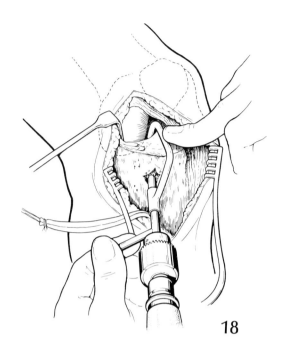

18

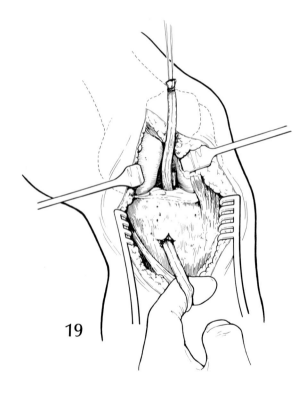

19

19

The conjoined tendons are then brought through the tibial tunnel. This is best effected by passing a malleable hook down the tibial tunnel and thereby bringing through the leading Bunnell suture. The conjoined tendons then follow.

Lateral dissection

20

The incision follows the line of the supracondylar and condylar regions of the lateral femur. The iliotibial tract is split along the same line.

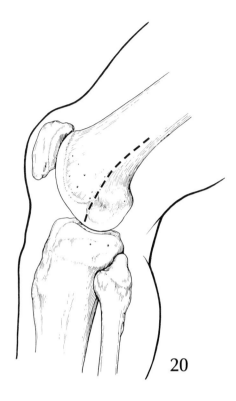

20

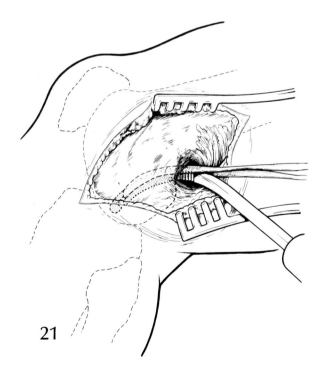

21

21

Dissection then proceeds beneath the lateral gastrocnemius, separating it from the lateral capsule. A curved director is passed through the intercondylar region and over the top of the lateral femoral condyle. A tape may be taken through the same path and the Bunnell suture attached. Alternatively, a long curved artery forceps may be similarly positioned and the conjoined tendon is brought through and over the top of the lateral femoral condyle.

22, 23a, b & c

The conjoined tendons are then strongly attached to the exposed supracondylar bone using two barbed staples. The whole procedure may be undertaken with arthroscopic assistance, and then smaller incisions are used.

Postoperative management

The wounds are closed in layers with appropriate drainage. A cast is then applied for 5–6 weeks in some 40° of flexion. If the repair is tight with excellent fixation, then early movement and controlled flexion using a brace may be considered. The constant passive motion machine is used to obtain a flexion range from 20° to 70°. A brace is then applied with movement block to allow a flexion range from 10° to 80° of flexion. The patient must not bear weight and must remain on crutches until the sixth week after operation.

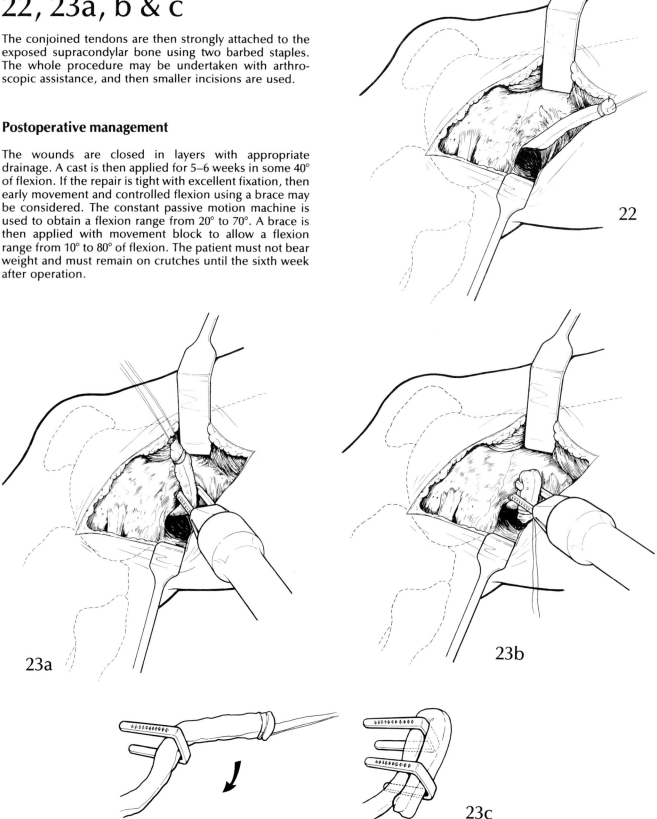

22

23a

23b

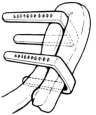

23c

POSTERIOR CRUCIATE REPAIR/RECONSTRUCTION USING TENDON TRANSFER FOR ACUTE INJURY

Incision

24

Surgical exposure will depend upon the extent of the posterior reconstruction. The lateral structures may require repair or reconstruction and this should be undertaken before the posterior cruciate procedure. A long medial incision is required for posterior cruciate ligament reconstruction.

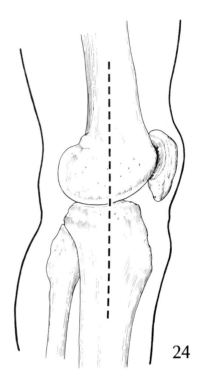

24

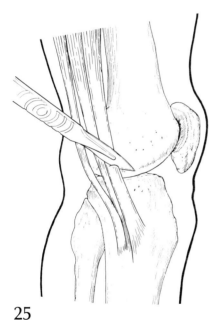

25

Posterior dissection

25

The knee is flexed and the pes anserinus defined. The semimembranosus tendon is then divided near its insertion, allowing easier access to the popliteal fossa. The tendons of semitendinosus and gracilis are then isolated and traced upwards. They are separated from muscle over their longest length and cut off as high as possible. They are best sutured together as a combined tendon transfer.

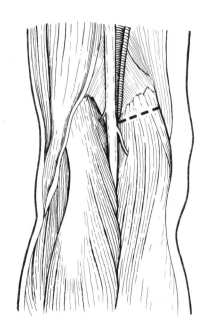

26

26 & 27

The origin of the medial gastrocnemius is then divided near its femoral attachment and the muscle belly is retracted laterally. The popliteal vessels are now easily visualized in the popliteal fat and areolar tissue. They are tethered to the site of the posterior tibial dissection by the middle genicular vessel and above by the superior medial genicular vessels. These two vascular leashes should be carefully identified, ligated and divided. Once these vessels are cut, the popliteal vascular bundle may be gently retracted laterally. The posterior capsule in the intercondylar region is palpated and divided vertically in the midline. Some of the upper border fibres of popliteus may obstruct the upper tibial bone at this site and they should be dissected laterally with a periosteal elevator.

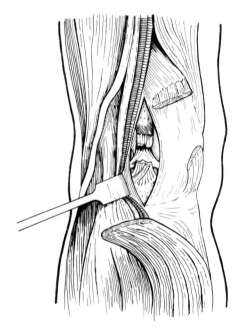

27

28

The tibial tunnel is drilled.

The drill enters the medial tibia above the pes anserinus insertion to exit at the upper posterior tibia in the midline at the normal insertion of the posterior cruciate ligament. A guide wire with cannulated drill is ideal in locating this site. The combined tendons are pulled through this tunnel on the end of a stout suture. This suture is then passed anteriorly and superiorly through the intercondylar region and into the knee joint cavity.

A medial parapatellar incision is then made and the suture is picked up as it emerges at the end of a director or a long curved artery forceps.

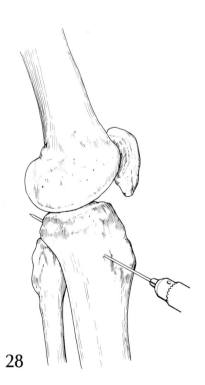

28

29 & 30

The femoral tunnel is drilled. This emerges at the apex of the intercondylar region at a point resembling 1.30 pm in the right knee and 11.30 am in the left knee. The combined tendons are then drawn through the knee to emerge at the apex of the intercondylar notch. They are taken through the femoral tunnel to emerge in the medial supracondylar region where the combined tendon is fixed to the bone with a double-barbed Richards staple technique after appropriate tensioning.

In chronic posterior cruciate laxity a prosthesis may be used and is routed in a similar fashion.

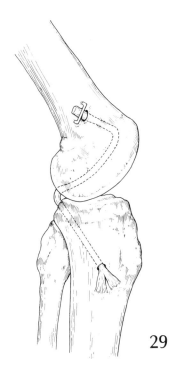

29

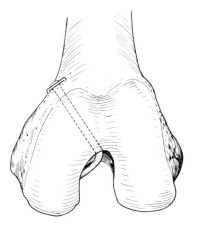

30

RECONSTRUCTION FOR CHRONIC ANTERIOR CRUCIATE DEFICIENCY (combined intra/extra-articular technique)

There have been many attempts at reconstruction of the chronic anterior cruciate-deficient knee. Tendons, iliotibial tract and prosthetic materials have all been used with various degrees of success. The extra-articular reconstruction of MacIntosh prevents anterorotary instability but stretches in time. It is, however, incorporated in this reconstruction and the long strip of iliotibial tract is tubulated and taken over the top of the lateral femoral condyle. (The 'over-the-top' route produces a more isometric positioning of the neoligament.) The tube then passes through the knee and into a tibial tunnel, accurately re-routing this structure. It has been found necessary, however, to augment this iliotibial tract with prosthetic material, and a Dacron prosthesis is thought to be best at the present time.

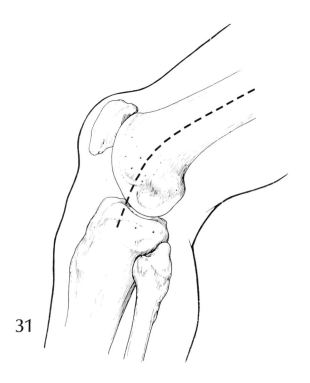

31

Incision

31

The lateral incision passes superiorly from a point 10 cm above the supracondylar region, laterally along the line of the shaft, through the midcondylar point, and finishes inferiorly at Gerdy's tubercle – the prominence on the upper, lateral tibial plateau where the iliotibial tract is inserted.

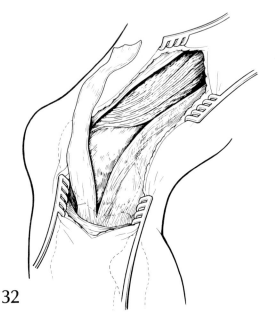

32

32

A strip of iliotibial tract is raised and detached, using appropriate skin retraction superiorly. The ribbon of iliotibial tract should be 2–2.5 cm broad and is left attached to Gerdy's tubercle inferiorly.

33

A MacIntosh extra-articular tenodesis procedure is now undertaken with the iliotibial tract passed beneath the lateral collateral ligament. The lateral collateral ligament must be isolated both anteriorly and posteriorly by extrasynovial dissection, and the iliotibial tract is placed beneath. With the knee in flexion and full lateral rotation, the iliotibial tract is kept very tight and four sutures are positioned to attach the iliotibial tract to this lateral collateral ligament. The sutures are positioned but are not tied at this stage.

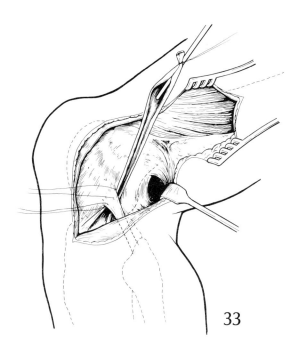

33

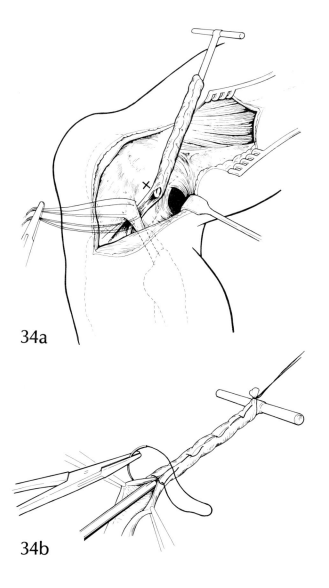

34a

34b

34a & b

The iliotibial tract is now tubulated from its end point to point 'X' (see also Illustration 33). This is best undertaken by bringing its two sides together over a T-shaped cannula. A fine but strong, absorbable suture is recommended and a running, interlocking stitch has been found preferable.

35

The leading loop of the prosthesis may be hooked and drawn through the iliotibial tract. Attached to this loop is a flexible probe which follows the loop into the tube of iliotibial tract from its distal to its proximal end. The end of the probe is now sutured to the free end of the iliotibial tract by an encircling stitch so that the tube and prosthesis may be pulled together over the top of the condyle by traction on the end loop.

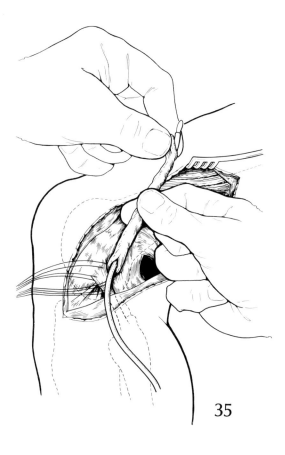

35

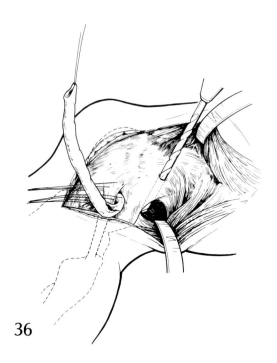

36

36

A drill hole is made in the supracondylar midpoint, emerging posteriorly just above the capsule at the origin of the lateral gastrocnemius muscle.

37

The ligament is now passed through this bony tunnel and a toggle is inserted in the loop.

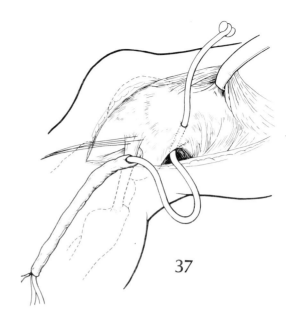

37

38

38

Attention must now be turned to the dissection of the posterior capsule extending into the intercondylar region. The fibres of the lateral gastrocnemius are identified, and dissection continues medially beneath this muscle, exposing the posterior capsule. Using sharp and blunt dissection, the intercondylar region is reached with instruments keeping close to the posterior capsule. A director is now passed through the intercondylar region and into the knee joint as indicated in *Illustration 39*. A routine medial parapatellar arthrotomy is made and extended inferiorly to the medial and inferior aspect of the tibial tubercle. The ruptured cruciate is noted in the intercondylar fossa.

The iliotibial tract tube, which is filled with prosthesis, is now ready to be passed behind the lateral femoral condyle, through the intercondylar region and into the knee joint cavity. The tube of iliotibial tract is tightened around the end of the prosthesis by a transfixion suture which encircles the tube and the prosthesis. The leading loop of the prosthesis is then attached to the director and passed into the knee joint cavity.

39

Using a tibial drill guide, a hole is made with the 6 mm drill through the anteromedial tibia. Superiorly it emerges in the normal tibial attachment for the anterior cruciate – between the two prominences of the anterior tibial spine. The upper end of the tibial hole on the tibial plateau surface should be opened and smoothed with a high speed burr and a fine curette. The prosthesis and iliotibial tract tube is now pulled through the intercondylar region and secondarily pulled through the tibial tunnel to the outside.

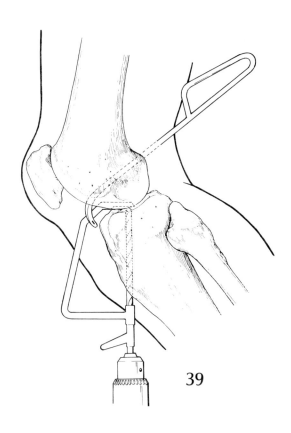

39

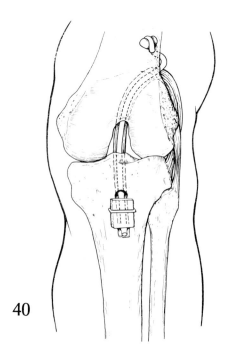

40

40

A bone block of cortical bone 1 × 2 cm in size is raised from the upper medial tibia, just below the exit hole of the tibial tunnel.

The toggle is positioned in the proximal loop of the prosthesis in the supracondylar position, and the prosthesis is pulled tight with the tibia rotated laterally on the femur and drawn posteriorly. The tubed prosthesis is put into the depression where the bone block was raised and the bone block is returned and stapled in position with the composite ligament under tension. The four stay sutures anchoring the iliotibial tract to the lateral collateral ligament are tightened and tied.

Postoperative management

The lateral wound is closed with drainage. The medial parapatellar wound is closed in the usual way.

The limb is then placed in the constant passive motion machine with a range of movement from 30° to 60°. At 1 week a brace is applied blocking movement from 30° to 70° of flexion. The brace is maintained until the sixth week after operation. After removal of the brace, increasing physiotherapy is given to mobilize and strengthen the knee joint to the maximum. The patient usually returns to some jogging, cycling and swimming at approximately 3 months. At 6 months some gentle recreational games may be considered, and at 1 year the patient may return to all field contact sports.

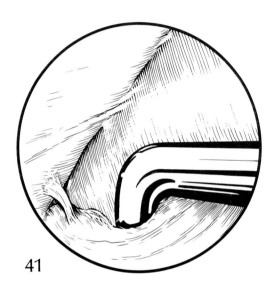

41

41

The 6-month arthroscopic appearance of the ligament is seen. The hook is prodding the midpoint of the ligament.

Recurrent dislocation of the patella

Paul Aichroth MS, FRCS
Consultant Orthopaedic Surgeon, Westminster Hospital and Westminster Children's Hospital, London; Queen Mary's Hospital, Roehampton, UK

Introduction

Dislocation of the patella occurs in both children and adults. Subluxation of this bone is more common in the teenager and frequently produces problems of diagnosis and management.

Patellar dislocations are most commonly lateral although medial and intra-articular positions have been recorded. The dislocation may be congenital or acquired, and the latter may be recurrent, or even persistent.

1

Anatomically there is a natural tendency towards lateral subluxation of the patella and to this may be added the following aetiological factors.

1. Abnormal weakness of the medial capsule following trauma.
2. An extreme valgus knee.
3. Flattening of the articular surface of the lateral femoral condyle and of the patella.
4. Lateral insertion of the patellar tendon, giving an increased Q angle.
5. Patella alta.
6. Anteversion of the femoral neck.
7. Contracture of vastus lateralis.
8. Familial joint laxity.

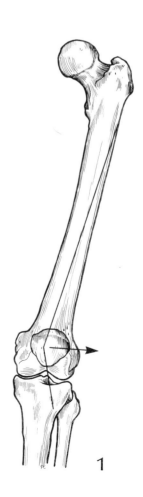

1

DISLOCATION IN CHILDREN

The dislocation may become recurrent and then habitual if the patella dislocates with every flexion and extension movement. Persistent dislocation is present when the patella is constantly displaced to lie lateral to the femoral condyle, and this may occur when there is gross vastus lateralis contracture – sometimes due to frequent neonatal antibiotic injections into the thigh.

Congenital dislocation is rare, but may be the cause of a flexion contracture of the knee in the newborn. An acquired dislocation may be totally painless, especially if it is persistent, but the child frequently falls, the joint 'gives way' and the knee cap may be described as being 'out of place'. Pain is less common in childhood.

Most children with recurrent dislocations in the first decade of life exhibit some generalized abnormalities such as familial joint laxity or local joint features, as described above.

Indications for operation

The above-mentioned symptoms associated with recurrent or persistent dislocation of the patella provide the indications for operative correction and repair. In doubtful cases, careful assessment of patellar instability under general anaesthesia must be performed. Recurrent dislocation of the patella may produce a loose body due to osteochondral fracture, chondromalacia patellae due to patellar malalignment and osteoarthritis in later life.

A soft tissue procedure is recommended in the child because any operation which disturbs the tibial tubercle will cause a genu recurvatum owing to disturbance of the anterior epiphyseal growth-plate.

Simple lateral patellar release is inadequate in the child and distal transplantation of the patellar tendon may produce severe chondromalacia patellae. A combined patellar release and medial repositioning of the patellar tendon is advocated.

Preoperative preparation

The physiotherapist should teach all the quadriceps-strengthening exercises. The presence of a loose body must be determined radiologically and if present should be removed arthroscopically.

PATELLAR RELEASE AND REPOSITIONING (GOLDTHWAITE–ROUX OPERATION)

After exsanguination of the limb by means of an Esmarch bandage, a very high pneumatic tourniquet is inflated. The skin is prepared from the tourniquet cuff to the ankle. An incise drape may be applied.

Incision

2

A lateral parapatellar incision starts well above the patella and proceeds inferiorly and then medially, crossing the tibial tubercle. If the operation is being performed for persistent dislocation or vastus lateralis contracture, a very high thigh incision will be required to allow adequate release of the vastus lateralis muscle.

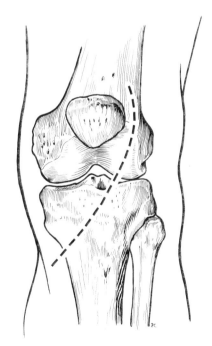

2

Lateral patellar release

3

The lateral capsule of the patellar expansion is incised in the same line, from the suprapatellar region to the tibial tubercle. When the knee is flexed and the lateral release is adequate, the two sides of this capsular incision will widely separate. The synovium may be left intact but in the persistent dislocation and in some recurrent dislocations this lateral synovium is so tight and thick that it must be similarly incised and released.

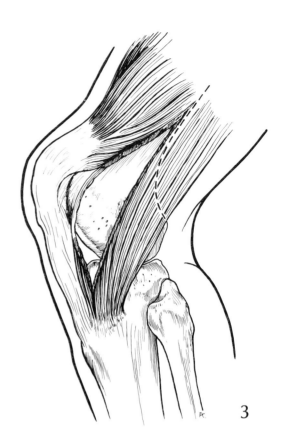

3

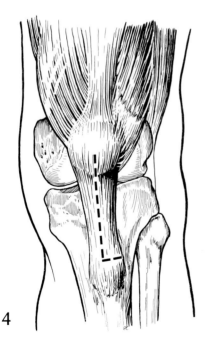

4

Longitudinal division of the patellar tendon

4

The patellar tendon is isolated throughout its length and divided longitudinally. The distal attachment of the lateral half is divided at the tibial tubercle.

Half-tendon transposition

5, 6 & 7

The lateral half of the patellar tendon is then transposed medially beneath the rest of the tendon, or sometimes superficial to it, thus pulling the patella over to the medial side.

The transposed half-tendon is then implanted beneath an osteoperiosteal flap. The flap is raised with an osteotome and the half-tendon is anchored with two or more thick polyglactin 910 sutures (Vicryl, Ethicon Ltd, Edinburgh, UK).

The tension is adjusted to prevent any lateral displacement of the patella on full flexion and the sutures are tied. In the adult a staple may also be added to anchor the patellar strand beneath the osteoperiosteal flap. However, this is not recommended in the child owing to the proximity of the upper medial growth-plate.

The medial patellar expansion is sutured with plication to the medial patellar tendon.

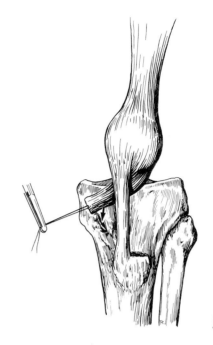

5

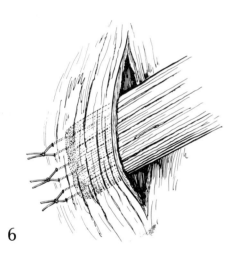

6

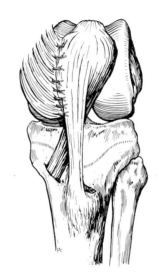

7

Closure

A vacuum drain is used and the wound is closed with an intradermal skin suture and adhesive tapes. A well-padded cylinder plaster is applied.

Postoperative management

The limb is elevated for 24 hours. Mobilization without weight-bearing may then commence and be followed after 2 weeks by weight-bearing with crutches or sticks.

The cylinder plaster cast is retained for 4 weeks with an optional change of plaster at 2 weeks to remove the sutures. The physiotherapist will be required to mobilize and strengthen the knee.

DISLOCATION IN TEENAGERS AND ADULTS

Symptoms and signs

The patient may present with a fully dislocated patella but more commonly there are episodes of 'giving way', with pain and subsequent knee effusion. Pain and tenderness over the medial capsule may be confused with a medial internal derangement of the knee. The most important signs are pain and apprehension of the patient when lateral movement of the patella is attempted: this apprehension causes the patient to tense his quadriceps, thus preventing the dislocation from occurring. With a very lax patella, substantial subluxation or dislocation may be demonstrated with only minor pain. In doubtful cases, assessment of patellar stability must be made under general anaesthesia.

Radiographic signs

8, 9 & 10

1. A tangential osteochondral fracture may be seen in the patellar sky-line view.
2. A loose body may be found or an area of osteochondritis dissecans may be present on the anterior aspect of the lateral femoral condyle.
3. Patella alta: the patella is high in most cases of dislocating or subluxing patellae. With the knee flexed at 30°, measurement A is greater than measurement B (Blackburne's method).
4. Hughston's view taken with the knee flexed at 45° shows the patella with a lateral tilt.
5. Patellar alignment in various positions of knee flexion is best assessed in the tangential view of the patella with the knee flexed at 30°, 60° and 90°. The lateral positioning of the patella is then easily seen and subluxation in flexion or extension may be assessed[1].

Treatment

The symptoms described above may occur so regularly that gross inconvenience is produced and correction is indicated. It is now known that degenerative changes are not as great as previously expected in recurrent dislocation of the patella; therefore, an occasional patellar dislocation does not constitute a definite indication for operation and a 'wait and see' policy may be adopted.

Multiple soft tissue operations have been suggested but the release/repositioning operation described above is recommended. A simple lateral patellar release (see *Illustration 3*) may be undertaken in patients with simple subluxation of the patella.

Bony procedures such as the Hauser operation have been used for many years. It is now known that the incidence of retropatellar osteoarthritis is increased markedly following this tibial tubercle transposition – especially if there is distal reimplantation of the tubercle, thus tightening the patellar tendon. In addition, there is an unacceptably high incidence of anterior compartment syndromes associated with this procedure, and it should be avoided.

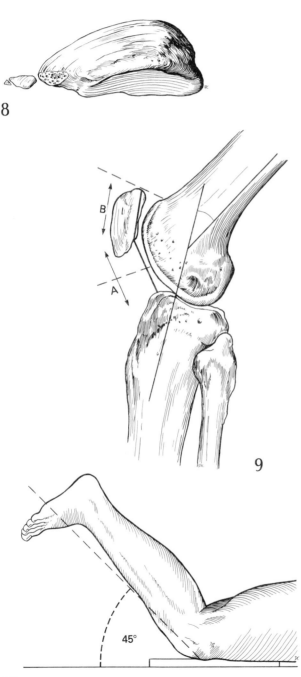

8

9

10

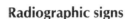

PATELLOFEMORAL OSTEOARTHRITIS

PATELLAR DECOMPRESSION AND REALIGNMENT (MAQUET OPERATION)

Retropatellar osteoarthritis associated with lateral subluxation of the patella may be relieved by the Maquet operation. This has the effect of correction of the malalignment together with decompression of the patellofemoral joint by forward and medial positioning of the tibial tubercle.

11

The skin incision is long and extends from the level of the lower patella, down the anteromedial aspect of the leg, passing 1 cm posterior to the tibial crest. Holes are drilled through the tibia which is then split with an osteotome along the lines connecting the drill holes. Care must be taken not to fracture across the distal end of this split tibia. A full-thickness bone graft is taken from the iliac crest or from the adjacent tibia.

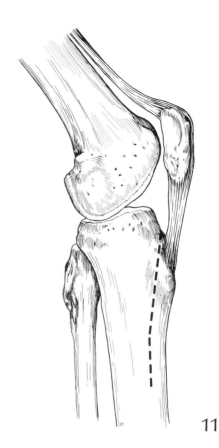

11

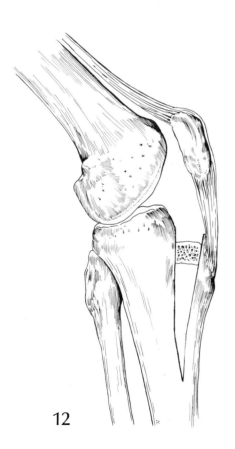

12

12

The anterior tibial fragment remains attached distally and the iliac crest graft is inserted behind this fragment, pushing it forwards and medially by a variable amount depending on the pathology. Care must be taken to avoid skin tension by mobilizing the edges if necessary. If tension is too great the thickness of the bone graft will be reduced. The wound is closed with adequate vacuum drains.

The leg is supported in a compression bandage for 1 week, and the patient begins walking after 48 hours. Knee flexion may be started within 7 days because fixation is firm but full weight-bearing is restricted for 1 month.

THE TRILLAT OPERATION

The distal insertion of the patellar tendon may be moved medially with a sliver of tibial tubercle bone and distal periosteum in the mature patient. This operation is not recommended in the child with an open tibial tubercle growth-plate.

13

A midline longitudinal skin incision is made and deepened to expose the extensor apparatus. Incisions are made along the medial and lateral borders of the patellar tendon, distally on each side of the tibial tubercle extending into the periosteum inferior to the tubercle. An osteotome then raises a sliver of tibial tubercle some 5–7 mm and the bone inferiorly is raised as an osteo-periosteal flap.

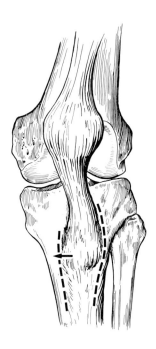

13

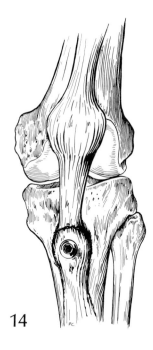

14

14

The patellar tendon and tubercle are then moved medially and a screw may be used to fix the position of the tibial tubercle in its definitive more medial position.

Postoperative management

The leg is enclosed in a plaster of Paris cylinder and elevated for 24 hours. Weight-bearing with crutches then begins with gentle quadriceps exercises daily. After 6 weeks mobilization under physiotherapy supervision is begun. Full activities are restricted for 3 months.

References

1. Dowd GSE, Bentley G. Radiographic assessment in patellar instability and chondromalacia patellae. *J Bone Joint Surg [Br]* 1986; 68-B: 297–300.

Illustrations by Gillian Oliver after G. Lyth

Synovectomy of the knee

W. Waugh MChir, FRCS
Emeritus Professor of Orthopaedic and Accident Surgery, University of Nottingham;
Honorary Consultant Orthopaedic Surgeon, Harlow Wood Orthopaedic Hospital, Nr Mansfield, Nottinghamshire, UK

Introduction

Indications

Synovectomy is indicated when there is a persistent chronic, or intermittent, synovitis (with effusion and thickening) which is producing pain and disability.

The pathological conditions in which this situation arises are as follows.

Rheumatoid arthritis

Synovectomy will relieve pain but there is no clear evidence that it will prevent further destruction of the knee joint. Operation should only be considered when medical treatment of at least 3 months' duration has failed to relieve pain and swelling. The best results will be achieved at a stage of the disease when the radiographs are normal (or show only peripheral erosions). Once there is extensive loss of articular cartilage and bony collapse, arthroplasty, using one of the modern designs of knee replacement, will be more likely to produce a painless, stable and mobile joint. Synovectomy may, however, be preferable in younger patients even in the more advanced stages of the disease.

Pigmented villonodular synovitis

Excision of localized nodules is satisfactory, but in the diffuse type of the disease recurrence is common and an extensive synovectomy is only justified when the symptoms are causing serious disability.

Tuberculosis

Operation may be considered when antituberculous treatment fails to produce resolution of the synovitis.

Preoperative considerations

There are four controversial points which should be discussed before the operation is described.

Amount of synovial tissue to be removed

It is technically impossible to carry out a total synovectomy, but through an anterior incision the synovium in the suprapatellar pouch, in the lateral recesses and in the intercondylar notch can be removed. Fortunately in rheumatoid arthritis this operation seems to produce regression of the remaining tissue, possibly as a response to injury.

One or two incisions?

It has been suggested that two short incisions (anteromedial and anterolateral) allow adequate exposure with less damage so that knee movement recovers more quickly. A long midline incision gives equally good access, and provided it is carefully closed, movements can be started after a few days; it also can be used for a subsequent knee replacement operation, which may eventually be necessary.

Should the menisci be removed?

Erosions frequently occur on the margins of the tibial condyles; if these are to be cleared, the menisci have to be removed. It is, however, important to remember that meniscectomy removes an essential part of the load-bearing mechanism of the knee and is likely to be followed by progressive degenerative changes. This has to be weighed against the theoretical advantages of a more thorough synovectomy. Generally it is better to retain the menisci.

Mobilization or immobilization?

Although the operation inflicts considerable damage to the knee joint, movement can be started after 3 or 4 days provided skin healing is satisfactory and there is no haematoma. Immobilization for 3 weeks seems to carry no special advantages; recovery of movement is delayed and manipulation is nearly always necessary.

Operation

A pneumatic cuff tourniquet is applied to the upper thigh after exsanguination.

Towelling

After skin preparation with chlorhexidine in spirit a plastic drape is applied. The foot can be completely isolated by wrapping it up in a large sheet of plastic drape. The leg is lifted so that the table below it can be covered with a towel. The rest of the body is excluded by towels applied from below and above and clipped around the thigh. The knee should then be flexed and extended to make sure that the towels are secure.

Incision

1 & 2

A midline incision is used and it should extend from at least 10 cm above the upper pole of the patella to 5 cm below the tibial tuberosity. The joint is entered on the medial side by division of the capsule opposite the patella (and about 1 cm from its medial border) in the line of the skin incision. The approach is extended proximally by separating vastus medialis from the rectus femoris with scissors. Distally the soft tissues and periosteum over the upper part of the tibia are divided and stripped laterally and medially by sharp dissection. It is important to preserve the soft-tissue flaps in this part of the incision to allow closure at the end of the operation.

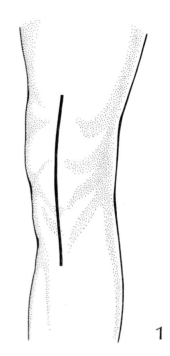

1

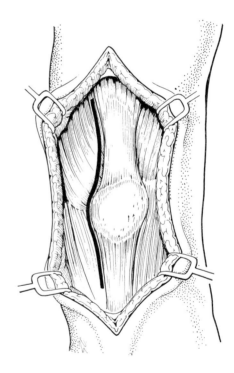

2

Dislocation of patella

3

Separation of vastus medialis from the rectus femoris is continued proximally and any adhesions in the joint divided until the patella can be turned so that its articular surface faces directly forward. It may be necessary to detach (by sharp dissection) the medial quarter of the patellar ligament before this can be done. The knee is then flexed to beyond a right angle and when this is done the patella can be turned over so that its articular surface faces outwards; the whole of the articular surface of the femur can now be seen. The joint is inspected with particular reference to the state of the synovial membrane and the articular cartilage.

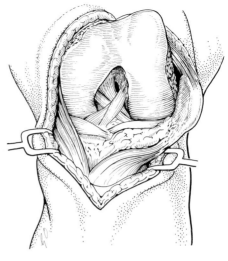

3

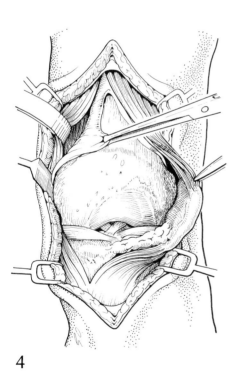

4

Excision of affected synovial membrane

4

The knee is straightened and the plane of dissection between the synovium and capsule found. This is begun most easily in the suprapatellar pouch; tissue forceps are applied to the capsule and synovium and the dissection carried out with Mayo scissors. The suprapatellar pouch is excised – the dissection starting from medial to lateral and then extending back across the femoral reflection. As much synovial membrane is removed from the paracondylar gutters as possible. The affected tissue is often removed piecemeal.

Special attention should now be paid to the articular margins around the patella and femoral condyles. The synovium must be carefully removed from these areas (particularly if there is any articular invasion) and all pannus should be stripped off the underlying cartilage. Erosions should be curetted and bone nibblers may be used to remove fragments of tissue. The intercondylar notch is often an area of active synovitis and affected tissue should be stripped off the cruciate ligaments in the hope of avoiding their subsequent destruction by the disease.

The joint should now be thoroughly examined and any remaining tags of tissue removed.

The tourniquet is removed and the wound packed with large swabs. After waiting for the reactive hyperaemia to subside, bleeding vessels (usually in the capsule) are sealed by diathermy.

Closure

One or occasionally two suction drains are inserted. The capsule should be closed with interrupted black silk stitches and the skin with interrupted nylon.

Dressings

5

If a standard pressure bandage is applied the knee will tend to flex over the mass of wool behind the knee. It is better to use a very thick (5 cm) strip of wool down the front of the leg and encircle this with a few turns of plaster wool. A crêpe bandage is applied from toes to groin followed by a plaster back splint (not including the foot).

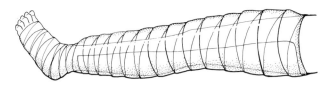

5

Postoperative management

This will vary with the amount of swelling in the knee and the response of the patient. Quadriceps and foot exercises are started immediately after operation. The splint and drains can be removed after 2 days and knee flexion exercises started after 4 or 5 days. The wound is then left exposed. Walking with crutches is allowed after 1 week. Manipulation should only rarely be necessary: it is best carried out (with due care) between the second and third weeks after operation.

Complications

Infection

The risks are decreased by careful operative technique, haemostasis and suction drainage.

Wound breakdown and skin necrosis

This is avoided by not undermining the skin more than necessary and careful suturing.

Haemarthrosis

The wound should be inspected at 48 hours after operation and any collection of blood aspirated.

Stiffness and extensor lag

These should be avoided by early movement and quadriceps exercises and, if necessary, manipulation. Primary wound healing is essential to achieve this.

Illustrations by Peter Cox

Tibial osteotomy for arthritis of the knee

J. P. Jackson FRCS
Emeritus Orthopaedic Surgeon, University Hospital, Nottingham, and Harlow Wood Orthopaedic Hospital, Mansfield, UK

Introduction

Indications

Tibial osteotomy is indicated for the relief of pain in osteoarthritis of the medial compartment of the knee in younger patients. The object of the operation is to realign the limb so that weight-bearing is transferred to the more normal part of the joint. Whilst the operation has been employed with some success in both valgus and varus knees, for the best and most consistent results to be obtained certain factors should be considered.

Contraindications

1. The degree of deformity There is a limit to the deformity that can be successfully corrected if a wedge is to be removed proximal to the tibial tuberosity. Correction of a tibiofemoral angle of more than 5° may weaken the proximal fragment so that fracture into the joint occurs.

2. Excessive collapse of the joint surface Bony collapse of more than 0.5 cm implies that the joint is too disorganized to benefit from the operation.

3. Limited movement The knee should flex to more than 90° and there should not be a flexion contracture of more than 10° before operation.

4. Valgus deformity Whilst many patients with a knock-knee deformity have benefited from this procedure, division through the tibia leaves a very oblique joint-line and a better result may be obtained by osteotomy of the femur. In general, patients with a valgus deformity present late when there is already considerable joint damage and a good result already compromised.

Assessment

The operation is best carried out by removal of a wedge of bone above the tibial tuberosity. This method has the advantage of being very stable and leading to early union. A curved osteotomy through the tibial tubercle may be required if for any reason, such as the presence of cysts, there is need for considerable correction.

The wedge size

1

This is calculated from the standing film. Full-length films which show both hip and ankle joints give a more accurate assessment. The object of the operation is to move the line of weight-bearing of the limb away from the affected side so that it passes across the more normal tibiofemoral compartment. In effect, this means moving the centre of the ankle joint so that it comes to lie beneath the opposite compartment from its preoperative position. The wedge removed should be sufficient in size to produce slight overcorrection of the deformity. The operation is carried out with the use of a tourniquet.

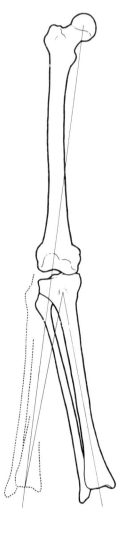

1

Operation

Division of the fibula

2

The limb is draped so that it is free and can be picked up and manipulated by the surgeon. The fibula can either be osteotomized in the shaft or the head can be excised. If the head is to be removed, then this is usually done as part of a lateral approach to the tibia. Section of the shaft of the fibula is easier and allows the tibia to be approached from the front, through a separate incision. The wedge can then be cut more easily and measured more accurately.

To approach the fibula the interval between the peronei and the calf muscles is defined. If the bulge of the peronei is felt, the intermuscular septum is just behind; this can be followed down to the bone without significant bleeding.

A vertical incision is employed and this should be centred on a point about 15 cm below the proximal tip of the fibula, or lower. The object of osteotomy at this site is to avoid precipitating a compartment syndrome, which has been found to be more common when bone division is above this level. The osteotomy should be oblique so that bone ends slide on each other and remain in contact, facilitating union.

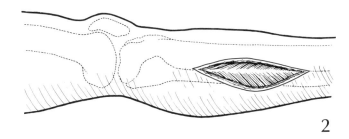

Incision

3

The tibia is best approached from the front by a transverse incision centred on the upper part of the tibial tubercle. If for any reason it is necessary to enter the knee joint (i.e. to remove loose bodies) a medial parapatellar incision is used.

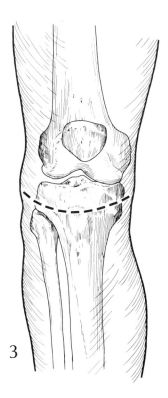

Incision of capsule and periosteum

4

The incision is deepened through superficial tissues and the tibial tubercle and anterior capsule are displayed.

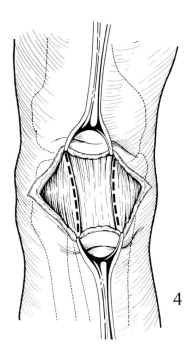

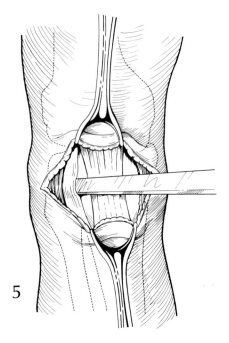

5

The tendon is isolated by two longitudinal incisions. The periosteum is then reflected medially round to the posteromedial border of the tibia and then to the posterolateral border. Care must be taken as the area just below the tibiofibular joint is entered, since the anterior tibial artery is very vulnerable. In addition, the recurrent branch of this vessel runs upwards to the patella and may also be injured. Bleeding from these arteries may cause increased compartmental pressure. A spike should not be placed behind the lateral border of the tibia as it may well cause damage to the vessels.

Insertion of Steinmann pins

6

Before the bone is cut, two Steinmann pins should be placed in position. The upper one must pass through the proximal fragment parallel to the proposed saw cut, but at a sufficient distance above it, so that there is no danger of cutting out, when compression is applied. The lower pin is positioned parallel to the proposed lower saw cut. The angle between the two pins will be that of the wedge which is to be removed. In fat patients particularly or if the surgeon is in any doubt, the two pins should be passed under X-ray control. It is essential that they are accurately placed, so that when the bone wedge is removed the pins will lie parallel, and compression can be evenly applied.

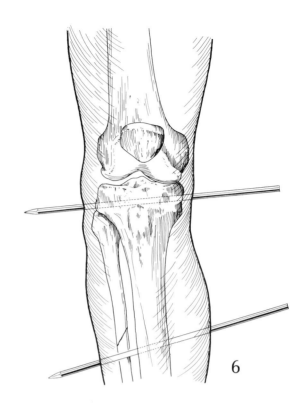

Division of the tibia

7

The tibial tendon is held forwards with the aid of a hook. The initial saw cuts are made with a keyhole saw, and will mark the exact dimensions of the wedge. In order to make the lower cut, it may be necessary to detach the tibial tendon insertion partially. Complete detachment is unwise, as this can jeopardize the success of the operation. The cuts are deepened as far as possible onto and through the posterior cortex. The structures behind the tibia can be protected by a Watson Cheyne dissector passed from the lateral side. Care must be taken to remove the cortex cleanly, as otherwise the bone ends may be held apart by small spicules of bone. Bone nibblers can be very helpful in smoothing off the posterior cortex. Once all bone has been satisfactorily removed, the wedge can be closed, and compression applied to the two Steinmann pins. When the bone is adequately compressed, the alignment of the tibia can be checked to see that correction has been obtained.

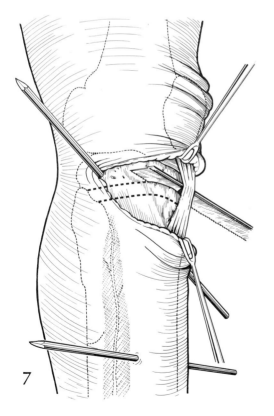

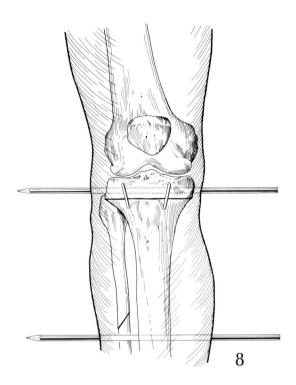

8

Insertion of staples

8 & 9

The final step is to insert two staples. On the medial side, the surface is sloping and an angled staple will fit best. The lateral surface usually has a step so that a stepped Coventry staple will fit more comfortably. Pre-drilling of the point of entry of the staple into the cortical bone of the distal fragment with a 3.5 mm drill will facilitate entry and prevent tilting of the staple. When the staples are judged to be correctly placed, the compression is released and the Steinmann pins withdrawn. Trial flexion and extension of the knee is now carried out to confirm that the osteotomy is firmly fixed. A third staple may sometimes be thought necessary. Finally, the wound is closed in layers. Suction drainage is advisable.

Postoperative management

A well-padded plaster cylinder is applied which should include the foot. Allowing the foot to fall into plantar flexion results in a significant rise of pressure in the anterior tibial compartment. The limb is elevated for 24 hours, or longer if the swelling is excessive. The patient is allowed up after the suction drainage is discontinued and swelling controlled. After 1 week the plaster is removed and changed for a lightweight cast-brace. This is applied with the limb in the corrected position. Once the patient is comfortable in the brace, full weight-bearing should be encouraged with knee flexion. With this regimen, satisfactory union is obtained at the end of 6 weeks. The brace is removed and the patient encouraged to walk normally.

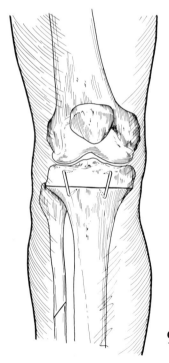

9

Illustrations by William Thackeray

Arthroplasty of the knee

Russell E. Windsor MD
Assistant Professor, Orthopaedic Surgery, Cornell University Medical College, New York; and Assistant Attending Orthopaedic Surgeon, The Hospital for Special Surgery and The New York Hospital, New York, USA

John N. Insall MD
Professor of Orthopaedic Surgery, Cornell University Medical College, New York; and Director, The Knee Service, The Hospital for Special Surgery, New York, USA

Introduction

Indications

Total knee arthroplasty is recommended for patients with severe *unremitting knee pain* due to: rheumatoid panarthritis (regardless of age), gonarthrosis, post-traumatic osteoarthritis, failure of high tibial osteotomy and arthritis associated with gout, psoriasis, or pigmented villonodular synovitis. A less common indication is *severe patellofemoral osteoarthritis* in an elderly patient. Usually, patchy articular degeneration is found at arthrotomy and the results of arthroplasty in this type of degenerative arthritis are better than any other method.

Total joint arthroplasty for a painful neuropathic joint is controversial, but it is feasible, provided that a surface replacement can be used, the joint is thoroughly debrided with a complete synovectomy and correct alignment and stability is achieved. Metal-backed components with long intramedullary stems are recommended for this situation.

Contraindications

A sound *painless arthrodesis* is an absolute contraindication to total knee arthroplasty. Long-term *painful ankylosis* in a young patient due to trauma or previous infection is also not recommended for arthroplasty. The chances of regaining movement and eradicating pain are unpredictable, and the high likelihood of postoperative complications in these patients make arthroplasty a poor choice. Arthrodesis in this situation is the preferred procedure. Gross quadriceps weakness, and genu recurvatum associated with muscle weakness and paralysis will severely compromise the function of the knee. Total knee arthroplasty in these knees, even if a constrained prosthesis is used, will fail early because of the excessive stresses placed upon the implants. The operation should also not be done in an actively *infected knee*. However, later arthroplasty is feasible after the infection is eradicated by thorough debridement and antibiotic therapy.

Preoperative

Planning

Before total knee arthroplasty is performed, the surgeon must appropriately plan the operation. This entails proper patient selection and choice of prosthetic design. If severe deformity is present, a custom-made implant may be needed, or consent for autologous bone grafting obtained.

Surgical preparation

A broad-spectrum antibiotic, such as cephalosporin, is administered preoperatively. General endotracheal or epidural anaesthesia may be used. The patient is placed in the supine position. A thigh tourniquet is applied and the knee is washed with antiseptic solution and draped thinly so as not to interfere with positioning of surgical instruments. The anterior superior iliac spine should be easily palpated through the drapes to allow assessment of alignment during surgery.

If a bilateral arthroplasty is required, the procedures should be done sequentially. After completion of the first arthroplasty, the dressings are applied and the second knee is prepared and draped. The instruments are re-sterilized. This method, in our opinion, is much safer than using the instruments simultaneously for both knees, as we feel the chances for infection are less.

1119

Operation

Incision

1

The limb is exsanguinated with an Esmarch bandage and the tourniquet is inflated to a pressure of 350–400 mmHg. A midline longitudinal incision should be used[1]. Although medial and lateral parapatellar incisions are acceptable, a midline incision generally offers a clear exposure and requires less dissection of the medial and lateral skin flaps. However, if other surgical scars are present, the incision should be modified so that the risk of skin necrosis is minimized.

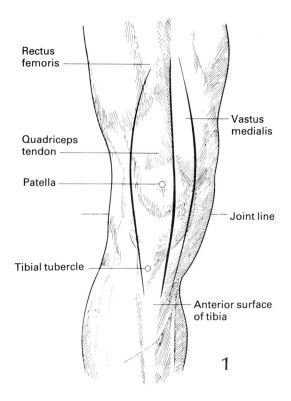

Capsular incision

2

A medial arthrotomy is performed in a straight line through the medial patellar retinaculum. The incision crosses the medial border of the patella, with care taken not to cut the patellar tendon. The distal aspect of the incision should lie 1 cm medial to the tibial tubercle to preserve a cuff of tissue so that inadvertent avulsion of the tibial tubercle will be prevented. Partial resection of the fat pad may be necessary to obtain sufficient exposure of the proximal tibia.

The proximal tibia is exposed by subperiosteal dissection of the pes anserinus and semimembranosus tendons. The latter tendon is not necessarily dissected off its insertion in cases of severe valgus deformity. A periosteal elevator or scalpel may be used. The patella is everted and the knee is flexed.

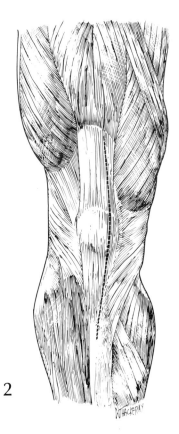

Correction of deformity and soft-tissue release

Usually, adaptive changes occur in the ligaments of the knee in cases of longstanding arthritis. Loss of cartilage and bone is symmetrical in rheumatoid arthritis, whereas it is frequently asymmetrical in osteoarthritis.

3a, b & 4

In a varus deformity, the medial collateral ligament is contracted and the lateral collateral ligament is stretched. In order to obtain normal mechanical alignment, the shortened collateral ligament must be released. The distal insertion of the medial collateral ligament and pes anserinus insertion are released by subperiosteal dissection along with the semimembranosus insertion. Medial osteophytes are removed and care is taken not to disrupt the ligament proximally. The release is done progressively as the situation requires, starting with osteophyte removal initially and proceeding to distal ligament release. It is sometimes necessary to release the deep fascia investing the soleus and popliteus muscles.

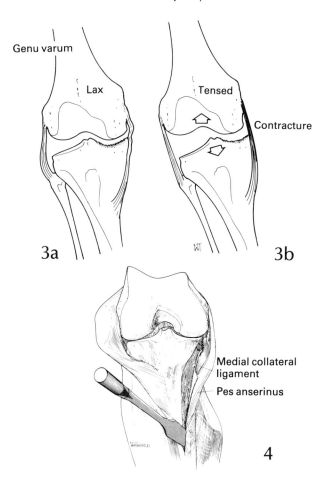

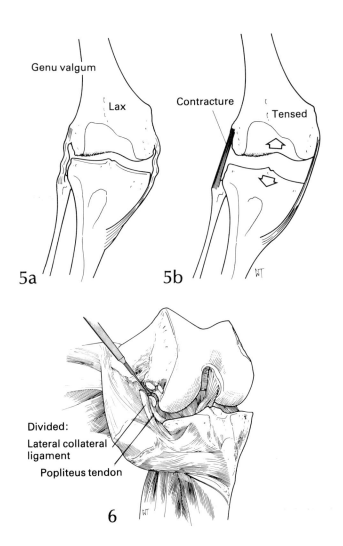

5a, b & 6

A fixed valgus deformity presents a shortened lateral collateral ligament and an attenuated medial collateral ligament. The lateral collateral ligament and popliteus tendon may be released proximally off the femur when the knee cannot easily be corrected to normal valgus alignment. In severe cases, the lateral head insertion of the gastrocnemius muscle is released subperiosteally and the iliotibial band is incised in a horizontal direction across its fibres. Stability will be achieved by obtaining a tight fit with the spacer in flexion to maintain tension on the medial collateral ligament.

Flexion contracture frequently accompanies fixed varus or valgus deformities and must also be addressed. This may be considerable in severe cases of rheumatoid arthritis. Resection of the posterior femoral condyles will correct mild contractures. However, posterior osteophytes should be removed initially and, in the severest cases, the femoral origins of the medial and lateral heads of the gastrocnemius muscles must be released. In cases of valgus deformity and flexion contracture, the surgeon and patient should be aware of the potential for a peroneal nerve palsy. If it occurs, it is best treated by removing the dressing and flexing the knee[2]. It is now rarely seen in cases which use continuous passive motion as the knee begins flexion immediately.

Implant design Given adequate soft-tissue release, most knees will not require a constrained prosthesis. We seldom use constrained devices except where the collateral ligaments have been totally destroyed by trauma or in a severe flexion contracture which requires bone resection above the femoral origins of the collateral ligaments. In the latter case, soft-tissue release may be inadequate, and a subsequently large femoral bone resection may compromise the collateral ligament insertions. Regardless of the implant design used, certain general principles should be followed to assure a successful surgical outcome[3]. Certain steps are the same whether a severe or mild deformity is present.

7a, b & 8a, b

The operation requires a transverse proximal tibial resection, followed by a resection of the posterior and anterior aspects of the femoral condyles to obtain a rectangular space in flexion. The rectangular space (flexion gap) may be obtained by collateral ligament release, or by lateral rotation of the cutting block on the femur. Further ligament release may be still necessary depending on the deformity of the knee.

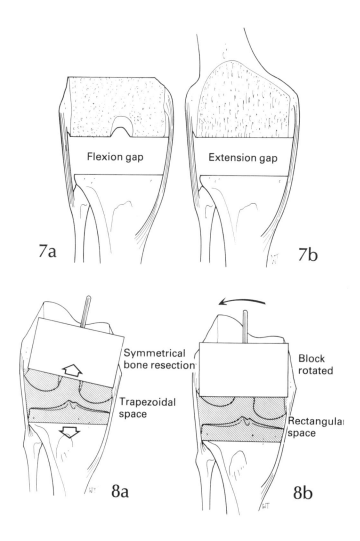

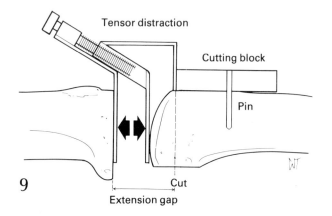

9

When the ligaments have been balanced, an extension gap is created by a tensor and distal femoral cutting block. The extension gap should equal the flexion gap; the distal femoral resection should be made in 7°–10° valgus while collateral ligament tension is kept relatively equal. Final chamfering and sculpting of the femur and tibia are performed according to the dimensions of the prosthetic design that is used.

Flexion gap

10, 11 & 12

The proximal tibia is transected perpendicular to the longitudinal axis of the shaft with the assistance of a cutting block and alignment bar which is affixed to bone. The lower end of the bar is placed on the lower tibia in line with the malleoli; the upper end of the bar is placed with the lateral edge in line with the centre of the tibial tubercle. The tibial surface is cut flat with an oscillating saw; no more than 5 mm of the proximal tibia should be resected in order to preserve strong trabecular bone stock. The femoral cutting block is placed and resection of the anterior and posterior aspects of the femoral condyles is performed. A rectangular space in flexion is obtained.

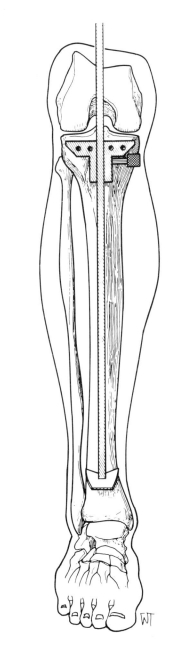

10

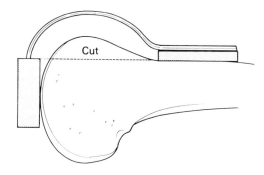

Cut

11

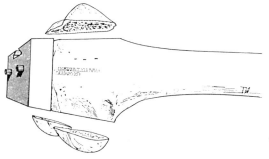

12

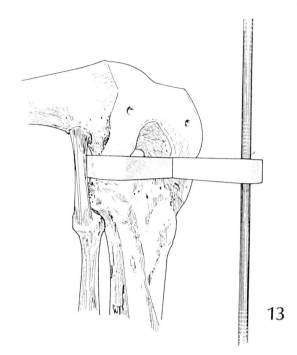

13

13 & 14a, b

A spacer block is placed in the rectangular gap with a suitable thickness to tense the collateral ligaments in flexion. The tibial resection is concurrently assessed by an alignment rod that is placed through the spacer. This rod should fall midway between the medial and lateral malleoli of the ankle joint if a transverse tibial resection is present. The surgeon must protect the collateral ligaments with retractors during these steps so that inadvertent transection of the collateral ligaments by the reciprocating saw is prevented.

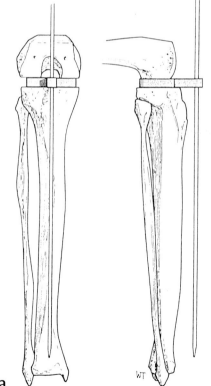

14a   14b

Extension gap

15a & b

After the surgeon has appropriately sized the flexion gap with a spacer, an extension gap must be created equal in dimension to the flexion gap. The collateral ligaments should be balanced. A tensor device (*see Illustration 9*) is used to tense the collateral ligaments[4]. An alignment rod which can be affixed to the device, should fall two to three fingers'-breadth medial to the anterior superior iliac spine in order to obtain 7°–10° of valgus. If the iliac crest is not easily palpable, a preoperative radiograph of the hip should be done so that an external marker can be applied over the centre of the femoral head. In this instance, the alignment rod should fall directly over this marker to assure correct alignment. The tensor must not be used to release the collateral ligaments any further. If the alignment rod falls medial to the femoral head, further lateral ligament release is required. If the rod is located lateral to the femoral head, the mechanical axis is in varus or neutral and more medial collateral ligament release should be performed.

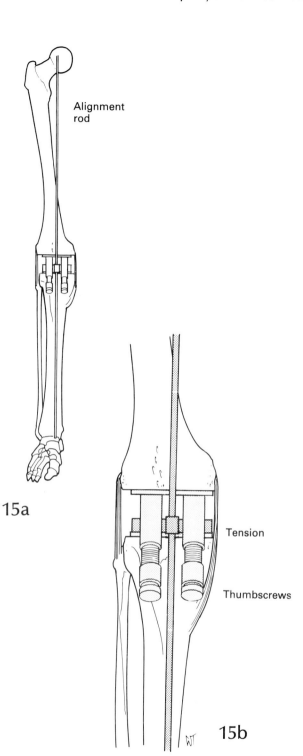

Alignment rod

15a

Tension

Thumbscrews

15b

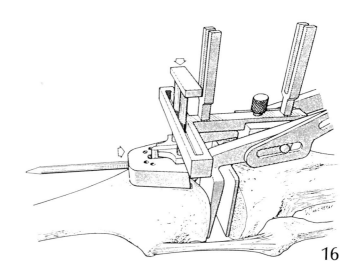

16

16, 17 & 18

When the correct alignment is obtained with appropriate ligament balance, a distal femoral cutting block is attached to the tensor and affixed by pins to the femur (see *Illustration 9*). The distal femur is transected with a reciprocating saw at an angle of 7°–10° of valgus. The same spacer block that was used to size the flexion gap is placed in the extension gap to check the fit, alignment and collateral ligament tension.

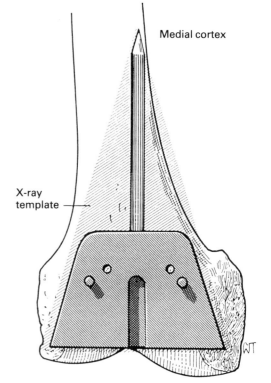

Medial cortex

X-ray template

17

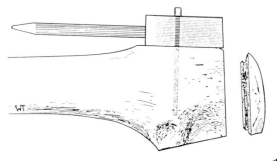

18

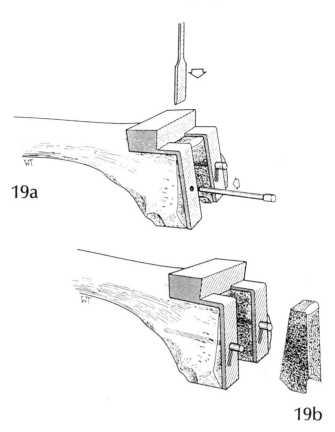

19a

19b

Final preparation of the femur, tibia and patella

19a, b, 20 & 21

The distal femur is prepared by placing a notch-cutting guide onto the distal femur, so that the intercondylar notch is resected to a depth equal to the dimension of the prosthesis. The anterior and posterior aspects of the distal femur are chamfered with the aid of a guide to complete the preparation of the femur.

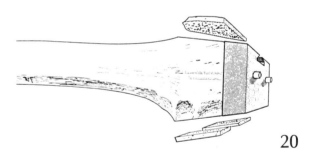

20

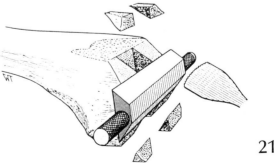

21

22a, b, 23, 24 & 25

A central fixation hole is made in the proximal tibia so that the central peg of the tibial component is correctly aligned with the tibial tubercle. Tibial component malrotation must be avoided by aligning the handle of the jig with the tibial spine, as excessive medial rotation will pose the risk of postoperative patellar dislocation.

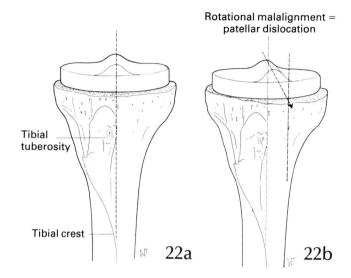

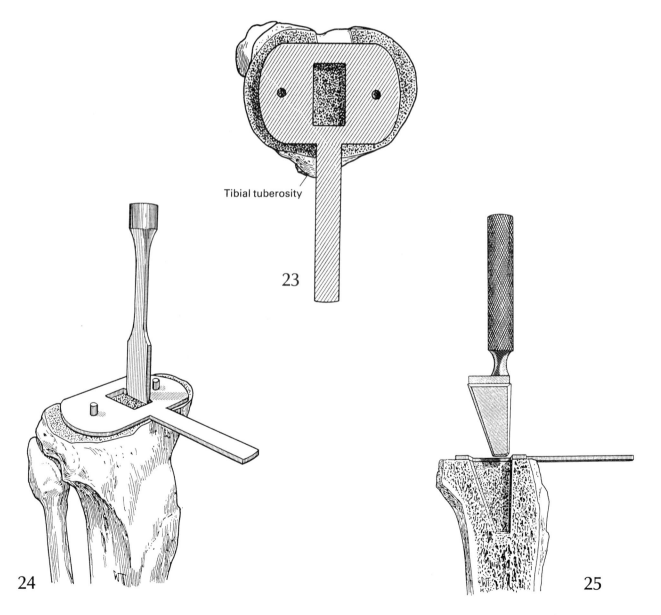

26

The patella is resurfaced in all cases where possible. The patella must be of sufficient size to accept a prosthesis, otherwise it is impractical to resurface it. The resection is done by eye, with the patella held everted. The resection is carried from the medial to lateral articular surfaces. A patellar thickness of 1–1.5 cm should remain to provide adequate fixation of the prosthesis. This may not be possible in rheumatoid knees because of loss of bone, and is then best avoided. A central fixation hole is made with a gouge.

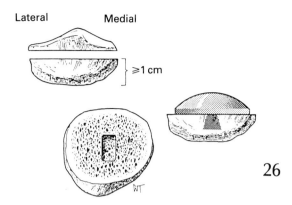

26

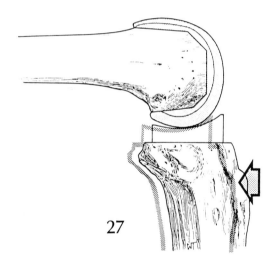

27

27 & 28

Trial prostheses are positioned onto each respective bony surface and the knee is reduced. Alignment and ligament balance are rechecked and the tibial component thickness should equal that of the spacer block that was used to size the flexion and extension gaps. Patellar tracking is evaluated and a lateral retinacular release is performed if there is a tendency for the patella to mistrack laterally.

The tourniquet is released, and haemostasis is maintained by means of cauterization. The limb is re-exsanguinated and the tourniquet re-inflated. The trabecular surfaces are cleansed by pulsatile saline lavage in order to remove blood and bone debris.

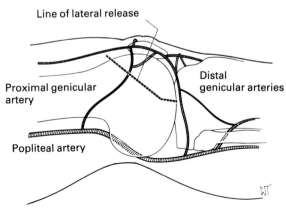

28

29, 30 & 31

The femoral and patellar components are affixed simultaneously to each respective dried surface with acrylic cement. Only sufficient cement is used to fill the gaps between the prosthetic components and the bone. Where there is loss of bone on the tibia this may be made up by bone grafts taken from the resected segments. (In this situation, weight-bearing is restricted by crutch-walking for 3 months after operation.) The tibial component is then inserted with a separate batch of cement. Excess acrylic is removed by scalpel or curette. The knee is reduced and brought into extension after the cement hardens and the wound is irrigated with an antibiotic saline solution and suction drains are placed in the knee. The wound is closed in layers with interrupted vertical mattress sutures. A bulky Robert Jones dressing is applied to the limb.

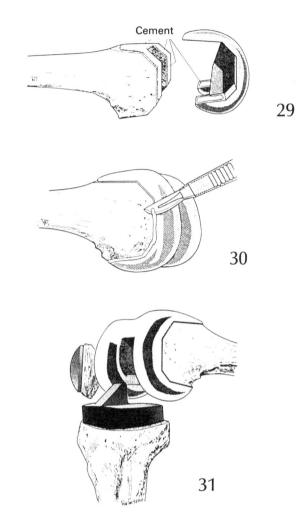

29

30

31

Postoperative management

Intravenous broad-spectrum antibiotics are continued postoperatively for 48 hours and suction drainage is used for 24 hours. Continuous passive motion, if available, is initiated in the recovery room, and a lighter postoperative dressing will then be required. If the situation dictates against early movement, a bulky Robert Jones dressing is used and kept in place for 2 days; active assisted flexion is begun on the second postoperative day. The patient stands and begins walking with assistance on the second or third postoperative day. The patient is discharged when he or she can climb stairs, walk with a stick and bend the knee to 90°. Active resisted quadriceps exercises are not recommended for 6 months to prevent inadvertent disruption of the extensor mechanism.

We consider that some form of postoperative prophylaxis against deep venous thrombosis should be given. We obtain a venogram on the fifth postoperative day. Warfarin prophylaxis is begun if there is a known risk of deep venous thrombosis. If thrombosis is present in the thigh or the patient is symptomatic, heparin therapy is started, followed by warfarin, and the patient remains on the latter medication for 2 to 3 months. Some surgeons, however, use salicylates postoperatively in a twice-daily dosage of 650 mg.

Complications

Complications may be divided into medical and mechanical. The medical complications include: deep venous thrombosis, pulmonary embolism, skin necrosis, and postoperative infection. Antibiotic prophylaxis, careful handling of soft tissues during surgery, and medical prophylaxis against clot formation will minimize these problems. Mechanical complications include: improper mechanical alignment (especially neutral or varus) owing to insufficient ligament release, malrotation of the tibial component with subsequent patellar dislocation, instability owing to inadvertent transection of the medial collateral ligament, component loosening, and peroneal

nerve palsy. Careful attention to proper surgical technique will minimize these difficulties and assure proper function of the knee.

References

1. Insall J. A midline approach to the knee. *J Bone Joint Surg [Am]* 1971; 53-A: 1584–1586.

2. Rose HA, Hood RW, Otis JC, Ranawat CS, Insall JN. Peroneal-nerve palsy following total knee arthroplasty. *J Bone Joint Surg [Am]* 1982; 64-A: 347–51.

3. Insall JN, ed. *Surgery of the knee.* New York: Churchill Livingstone, 1984.

4. Freeman MAR, Insall JN, Besser W, Walker PS, Hallel T. Excision of the cruciate ligaments in total knee replacement. *Clin Orthop* 1977; 126: 209–12.

Acknowledgement

Illustrations 12–14, 16–21, 23–27 and 29–31 are reproduced with permission from Insall JN, Burstein AH, Freeman MAR. *Principles and Techniques of Knee Replacement,* published by the New York Society for the Relief of the Ruptured and Crippled.

Compression arthrodesis of the knee

The late Sir John Charnley   *CBE*, FRS, FRCS, FACS
Formerly Emeritus Professor of Orthopaedic Surgery, University of Manchester, Honorary Orthopaedic Surgeon, Centre for Hip Surgery, Wrightington Hospital, Wigan; Consultant Orthopaedic Surgeon, King Edward VII Hospital, Midhurst, Sussex, UK

Introduction

Indications

The pathological conditions suitable for treatment by knee fusion are varied though the procedure is now rarely performed. They range from painless mechanical instability in paralytic and traumatic conditions, to painful and stiff knees in chronic arthritis and destructive processes such as tuberculosis and failed prosthetic replacement. Cancellous bone graft may be required to fill any gaps between the bone ends after failed prosthetic replacement.

Contraindications

The involvement of other joints in chronic arthritis, especially the opposite knee and one or both hips, makes it difficult for a patient to cope with a stiff knee. Ideally knee fusion should therefore be done only in patients whose other joints in the lower extremities are normal. There are many cases where a knee disability so dominates the clinical picture that there is no alternative but to fuse the knee in the presence of other abnormal joints, and in these cases the patient will be greatly benefited though still remaining disabled to some extent.

In very rare instances bilateral fusion of the knees can produce remarkable benefit if both hips are normal, and if the patient fully understands all that this operation entails. Usually a combination of an arthrodesis of one knee and an arthroplasty of the other produces a better result.

Preoperative

Anaesthesia

Any form of anaesthesia can be used for this operation except a local anaesthetic, since a tourniquet on the thigh is essential.

Position of patient

The patient lies supine on an ordinary operating table.

Tourniquet

This should be applied high in the thigh. It can be applied, unsterile, before skin preparation and draping.

Draping

The skin is prepared with Hibitane in spirit (ICI Pharmaceuticals, UK). Adhesive plastic drape is then applied.

Operation

Incision

1

Generally, a transverse incision is the best. When in tuberculosis excision of the suprapatellar pouch is needed then a longitudinal incision is better. It is unnecessary to excise the suprapatellar synovia of non-tuberculous chronic arthritis.

The knee should be flexed to 90° with the heel on the table. The skin incision is made exactly at the level of the joint line in the plane of the head of the tibia. The incision should be carried medially and laterally about 1 cm posterior to the central axis of the limb.

Incision of capsule

The capsule of the joint should be incised in the same line as the skin without undercutting. The capsular incision should go down to the bone of the tibia all the way round just below the level of the menisci. The patellar tendon is divided at this level.

The front of the capsule should be reflected upwards as a flap containing the patella. This may require short relaxing incisions at the lateral and medial extremities of the capsule.

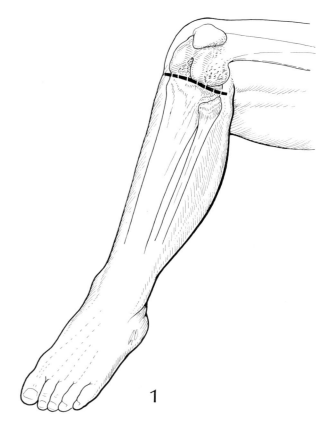

1

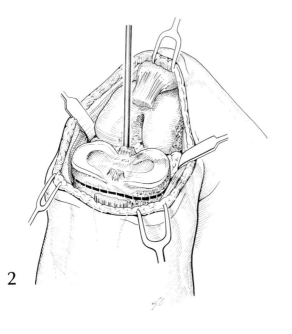

2

Subluxating the joint

2

Division of the capsule and the medial, lateral and cruciate ligaments is complete when the knee can be fully flexed with the heel touching the buttock. The head of the tibia is thereby slightly subluxated forwards. A bone lever passed behind the head of the tibia, using the lower end of the femur as a fulcrum, will help in this forward subluxation of the tibia and will also protect the popliteal structures when the saw is used on the upper end of the tibia. It should be emphasized that to present the upper end of the tibia easily to the saw: (a) the skin incision should not be at a higher level than the upper end of the tibia, and (b) full flexion of the knee should be secured.

Patella

A decision must be made on the fate of the patella. Ideally it is best excised since residual pain sometimes can arise in patellofemoral arthritis but the majority of cases do well with the patella left *in situ*.

Inserting the femoral pin

The Charnley compression clamps are now applied to the distal pin to act as a guide for the second pin in the femur. The blocks in the clamps should be separated the full distance of 10 cm. Care should be taken to place the pin in the femur half-way between the anterior and posterior cortices.

Tightening the clamps

An assistant holding the foot should put the posterior edges of the cut bone surface in contact by pushing in the axis of the tibia, while leaving the anterior edges gaping slightly so that the surgeon can be sure that no soft parts are trapped posteriorly between the bone surfaces.

As soon as the tightening of the clamps has reached the point where the cut surfaces are first drawn into full apposition, the process of applying mechanical compress-ion can be started. With 4 mm Steinmann pins, and with the clamps separated laterally from each other by 15 cm the Charnley clamps will give 50 kg of compression force if both are tightened 12 half turns. This is because the screw threads are 6.2 mm (0.25 inch) Whitworth; any other type of thread would need a different calibration. If the bones are of normal density, and if the pins are well placed, the tightening of the clamps should give sufficient rigidity for the fixation to hold with nothing more than a compression bandage.

Checking rotation

If any error in rotation has been incurred, as indicated by the position of the foot, this is easily altered at this stage by the ability of the simple Charnley pattern of clamps to permit rotary adjustment. The compression is released, the rotatory error corrected and the clamps are retightened.

Additional fixation

8 & 9

If the rigidity of the fixation is not considered satisfactory, or if the bone is osteoporotic, additional fixation against movement in the plane of flexion–extension may be considered advisable and can be obtained either by (a) external support or (b) additional fixation. External support by means of a Thomas' splint is mechanically superior to a plaster cylinder. Additional internal fixation is most conveniently added by using two more 4 mm Steinmann pins and mounting a second pair of Charnley compression clamps to make a 'side-pin compression unit'. The two pins are driven into the tibia and femur from the front, making sure that the points merely penetrate the posterior cortices without projecting into the popliteal fossa. The first clamp is then slid along the pins to within about 1.2 cm of the skin and fixed by tightening the set-screws on the clamp. The second clamp is now re-assembled to act as a 'pusher' rather than a compressor, as indicated in the diagram. The 'pusher' clamp is applied to the free ends of the pins and adjusted to hold the free ends apart. Tightening the compression clamp near to the knee will then apply compression as well as lock any tendency of the knee to move in the flexion–extension plane.

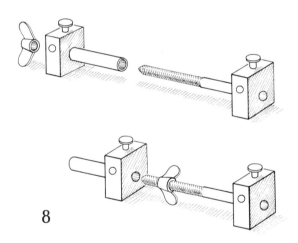

8

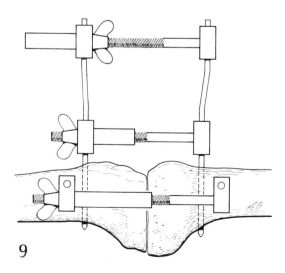

9

Closing the wound

A few interrupted stitches of polyglactin 910 are inserted into the capsule and the patellar tendon.

The skin punctures round the pins should be inspected to avoid unequal tension. If unequal tension in the skin is present appropriate incisions should be made, and if necessary one or two fine skin sutures inserted.

Dressings

10

A pressure dressing is applied, completely burying the whole compression unit in 'fluffed up' wool, and then compressing everything with a crêpe bandage applied over all.

The tourniquet is then removed.

It is important never to strain the arthrodesis by lifting the limb by the foot during this bandaging. Lifting the foot can allow the knee to sag backwards and crush the cancellous bone. The limb should be lifted at the centre of gravity, by a hand under the upper part of the calf.

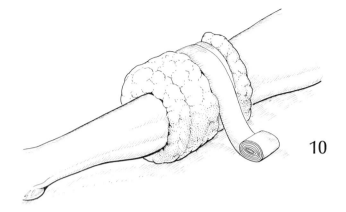

10

Postoperative management

The compression unit should be left in position for 1 month. It is usually unnecessary to retighten the clamps if the bone is soft, because retightening will merely cause the pins to cut through the bone with further loss of pressure. A check radiograph of the anteroposterior plane should be taken at 10–14 days and this should show the pins deflected by the same amount that they were at the end of the operation if the bone is of good quality. If the deflection has diminished at 10–14 days, in the presence of good bone, then the clamps should be retightened, which can be done without anaesthesia.

The patient is confined to bed for 4 weeks while the compression unit is in position.

At the end of 4 weeks the clamps should be removed from the nails and the knee tested for movement with the nails in position. The accuracy of detecting movement is increased by leaving the pins to act as pointers.

If fibrous movement should be present the clamps should be reapplied for another 2 weeks. In most cases the knee will be quite solid at 4 weeks.

A close-fitting plaster cast is applied for another 4 weeks after the pins have been extracted, and the patient is allowed to take full weight on the foot. This cast prevents excessive external leverage being exerted on the fusion site.

Patients are usually able to rehabilitate completely in the 4 weeks following removal of the plaster. The total time of disability is 3 months (4 weeks of compression, 4 weeks of walking in the plaster cylinder and 4 weeks of walking without plaster).

Complications

The author never found it necessary to use suction drainage after this operation. Occasionally the dressings may drip blood soon after the tourniquet has been removed. If this should happen it is not necessary to take the dressings down; the limb should be steeply elevated, an extra pressure bandage applied over the existing dressings, and the foot of the bed should be raised.

Sepsis in pin tracks was never any trouble in the author's experience. If the patient is confined to bed during the whole time the pins are *in situ*, and if the pins are not *in situ* for more than 6 weeks, superficial sepsis clears up in a few days.

Illustrations by Gillian Lee

Massive replacement for tumours of the lower limb

H. B. S. Kemp MS, FRCS
Consultant Orthopaedic Surgeon, The Middlesex Hospital, London, and The Royal National Orthopaedic Hospital, Stanmore, UK

John T. Scales OBE, FRCS, CIMechE
Emeritus Professor of Biomedical Engineering, The Royal National Orthopaedic Hospital, Stanmore, UK

Introduction

Benign tumours of the appendicular skeleton can generally be treated by curettage with or without adjuvant therapy such as cryosurgery, and by marginal excision. Nevertheless, extensive or recurrent benign tumours may require wide resection and conservative reconstructive surgery.

In the field of malignant tumour surgery, where amputation was originally accepted as the only method of treatment, considerable advances have been made in conservative management. Although initially this was limited to such tumours as chondrosarcoma, the introduction of cytotoxic therapy and, in particular, the regime advocated by Rosen et al.,[1] not only led to a marked improvement in the prognosis but also facilitated the surgery required to preserve the affected limb. In contemporary surgical management of malignant tumours of the lower limb there are four generally accepted methods of treatment.

1. Resection and autogenous bone grafting
2. Resection and allografting (using cadaveric bone)
3. Resection and rotational approximation of the femur and tibia
4. Resection and prosthetic replacement.

In the UK, as a sequel to the pioneering work of Burrows, Wilson and Scales[2], the method of choice and the management of such lesions is that of prosthetic replacement.

Indications

In the lower limb, massive replacement is indicated for tumours of the proximal femur, the distal femur and the proximal tibia. Benign tumours and osteoclastomas that are too extensive for local curettage or have been affected by a pathological fracture and malignant tumours such as osteosarcomas, parosteal osteosarcomas, periosteal osteosarcomas, chondrosarcomas, malignant fibrous histiocytomas and Ewing's sarcomas may all be suitable for such replacements.

Contraindications

Tumours that have widely infiltrated locally and, in particular, those that have invaded subcutaneous tissue and skin are rarely suitable for such treatment, though there are instances where a vascularized musculocutaneous pedicle may be rotated to cover a skin defect.

Occasionally, patients are shown to have extensive medullary involvement. Such patients are probably most suitably treated by disarticulation, though the occasional individual may be suitable for total replacement of the affected bone. However, such surgery is only applicable to tumours affecting the femur or humerus.

Preoperative

Assessment

Patients presenting with tumours suitable for conservative resection and prosthetic replacement, regardless of whether they require cytotoxic therapy, should have a full medical and dental assessment in order to exclude or treat any pre-existing infection. Routine radiographs of the lesion and the lungs should be obtained. In addition, computed tomographic (CT) scans of the lesion and the lungs, radionuclide skeletal scans and magnetic resonance imaging (MRI) scans of the affected limb should be performed. The reasons for such detailed radiological investigations are to determine the local extent of involvement of the affected bone, to exclude the extremely rare occurrence of a 'skip' lesion and to assess whether the tumour is contained within the periosteum. In addition, it is necessary to determine the presence of pulmonary and other secondaries and to exclude the rare manifestation of multiple skeletal metastases. If it is considered that the tumour is resectable, measurement films are then taken so that a custom-built prosthesis can be manufactured.

Biopsy

A biopsy should always be performed as the last procedure before a tumour is resected, in that, at least theoretically, such a procedure may convert an intracompartmental lesion into an extracompartmental lesion. However, a biopsy is essential to determine the precise histological nature of the lesion. In the majority of patients, adequate material can be obtained by needle biopsy, though very occasionally core biopsy is necessary. Positioning of the biopsy site is critical to enable the biopsy scar to be excised *en bloc* when definitive surgery is performed. All too frequently, biopsies performed by the referring hospital seriously prejudice the surgical management. Bone biopsy, if incorrectly performed, carries a considerable morbidity. Consequently it is preferable that the biopsy should be performed by an individual aware of the implications of surgical resection and prosthetic replacement (*see* chapter on 'Techniques of bone biopsy' pp. 91–99).

Prosthesis

Design and manufacture

Major prostheses are individually designed and custom-built for each patient. In order to manufacture these prostheses measurement films, CT and MRI scans are required. Routine radiographs produce a variable degree of magnification. Radiographs of the appendicular skeleton enlarge the image between 10 and 15 per cent. To correct for this error a radio-opaque linear scale is placed alongside the limb that is to be radiographed. Anteroposterior and lateral views of the affected bone including the articular surfaces and views of the unaffected contralateral bone are required for accurate measurement and design. The CT and MRI scans are necessary in order to determine the soft tissue and intramedullary extent of the tumour.

Stainless steel is a suitable material for prosthetic manufacture, though for technical reasons it is now rarely used. Cobalt–chromium–molybdenum alloys, titanium (T1–T5), and titanium alloy (TAI) are preferred, for only these alloys possess adequate fatigue and endurance properties required for the manufacture of the highly stressed, shaped and cross-sectionally contoured intramedullary stem employed in the fixation of the prosthesis to the bone. The optimal length of the intramedullary stem is 14 cm, and it is grouted into the prepared medullary cavity using injected polymethylmethacrylate bone cement. In preparing the cavity, reaming must be minimal and the resultant cavity should not exceed the diameter of the pin by more than 2 mm. Antibiotic cement should be used where there have been previous surgical procedures or if the patient is on cytotoxic drugs. Titanium alloys possess the additional advantage that, to date, no adverse tissue responses have been reported in implants.

The weight-bearing surfaces of orthopaedic components usually have a concavo-convex configuration. Ultra-high-density polyethylene (RCH 1000) is the most commonly used material for the concave component, while the convex component is made of metal or ceramic alumina.

All prostheses eventually become surrounded by a sheath of fibrous tissue. The various muscles detached in the process of dissection become adherent to this capsule. However, in certain situations, it is necessary to obtain a more accurate fixation of the tendons: for instance, in reconstituting the rotator cuff at the shoulder, the prosthesis is sheathed in a polyester locknit mesh which facilitates the reattachment of the muscles of the rotator cuff. At the hip, the abductors are attached to the prosthesis; and at the knee, the patellar tendon is reconstituted using artificial tendons of several layers of folded mesh. It is also possible to use such material to extend tendons and to repair muscle and fascial defects.

Extending or growing prosthesis

The rationale behind the use of an extending prosthesis is that the loss of growth of the relevant growth-plate can be compensated for by the periodic lengthening of the prosthesis. These prostheses have a specific complication: occasionally abundant soft tissue scarring in the adolescent may in some instances produce contractures and limit repeated extension. In addition, the size of the prosthesis used in a child may be inadequate to maintain the mature adult weight. Consequently a further prosthetic replacement sometimes becomes necessary prior to or with the completion of growth. However, such a prosthesis is of particular importance in the lower limb in order to maintain equal length of the two legs.

1

The prosthetic component that replaces the bone deficit is similar in design to that used in adult prostheses. The articulating portion of the prosthesis is connected to the shaft segment by a piston which contains an anti-rotation device so that only extension can take place. At present, two methods are employed to extend the piston. In one method, a distraction tool is used to draw the piston out of the shaft; then tungsten–carbon ball-bearings are introduced through a port at the side of the prosthesis, which is normally closed by a threaded plug. The disadvantage of tungsten–carbon ball-bearings is that maximum loading will occur over a minimal contact area. In consequence, even such a hard material is subjected to stress fracturing. The alternative method of maintaining extension is the use of C-ring sections which can be fitted round the piston between the jaws of the distraction tool.

On the opposite side of the joint, where, for instance, the growth-plate has been preserved in the proximal tibia, the tibial spines are removed, the plateau is reamed and the reamer is carried through the epiphysis, the growth-plate and into the metaphysis. The cavity is progressively enlarged to allow the insertion of a polyethylene sleeve. This lies distal to the growth-plate in intimate contact with the medullary bone. In this particular instance, the component which is inserted into this sleeve is similar to the tibial component of the constrained hinge joint, but it is mounted on a floating table with lugs which fit into grooves cut into the tibial plateau. Under the table there is a medullary rod which fits into the polyethylene sleeve. Subsequently, as growth occurs, this intramedullary rod is progressively extruded. Despite the creation of a defect in the growth-plate there is no clinical evidence of a synostosis occurring between the epiphysis and metaphysis, and unconstrained growth occurs.

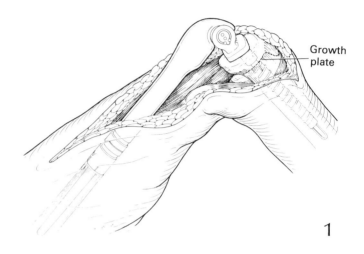

1

Preoperative management

Patients with malignant tumours are initially treated by the oncologist and admitted to a randomized therapeutic trial[3]. The patients usually receive three cycles of treatment prior to surgery. The rationale for this is that the tumour response to chemotherapy can then be assessed by the histopathologist and an alternative drug regime can be administered, when appropriate, to patients with resistant tumours.

The major risk of massive prosthetic replacement is infection. This applies particularly to the patient who is immunologically suppressed as a sequel to chemotherapy. For this reason patients are given antibiotics intravenously prior to surgery and this regime is continued until the wound has healed. The reason for giving antibiotics intravenously is to maintain a constant blood level. If the patient receiving chemotherapy has a tunnelled central line *in situ*, these lines may have been previously colonized by pathogens, so a separate intravenous line should be used for the antibiotics.

Principles of tumour surgery

Enneking *et al.*[4] have propounded the guidelines for the resection of tumours based on a staging system.

1. Intracapsular excision: a debulking procedure performed within the pseudocapsule
2. Marginal excision: *en bloc* resection performed extracapsularly within the reactive zone (not applicable to bone tumours)

3. Wide excision: *en bloc* excision performed through normal tissue beyond the reactive zone but within the compartment of origin
4. Radical excision: an *en bloc* resection including the compartment of origin.

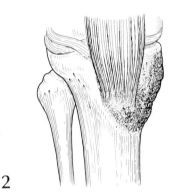

2

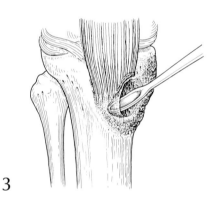

3

Marginal excision

2

Marginal excision of bone is not feasible. A benign tumour is removed by curettage and subsequent resection is made of the reactive bone that surrounds it.

3

Curettage through a small window inevitably leaves a residual tumour behind.

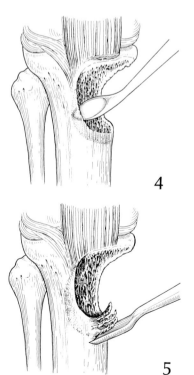

4

5

4 & 5

The fenestration of a bone should be as extensive as the parameters of a lesion. The reactive margin of a lesion should then be removed with gouges.

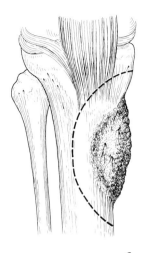

6

Wide excision

6

Occasionally, even relatively malignant tumours, such as periosteal osteosarcomas, may be resected by wide excision provided the patient is treated by adjuvant chemotherapy.

7

Large defects are partially or completely replaced by new bone formation.

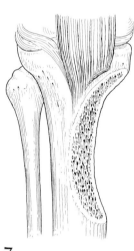

7

Malignant bone tumours

Only Enneking's last two methods are applicable to malignant bone tumours, though at best the surgeon can only achieve a wide margin of resection. The approach to malignant bone tumours in the UK differs in two aspects to Enneking's principles. First, it is believed that in almost all sarcomas the periosteum constitutes a distinctive barrier to tumour spread. In consequence an intact periosteum modifies the staging of the tumour. This does not apply to Ewing's sarcoma which freely permeates the periosteum to involve the soft tissues. Second, in performing a wide resection, if Enneking's principles are followed, a margin of 2 cm of normal tissue is removed with the tumour. While this represents the ideal, it cannot necessarily be obtained in that bone anatomically has 'bare areas' as instanced by the distal femur in its relation to the popliteal fossa. Consequently, an attempt to achieve such a margin posteriorly would result in the resection of the neurovascular bundle, subcutaneous tissue and skin. Sarcomas rarely involve the neurovascular bundle by direct spread; fascial layers, periosteum, epineurium and the adventitia of major arteries are relatively resistant to invasion and, as a result, arterial resection and replacement is only rarely required[5].

Operation

Limb salvage surgery should be performed in an ultra-clean air theatre. The surgeon and his assistants should be hooded and fully gowned in impervious material.

REPLACEMENT OF PROXIMAL FEMUR

Position of patient

The patient is placed on the operating table with the affected side uppermost. The skin should be scrupulously prepared and the patient should be doubly draped with impervious towelling. The incision site is covered with an adhesive drape once the skin has been effectively dried.

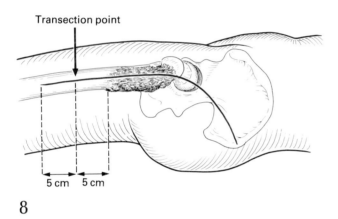

Transection point

5 cm   5 cm

8

Incision

8

Although any of the standard approaches are acceptable, whenever possible we favour the posterior or lateral approach. The proposed point of transection is marked on the skin. The incision is made over the gluteus maximus in line with the muscle fibres, passing downward and forward to the anterior border of the greater trochanter. It is then carried downward in line with the femur to 5 cm beyond the point where it is intended to transect the affected bone.

9 & 10

Using a muscle-splitting technique, the incision through the gluteus maximus is deepened and the fascia lata is incised along the line of the femur anteriorly. The insertion of gluteus medius and minimus into the greater trochanter, when the latter is unaffected by tumour, can be detached in continuity with the fascia lata by removing a thin sliver of the trochanter with an osteotome. If the insertion has to be sacrificed the tendinous insertions of these muscles are transfixed with stay sutures. The underlying musculature is systematically excised so that some 2 cm of normal tissue surrounds the tumour.

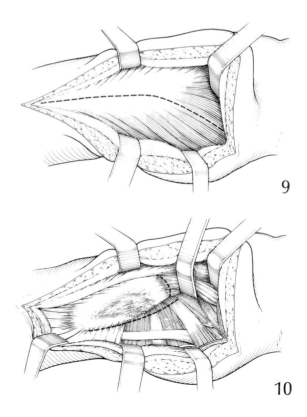

9

10

11

When the tumour has been completely freed, the femur is divided at the site of election. It is sometimes easier to divide the femur at an early stage and complete the dissection in a retrograde manner. The capsule of the hip joint is incised circumferentially. The femoral head is gently distracted and the ligamentum teres is divided. When the femur has been transected a sample of the distal medullary contents is taken so that an imprint can be examined to determine that full clearance of the affected bone has been obtained.

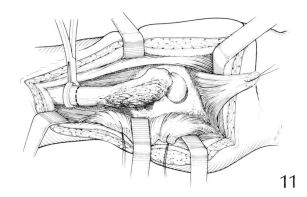

11

Insertion of prosthetic replacement

12

The acetabulum is prepared as for a routine hip replacement. Although it is necessary to remove the normal cartilage, the subchondral bone is preserved. Key holes are shaped in the body of the ilium, ischium and occasionally the pubic bone. The acetabular component is then cemented *in situ*. The residual femoral shaft is curetted and then thoroughly cleared by irrigation and brushing. The femoral component is inserted and a trial reduction is carried out. Occasionally it is necessary to ream the intramedullary bone using graduated AO flexible reamers.

When it has been shown by trial reduction that the desired length of femur has been resected, cement is injected into the femoral canal. Because of the length of the canal, in order to achieve adequate filling, it is necessary to use a cement gun with a long nozzle of the appropriate diameter. The nozzle that is normally used corresponds to the diameter of the medullary lumen so that cement insertion is under pressure. For this reason, the prosthesis needs to be inserted as soon as the cement is of appropriate consistency because such a long column of cement offers a mechanical resistance as the stem is introduced. As far as the orientation of the prosthesis is concerned, this is normally done by relating the prosthesis to the linea aspera. When the linea aspera is defective it is advantageous to put a small drill hole anteriorly in the residue of the femur for orientation. When the cement has polymerized, the prosthesis is articulated with the acetabular cup.

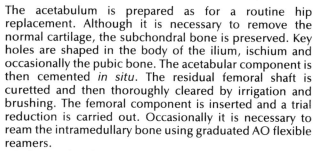

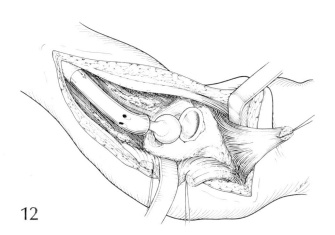

12

13 & 14

Originally the wound was closed in layers, the tendinous insertions of the gluteus medius and minimus being stitched in to the fascia lata with the hip in abduction, but this presented problems in terms of function. Now, a hole drilled through the neck of the femoral component allows a polyester tape to be stitched to the tendons of the muscles, providing more adequate fixation. The wound is closed in the normal manner after obtaining haemostasis. The wound should be drained using a superficial and deep drain.

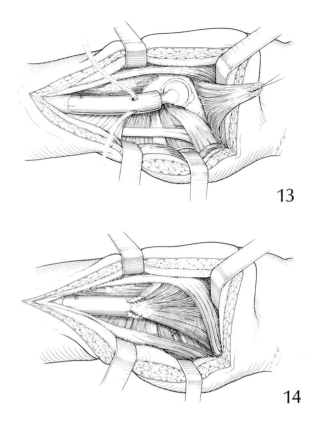

13

14

Postoperative management

The patient is nursed with the leg in abduction and supported on balanced slings. Physiotherapy is commenced on the second postoperative day and consists essentially of isometric contractions. Eventually, when adequate muscle tone has been achieved the patient is mobilized in an anti-rotation and anti-adduction splint for 12 weeks using crutches. At this stage all active movements are encouraged by intensive physiotherapy.

Function

Lateral rotation without the reattachment of the rotators is increased to some 60°. Because there is no control over the prosthesis at the point where the greater trochanter was, these patients will walk, in the majority of cases, with a positive Trendelenburg gait. However, with the reattachment of the abductors, most patients can walk with a negative gait or a slight lurch; many patients will be able to run with a negative Trendelenburg gait.

REPLACEMENT OF DISTAL FEMUR

Position of patient

The patient is normally placed in a supine position on the table, with a sandbag under the ipsilateral buttock. If the transection point is at a suitable position, the operation is done under a tourniquet. The patient is towelled in the normal manner, the foot is preferably enclosed in a rubber glove so that the peripheral pulses can be palpated as required.

Incision

15

The proximal point of transection is marked on the skin and a medial parapatellar incision is usually made from 5 cm proximal to this point, passing distally to a level of 5 cm below the joint line. The incision on occasion is modified to encompass the biopsy scar where this is feasible, though in certain circumstances it is necessary to make a lateral parapatellar incision in order to do this.

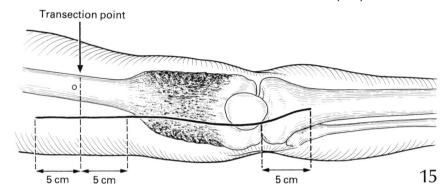

Transection point

5 cm   5 cm   5 cm

15

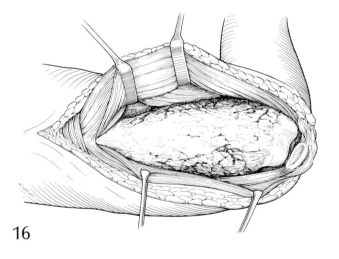

16

16

The incision is deepened in the midline through the tendon of the quadriceps muscle. Depending on the nature of the tumour the lesion is then marginally or widely excised, malignant tumours being resected with an adequate margin of the three vasti muscles. This resection is extended both medially and laterally.

17

At this stage the distal femur and the proximal tibia are disarticulated. This is performed by detaching the medial and lateral collateral ligaments from their tibial attachments. The patella and the quadriceps tendon are then displaced laterally. The knee is progressively flexed and the cruciate ligaments are divided. At this stage the posterior capsule is easily visualized and divided or resected at its attachment to the tibia. The manoeuvre is facilitated if preceded by gentle blunt dissection behind the capsule. The origins of popliteus and gastrocnemius are exposed and divided from their origins or resected leaving a wide margin.

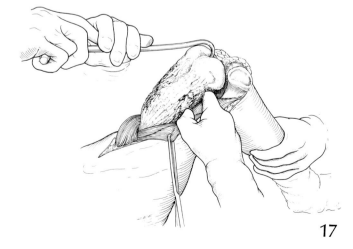

17

18

The dissection behind the femur is then continued in a retrograde manner. On occasion the involvement of the soft tissues is extensive and the resection can be made easier by dividing the femur and carrying the dissection distally. The neurovascular bundle is rarely involved when the tumour is otherwise removable. However, if the vessels are invaded by tumour they are resected and replaced by a graft taken from the ipsilateral saphenous vein.

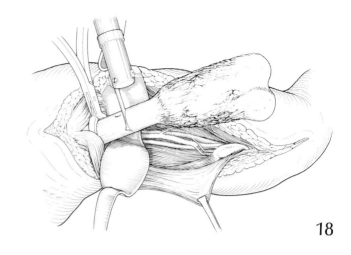

18

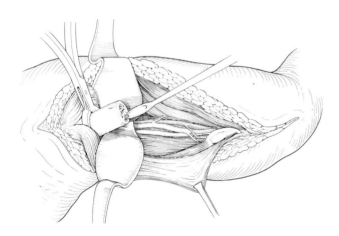

19

19

As with tumours of the proximal femur, marrow is removed at the time of resection and imprints made to confirm that no residual tumour is present.

Insertion of prosthesis

20

The content of the femoral canal is cleared by curettage and brushing and where necessary the canal is enlarged by the use of flexible reamers. The tibial table is prepared by removing the tibial spines so that the surface is flattened in order to receive the tibial component. Using Capener gouges, the table is breached sufficiently to accept the prosthetic stem.

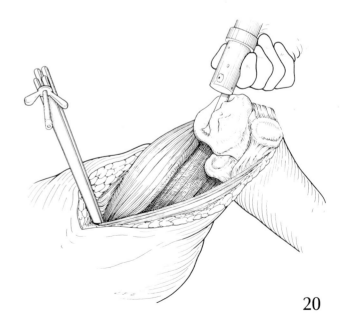

20

21 & 22

The medullary canal is cleared of all debris by curettage and brushing. Subsequently a cement restrictor is inserted. The two prosthetic components are then introduced and a trial reduction is made. The peripheral vessels are palpated with the knee in extension to determine that there is normal pulsation. If it is necessary to perform further resection this is normally taken from the residual femoral shaft. When a trial reduction is satisfactory, both the femoral canal and the tibia are irrigated and the two components of the prosthesis are cemented into position.

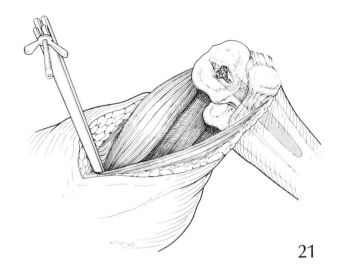

21

Closure

Wound repair is essentially routine though no attempt is made to close a lateral release if a lateral approach has been made. However, if a standard medial approach has been made a lateral release is performed so that subsequent subluxation of the patella does not occur. The wound is closed in layers and drained.

Postoperative management

The patient is placed on a continuous passive motion (CPM) machine as soon as drainage has ceased. The knee is then progressively passively flexed within the tolerance of the patient. The skin is carefully observed during the initial stages to confirm its viability. As soon as the patient can tolerate active movement, intensive quadriceps and hamstring exercises are instituted. Walking with crutches is begun when the wound is healed, and the crutches and sticks discontinued as muscle control is achieved.

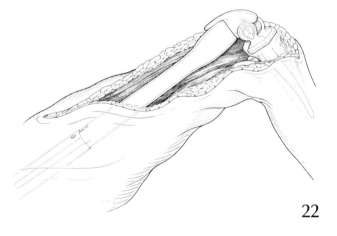

22

REPLACEMENT OF PROXIMAL TIBIA

Position of patient

The patient is supine on the operating table and the operation is normally carried out under tourniquet control without exsanguination; towelling is performed as previously described.

Incision

23

The incision is preferably a lateral parapatellar incision though it may be modified to encompass a biopsy scar. Starting 15 cm proximal to the knee joint it runs distally to 5 cm distal to the point of transection of the tibia. The incision should avoid the crest of the tibia.

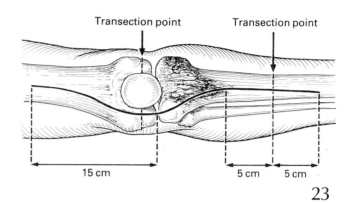

23

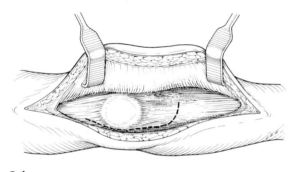

24

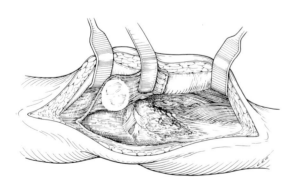

25

24 & 25

The affected tibia is exposed and the distance from the inferior pole of the patella to the point of transection is determined. The patellar tendon is appropriately reflected from the tibial tuberosity, preserving where possible the medial patellar expansion. The knee joint is disarticulated following the procedure described above.

The medial popliteal nerve and the associated popliteal artery and vein are identified. The origins of gastrocnemius and popliteus are defined prior to disarticulation of the knee. (The origin of soleus is identified and the muscle belly divided at a suitable distance from the tibial lesion.) The neurovascular bundle is traced distally to the point where the artery and vein enter the anterior compartment. The common peroneal nerve is only identified when the tumour encroaches or surrounds the proximal fibula, when it may be necessary to resect this portion of the fibula with the tumour. Normally, the proximal tibiofibular joint is disarticulated.

Muscles of the anterior and posterior compartments and the interosseous membrane are divided at an appropriate distance from the tumour, dissection being carried distally to the point of transection of the tibia. After transection, medullary content is removed for imprint examination. On occasion it is necessary to divide the anterior tibial artery; this can be performed without prejudicing the vascular supply.

Insertion of the prosthesis

26

The marrow cavity in the femur is opened by drilling into the intercondylar notch at the apex of the concavity. Drills of appropriate diameter are then used until the femoral canal accommodates the Stanmore femoral cutting jig (correctly adjusted for left or right knee). The condyles are marked for transection. They are excised using either a power or an amputation saw, the jig being removed at an appropriate point in the transection.

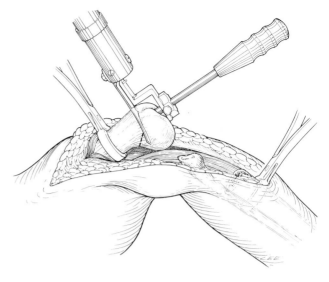

26

27

The femoral component is prepared, the bushes are impressed and it is inserted into the femoral shaft. Seating of the component is checked. The residual condyles are marked posteriorly and resected. The tibial component is subsequently inserted into the residual medullary cavity. Initially, it may not be accommodated, so the cavity will require reaming with flexible AO reamers until the diameter of the cavity is 1–2 mm greater than the intramedullary stem.

At this stage a trial reduction is performed and the components articulated using a test axle. It is the usual practice to employ a femoral and a tibial plateau plate so that end-bearing of the components is evenly distributed. The articulated prosthesis is extended and if there is limitation of extension it may be necessary to resect the femur further. Even when extension is free, it is essential to check for peripheral pulses and, if they are absent in extension, further resection should be performed. Occasionally the vessels will be in spasm as a sequel to surgery; if this is the case, topical lignocaine may be used. The components are removed when reduction is adequate.

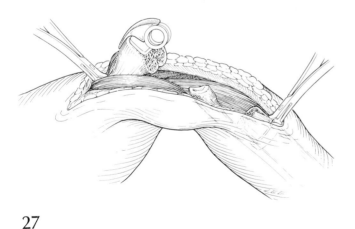

27

28

The medullary cavity is thoroughly irrigated and any residual debris removed using an intramedullary brush. A cement restrictor is inserted into the femoral medullary cavity. The femoral component is cemented into position using a cement gun containing radio-opaque antibiotic cement. While this is setting and compression is maintained by an assistant, the tibial cavity is filled using a Stanmore cement gun with an appropriate nozzle diameter. The tibial component is inserted, orientating the prosthesis in relation to the malleoli or, alternatively, the second toe. When the cement is set the tourniquet is removed and haemostasis obtained. The wound is irrigated to remove residual debris. A polythene tape is threaded into the tibial component and stitched to the patellar tendon with the correct amount of tension. The flexion of the knee is checked and should be in the region of 120°. A drain is inserted and the wound closed in layers with interrupted sutures.

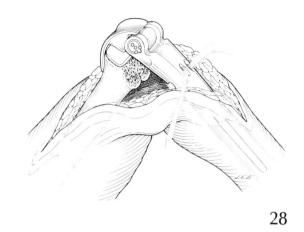

28

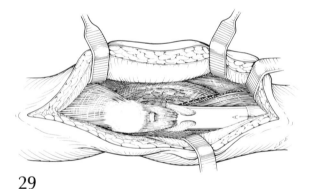

29

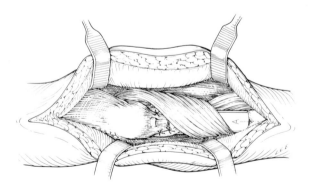

30

Closure

29 & 30

Closure following replacement of the proximal tibia may present problems. If there is a deficit in the fascia it is occasionally possible to approximate this using a polyester mesh. Alternatively, the medial belly of gastrocnemius can be turned forward as a vascularized muscle flap. Because of the tension which so frequently occurs after replacement of the proximal tibia, the skin should be closed with interrupted sutures or clips. The wound is dressed and a wool and a crêpe spica applied.

Postoperative management

The leg is placed on a supporting pillow and the pulses checked regularly. Once drainage has ceased progressive mobilization using a CPM machine is commenced. Walking starts when the wound is healed, and crutches and sticks dispensed with as muscle control is achieved.

Complications

Infections

The most serious complication of prosthetic replacement is infection. The individual who is immunologically compromised by cytotoxic drugs before operation is particularly vulnerable. Biopsy must always be performed using scrupulous surgical techniques and sources of sepsis, such as dental caries, should be treated initially.

The overall infection rate, in over 1000 cases, is approximately 5.5 per cent. This relatively high figure was initially due to the fact that some cases were operated upon when they were too advanced for conventional surgery. The majority of patients who have manifested postoperative problems have had superficial soft tissue infections that have responded to or have been controlled by long-term antibiotics. Approximately 2 per cent have manifested osteomyelitis either of early or late onset and of these 0.5 per cent have required an amputation.

Loosening

As with routine prosthetic replacements, loosening may occur with massive prosthetic replacements. The incidence, however, is surprisingly low at 2.1 per cent per decade. There are possibly two reasons why this is so. First, the patients are relatively young and, in consequence, have good bone stock. Second, the prostheses are custom-built for the individual and the medullary pin is shaped to conform to the canal.

Prosthetic fracture

Initially, when prostheses were manufactured from materials that were not of a uniform quality, the risk of fracture due to metal fatigue or excessive loading was relatively high. Now that prostheses are manufactured of materials that conform to the requirements of the British Standards Institute, the incidence of such breakages is negligible. The overall incidence in the series is 1.9 per cent, and it has been possible to revise all such cases apart from the prostheses in two patients.

Local recurrences

There are two factors responsible for local recurrences:

1. The inability to excise the primary tumour with an adequate margin of soft tissue
2. Injudicious biopsy causing soft tissue contamination.

Both factors predispose to local recurrence particularly if chemotherapy fails to control the tumour. It is frequently possible to excise such recurrences and sterilize the area with local radiotherapy. Rarely is it necessary to amputate the affected limb.

Conclusions

The management of bone tumours and, in particular, malignant bone tumours, is dependent on collective management by the radiologist, oncologist, radiotherapist, pathologist, and surgeon in conjunction with a supporting nursing and paramedical team.

As a result of adequate chemotherapy coupled with surgery, Rosen[6,7] claimed an 85 per cent survival rate for osteogenic sarcoma and a 90 per cent survival rate for Ewing's sarcoma of the appendicular skeleton. In the UK the 5-year survival for osteosarcoma would appear to be in the region of 65 per cent, whereas Ewing's sarcoma is approximately 50 per cent. Although there are obvious risks to prosthetic replacement, there are also distinct advantages over other methods of replacement. These are:

1. Early mobilization: the average time for a patient to be fully ambulant is 8 weeks postoperatively
2. Apart from the surgical scar, the body image is maintained
3. Children, adolescents and young adults in whom the prognosis is poor may be rapidly returned to a reasonably normal existence even though their life span is limited
4. Extending prostheses are the only way of combating the loss of growth potential in the lower limb of a child
5. Twenty-five years of experience in this field coupled with a probability survival of 60 per cent at 20 years suggest that massive prosthetic replacement is more successful than any other form of limb salvage surgery.

References

1. Rosen G, Suwansirikul, Kwon C. et al. High dose methotrexate with citrovorum factor rescue and adriamycin in childhood osteogenic sarcoma. Cancer 1974; 33: 1151–63.

2. Burrows HJ, Wilson JN, Scales JT. Excision of tumours of humerus and femur, with restoration by internal prosthesis. J Bone Joint Surg [Br] 1975; 57-B: 148–59.

3. Bramwell VHC. Chemotherapy of operable osteosarcoma. Baillière's Clinical Oncology. Bone Tumours. London: Baillière Tindall, 1989: 175–203.

4. Enneking WF, Spanier SS, Goodman MA. A system for the surgical staging of musculo-skeletal sarcoma. Clin Orthop 1980; 153: 106–20.

5. Westbury G. The management of soft tissue sarcomas. J Bone Joint Surg [Br] 1989; 71-B: 2–3.

6. Rosen G, Nirenberg A, Caparros B. et al. Osteogenic sarcoma: eight per cent, three-year, disease-free survival with combination chemotherapy (T-7). Nat Cancer Inst Monogr 1981; 56: 213–20.

7. Rosen G. Current management of Ewing's sarcoma. Prog Clin Cancer 1982; 8: 267–82.

Illustrations by Robert Lane

Treatment of leg length inequality

Andrew M. Jackson FRCS
Consultant Orthopaedic Surgeon, University College Hospital, and The Hospital for Sick Children, Great Ormond Street, London, UK

Introduction

Leg length discrepancies of less than 2 cm are commonplace, seldom cause a problem and, if they do, a small shoe-raise is the treatment. A greater difference in leg length will cause postural imbalance and an uneven gait. Patients seek primarily a cosmetic improvement and invariably reject a cumbersome shoe-raise or extension orthosis if there is a more attractive alternative. However, there are also solid orthopaedic reasons which justify the correction of significant leg length discrepancies. The avoidance of backache in later life and osteoarthritis of the hip and knee of the longer leg are obvious. Scoliosis frequently becomes fixed with age. Stiffness in the spine and major joints may make it difficult for an individual to tolerate even a minor discrepancy.

Aetiology

The discrepancies that require correction usually have a congenital basis or are caused by premature epiphyseal arrest. The congenital group includes the whole spectrum of lower limb dysplasias, hemi-atrophy and hemi-hypertrophy, vascular malformations and a variety of syndromes such as neurofibromatosis, Ollier's disease, Klippel–Trenaunay syndrome and Silver's syndrome.

Premature growth-plate arrest may be iatrogenic as happens, for example, when avascular necrosis complicates the treatment of congenital dislocation of the hip, or may be secondary to trauma, infection or radiotherapy. Both infection and trauma can also cause overgrowth of the affected limb. Rarely, midshaft fractures heal with excessive shortening, sometimes combined with angular and rotational deformities, and these need correction. Neurological disorders such as spina bifida, spinal dysraphism and cerebral palsy account for a large number of patients with limb length discrepancies but relatively few of them are candidates for equalization procedures. Leg lengthening techniques have been performed in certain types of dwarfism where short stature alone is the problem, but the advisability of this sort of surgery is debatable and the surgeon must be highly selective.

The short paralytic limb of poliomyelitis is much less common than it used to be. Two or three centimetres of shortening in a paralysed limb is advantageous if it is associated with weak hip flexors or a foot drop since it enables the foot to clear the ground easily during the swing phase of gait. In such patients larger discrepancies can be reduced but should never be totally corrected.

Preoperative

Assessment of the patient with a leg length discrepancy

True and apparent shortening

It is fundamental to distinguish between true and apparent shortening and to bear in mind that some patients have both. Fixed deformities of the hips should be corrected before considering other equalization procedures. If an upper femoral osteotomy is required to adjust the neck–shaft angle, then the true leg length may well be altered by about 1.5 cm; this must be allowed for in determining the correction required for apparent deformity. Occasionally it is appropriate to add a formal femoral shortening to such a procedure.

A special problem arises in the child with a short leg secondary to a poor outcome of treatment for congenital dislocation of the hip. Osteotomies in this instance need to be carefully planned since the future of the hip joint is of equal importance to the correction of the leg length discrepancy. A preoperative arthrogram is often helpful; an abduction osteotomy may uncover the femoral head and need to be combined with some sort of acetabular shelf procedure, and perhaps a trochanteric epiphysiodesis should be added to the operation. A Salter osteotomy may improve the cover of the femoral head and add a little to leg length. On occasion, a more ambitious trans-iliac lengthening may be contemplated.

A true leg length discrepancy associated with fixed pelvic obliquity and scoliosis needs to be regarded with caution. It may well be to the patient's advantage to have a short leg on the 'downhill' side of the pelvis. Correction of true leg length in such a patient may render it difficult for them to compensate for an unbalanced scoliosis and may interfere with walking.

Measurement of the discrepancy

By tape It is traditional to measure true leg length with a tape measure as the distance from the anterior superior iliac spine to the medial malleolus, but this can be misleading. First, pelvic asymmetry occurs if the triradiate cartilage is damaged early in life by infection or radiotherapy, and as a consequence the anterior spines are at different levels. Second, in patients treated for congenital dislocation of the hip, the anterior spine may have been removed. Third, deformities of the hindfoot can alter leg length. The distance between the medial malleolus and the sole will be increased if the hindfoot is in calcaneus or decreased if there is a congenital hindfoot coalition.

Blocks The estimation of leg length discrepancy using blocks may seem crude but in the absence of pelvic obliquity or fixed deformity of the hips it is the most accurate guide to the amount of correction required. The effect of leg length equalization on the hip joints can be studied on a standing radiograph of the pelvis taken using appropriate blocks.

Scanogram This gives a very accurate measurement from hip to ankle providing both legs will lie flat on the X-ray table. It is a useful method for monitoring limb growth and discrepancy and determining exactly how much shortening is in the femur and how much is in the tibia. In the presence of complex deformities it can be very helpful to see the whole of both lower limbs on one film. More recently CT scanograms have proved quicker to perform and easier to measure and store.

In practice all three methods of measurement are used and should there be a discrepancy in the results obtained from different methods an explanation must be sought.

Assessment of associated abnormalities

It is strongly recommended that a systematic list is made of all the features which adversely affect the patient's stance and gait (*see Table 1*). If leg length discrepancy does not stand out as being a major contributor to the problem, then an equalization procedure will not on its own result in much improvement. Furthermore, there are some specific abnormalities that will rule out one or more of the treatment options. For example, instability of the hip owing to acetabular dysplasia and instability of the knee owing to congenital ligament deficiency are both contraindications to femoral lengthening on the grounds that a major joint dislocation is liable to occur.

Patients with severe limb dysplasias will not be candidates for leg equalization procedures. If the foot is deemed to be useless an early Syme's amputation may be the correct decision; if the length at maturity will be out of range of leg lengthening techniques then there is no alternative but to treat the problem with a suitable orthosis or prosthesis.

Monitoring the patient and predicting the discrepancy

If patients are referred early, which is advisable, their maturation and leg length discrepancy can be monitored on an annual basis. The parental height is noted and the child's height standing on the normal leg is recorded on a growth chart. Skeletal age should be estimated between the age of 10 and 12 years to rule out any serious abnormality of skeletal development. Predicting the patient's overall height at maturity is necessary in choosing a sensible course of action.

An accurate prediction of the discrepancy at maturity is also fundamental if epiphysiodesis is to be performed at the correct time or if leg lengthening is to be performed much before the end of growth. In the latter instance, an over-lengthening may be indicated. The methods of prediction all assume that growth proceeds in a linear fashion. There are three main methods of prediction: (1) the White/Menelaus method; (2) the Anderson–Green method; and (3) Moseley's straight-line graph.

As well as monitoring growth, the annual visit allows the surgeon to check on the progress of any associated deformities, perhaps offer a shoe-raise as an interim measure, and to get to know the patient and parents. An assessment of character, emotional stability and motivation are important because leg lengthening should not easily be recommended for the faint-hearted or the uncooperative. The realistic expectations of surgery and a knowledge of the complications that can occur must be imparted to the patient.

Table 1 Associated abnormalities to be looked for in the spine and involved leg

Spine	Structural scoliosis
	Mobility
Pelvis	Fixed pelvic obliquity
	Asymmetry
Hip	Soft tissue contracture
	Bony deformity
	Dysplasia
	Muscle weakness (Trendelenburg-positive)
Femur	Deformity (angular or rotational)
Knee	Soft tissue contracture
	Bony deformity
	Dislocation of patella
	Ligamentous instability
Tibia	Deformity (angular or rotational)
Ankle	Soft tissue contracture
	Bony deformity
	Absent fibula
	Ball-and-socket joint
Foot	Soft tissue contracture
	Bony deformity
	Dysplasia
General	Muscle – wasting
	– weakness
	– fibrosis
	Neurovascular abnormalities
	Congenital fibrous bands

Possible procedures and indications

Shortening the long leg

These procedures are ideal if the long leg is the abnormal one. If the patient tends to stand and walk with the knee of the long leg slightly flexed, then procedures that shorten the long leg will not significantly reduce the effective height of the patient.

Epiphysiodesis

Permanent epiphysiodesis is preferable to stapling. Only one operation is required and the complication rate is lower. Staples can displace or break and removal of staples is not always followed by the normal resumption of growth. As already stated, the timing of epiphysiodesis is critical and depends on predictions that the short leg will continue to grow at a specific rate until maturity. The operation that is described has the advantage that it is the smallest and least disruptive of all the leg equalization procedures. It requires the shortest hospital admission and recovery should be complete in 6 weeks. It may be superseded in the future by a reliable method of performing transcutaneous epiphysiodesis.

The disadvantages are that the predictions are not always realized in practice and it is therefore the least accurate method of correcting a discrepancy. Because of this inaccuracy it is wise to aim at reducing the discrepancy to 1 cm since the patient is usually displeased if the procedure converts the longer leg into the shorter one. From a cosmetic point of view the scarring is sometimes obvious and there may be a delay between the time of operation and the cessation of growth. Parental worry occurs because the operation is usually performed on the normal leg and the surgery must be followed by careful follow-up.

The indications for epiphysiodesis follow.

1. If there is sufficient growth left to effect a correction
2. If the patient is growing on or above the 50th centile and will be taller than average height
3. If the discrepancy is 6 cm or less; with increasing discrepancy, the potential for error is magnified.

Femoral and tibial shortening

These procedures are precise if applied once skeletal maturity has been reached. Good internal fixation allows early mobilization; and using the method to be described for the femur, postoperative muscle weakness and non-union are most unlikely. Shortening necessarily leads to an increase in soft-tissue bulk, but if the femur is shortened proximally, this bulkiness and the scarring are not visible when normal clothes are worn.

Tibial shortening gives a poor cosmetic result, and the muscles may never take up the slack. If more than 2 or 3 cm are resected there is liable to be a problem with skin closure and the vascularity of the limb may be threatened. There can be few indications for this procedure and it will not be described.

The indications for femoral shortening follow.

1. If the patient is skeletally mature
2. If the discrepancy is less than 6 cm

3. If the discrepancy is principally in the femur
4. If the patient is on or above the 50th centile.

Operations on the short leg

Femoral and tibial lengthening

Many methods of leg lengthening have been described and currently there is great interest in improving the distraction techniques. Advances in the design of distraction apparatus have allowed the lengthening to be performed on an ambulatory basis. The demonstration that a bone gap can consistently be bridged with callus without the need for bone grafting, and also the development of epiphyseal distraction, have revolutionized the approach and shortened the duration of treatment. Decisions have to be made about the choice of apparatus and the technique of lengthening to be employed. It is beyond the scope of this chapter to cover all these developments but the choices will be considered briefly.

Choice of apparatus The basic choice is between a single-bar distractor such as the Wagner or Orthofix (Biomet Ltd, Bridgend, UK) devices and a frame with all-round support such as the Ilizarov or Monticelli frames. The single-bar fixators are sturdy and compact and a minimum of soft tissues are transfixed by the pins. However, they fail frequently to keep perfect alignment during the lengthening. The Monticelli frame, on the other hand, will consistently produce a beautifully straight lengthened segment but it is bulky and more easily applied to the tibia than the femur.

Choice of site Diaphyseal lengthening allows both the upper and lower pins to be placed through solid cortical bone. Should internal fixation be necessary at a later date, then there is good bone stock on either side of the lengthened segment. One should bear in mind that plating is probably the easiest way to correct significant angular deformity at the end of lengthening, if the frame itself does not possess the capability.

Metaphyseal lengthening has the advantage that the callus response is more readily achieved when the lengthening is made through cancellous bone, but the pin fixation can be less reliable. Metaphyseal lengthening is the method of choice if deformity at this site is to be corrected concurrently with lengthening.

Epiphyseal lengthening has the advantage that no osteotomy is required. The lack of incisions is cosmetically attractive but the lengthening can be unusually painful. Nevertheless, a strong and wide lengthened segment can be produced which consolidates quickly. One has to assume that even if the distraction is performed slowly, at half a millimetre a day, and the growth-plate does not rupture, it still may not function normally at the end of the procedure.

A few surgeons have gained experience in synchronous lengthening of the femur and tibia of the same leg and of epiphyseal lengthening synchronously at the upper and lower end of the tibia. We have tended to tackle the bigger discrepancies by a combination of lengthening of one leg and shortening of the other.

LEG SHORTENING

EPIPHYSIODESIS

A preoperative radiograph is necessary to check the anatomy of the physis to be fused. The growth-plates are usually slightly convex towards the joint. Image intensification enables the surgeon to make small vertical incisions, 3.5 cm in length, centred at the correct level with certainty. Each growth-plate is approached from medial and lateral aspects; if femur and tibia are to be tackled, four separate incisions will give the most satisfactory cosmetic result. With the patient supine the limb is exsanguinated, draped and positioned on a thigh rest in 30°–40° of flexion.

Surgical approach

1a & b

Lower femoral physis

The lateral incision splits the fascia lata. The vastus lateralis is retracted forwards from the lateral intermuscular septum to expose the periosteum which overlies the physis. In a similar fashion, the medial incision splits the deep fascia 1 cm in front of the adductor tubercle and the vastus medialis is retracted forward from the medial intermuscular septum to expose the relevant portion of the femur. The origin of the medial ligament lies posteriorly and must not be disturbed. On both sides the superior geniculate arteries may have to be divided.

Upper tibial physis

The lateral incision is made just in front of the fibular head and the anterior aspect of this bone is exposed. The dissection is not carried posteriorly nor are retractors placed behind the fibular head for fear of damaging the common peroneal nerve. The tibia is exposed and the origins of peroneus longus and tibialis anterior are reflected downwards for 1 cm.

The anteromedial aspect of the growth-plate lies subcutaneously and its exposure poses no problems. The pes anserinus is retracted backwards as is the anterior margin of the medial ligament.

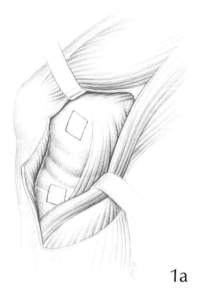

1a

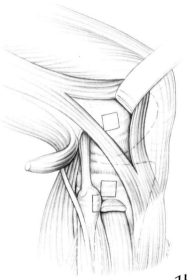

1b

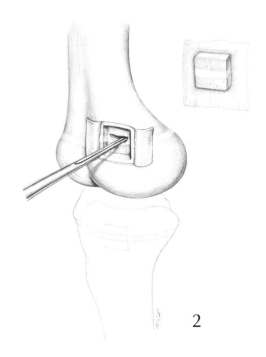

2

Technique

2 & 3

An I-shaped incision 2 cm long is made in the periosteum and the anterior and posterior osteoperiosteal flaps elevated with an osteotome. The physis is seen as a white line traversing the window that has been opened in the periosteum. Using a 1.5 cm osteotome, a square block of bone as deep as possible is removed with care; a curved osteotome will help to ease the block out. Then, with a small gauge or curette, as much of the growth-plate as possible is removed from the depths of the hole anteriorly, posteriorly and towards the centre of the bone. The same procedure is performed on the opposite side. The excavation of the growth-plate on medial and lateral sides should meet centrally.

When this has been achieved the bone blocks are rotated through 90° and punched back into the holes from which they were taken. The osteoperiosteal flaps are sutured back in position over the bone blocks. The skin is sutured with a subcuticular suture and for comfort the limb is immobilized in a plaster of Paris cylinder for 2 weeks.

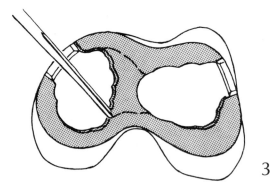

3

Postoperative management

Weight-bearing is allowed as comfort dictates and physiotherapy is commenced when the cast is removed. It usually takes 6 weeks for the knee to regain a full range of pain-free movement. Careful follow-up will determine if the expected correction is being achieved without the development of deformity. If only the femoral physis has been fused and the expected correction is not being achieved, fusion of the upper tibial physis may be performed at a later date.

FEMORAL SHORTENING

The patient is positioned on an orthopaedic table as for pinning of a fractured hip. The image intensifier is placed to give an anteroposterior view of the hip and the operated leg is held in neutral rotation and under slight traction.

The lateral aspect of the greater trochanter and upper femoral shaft are exposed in the standard way through a lateral incision which has to be lengthened, bearing in mind the size of the segment of femur to be removed (see chapter on 'Total hip replacement arthroplasty' pp. 943–964). The vastus lateralis is reflected off the bone anteriorly and the lesser trochanter identified. The exposure is maintained with two deep self-retaining retractors.

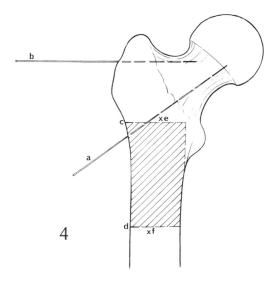

4

A guide wire (a) is inserted along the front of the femoral neck as a marker and advanced into the femoral head so that it stays in place. A second marker wire (b) is inserted in the mid-lateral line through the greater trochanter and onwards into the upper femoral neck at right angles to the femoral shaft. The bone to be resected is now marked out. The upper osteotomy is planned so that the lesser trochanter remains attached to the proximal fragment, and iliopsoas function will therefore be unimpaired. The level of the proximal osteotomy is opposite the upper margin of the lesser trochanter and a line (c) is made on the bone with an osteotome. The length of bone to be resected is measured with a ruler and the level of the lower cut (d) is marked. This length is checked. Two further longitudinal marks (e) and (f) are made so that rotational alignment (x–x) is not lost after the bone has been resected.

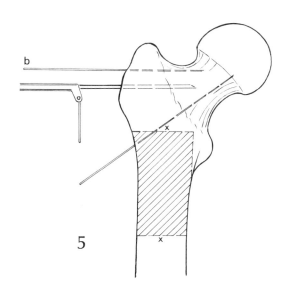

5

The seating chisel enters the greater trochanter 2 cm above the proximal osteotomy line. Its entry into the bone is facilitated by drilling the cortex with four or five small drill holes. The chisel fitted with the chisel guide is hammered into the centre of the femoral neck, parallel to and just below the guide wire (b), usually to a depth of 4–5 cm. The depth of insertion will dictate the size of the blade–plate. The seating chisel is eased back a little with the extractor to make its later removal easier but it is left in place as it will prove useful in controlling the proximal fragment, and it also gives the line of the proximal osteotomy.

6

It is important that the distal osteotomy is performed first. The cut is made at right angles to the shaft with a power saw, the blade being cooled with saline. This allows the proximal fragment to be abducted from the wound whilst the soft tissues are stripped from the medial aspect up as far as the lesser trochanter. It also makes it easier to cut the vertical limb of the proximal osteotomy. The proximal cut is made and the segment of bone removed.

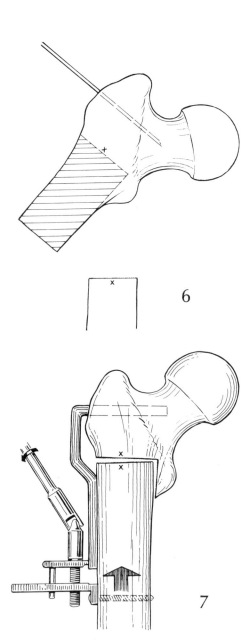

6

7

Traction on the limb is released and the two fragments brought together with due attention to the rotational markers. The seating chisel is removed and the right-angled blade–plate held on the driving device is hammered into the channel cut by the chisel. The plate is clamped to the shaft with a bone clamp and, if the cuts have been made correctly, the osteotomy should be open a little on its lateral aspect. This gap will close as compression is applied with the tensioning device.

7

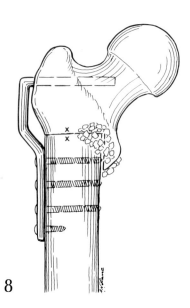

8

8

Once the osteotomy is compressed the plate is screwed to the bone and the tensioning device removed. Bone graft obtained from the medullary cavity of the excised segment is placed around the osteotomy. The wound is closed in layers over a suction drain.

Postoperative management

The leg is mobilized for 3 or 4 days in 'slings and springs' or on Hamilton Russell traction and the patient is then allowed partial weight-bearing on crutches. Union usually occurs by 8 weeks when full weight-bearing is allowed. The high level of bone resection should not give rise to any muscular weakness and the plate should not be removed for at least 1 year.

LEG LENGTHENING

On admission to hospital these patients should be assessed by a physiotherapist and taught shadow walking – how to walk with crutches without bearing weight. In the case of tibial lengthening, a foot-drop appliance is made which can be connected to the fixator.

FEMORAL LENGTHENING

The preferred method is a midshaft lengthening using a single-bar leg-lengthening device applied to the lateral aspect of the femur. Details specific to the type of fixator employed are not included in the description but are available from the manufacturers. The method of bone division is an oblique diaphyseal corticotomy.

Stage 1: Application of the apparatus

The patient, under general anaesthesia, is placed in the lateral position and the leg to be operated on is separately draped. An image intensifier is arranged so that it can be moved into place during the operation: with the C-arm above the operating table a horizontal beam will give an anteroposterior view of the femur which is essential for checking the placement of the pins.

Pin insertion

The four pins are placed in line 1 cm anterior to the mid-lateral line and the upper pin is inserted first. The technique of pin insertion is important. Large 6 mm cortical threaded pins are required.

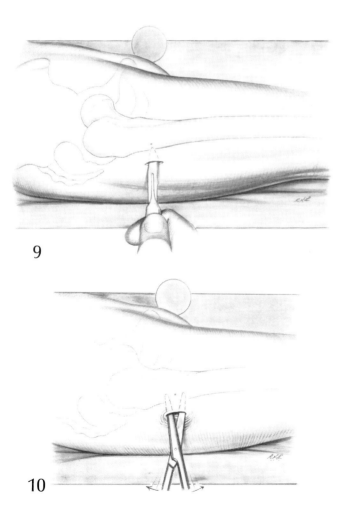

9

10

9 & 10

A deep longitudinal incision 1 cm long is made down to bone. A pair of blunt-tipped scissors are inserted into the track created and the blades opened to stretch the soft tissues.

11

A trocar and cannula are next inserted into the hole and by careful palpation the midline of the cortex is identified. This is important because the screw must pass through the middle of the bone and fix well to both cortices. The trocar must be held perpendicular to the long axis of the femur. The cannula is removed maintaining pressure on the trocar which is tapped gently with a hammer so that its teeth engage on the cortex.

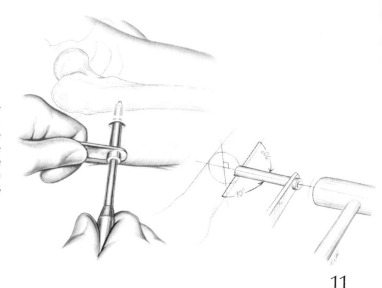

11

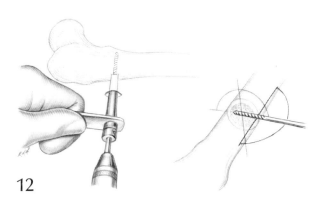

12

12

The femur is then drilled using the correct size drill bit. A low-speed power-drill gives good control and minimizes the risk of thermal necrosis. It is crucial that the drill is at a right angle to the long axis of the bone and this should be checked both by eye and with the image intensifier, especially when the first and most critical hole is made.

13

If the first pin is not inserted correctly then the template which is to be used next, and ultimately the external fixator, will not be parallel to the femoral shaft. It is important that the second cortex is completely penetrated. The pin of appropriate length and with a self-tapping tip is then inserted by hand. The screw should be tightened until at least two threads are seen to protrude beyond the far cortex. Should there be any heaping up of soft tissues around the pin, the skin incision must be extended to relieve this problem.

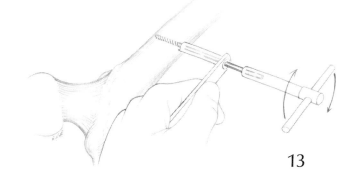

13

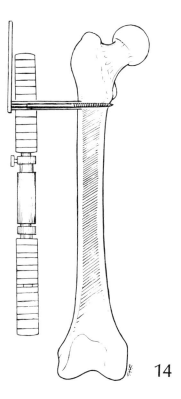

14

14 & 15

The template is passed over the proximal pin and if this has been correctly placed the template will lie parallel to the femoral shaft. The lowest pin is inserted next through the cortical bone that lies just above the femoral flare. The two remaining pins are now inserted and the template is removed. The knee is flexed fully to confirm that the soft tissues impaled by the pins will allow this movement. It is wise at this stage to adjust the leg-lengthening device so that it fits exactly over the pins in the position in which they have been inserted.

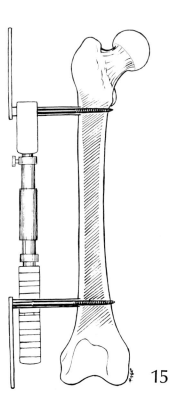

15

Stage 2: Soft tissue release and corticotomy

16

The midshaft of the femur is approached through a short posterolateral incision. The tensor fasciae latae is split longitudinally to expose the vastus lateralis. At the proximal end this split is carried anteriorly and at its distal end posteriorly, in effect forming a Z-cut in the fascia which will facilitate the lengthening.

17

The vastus lateralis is then reflected forwards and the lateral intermuscular septum is divided. A perforating branch of the femoral artery invariably needs to be secured as the femoral shaft is exposed. The periosteum must be treated with great care. It is incised longitudinally and stripped carefully off the bone. The intention is to divide the femur with a minimum of trauma and then to re-suture the periosteum. Four retractors are inserted subperiosteally to maintain the exposure.

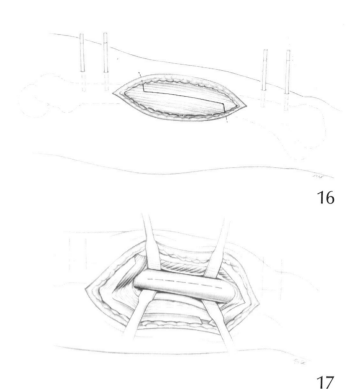

16

17

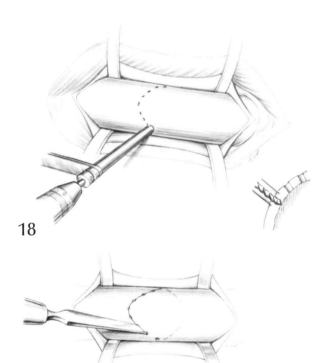

18

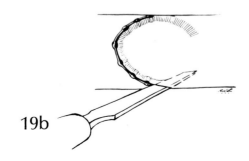

19a

19b

18, 19a & b

The bone is divided in an oblique fashion to present a greater surface area for callus formation. The oblique corticotomy is performed by, first, placing a small drill through a drill sleeve so that only 5 mm of the drill protrudes beyond the tip of the guide; drill holes are then made along the line of the proposed corticotomy. These are then joined together with a small osteotome without entering the medullary cavity. It is then possible to cut some way round the back of the bone beyond the limits of vision with the same instrument.

20

The osteotomy is completed by gently flexing the thigh until the far cortex cracks. The pins must not be used for leverage.

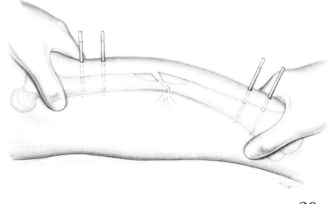

20

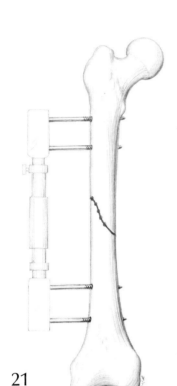

21

21 & 22

The leg lengthening device is then applied and the alignment at the femur checked. The periosteum is sutured back over the corticotomy and the wound closed in layers over a suction drain.

At the end of the procedure the fixator should be 2 cm clear of the skin to allow for postoperative swelling of the thigh. No distraction is performed at this stage. A Marcain (Astra Pharmaceuticals Ltd, Kings Langley, UK) femoral nerve block will reduce postoperative pain.

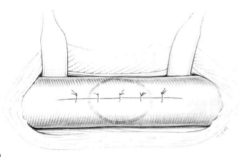

22

Stage 3: Distraction

A postoperative anteroposterior radiograph of the femur is taken to check the alignment and pin insertion. The drain is removed at 48 hours. Analgesia is prescribed as required and physiotherapy to encourage hip and knee flexion are commenced on day 1. As the pain subsides the patient is encouraged to shadow walk with crutches.

The lengthening device is left undisturbed for 2–3 weeks depending on the age of the patient. By then callus formation has commenced and the vascularity between the proximal and distal fragments should be re-established. The lengthening is commenced at the rate of 0.5 mm twice daily and alignment radiographs should be taken at 2-week intervals. The first film will confirm the separation at the corticotomy site and subsequent films will also show the quality of the callus response. If this response is poor the distraction should be discontinued for a week.

The pin sites are cleaned daily with an alcohol solution and redressed. Any crusts are removed. Should the skin heap up around the pins as lengthening proceeds it is a small procedure under local anaesthesia to make a relieving incision.

The distraction is continued until the desired length is achieved, but if complications intervene the distraction may have to be abandoned short of the objective. The distraction phase needs close supervision and should only be performed as an outpatient procedure if the patient is completely reliable.

Stage 4: Consolidation

Once the distraction is complete the bone must be protected from undue stress whilst the callus segment matures. Bone grafting at this stage is seldom necessary. There are three approaches to this problem (*see Illustrations 23, 24 and 25*).

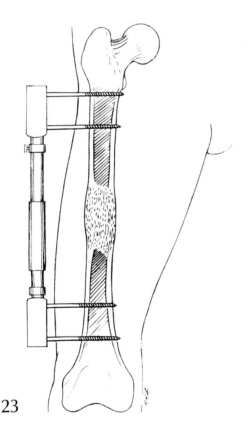

23

23

If the fixator is well tolerated and providing there is no angular deformity, it is preferable to leave the fixator in place for 5 or 6 weeks while the patient continues shadow walking. By then the callus will be strong enough to resist compressive forces and full weight-bearing is allowed. If the device allows the callus to be subjected to axial compression forces, the necessary adjustment to the device is made at this time. Full weight-bearing is continued until the callus begins to differentiate into cortex and medulla. It is then safe to remove the device but it is wise to revert to partial weight-bearing for 2 months and then gradually increase activities again.

24

If there is significant deformity at the end of lengthening, the best way of correcting this is by plating the femur through a posterolateral approach while removing the external fixator. At least four screws are required above and below the lengthened segment together with special heavy duty bridging plates which are not weakened in their central section by screw holes.

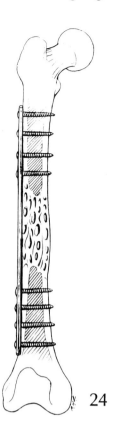

24

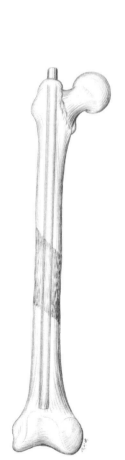

25

25

The third alternative is to stabilize the bone by means of closed femoral nailing. This can be performed at the stage when the callus is mature enough to resist axial compression forces. Nailing gives immediate whole-bone protection and facilitates the recovery of stiff joints as well as allowing early and safe weight-bearing. The risk is obviously that of infection and for this reason the fixator must be removed and the leg maintained on traction for 1–2 weeks so that the pin tracks are healed before closed nailing is performed.

TIBIAL LENGTHENING

The principles of lengthening the tibia are exactly the same as for the femur. For simplicity the diagrams are drawn with a single-bar fixator. As already stated, the Monticelli frame has the advantages of all-round support to which I have already referred.

Stages 1 and 2: Application of apparatus and corticotomy

26

The pins are inserted in the standard way through the subcutaneous border of the tibia. Under X-ray control an oblique midshaft corticotomy is made under vision exactly as for femoral lengthening.

Through a separate lateral incision at the same level 1 cm of fibula is excised and the interosseous membrane is also divided.

A third incision 1 cm long is made over the distal fibula and a diastasis screw is inserted in order to neutralize any distraction forces that may be imposed on the lateral malleolus. If the heel cord is tight preoperatively, it will have to be lengthened; and after passage of the diastasis screw, dorsiflexion of the foot is checked.

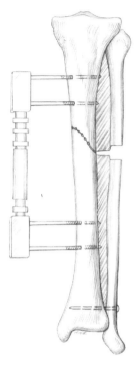

26

Stage 3: Distraction

The limb is elevated postoperatively and physiotherapy commenced. From day 1 the foot-drop spring-splint is worn. When pain and swelling subside the patient is allowed up on crutches, shadow walking. Lengthening is commenced at 2–3 weeks as for femoral lengthening and regular radiographs are taken to check alignment and the quality of callus formation.

Stage 4: Consolidation

27

The management during this phase depends on the callus response. It is invariably possible to maintain the fixator in place without the need for bone grafting or internal fixation. After 5–6 weeks of shadow walking, weight-bearing is increased and the lengthened segments subjected to axial compression forces if this is appropriate. As a rule of thumb, the device is left on for a further 1 week per centimetre lengthened. When this time has expired and if the radiograph shows good consolidation with the beginning of differentiation into cortex and medulla, the device is removed. Before the pins are removed it is wise to test the strength of the lengthened tibia.

The pin tracks are cleaned and a long-leg cast applied. Full weight-bearing is allowed and 2 weeks later the cast is removed. A cast-brace is applied for a further 6 weeks.

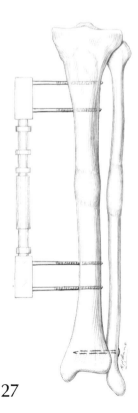

27

Complications

Complications are to be expected when leg lengthening is undertaken. Vigilance on the part of the surgeon will often lead to the recognition of problems as they emerge, and appropriate action at this stage will prevent serious trouble. Some of the more common complications are listed below.

Loss of patient compliance

Patients may tamper with the distraction device and make highly inappropriate adjustments. Some are unable to control their youthful exuberance for the duration of the lengthening, and foolish behaviour can result in unnecessary trauma to the limb.

Pin-track infection

This can be minimized by removal of crusts and regular cleansing of the skin around the pins with an alcoholic solution. A relieving incision is mandatory if the skin begins to heap up on one side of a pin. If there is surrounding erythema, antibiotics should be prescribed. Failure to control infection will lead to loosening of the pins and is a cause for their premature removal.

Loss of alignment

This will occur if the single-bar external fixator is not parallel to the bone, if the pins bend or if the attachment of the pin to the fixator fails. If the angulation is not corrected, further distraction tends to increase the deformity rather than increase the length.

Muscle contractures

Most of these problems are encountered in patients with congenital discrepancies. A slight preoperative contracture will become more pronounced during lengthening. Therefore prophylactic open adductor tenotomies, anterior hip releases, and lengthening of the hamstrings and heel cord are all occasionally indicated. Similar procedures are sometimes required at the end of lengthening. The importance of physiotherapy in minimizing contractures and keeping the joints as mobile as possible should not be underestimated.

Joint damage

Dislocation of the hip or knee is usually a forseeable complication and will seldom be encountered if femoral lengthening is avoided in patients who are at risk. A sudden increase in joint pain and stiffness should always arouse suspicion.

Pain

This can be a difficult problem and the cause must always be sought and not simply suppressed with analgesics. Epiphyseal lengthening is probably the most painful form of distraction, but pain is often encountered towards the end of lengthening and may be a reason to 'go slow'.

Neurovascular damage

This may complicate pin insertion but is remarkably rare during distraction performed at the correct rate.

Tibiofibular joint displacement

Downward migration of the head of the fibula will tighten up the lateral collateral ligament of the knee and cause fixed flexion deformity, whereas upward migration of the lateral malleolus will de-stabilize the ankle mortise. A correctly placed osteotomy and a diastasis screw should prevent these complications.

Complications of internal fixation

All the well-known complications can occur if internal fixation is employed. This includes infection, bent plates, screws pulling out, and fractures at one or other end of the plates.

Delayed union

If there is poor callus response, bone grafting is best performed early, using cancellous bone from the iliac crest. Non-union after leg lengthening is extremely rare.

Fractures

Fractures may occur at a variety of sites and times and include the following.

1. Early fracture at one end of the lengthened segment when the fixator is removed
2. Fracture at the level of the end of a plate
3. Fracture away from the site of lengthening related to disuse osteoporosis
4. Late stress fractures through a lengthened segment usually in the presence of a slight deformity.

Further reading

General

Symposium. Equalization of leg length. *Clin Orthop* 1978; 136: 1–312.

Coleman SS. Lower limb length discrepancy. In: Lovell WW, Winter RB, eds. *Pediatric orthopaedics,* 2nd ed. Philadelphia: Lippincott, 1986: 781–863.

Growth prediction

Anderson M, Messner MB, Green WT. Distribution of lengths of the normal femur and tibia in children from one to eighteen years of age. *J Bone Joint Surg [Am]* 1964; 46-A: 1197–1202.

Anderson M, Green WT, Messner MB. Growth and predictions of growth in the lower extremeties. *J Bone Joint Surg [Am]* 1963; 45-A: 1–14.

Menelaus MB. Correction of leg length discrepancy by epiphyseal arrest. *J Bone Joint Surg [Br]* 1966; 48-B: 336–9.

Moseley CF. A straight line graph for leg length discrepancies. *J Bone Joint Surg [Am]* 1977; 59-A: 174–9.

Leg lengthening

Armour PL, Scott JHS. Equalisation of leg length. *J Bone Joint Surg [Br]* 1981; 63-B: 587–92.

De Bastiani G, Aldegheri R, Brivio LR, Trivella G. Chondrodiatasis – controlled symmetrical distraction of the epiphyseal plate: limb lengthening in children. *J Bone Joint Surg [Br]* 1986; 68-B: 550–6.

Hood RW, Riseborough EJ. Lengthening of the lower extremity by the Wagner method: a review of the Boston children's hospital experience. *J Bone Joint Surg [Am]* 1981; 63-A: 1121–31.

Monticelli G, Spinelli R. Distraction epiphysiolysis as a method of limb lengthening. III. Clinical applications. *Clin Orthop* 1981; 154: 274–85.

Wagner H. Surgical lengthening or shortening of femur and tibia: technique and indications. In: Hungerford DS. *Progress in orthopaedic surgery.* Berlin: Springer-Verlag, 1977.

Illustrations by Peter Cox after F. Price

Distal gastrocnemius release

W. J. W. Sharrard   MD, ChM, FRCS
Emeritus Consultant Orthopaedic Surgeon, Royal Hallamshire Hospital and Children's Hospital, Sheffield;
Professor of Orthopaedic Surgery, University of Sheffield, UK

Preoperative

Indications and assessment

There is a limited indication for this operation for specific shortness of the gastrocnemius muscles in cerebral palsy and occasionally in other paralytic conditions. Shortness of the gastrocnemii is assessed by determining the range of dorsiflexion of the ankle with the knee extended compared with the range with the knee flexed. If there is a full or adequate range of dorsiflexion with the knee flexed but it is less than a right angle with the knee extended, shortness of the gastrocnemii is present. The condition is particularly likely to present in diplegic cerebral palsy, when it usually develops bilaterally. Gastrocnemius release is not indicated when there is equinus deformity which does not alter when the knee is flexed.

Anaesthesia and position of patient

General anaesthesia is needed. The shortness of the gastrocnemius is confirmed with the patient anaesthetized. The limb is exsanguinated by elevation for a minute and inflation of a cuff tourniquet on the upper thigh. The patient is placed prone with a sandbag under the anterior aspect of the thigh to lift the limb away from the operating table so that the ankles can be dorsiflexed. The skin is prepared and the lower limbs are covered to the level of the mid-thigh by sterile stockinette stuck to the posterior aspect of each calf with adhesive solution, or an oval is cut out of the stockinette in the region of the calf and the operative area is covered by an adhesive transparent drape.

Operation

Incision

1

A posterior longitudinal incision 8–12 cm long is made in the midline of the calf centred half-way between the knee and the ankle. The incision is deepened through the subcutaneous fat. Immediately beneath the fat layer the sural vein and the sural nerve need to be identified and retracted medially or laterally.

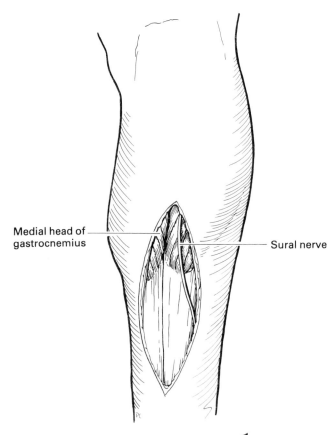

Medial head of gastrocnemius

Sural nerve

1

Exposure and division of the gastrocnemius tendons

2a & b

The two bellies of the gastrocnemius muscle and their flattened aponeurotic tendons are exposed by a vertical incision through the deep fascia.

The midline gap between the distal ends of the bellies of the muscle and the tendons arising from them is identified by blunt dissection. The medial side of the tendon of the medial gastrocnemius is identified by blunt dissection and a MacDonald blunt dissector passed transversely beneath the tendon to the midline. Care must be taken to separate the gastrocnemius tendon from the soleus aponeurosis deep to it, with which it blends distally. The gastrocnemius tendon is divided transversely by cutting down onto the blunt dissector. The tendon is mobilized upwards, separating some weak fascial attachments laterally.

The lateral gastrocnemius tendon is similarly identified on its lateral side, separated from the soleus by a MacDonald blunt dissector, divided and mobilized upwards. At this point, the whole of the gastrocnemius insertion should be freely mobile so that, when the ankle is dorsiflexed keeping the knee straight, the soleus aponeurosis and the distal stumps of the gastrocnemius tendon can be seen to move distally whilst the proximal tendons and muscle bellies of the gastrocnemius remain static and, in effect, retract upwards.

The proximal tendons can be sutured with one or two fine non-absorbable sutures to the underlying soleus aponeurosis but this is not strictly necessary since the tendons will remain proximally displaced when the knee is extended and the ankle dorsiflexed.

Wound closure

The wound is closed by interrupted or continuous non-absorbable sutures to the deep fascia and interrupted absorbable sutures to the subcutaneous fat. The skin is sutured by a subcuticular absorbable suture or by interrupted non-absorbable sutures.

The patient is turned into the supine position, the tourniquets removed and plaster cast applied from the groin to the toes with the knee fully extended and the ankle dorsiflexed as fully as possible. Overcorrection does not occur.

Postoperative management

The circulation to the toes needs to be observed for the first 24 hours. The patient can then return home. Plaster fixation is maintained for 3½ weeks, the patient being allowed to bear weight on the plaster after the tenth day. After the plaster is removed, physiotherapy is given to encourage activity and walking function.

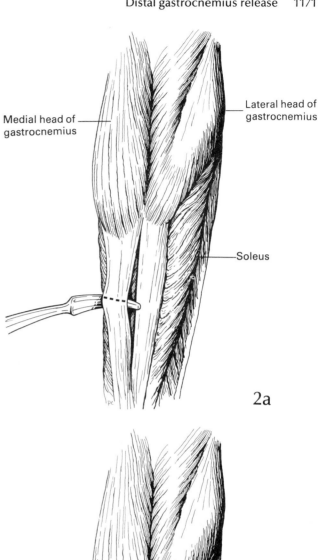

Medial head of gastrocnemius

Lateral head of gastrocnemius

Soleus

2a

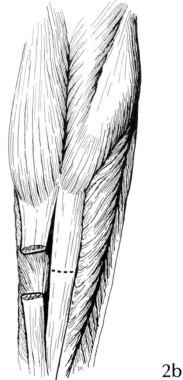

2b

Further reading

Strayer LM. Recession of the gastrocnemius: an operation to relieve spastic contracture of the calf muscles. *J Bone Joint Surg [Am]* 1950; 32-A: 671–6.

Lengthening and repair of the tendo Achillis

B. Helal MChOrth, FRCS
Honorary Consultant Orthopaedic Surgeon, The Royal London Hospital and The Royal National Orthopaedic Hospital, London, and Enfield Group of Hospitals, UK

S. C. Chen FRCS
Consultant Orthopaedic Surgeon, Enfield Group of Hospitals, UK

Introduction

The tendo Achillis may be tight as a result of upper motor neurone problems or secondary to muscle contracture. Degenerative changes due to overuse, injury, or urate deposits in gout give rise to peritendinitis and possibly partial or total rupture. Injections of steroid may also cause rupture. The methods described below deal with these problems.

LENGTHENING

This procedure is used to correct an equinus deformity of the ankle which may arise from a variety of conditions such as cerebral palsy, longstanding lateral popliteal nerve injury or inadequate splintage following ankle injuries. If the equinus deformity is severe or longstanding then release of the posterior ankle joint capsule and tibialis posterior may be necessary. In addition, gastrocnemius release can be performed to achieve further lengthening.

INCOMPLETE TENOTOMY[1]

The advantage of this technique is that a large incision is avoided. It is of limited use in severe contractures as no exposure is made of other tight structures such as tibialis posterior and the posterior joint capsule.

In performing this procedure, it must be remembered that the fibres of the tendo Achillis spiral through almost 90° from their insertion to their origin. Viewed from behind, the rotation is from medial to lateral.

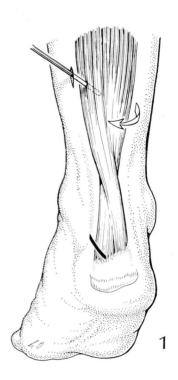

Incisions

1

A tiny skin incision is made on the medial side of the tendo Achillis at its insertion. The anterior two-thirds of the tendo Achillis is cut. This is best done by inserting a tenotome into the substance of the tendo Achillis at the junction of the middle third and posterior third of the tendon and cutting forwards.

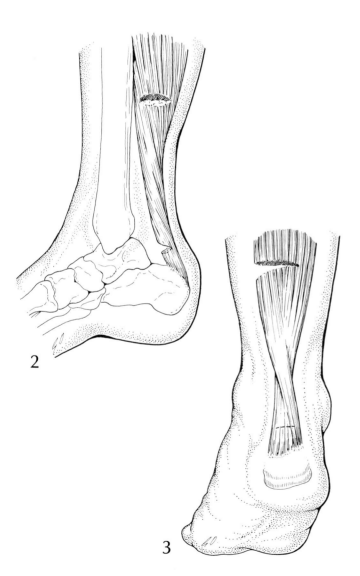

2 & 3

Another short incision is made on the medial side of the tendo Achillis at its musculotendinous junction. With the ankle in dorsiflexion the medial two-thirds of the tendon is divided at the musculotendinous junction. Dorsiflexion of the ankle lengthens the tendo Achillis and stitches are not necessary.

Postoperative management

A below-knee plaster cast is applied with the ankle in neutral position. At the end of 6 weeks the plaster is removed and ankle exercises commenced.

Z-PLASTY OF TENDO ACHILLIS

In severe contractures of the tendo Achillis it is necessary
to lengthen it by complete division of the tendon.

Incision

4

A straight vertical incision is made down the back of the
ankle. A Z-shaped incision is made in the tendo Achillis so
that the lateral half of the tendon is attached to the
calcaneum.

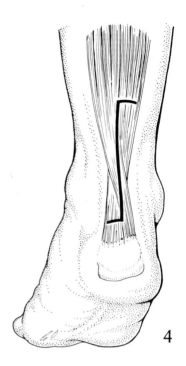

4

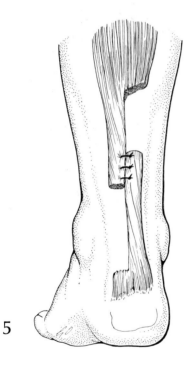

5

Repair

5

The foot is brought up to the neutral position and the
tendo Achillis sutured together with three thick synthetic
slowly absorbable sutures (polydioxanone-PDS). The deep
fascia is sutured carefully and the skin wound closed.

Postoperative management

A below-knee plaster cast is applied with the ankle in
neutral position. It is removed after 6 weeks and ankle
exercises started.

Gastrocnemius contracture

The calf muscles consist of the gastrocnemius which arises proximal to the knee joint, and the soleus which is attached distal to the knee.

Usually both muscles contribute to the equinus deformity, but occasionally the gastrocnemius is mainly affected. It is relatively easy to distinguish between the two types. Where the gastrocnemius only is affected, the equinus deformity disappears when the knee is flexed; whereas where both muscles are affected, knee flexion does not influence the equinus deformity.

The functional result is better when the soleus is not lengthened. The gastrocnemius can be detached from its proximal attachment to the posterior part of the femoral condyles (Silfverskiöld operation) or divided distally (Strayer operation).

PROXIMAL DETACHMENT OF THE GASTROCNEMIUS (Silfverskiöld operation[2])

Incision

6

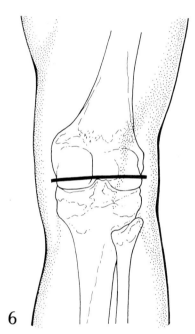

The patient lies prone, and the operation performed under tourniquet control. A transverse incision is made across the popliteal space along the joint crease, extending from the medial hamstring to the lateral hamstring muscles. Care must be taken not to damage the lateral popliteal nerve as well as the tibial nerves and vessels.

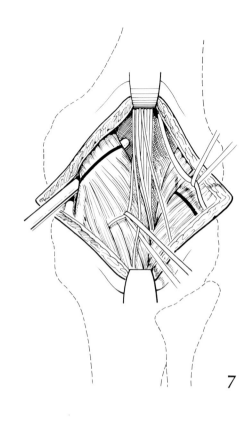

7

Dissection

7 & 8

The deep fascia is incised, and the two heads of gastrocnemius are identified. It may be necessary to divide the motor branches to the gastrocnemius from the tibial nerve if the gastrocnemius is grossly hypertonic. The heads of gastrocnemius are elevated from the posterior aspect of the femoral condyles by blunt dissection, and divided close to bone. The deep fascia, fat and skin are sutured in layers.

Postoperative management

An above-knee plaster cast is applied with the ankle in dorsiflexion, and the knee fully extended. The plaster cast is removed at the end of 4 weeks and physiotherapy commenced.

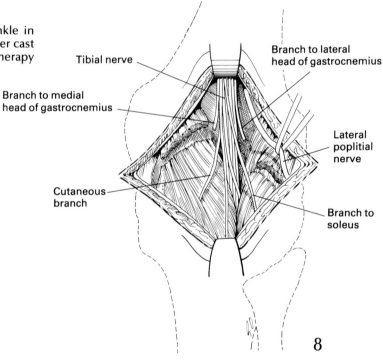

Tibial nerve

Branch to lateral head of gastrocnemius

Branch to medial head of gastrocnemius

Lateral poplitial nerve

Cutaneous branch

Branch to soleus

8

DISTAL DIVISION OF THE GASTROCNEMIUS (Strayer operation[3])

Incision

9

The patient lies prone, and the operation is performed under tourniquet control. A vertical incision is made down the middle of the calf. The sural nerve medially, and the superficial peroneal nerve laterally, are identified and protected.

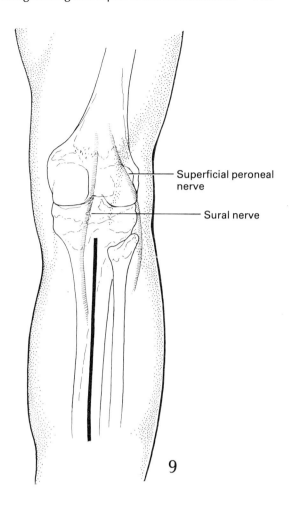

Superficial peroneal nerve

Sural nerve

9

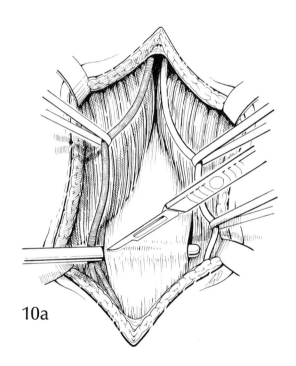

10a

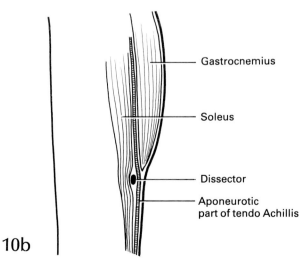

Gastrocnemius

Soleus

Dissector

Aponeurotic part of tendo Achillis

10b

Dissection

10a & b

The deep fascia is incised in line with the skin incision, and the calf muscles exposed. The gastrocnemius is separated from the deeper soleus muscle by blunt dissection which is extended distally to the common tendo Achillis.

11

The gastrocnemius is divided at its musculotendinous junction. The ankle is dorsiflexed to separate the cut gastrocnemius. The muscle bellies of the gastrocnemius may have to be dissected off the deeper soleus to obtain adequate dorsiflexion of the ankle. Sometimes the aponeurosis of the soleus may be contracted and has to be incised, taking care not to damage the soleus muscle itself.

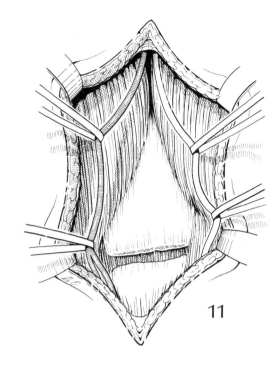

11

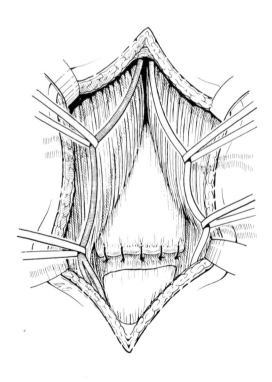

Closure

12

The proximal cut end of the gastrocnemius is sutured to the underlying aponeurosis of the soleus with interrupted sutures, whilst the ankle is kept fully dorsiflexed. The wound is closed in layers.

Postoperative management

An above-knee plaster cast is applied with the ankle in dorsiflexion, and the knee fully extended. The plaster cast is removed at the end of 4 weeks and physiotherapy started.

REPAIR

Ruptures of the tendo Achillis usually present acutely. However, the diagnosis is not always easy and some patients present with chronic ruptures weeks or months after the injury. The operative techniques will be considered separately.

Acute rupture of the tendo Achillis

This condition usually occurs following an acute injury to a degenerate tendon and is therefore most common after the age of 40 years.

The history is typical: the patient experiences sudden severe pain behind his ankle and, thinking that he has received a kick or blow, may strike out at any unfortunate individual who might happen to be behind him.

Diagnosis

Diagnosis of this condition can be difficult as the flexors of the toes can still plantarflex the ankle. Two clinical signs are very useful.

1. The patient cannot stand on tiptoe on the affected leg.
2. When the patient is lying prone with the feet over the end of the examination couch, squeezing of the relaxed calf muscles will not cause plantarflexion of the ankle if the tendo Achillis is ruptured, whereas the ankle will plantarflex if the tendo Achillis is intact (Simmonds' and Thompson's test[4, 5]).

A gap in the tendo Achillis is not always palpable due either to incomplete separation of the frayed and ruptured ends or to congealed blood in the gap.

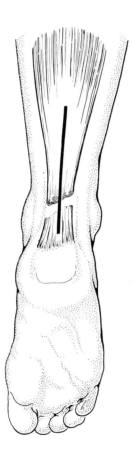

13

OPEN REPAIR

Incision

13

A vertical incision is made straight down the back of the lower leg, taking care not to extend down to the calcaneum. The deep fascia is divided to expose the ruptured tendo Achillis. (Skin healing is a problem and it is important not to curve the skin incision or extend it too far distally.)

Repair

14

The ruptured tendo Achillis usually frays, and it is not possible to insert any sutures which will take tension. However, by plantarflexing the ankle, the frayed ends of the tendo Achillis can be brought together with one non-absorbable suture using the Kessler technique[6]. The frayed ends are approximated as well as is possible with several chromic catgut sutures.

Closure

The deep fascia is stitched carefully and the skin closed with interrupted sutures taking care not to invert the skin edges.

Postoperative management

A below-knee plaster cast is applied from the toes to the tibial tuberosity with the foot in equinus. At the end of 3 weeks the skin sutures are removed and another plaster cast reapplied but with the foot in as near a neutral position as possible. After 6 weeks the plaster cast is removed and ankle exercises started. Full weight-bearing is started when the ankle can dorsiflex to neutral.

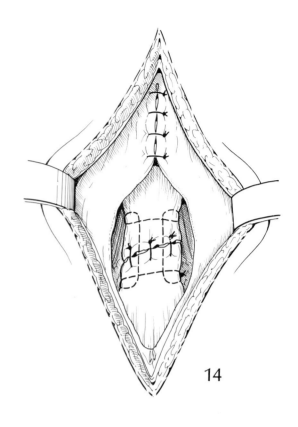

14

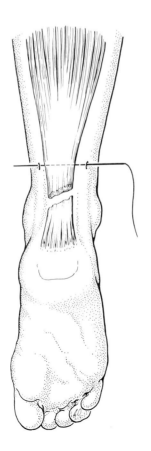

15

CLOSED REPAIR (Ma and Griffith[7])

The problem with open repair of an acutely ruptured tendo Achillis is skin healing. The vascularity of the skin in this area is poor, and injudicious skin incisions and rough retraction compromise an already poor blood supply.

Position of patient

The patient lies prone, and the operation is performed under tourniquet control. The gap in the tendo Achillis is assessed. The ankle is held plantarflexed throughout the procedure so that the tendon ends are approximated, and the subcutaneous tissue and skin are relaxed. This allows for the various manoeuvres to be carried out.

Stab incisions

15

A stab incision is made on the lateral side of the tendon about 3 cm proximal to the rupture. A No. 1 non-absorbable suture on a straight needle is passed transversely across in the substance of the tendon. As the tip of the needle comes out through the skin on the medial side it makes another stab wound in the skin.

16

The two ends are mounted on straight cutting needles and passed obliquely across to the other side, to come out just proximal to the ruptured end, making sure that the needles are still in the substance of the tendon. Two stab wounds are made in the skin at the point of exit on either side, distal to the other end of the rupture – that part of the tendon which is still attached to the calcaneum.

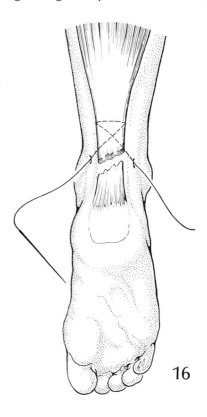

16

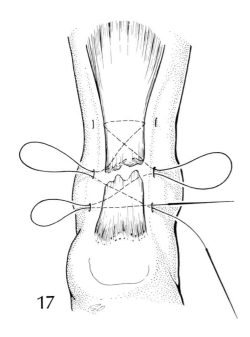

17

17

The straight needle on the medial side is driven transversely across the substance of the distal tendon stump about 2–3 cm away from the ruptured end. This comes out through the previously made stab wound on the lateral side.

It must be ensured that the suture is freed from the subcutaneous tissue and lying tightly within the substance of both parts of the ruptured tendon.

Suture of wounds

18

The suture is then knotted on the lateral side, making sure that the tendon ends are brought together. This can be observed through the medial stab wound. The several stab wounds are sutured with one stitch to each wound.

Postoperative management

A non-weight-bearing below-knee plaster cast is applied with the ankle plantarflexed for 4 weeks. This is followed by a further 4 weeks in a weight-bearing cast with the foot brought up, as near as possible without force, to a plantigrade position. Physiotherapy is then started.

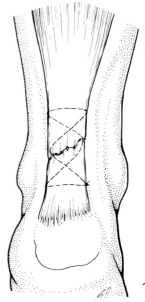

18

Old ruptures

The calf muscles retract in old ruptures and a gap is almost always present in the tendo Achillis.

Incision

19

As before, a straight vertical incision is made down the back of the leg, taking care not to extend it too far distally onto the calcaneum.

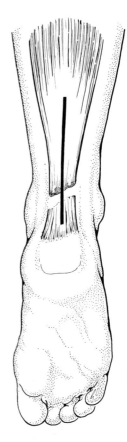

19

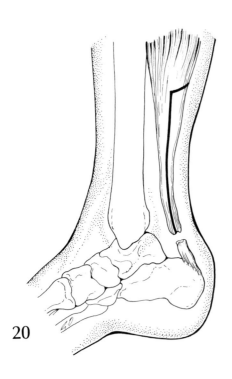

20

Division and slide

20

The ruptured ends of the tendo Achillis are identified – these are usually rounded off and thickened. They should be freshened.

An incision is made across the proximal segment of the tendo Achillis at the musculotendinous junction, directed downwards and forwards and cutting through the posterior half of the tendon.

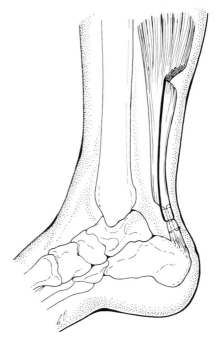

21

21 & 22

The posterior half of the tendon is slid downwards to approximate the tendon ends. The ends are sutured together using non-absorbable suture material. A Kessler grasping stitch is inserted and supplemented with several chromic catgut sutures, with the ankle in full plantar-flexion.

The tendon slide in the proximal segment of the tendo Achillis is also reinforced with chromic catgut sutures.

Postoperative management

A below-knee plaster cast is applied with the foot in equinus. The plaster cast is changed at 3 weeks, placing the ankle as near to the neutral position as possible. The plaster cast is removed at 6 weeks and passive and active exercises started.

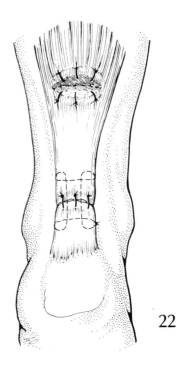

22

References

1. White JW. Torsion of the Achilles tendon; its surgical significance. *Arch Surg* 1943; 46: 784–7.

2. Silfverskiöld N. Reduction of the uncrossed two-joint muscles of the leg to one-joint muscles in spastic conditions. *Acta Chir Scand* 1923; 56: 315.

3. Strayer LM. Recession of the gastrocnemius: an operation to relieve spastic contracture of the calf muscles. *J Bone Joint Surg [Am]* 1950; 32-A: 671–6; 712.

4. Simmonds FA. Test for rupture of tendo Achillis. In: Apley AG. *A system of orthopaedics and fractures.* London: Butterworths, 1959.

5. Thompson TC. A test for rupture of the tendon Achillis. *Acta Orthop Scand* 1962; 32: 461–5.

6. Kessler I. The "grasping" technique for tendon repair. *Hand* 1973; 5: 253–5.

7. Ma GW, Griffith TG. Percutaneous repair of acute closed ruptured Achilles tendon: a new technique. *Clin Orthop* 1977; 128: 247.

Illustrations by Gillian Oliver after B. Hyams

Transfer of tibialis posterior tendon to the dorsum of the foot

B. Helal MChOrth, FRCS
Honorary Consultant Orthopaedic Surgeon, The Royal London Hospital and The Royal National Orthopaedic Hospital, London, and Enfield Group of Hospitals, UK

S. C. Chen FRCS
Consultant Orthopaedic Surgeon, Enfield Group of Hospitals, UK

Introduction

In poliomyelitis, leprosy, peripheral neuropathy or injury to the lateral popliteal nerve, the peroneal muscles and tibialis anterior may be paralysed leading to a foot drop deformity, but the tibialis posterior muscle may be normal. The tendon of this muscle can be transferred through the interosseous space onto the dorsum of the foot to restore dorsiflexion.

Operation

1

Two small skin incisions are made on the medial aspect of the foot and ankle: (*1*) posterior to the medial malleolus; and (*2*) at the attachment of the tibialis posterior to the navicular.

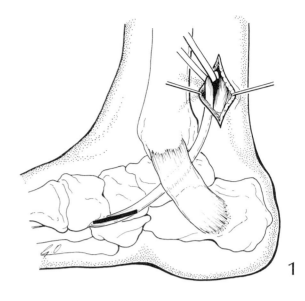

2

The tibialis posterior tendon is divided as near to the navicular attachment as possible and withdrawn into the proximal skin incision by pulling on it. The lower incision is closed.

A non-absorbable suture is attached to the end of the tendon using a Kessler stitch.

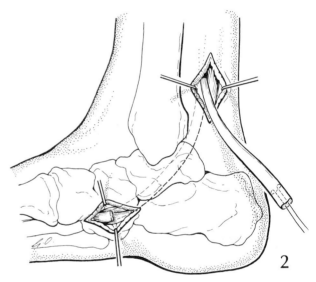

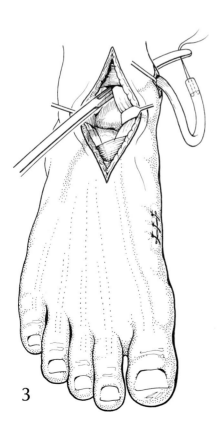

3

A third incision is then made on the front of the ankle.

The tendons and neurovascular bundle are retracted laterally and curved artery forceps are passed through the interosseous membrane. The artery forceps are opened in order to enlarge the hole in the interosseous membrane.

Next, the artery forceps are directed into the wound behind the medial malleolus. The end of the suture attached to the tibialis posterior tendon is grasped.

4

The tendon is pulled taut and the tibialis posterior muscle and tendon in the posterior compartment of the leg inspected to ensure that the tendon is not twisted and that the line of pull upon the intermediate cuneiform is straight. The tibialis posterior muscle is freed by blunt dissection if necessary.

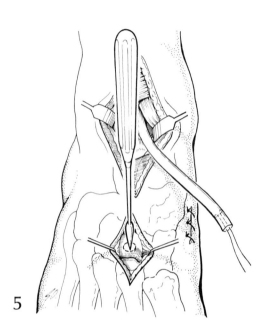

5

A final skin incision is made over the intermediate cuneiform. The bone is exposed and, with a Paton's burr, a hole is made in the centre of this bone large enough to thread the tibialis posterior tendon through.

6

The sutures are threaded through a large straight needle and this is passed through the hole in the intermediate cuneiform and through the sole of the foot. There is usually just sufficient length of posterior tibial tendon to pass into the cuneiform bone. The sutures are tied over a large button on the sole of the foot with the ankle in neutral position and with the tendon taut. The remaining skin incisions are closed.

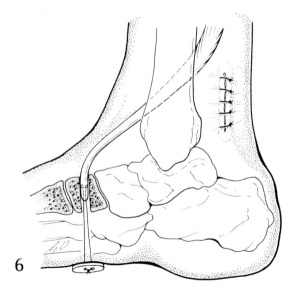

Postoperative management

A below-knee plaster cast is applied from the toes to the tibial tuberosity with the ankle in neutral position. No weight-bearing is allowed for 6 weeks. The plaster is removed at the end of 6 weeks and the sutures over the button undone. The button is removed and the sutures cut just deep to the skin. Passive and active ankle exercises are commenced.

Multiple tendon transfers into the heel

E. W. Somerville   FRCS (Ed), FRCS
Emeritus Consultant Orthopaedic Surgeon, Nuffield Orthopaedic Centre, Oxford, UK

Introduction

Indications

This operation is performed for the correction of calcaneocavus deformity of the foot in patients between the ages of 5 and 18 years. The deformity of calcaneocavus results from a pure muscle imbalance. In young people, where there is an isolated paralysis of the muscles inserted into the tendo Achillis, with all the other muscles of the calf acting normally, this deformity will always develop. The mechanism of the deformity is shown in *Illustrations 1 and 2*.

1

Plantarflexion of the foot is achieved by: the heel being drawn up by the gastrocnemius and soleus muscles; and the forefoot being pulled down by the other muscles of the calf which pass behind the malleoli and are attached to the plantar surface of the forefoot.

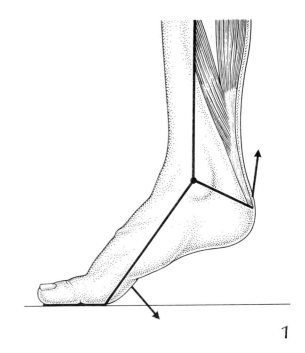

1

2

If the gastrocnemius and soleus muscles are paralysed or the tendon is cut and not repaired during the growth period, attempts to plantarflex the foot will result in the forefoot being pulled down without the heel being pulled up. The heel assumes an increasingly calcaneus position and the forefoot becomes increasingly plantarflexed until this position becomes fixed.

The hypertrophy of the tibialis anterior which is often seen in this condition is not related to the development of the deformity; rather, the hypertrophy results from dorsiflexion against a severe mechanical disadvantage.

Principle of treatment

The aim of surgical treatment is to remove the deforming force by taking the tendons which are inserted into the forefoot and transferring them to the heel where they will pull the tuberosity of the calcaneum upwards, thereby acting as a correcting force.

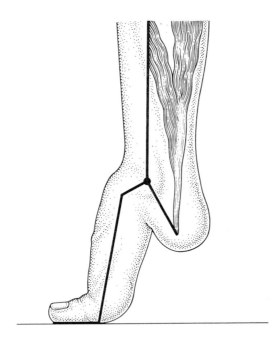

2

Operation

Position of patient

The patient is placed on the operating table in the prone position with a sandbag under the ankles so that the toes will not rest on the table when the foot is dorsiflexed.

Incision

3

A right-angled incision is made, the vertical limb of which extends from above and behind the medial malleolus downwards to the lower border of the calcaneum. It is situated one-third of the distance between the tendo Achillis and the medial malleolus. At the lower border of the calcaneum it turns at 90° posteriorly and laterally to pass round the back of the heel, finishing below the lateral malleolus at the level of the lower border of the calcaneum.

The skin flap, which must be kept as thick as possible, is turned up the smallest amount that will allow access to the tendons behind the medial malleolus and the peroneal tendons on the other side. The tendo Achillis is divided as its lower end is turned up, exposing the upper border of the calcaneum.

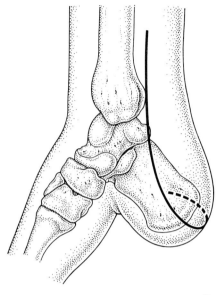

3

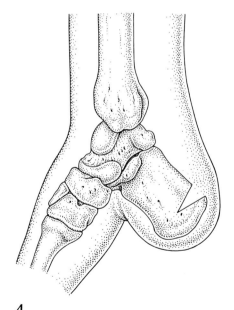

4

4

A groove is cut in the end of the calcaneum to a depth of 2.5 cm with an osteotome.

5a & b

The tibialis posterior, the flexor digitorum longus and the flexor hallucis longus tendons are divided behind the medial malleolus with as much length as possible and are stripped upwards so that they can be brought without kinking to the midline. The peroneal tendons are similarly treated. A strong catgut suture is introduced into each tendon, the ends being left very long. Holes of 0.8 mm (1/32 inch) are drilled from the posterior aspect of the calcaneum into the bottom of the groove. Using a Mayo trocar-ended needle each suture end is passed through one of these holes.

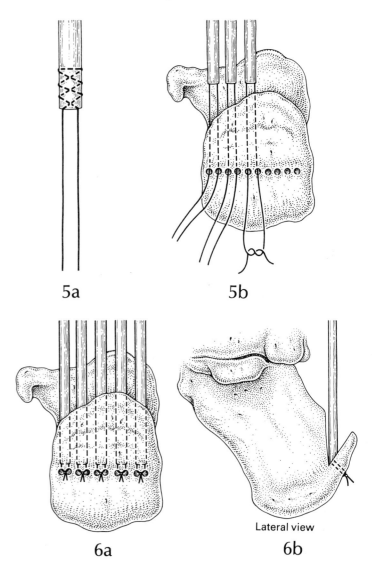

5a   5b

6a & b

When they have been passed through the heel is pushed upwards, which is quite different from the forefoot being pulled down, the tendons are pulled down as tightly as possible into the bottom of the groove and the sutures are tied over the bone.

Care must be taken to ensure that the tendons have been cut previously to a length which will only just allow them to reach the bottom of the groove. The skin flap is sutured back into position with as few interrupted sutures as possible.

Lateral view

6a   6b

Postoperative management

A well-padded below-knee plaster cast is applied with the heel pushed well upwards and extending distally to the end of the toes.

The leg is kept elevated until the postoperative swelling has settled, which may take a week. The leg should not be lowered too soon. The patient is then allowed to walk with crutches, but weight-bearing is not allowed until the plaster is removed at 6 weeks.

Comment

This operation is really the second half of the Jones' operation in which the tendon transfers are preceded by a formal stabilization of the foot to bring the forefoot in line with the calcaneum. When bony union is established the tendon transfers are carried out. The results of the tendon transfers alone in children up to at least the age of 18 years are so good that the bone operation is contraindicated. In adults, however, in whom the operation is rarely necessary, bone resection may be required. After the tendon transfer the restoration of the foot to a normal appearance is remarkably rapid and function is also rapidly restored.

Illustrations by Philip Wilson after G. Lyth

Arthrodeses of the ankle

E. W. Somerville FRCS(Ed), FRCS
Emeritus Consultant Orthopaedic Surgeon, Nuffield Orthopaedic Centre, Oxford, UK

Introduction

Arthrodesis of the ankle provides pain relief and stability in patients with a disorganized joint following ankle fractures, fractures of the talus or infections. Deformity and weakness secondary to neuromuscular diseases can be greatly alleviated by ankle stabilization. The best results occur in the young and those with healthy subtalar and tarsal joints.

Indications

1. To relieve pain in arthritic conditions or following severe trauma.
2. To stabilize the ankle in cases of drop foot where there is no deformity in the distal joints.

This is a better operation than the Lambrinudi operation, which is described in the chapter on 'Arthrodeses of the foot' (pp. 1199–1207), because it allows greater correction and there is no tendency to relapse. However, only small degrees of varus can be corrected at the ankle joint and marked varus is better corrected by the Lambrinudi procedure.

Operations

ANKLE ARTHRODESIS BY THE ANTERIOR APPROACH (WATSON-JONES)

Position of patient

The patient is placed on the operating table in the supine position with a small flat sandbag underneath the buttock.

Incision and exposure

1a & b

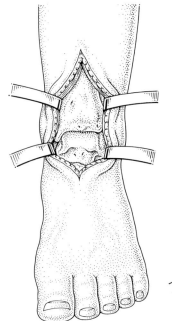

1a

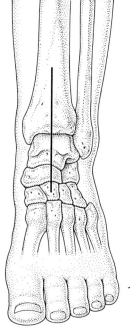

1b

An anterior incision is made 10 cm above the ankle joint extending to 5 cm below. The tibialis anterior tendon is exposed and, together with the tendon of the extensor hallucis longus, is retracted medially, the tendons of the extensor digitorum communis being retracted laterally. The tendon sheaths are preserved if possible. The dorsalis pedis artery will often have to be divided between ligatures but can sometimes be retracted out of the way. The anterior capsule of the ankle joint is then exposed.

The capsule is excised across the front of the joint to the tips of the malleoli which will allow the joint to be opened up widely with forced plantar flexion. Using a sharp chisel, rather than an osteotome, the articular surfaces are excised from the lower end of the tibia, the upper surface of the talus and from the lateral surfaces of the talus and the medial and lateral malleoli, if possible down to cancellous bone. Care must be taken to prevent the chisel from damaging important structures lying posterior to the ankle joint and the medial malleolus. The lower surface of the tibia and the upper surface of the talus are fitted together in the selected position for the foot, and the site for the graft in the talus is defined. The graft is outlined on the anterior surface of the tibia. The joint is again opened up so that the notch for the graft may be cut in the body of the talus. This notch will measure 13 mm wide, 19 mm deep and 10 mm anteroposteriorly. The bone removed is preserved for later use.

2

A graft 13 mm wide at the bottom, very slightly wider at the top and 7.5 cm in length, is cut from the anterior surface of the tibia with a circular saw and when freed is driven hard down into the talus. If it has been tapered correctly it will fit tightly into the lower part of the groove and into the notch. While the graft is being driven down heavy counterpressure must be applied to the undersurface of the heel to prevent distraction of the talus and tibia. Since excising the articular surfaces will have made the talus smaller and the joint mortise bigger there will be gaps on one or both sides which must be filled with the bone which was previously removed and with other cancellous bone from the tibia.

Wound closure

The tendons are allowed to resume their normal position and are held in place by lightly suturing the extensor retinaculum. The wound is closed in layers.

Postoperative management

A long leg plaster cast is applied with the knee slightly bent to control rotation. For this reason a short plaster must not be used. The leg is elevated for several days until the postoperative reaction is over, when the patient is allowed up on crutches without weight-bearing. A walking heel is applied at 6 weeks but the plaster should not be reduced to below-knee before 10 weeks. Union should be sound in 4 months but may sometimes be slower.

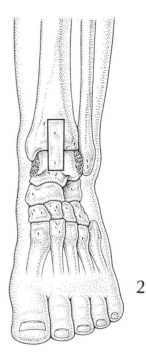

2

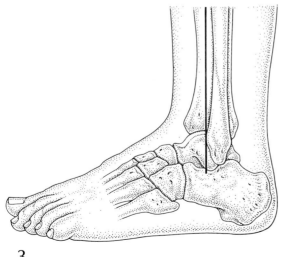

3

ANKLE ARTHRODESIS BY THE LATERAL APPROACH

Position of patient

The patient is placed on the operating table in the supine position with a large sandbag under the buttock on the operation side so that he is tilted into the semilateral position.

Incision and exposure

3

A straight incision 13 cm in length is made over the anterior border of the lower fibula extending to just below the tip of the lateral malleolus. The fibula is exposed subperiosteally and anteriorly and posteriorly within the limits of the incision but anteriorly the exposure is carried to the middle of the tibia.

4

With a small circular saw the adjacent surfaces of tibia and fibula are excised including the inferior tibiofibular joint, the articular surfaces of the lateral malleolus and the lateral side of the talus. This excision is carried 6.5 cm above the ankle joint at which level the fibula is divided. The fibula, together with the excised bone, is removed, exposing the lateral aspect of the ankle joint. A small bone lever is passed behind the joint to keep the tendons out of the way and with a sharp chisel the articular surfaces of talus and tibia are excised in parallel while the foot is held in the required position. Care must be taken not to remove too much bone from the lateral side of the joint unless it is intended to correct some varus.

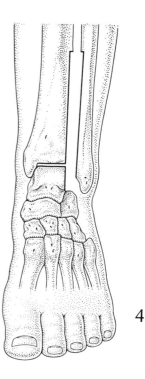

4

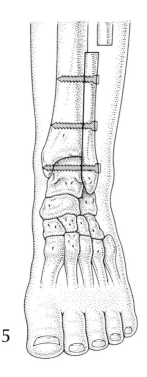

5

5

With the tibia and talus held in close apposition, the removed lower end of the fibula, the medial side of which will already be raw from the circular saw, is applied to the lower end of the tibia and talus, which will be similarly raw, and is fixed in position with two screws above and one screw below the joint.

Wound closure

The peroneal tendons are replaced in position behind the lateral malleolus and held there by repair of the retinaculum. The soft tissues are drawn lightly together and the skin is closed.

Postoperative management

This is as for the anterior approach.

COMPRESSION ANKLE ARTHRODESIS (CHARNLEY)

The patient is placed on the operating table in the supine position.

Incision and exposure

6a

An incision is carried across the front of the ankle joint from the tip of the medial malleolus to the tip of the lateral malleolus. All the anterior tendons are divided between stay sutures and retracted and the dorsalis pedis artery is divided between ligatures. The capsule of the joint is incised in its entirety and both malleoli are osteotomized through their bases.

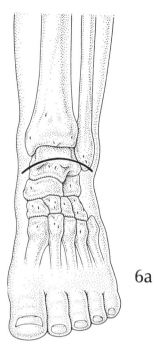

6a

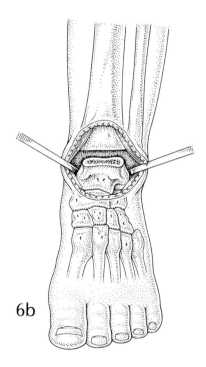

6b

6b

The ankle joint is completely dislocated by plantarflexion of the foot and the malleoli are excised. The lower 13 mm of the tibia is cleared of soft tissue as far as possible. Two small bone levers are placed behind the lower end of the tibia, being passed through the ankle joint with the foot plantarflexed. These are to protect the posterior tibial nerve and blood vessels from damage. With soft tissue retraction the lower end of the tibia is divided with a handsaw 6 mm from the articular surface and at 90° to the long axis of the bone. The foot is lined up into the required position and a cut is made with the saw in the body of the talus parallel to the cut end of the tibia. The foot is again dislocated, the two bone levers are reversed to lie behind the talus and the excision of the upper surface of the talus is completed with the saw.

7a & b

A stout 15 cm Steinmann pin is passed through the centre of the lower end of the tibia 5 cm from the cut surface and parallel to it. The cut surfaces are placed in close apposition and a similar Steinmann pin is passed through the body of the talus parallel to the first pin. This pin should be placed so that it lies just anterior to the centre of the bone. Where the pins pass through the skin a small incision is made with a tenotomy knife so that the skin edges will not slough from pressure. While this is being done the skin edges of the main wound should be held lightly together to ensure that the wound can be closed with the pins in position. Compression clamps are applied to the pins with the butterfly nuts downwards so that they can be tightened equally until there is good compression with some bending of the pins.

Wound closure

The tendons are sutured together under slight tension, the tendon sheaths and subcutaneous tissue are sutured as a single layer over them and the skin is lightly closed.

Postoperative management

Opinions differ as to the necessity for plaster postoperatively. If the bones are porotic, plaster should always be applied to reduce the risk of the pins cutting out. The author prefers always to apply a plaster for the patient's comfort but it need only be below-knee.

The foot is kept elevated until the postoperative swelling has settled when the patient is allowed up on crutches. At 5 weeks the plaster and pins are removed and a below-knee walking plaster is applied and retained until union is sound at 8–10 weeks.

Complications

Since this operation always involves division of the dorsalis pedis artery there must be no doubt that the posterior tibial artery is patent. In post-traumatic conditions this may not always be so, in which case it is possible to perform compression arthrodesis through two lateral incisions without disturbing the dorsalis pedis artery.

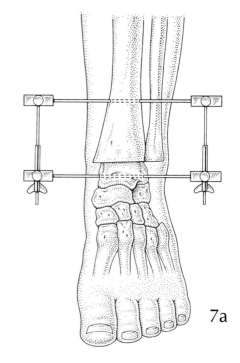

7a

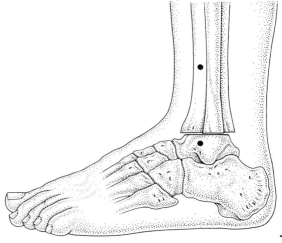

7b

'TREPHINE' ANKLE ARTHRODESIS (THOMAS)

This is a simple, neat operation with minimal postoperative reaction but with the difficulty that if there is deformity of the joint it cannot easily be corrected. This operation is best confined to those ankles where no change of position is required.

Position of patient

The patient is placed on the operating table in the supine position.

8a

Incision and exposure

A 5 cm vertical incision is made over the medial malleolus which is then exposed subperiosteally.

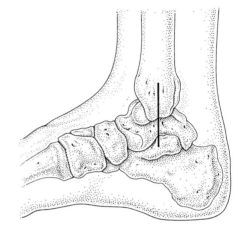

8a

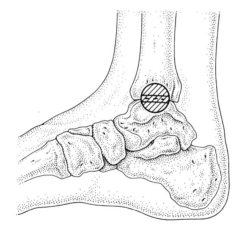

8b

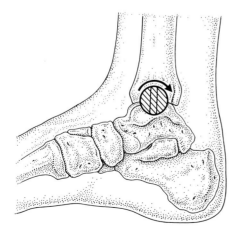

8c

8b & c

The exact position of the ankle joint is determined by direct vision. A 19 mm trephine is centred over the joint on the medial side of the medial malleolus and is passed across the joint to the lateral side, taking out a core with the joint in the centre of it. This core is rotated through 90° and is then hammered in to make it spread. Alternatively the core may be removed completely and replaced by a piece of cancellous bone from the iliac crest which is similarly hammered in.

Wound closure

The periosteum and skin are closed with chromic catgut sutures.

Postoperative management

A below-knee walking plaster is applied. As soon as the postoperative reaction has settled the patient may start to walk with weight-bearing. Union is a little slow after this operation, usually taking 4 months.

OPTIMUM POSITION FOR ANKLE ARTHRODESIS

Opinions differ as to the position in which the foot should be placed. Some believe it should be related to the height of heel worn, particularly in women. However, this presents problems when shoes are not worn, and callosities may develop under the metatarsal heads if it is too extreme. A more sensible position for both men and women is sufficient plantarflexion, i.e. 5°–10°, to allow for a small heel and at the same time to compensate for the 13 mm shortening resulting from the excision of the joint.

A position of 5°–10° dorsiflexion is less often advocated though it has many advantages. In this position the patient stands well, has a more normal gait and will run better, which is of great importance in the younger patient. There is no risk of callosities developing on any part of the foot. Although not applicable in all cases serious consideration should be given to it when determining the position preoperatively.

In the presence of weakness or paralysis of the quadriceps, arthrodesis in dorsiflexion is absolutely contraindicated. In this condition the foot must always be placed in some equinus.

PANTALAR ARTHRODESIS

In certain patients where trauma to the ankle and foot has been extensive, resulting in painful deformity of both, it may be necessary to perform arthrodesis of the ankle, subtalar and mid-tarsal joints. This is, however, not a good operation because it leads to so much rigidity of the foot that persistent painful callosities are a not infrequent sequel. It should therefore be avoided whenever possible. For this reason the author recommends that, where there is a possibility that pantalar arthrodesis will be necessary, a subtalar stabilization of the foot with correction of the deformity should be performed. This will relieve the symptoms sufficiently often so that no further surgery will be required. However, if symptoms persist to a degree that arthrodesis of the ankle is necessary there is no difficulty in doing this as a second stage by one of the techniques already described above.

Arthrodeses of the foot

E. W. Somerville FRCS, FRCS(Ed)
Emeritus Consultant Orthopaedic Surgeon, Nuffield Orthopaedic Centre, Oxford, UK

Introduction

Arthrodesis has been supplanted in many of the larger joints by replacement arthroplasty, but in the foot it remains an important technique.

Indications

Arthrodeses of the foot are indicated for (1) correction of valgus and varus deformity, (2) stabilization in paralytic conditions, and (3) fixation of painful and arthritic joints. Not infrequently two of these factors may be combined in the same foot.

Stabilization of the foot and the correction of varus

NAUGHTON DUNN'S OPERATION (TRIPLE ARTHRODESIS)

This was the first operation of its kind to be described. Since then there have been many modifications but the original is still the most commonly used and in the author's opinion is the one to be preferred. It consists of fusion of the subtalar, talonavicular and calcaneocuboid joints.

The operation aims to correct varus of the heel by removal of a suitable wedge from the subtalar joint, to correct adduction and varus of the forefoot by excision and fusion of the calcaneocuboid joint, which will shorten the foot, and to produce backward displacement of the foot at the talonavicular joint, which will improve stability.

Indications and contraindications

This operation is indicated for the correction of equino-varus deformity such as often follows the incomplete correction of club foot but which may also be found in paralytic conditions and as a post-traumatic lesion when it will be accompanied by osteoarthritis in one or more of the joints. This deformity is also quite commonly found in rheumatoid arthritis.

The operation should not be performed under the age of 13 years because of the risk of damaging the growth of the foot.

Position of patient

The patient is placed in the supine position on the operating table with a sandbag beneath the buttock on the operation side to give a tilt of about 30°.

Incision

1

A curved incision begins just above and behind the lateral malleolus, curving downwards and forwards to pass about 2.5 cm below the tip of the malleolus and up towards the dorsum of the foot to finish over the base of the second or third metatarsal.

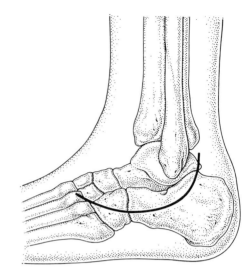

1

Exposure and excision

2

The peroneal tendons are exposed by splitting the tendon sheaths from behind the lateral malleolus down to the calcaneocuboid joint. The belly of the extensor digitorum brevis is defined, separated from the talus and turned down to expose the sinus tarsi. The calcaneocuboid joint is excised using a 3.8 cm (1½ inch) osteotome or chisel so that the excision on each side of the joint will be clean. The two cuts should be either parallel or slightly more separated below than above, never the reverse, since this will lead to boating of the sole of the foot which will cause a painful callosity under the prominence.

A small bone lever is passed over the neck of the talus to expose the talonavicular joint. With a 3.8 cm (1½ inch) gouge the navicular is divided obliquely from above downwards and before backwards, excising the concave surface articulating with the head of the talus. The talocalcaneal ligaments are incised and the sinus tarsi cleaned of all soft tissue.

With the knee bent to 90° and controlled by an assistant the surgeon takes the heel in one hand and forcibly inverts it, dislocating all three joints. The separated fragments of bone in the mid-tarsal joints are easily excised with a scalpel. A bone lever is passed over the medial side of the calcaneus to protect the important structures there while the articular surface is being excised. A 5 cm (2 inch) chisel is used to excise the articular surface from the anterior to the posterior extremity, with care being taken to include the sustentaculum tali.

Reversing the bone lever the articular surface of the talus is similarly excised. Usually more bone will unconsciously be removed from the outer than from the inner

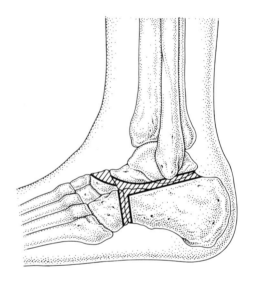

2

side so that it is often unnecessary to remove a wedge consciously, but care must be taken to ensure that sufficient bone is removed so that the heel will lie in some slight degree of valgus at the end of the operation. The articular surface of the head of the talus is removed with bone cutters to the shape of the raw surface of the navicular with which it will lie in contact. The use of a chisel for this will run the risk of fracturing the neck of the talus if it is soft or brittle.

Reduction

3

When all the joint surfaces are prepared the foot is reduced. If the excision has been carried out well the surfaces will fit together accurately with the heel in slight valgus – never varus. If the operation has been correctly performed it should not be necessary to use wires or staples to hold the position. Wires and staples increase the risk of infection and the use of them is an admission of failure.

Wound closure

With the foot held in the reduced position the peroneal tendons are replaced and held in position by lightly suturing the retinaculum. The extensor digitorum brevis is reattached to the talus and the subcutaneous tissues lightly approximated. The skin closure is important. It should be done with the fewest possible everting stitches even if gaps are left between them. The skin edges of this incision are apt to slough, but this can be reduced to a minimum by very loose closure. This sloughing should not be mistaken for infection and even though it may at times be extensive it can be largely ignored, needing only to be covered with a dressing and enclosed in plaster. When the plaster is removed it will be healed.

Postoperative management

A full-length plaster cast should always be applied to control rotation for the first 6 weeks. If the plaster is carried to the tips of the toes on the dorsal and plantar surfaces so that only the tips are showing it should not be necessary to split the plaster, but this does not in any way exonerate the surgeon from ensuring that the circulation is satisfactory at all times.

The foot is kept elevated until the postoperative reaction has passed. The patient is then allowed up on crutches and at the end of 6 weeks the plaster is reduced to below-knee. If possible it is better not to remove and replace the plaster. A walking heel is applied and the patient is allowed to start weight-bearing. This plaster must be retained until 4 months after the operation. When the plaster is finally removed swelling is to be expected and this may persist for several months.

LAMBRINUDI OPERATION

Indication

This operation is a stabilization of the foot in paralytic conditions to correct drop foot where there is a varus deformity making an arthrodesis of the ankle inadvisable.

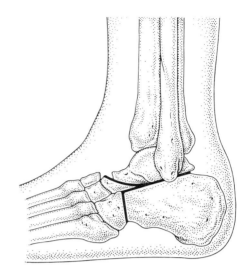

3

Principle

In doing the stabilization a wedge is removed with its base forward at the mid-tarsal joint so that when the wedge is closed the forefoot will be dorsiflexed about 25°, thus reducing the drop foot by this amount as well as correcting the deformity in the foot. It is not safe to try to reduce the drop foot by more than 25° because the base of the wedge would be so great that there would be risk a of non-union at the mid-tarsal joint.

Usually this operation produces an improvement rather than full correction and it will unfortunately be found that in many cases there will be a gradual recurrence of deformity due to stretching of ligaments. If it is apparent that the patient will need to wear a caliper and that this will correct the deformity, the operation should not be done; but there are occasions when it will not be possible for the patient to wear the caliper unless deformity has been corrected surgically.

The best results are in those patients in whom the paralysis is incomplete and in whom the ligaments are strong and tight.

Position of patient

The patient is placed on the operating table in the supine position with a sandbag under the buttock on the operation side to give a 30° tilt, as in the Naughton Dunn procedure.

Incision

The incision is also similar, curving below the lateral malleolus from behind and extending to the centre of the dorsum of the foot (see Illustration 1).

Exposure and excision

The peroneal tendons are exposed by splitting their sheaths from behind the malleolus to the calcaneocuboid joint. The belly of the extensor digitorum brevis is defined, separated from the talus and turned down.

The calcaneocuboid joint is excised, making sure that the excision is slightly wider below than above to avoid boating of the outer border of the foot which can be a problem with this operation. A small bone lever is passed over the neck of the talus to expose the talonavicular joint. The ligaments of this joint are divided, the sinus tarsi is cleared of all soft tissue, the talocalcaneal ligaments are

divided and the foot is dislocated at the subtalar and mid-tarsal joints.

A small bone lever is passed across the subtalar joint and over the medial side of the calcaneum. The articular surface of the calcaneum is excised throughout its length with a very broad chisel, removing more bone anteriorly than posteriorly. Any temptation to increase the size of the wedge by taking too much bone from the anterior end must be resisted because if the contact between calcaneum and cuboid is too small non-union may result with subsequent boating, which will be very difficult to correct. Most of the wedge is obtained by excision from the talus.

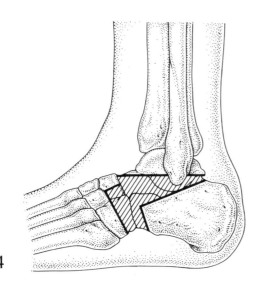

4

4

The line of excision for the talus should be carefully marked out, extending anteriorly from the edge of the articular cartilage of the upper part of the head of the talus and posteriorly to the posterior lip of the body of the talus. The whole of this piece of bone is excised, making due allowance for whatever lateral wedge has to be removed to give slight valgus to the heel. The navicular is then divided at the junction of its lower and middle thirds, the line of division being slightly upwards and backwards, and the lower third is removed. The upper surface of the neck of the talus is roughened.

Reduction

5

Any loose fragments of bone are excised and the dislocation is reduced, the upper surface of the calcaneus being pushed upwards into contact with the undersurface of the navicular. The calcaneocuboid joint is reduced, ensuring that there is no boating at this level, and the forefoot is displaced backwards so that the cut surface of the navicular is in contact with the roughened area on the superior surface of the neck of the talus. Again, the use of pins or wires to hold the position should be avoided.

Wound closure

The peroneal tendons are replaced and held in position by light suturing of the retinaculum. The belly of the extensor digitorum brevis is reattached to the talus, the subcutaneous tissues lightly approximated and the skin closed with a minimum of interrupted sutures.

Postoperative management

With the foot carefully held in the correct position a leg plaster cast is applied.

The leg is kept elevated until the postoperative swelling has settled, when the patient is allowed up on crutches. At 6 weeks the plaster is reduced to below-knee and a walking heel is applied. The plaster is retained for a minimum of 4 months.

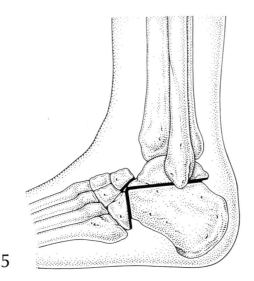

5

Arthrodeses for the correction of valgus

Valgus deformity of the foot is caused by:

1. *Paralysis* – due to muscle imbalance
2. *Spasticity* – due to cerebral palsy or local lesions in the subtalar joint, e.g. spastic valgus foot
3. *Abnormal posture* – mobile flat foot where collapse of the arch in weight-bearing is closely associated with instability of the heel or valgus of the foot resulting from a tight tendo Achillis but with irreversible stretching of the medial ligaments of the foot
4. *Trauma* – fractures of the os calcis.

Operations for spastic and paralytic valgus deformities

These deformities may be corrected by a triple arthrodesis such as the Naughton Dunn operation, but this will be much more difficult than in feet with varus deformities. The dislocation of the foot and the removal of a medial wedge is always more difficult than is the removal of a lateral one. Apart from these difficulties the operation is the same.

GRICE–GREEN OPERATION

This is an extremely useful operation which can be employed any time after the age of 7 years. It can be done earlier but the small amount of bone may lead to non-union of one end of the graft, and it is better to postpone the operation. There is no upper age limit.

Indications

This operation is indicated for (*1*) symptomatic flat feet; (*2*) valgus feet due to a tight tendo Achillis; (*3*) the valgus of

cerebral palsy, provided the heel can be manipulated to the neutral position; (*4*) for relieving pain due to damage to the subtalar joint by fracture of the calcaneum; and (*5*) for poliomyelitis.

Principle

The Grice–Green procedure is a simple operation for fusion of the subtalar joint without interference with any of the other joints. Fusion of the subtalar joint in isolation by excision will cause malalignment of the rest of the mid-tarsal mechanism, leading to degenerative changes and pain. The Grice–Green operation causes no change in the relationship between the talus and the calcaneum so there is no disorganization of the mid-tarsal mechanism.

Position of patient

The patient is placed on the operating table in the supine position with a sandbag under the buttock on the operation side.

Incision

An incision is made from the lateral aspect of the head of the talus obliquely backwards and downwards to below the tip of the lateral malleolus.

Preparation of the graft bed

The belly of the extensor digitorum brevis is identified, detached from the talus and turned down, exposing the sinus tarsi. All the soft tissue is cleared from the sinus tarsi, exposing the neck of the talus, the non-articular area on the upper surface of the calcaneum and the anterior part of the subtalar joint. A groove is cut in the undersurface of the neck of the talus as close to the articular surface as is possible.

6

An osteotome of suitable size is wedged, angled forwards, between this groove and the anterior part of the non-articular area of the calcaneum. If, when the heel is forcibly everted, the osteotome becomes wedged more tightly and does not displace then the angulation is correct. A second groove is cut in the base area where the osteotome became embedded. The appropriately sized osteotome which will hold the heel in the correct position, i.e. very slight valgus, is wedged in the grooves to assess the size of the graft required. The osteotome is removed and the wound closed with a towel clip.

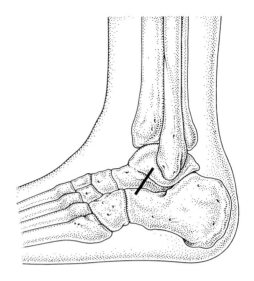

6

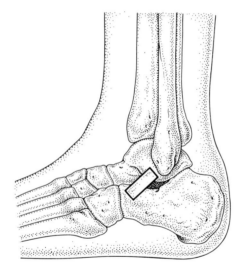

7

Insertion of graft

7

A second incision is made over the subcutaneous surface of the tibia in its upper third. The periosteum is split and the bone exposed. A graft, the length of which is equal to the width of the osteotome and 13 mm wide, is removed with a saw. The graft is at once introduced into the two grooves and tested to ensure it is the right length. When it is firmly jammed in position the heel should be in slight valgus. If the graft is a little too long one of the grooves is slightly deepened. This is easier than shortening the graft. Behind the graft the articular surface is removed from the calcaneum and the space between it and the graft packed with cancellous bone from the tibia.

Wound closure

The belly of the extensor digitorum brevis is reattached by sutures and the wound is loosely closed.

Postoperative management

A padded below-knee plaster is applied. The leg is kept elevated until the postoperative reaction is over when the patient is allowed up on crutches. After 2 weeks a walking heel is applied and the plaster is retained for 3 months.

MODIFICATIONS TO GRICE–GREEN OPERATION

Two useful modifications have been suggested which are worth consideration.

Fibular graft

8

A 5 cm incision is made over the neck of the talus. The extensor tendons are exposed and separated and the neck of the talus defined with a small bone lever on either side. A 6 mm (¼ inch) hole is drilled through it and this is then enlarged to 13 mm (½ inch). With the heel held in the required position the 13 mm drill is passed into the calcaneum to a depth of at least 2.5 cm. A piece of fibula is taken of the appropriate length, which will usually be about 6 cm. It is trimmed to fit the hole and driven in. Plaster immobilization is required for at least 3 months.

Because (a) the fibula, being sclerotic, is not a good bone for grafting and (b) the graft is not under compression, union may be slow or even uncertain. Also the neck of the talus is somewhat brittle and there is a risk of fracture. For these reasons this operation is best avoided.

Screw fixation

9

The sinus tarsi is approached and cleared of all soft tissue. The exposed bony surfaces are decorticated. Cancellous bone is removed from the iliac crest and packed into the sinus tarsi. A second small incision is made over the upper surface of the neck of the talus and the neck is exposed and drilled for a screw. With the heel held in the correct position the screw is introduced, extending well into the calcaneum. Since the calcaneum is soft bone, it is undesirable to drill it if a firm grip with the screw is to be obtained. Plaster immobilization should be for 3 months but union may be complete before this. The fixation with this screw is poor.

Postoperative precautions

Operations around the ankle and foot where there is little room for subcutaneous swelling are frequently very painful postoperatively when swelling takes place. For this reason the plaster, including the underlying dressing, is often split in its entire length in the anterior midline. This will involve the plaster being changed quite early which is often a disadvantage. Elevation alone is not enough to control this swelling. Two simple measures will often help greatly.

The tourniquet can be removed before the plaster is applied. This, however, may involve bleeding which will spoil the plaster and cause subsequent softening. It is

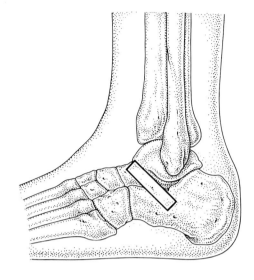

8

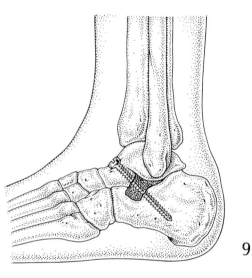

9

usually sufficient to remove the tourniquet while the first plaster bandage is being applied. This will give time for the swelling resulting from the removal to occur before the plaster is complete.

The second measure, whose rationale is less obvious, is more effective. If the plaster is taken only to the base of the toes, even though there may be a toe platform, the toes become very swollen and cause much pain, necessitating the urgent splitting of the plaster. However, if the plaster is taken to the tips of the toes, both on the plantar and dorsal surfaces, so that only the tips are visible, swelling will not occur and pain will be greatly reduced. Splitting of the plaster will rarely be necessary and the plaster may remain intact until union is complete. This immobilization does not cause stiffness, since it is the postoperative swelling and oedema which are the cause of stiffness.

It cannot be over-emphasized that none of these measures in any way exonerates the surgeon from keeping a close watch to ensure that the circulation is satisfactory.

CALCANEONAVICULAR SYNOSTOSIS

10

This is a congenital abnormality in which the postero-inferior part of the navicular is joined to the anterosuperior part of the calcaneum by a bridge of bone. During early life this usually produces no symptoms and on examination there is a full range of movement in subtalar and midtarsal joints. Symptoms and signs of spastic flat-foot develop, usually during teenage but sometimes not until adult life. It seems that the synostosis itself is not responsible for the signs and symptoms but gives rise to arthritic changes which are responsible.

Lateral radiographs show the bar quite clearly. If the radiographs are taken before ossification is complete, the appearance will suggest a fibrous union between the two bones which, if followed up, will go on to show bony union.

Operative excision of the bar will only be successful if carried out before the rigidity has developed. Even then, results are not always satisfactory and frequently a triple arthrodesis will be necessary.

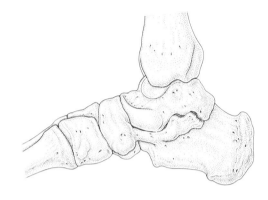

10

Operation

The patient lies in the supine position with a sandbag under the buttock on the affected side. A straight incision is made over the outer side of the talonavicular joint, which is then exposed. It will be found that what appeared radiologically to be a bar is in fact a sheet of bone 0.5 cm thick joining the navicular to the calcaneum across the whole width of the joint. This sheet of bone must be excised widely so that it can be clearly demonstrated that there is no contact between calcaneum and navicular in any position when the foot is put through a full range of movement. The skin of the wound is closed with interrupted polypropylene sutures.

Postoperative management

A below-knee plaster is applied with the foot in the neutral position. After 10 days the plaster is removed and active movements are encouraged, but a broad heel should be worn on the shoe to prevent sudden and unexpected strains.

TALOCALCANEAL SYNOSTOSIS

11

In this condition the two bones are joined by a strong synostosis in the region of the sustentaculum tali. Symptoms rarely arise until teenage and some not until adult life. The symptoms are similar to spastic flat-foot. They arise from the development of arthritic changes in the midtarsal joint. This lesion is not visible in either lateral or anteroposterior radiological views. To see it radiologically a special view must be taken from the back with the foot in full dorsiflexion.

Excision of the bar is useless and should not be attempted. It is necessary to fuse the talonavicular and calcaneonavicular joints. The subtalar joint is already fused and nothing need be done to it.

Operation

The operation is carried out as already described.

Postoperative management

A below-knee plaster of Paris cast is applied and the foot is elevated high on two pillows for 24 hours postoperatively. The patient then walks without bearing weight with crutches for 4 weeks. Then a new well-fitting plaster is applied and weight-bearing commences. The plaster is bivalved and a radiograph taken of the foot out of plaster at 3 months from operation. If fusion has occurred the patient progresses to unprotected walking, but further protection in a cast may be necessary if fusion is not solid.

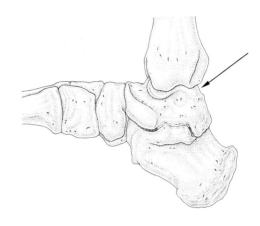

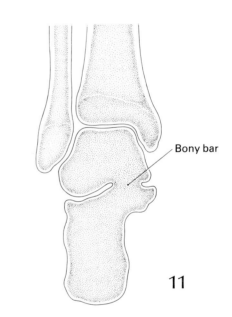

Bony bar

11

Illustrations by Philip Wilson after G. Lyth

Wedge tarsectomy

E. W. Somerville   FRCS (Ed), FRCS
Emeritus Consultant Orthopaedic Surgeon, Nuffield Orthopaedic Centre, Oxford, UK

Introduction

Indications

This operation is performed in cases of pes cavus where the deformity is rigid and beyond relief by conservative measures or in which the deformity is obviously getting worse as in certain neurological conditions such as Friedreich's ataxia. When there is deterioration in the presence of neurological changes it is advisable to carry out bony correction and stabilization before the deformity is too severe. If the correction is left too late, there may be difficulty in getting the patient to walk again and he may even remain chairbound. When the deformity is a simple but severe cavus a formal foot stabilization will not be necessary. Correction can be obtained in the mid-foot by a wedge tarsectomy.

Operation

Position of patient

The patient is placed on the operating table in the supine position.

First stage

It is necessary to flatten the foot as much as possible. With the tight structures in the sole of the foot put on the stretch to the greatest extent possible, a subcutaneous tenotomy is carried out. In a line below the medial malleolus just anterior to the medial tubercle of the tuberosity of the calcaneum a short-bladed tenotomy knife is introduced through the skin with the blade parallel to the skin surface. The blade is passed between the skin and the tight plantar fascia and is then rotated with its sharp edge towards the fascia. Maintaining as much tension as possible the fascia is completely divided in its full width down to the bone. The division of the fascia must always be away from the skin. It is in such a case that the tension can be maintained by a Thomas' wrench. Tenotomy of the flexor tendons to all the toes will often improve the degree of correction.

Incision

1

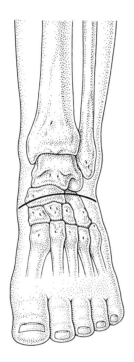

1

This is made transversely across the dorsum of the foot from one side to the other at the point where the deformity is greatest.

The tendons are exposed and divided with the exception of the tibialis anterior. Disregarding the joints, a wedge estimated to be the correct size is removed. It will usually be smaller on the lateral side of the foot than on the medial.

2

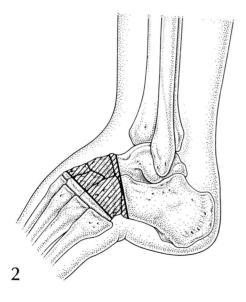

2

Depending on the success of the soft tissue release it may be necessary to remove a trapezoid, even though this will shorten the foot considerably, as otherwise the wedge will not be closed.

Wound closure

With the forefoot strongly dorsiflexed to close the gap the remains of the capsule are sutured. The tendons are left unsutured. The subcutaneous tissues are lightly sutured and the skin lightly closed with interrupted sutures. If the toes remain clawed dorsal capsulotomies are carried out to achieve extension.

Postoperative management

A moderately padded below-knee plaster of Paris cast is applied, extending to the tips of the toes on the dorsal and plantar aspects with the forefoot pushed well up into dorsiflexion.

The foot is kept elevated until postoperative swelling has settled, after which the patient may walk with crutches and at 4 weeks bear weight on a walking heel. The plaster should be retained for 4 months because union is often slow.

The neurological pes cavus is a severe problem. There is loss of soft tissue from the sole of the foot particularly under the metatarsal heads so that callosities are present. After the operation the distribution of weight will improve but the foot will still be stiff, perhaps even stiffer than before, so that callosities can still be a problem. The foot will be short, necessitating special footwear. Clawing of the toes may be such that further surgery will still be required to prevent callosities resulting from pressure on the uppers of the shoes.

Illustrations by Philip Wilson

Operations for flat foot and pes cavus

Leslie Klenerman ChM, FRCS
Professor and Head of University Department of Orthopaedic and Accident Surgery, Royal Liverpool Hospital, Liverpool, UK

Introduction

Flat foot and pes cavus are the extremes of a range which extends from a foot which is unstable because of collapse of the longitudinal arch to one which is mechanically inefficient because of an exaggerated high arch. Despite the obvious abnormal appearance of these feet, treatment must always be related to symptoms.

PES PLANUS

The hypermobile flat foot in children or adolescents may require operative correction because of difficulty in walking or, more rarely, pain. The absence of a positive great toe extension test[1], which demonstrates that the 'windlass' mechanism of the plantar fascia is ineffective, indicates the need for surgery.

In the growing child, two options are available. In the younger child (below 5 or 6 years), the treatment of choice is the reversed Dillwyn Evans procedure[2,3]. Where the heel is better developed, a medial displacement rotation osteotomy of the calcaneum will be equally effective[1]. Most flat feet are mobile. If the foot is rigid and painful, this is due to the presence of an underlying tarsal anomaly, of which the calcaneonavicular bar is the commonest variety.

Preoperative preparation

Preoperative assessment of a flat or rigid foot is made primarily on clinical grounds. Radiographs are essential for the diagnosis of tarsal anomalies. Calcaneonavicular bars are seen on oblique views of the foot but for talocalcaneal bars computed tomography is necessary. Lateral weight-bearing radiographs are useful as a record of the preoperative state of the foot. The relationship between the axis of the first metatarsal and that of the talus is used to show the extent of a flat foot, and the relationship of the axis of the first metatarsal and the axis of the calcaneum is used for the cavus foot.

General anaesthesia and a high thigh tourniquet are necessary. In operations on the dorsum of the foot, skin flaps should be kept as thick as possible. Care is necessary to avoid damage to skin nerves. The sural nerve behind the lateral malleolus and the branches of the musculo-cutaneous nerve on the dorsum of the foot are especially at risk of damage.

REVERSED DILLWYN EVANS PROCEDURE

The principle underlying the operation is the concept that the lateral side of the longitudinal arch of the foot is too short. The operation was designed to lengthen this by the insertion of a tibial bone graft immediately proximal to the calcaneocuboid joint.

Technique

1 & 2

An oblique incision is made over the lateral surface of the calcaneum above and parallel to the peroneal tendons. The sural nerve is protected and the anterior end of the calcaneum is divided through its narrow part in front of the peroneal tubercle using an osteotome. The osteotomy is parallel with and 1.5 cm proximal to the articular surface of the calcaneocuboid joint.

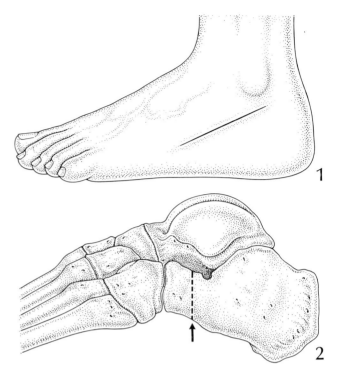

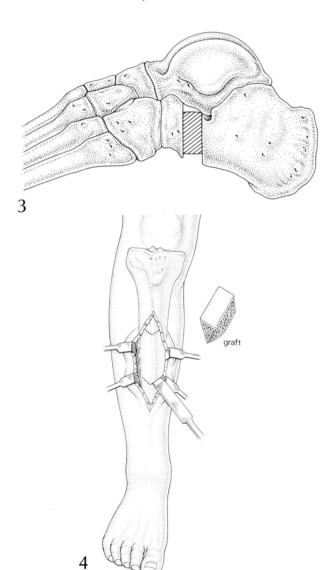

3

A graft of cortical bone is taken from the crest of the ipsilateral tibia and inserted into the osteotomy site. Further grafts are inserted above and below the first graft to ensure that the two surfaces of the calcaneum remain apart. Occasionally it may be necessary to lengthen the peroneal tendons.

4

The graft is taken from the crest of the tibia of the operated leg. A skin incision is made two fingers'-breadth distal to the tibial tuberosity, to ensure that the graft will be well clear of the epiphysis. The graft needs to be sufficiently long to extend from the superior to the inferior surface of the calcaneum. It should include the anterior third of the tibial crest. It is best to mark out the dimensions of the graft with an osteotome and then with a fine drill follow the linear markings so that the graft does not shatter when it is removed with an osteotome.

Postoperative management

At the end of the operation it is advisable to release the tourniquet and to secure haemostasis before the wound is closed. Suction drainage is helpful to reduce swelling. Wool and a crêpe bandage provide a firm dressing to reduce oozing. A second layer of wool and a plaster of Paris backslab are applied to immobilize the foot. It is unwise to use a complete plaster cast immediately after the operation because of the danger of a compartment syndrome. At the end of 2 weeks when the slab is removed a complete plaster can be applied, which is retained for 8 weeks and partial weight-bearing is allowed.

MEDIAL DISPLACEMENT ROTATION OSTEOTOMY OF CALCANEUM

The primary function of a calcaneal osteotomy is to shift the posterior weight-bearing pillar of the foot medially and, in doing so, to place the line of tibial thrust through the subtalar joint, so that there is neither a medial nor lateral moment of rotation, and to distribute the weight evenly over the support area of the sole. It modifies the action of triceps surae from eversion to inversion. A closing wedge combined with displacement is best.

Technique[1]

5

A longitudinal incision is made over the lateral aspect of the heel in the line of the peroneal tendons, which extends from the tendo Achillis to the plantar surface of the foot. The skin flaps are not undermined, but it is necessary to identify the peroneal tendons superiorly, to act as a guide for the line of the osteotomy. A bone spike is inserted anterior to the tendo Achillis at the upper end of the wound and onto the plantar surface of the calcaneum at the lower end.

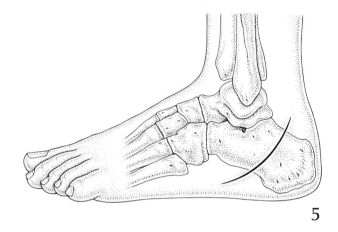

5

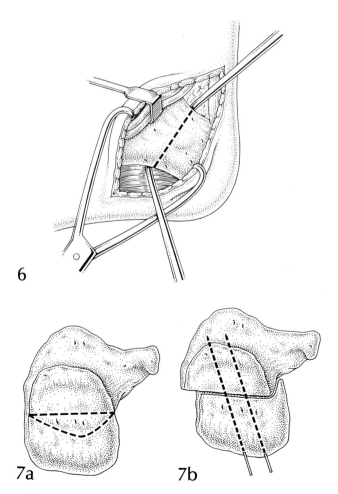

6

7a   7b

6, 7a & b

The periosteum is reflected in the line of the incision. The osteotomy is carried out as indicated in the diagram so as to produce a small medial spike, which can be used to lock the displaced posterior part of the calcaneum. Two percutaneous Kirschner wires are used to hold the posterior segment in place.

Postoperative management

The wound is closed in layers and a padded plaster of Paris backslab applied. This is converted to a full below-knee plaster after 10 days, when the operation wound is healed. The patient should remain non-weight-bearing for 4 weeks, when the Kirschner wires should be removed and a below-knee walking plaster applied for 2 weeks.

Full weight-bearing in plaster is allowed when the wound is healed and when Kirschner wires have been removed. The foot functions more effectively under load.

Once the plaster cast has been removed and although the postoperative appearances are satisfactory on radiographs, swelling of the foot may be a major problem. Encouragement to walk with a supporting elastic bandage, with instructions to elevate the leg when resting, help reduce the oedema. Physiotherapy does not play a major role in the rehabilitation of the patient after foot surgery.

EXCISION OF CALCANEONAVICULAR BAR FOR TREATMENT OF RIGID FLAT FOOT

The cause of rigidity is a tarsal anomaly, of which the most common is a calcaneonavicular bar. In children under 14 years of age, excision of the bar is a useful procedure[4]. The results are much less effective for older adolescents and adults, where it may be necessary to carry out a formal triple arthrodesis.

Technique

8

An incision is made 1 cm below the tip of the lateral malleolus, and is curved forward onto the muscle belly of the extensor digitorum brevis. The skin flaps are retracted and care is taken to avoid damage to the sural nerve.

9 & 10

Extensor digitorum brevis is divided in the line of its fibres to reveal the underlying bony bar. This is cleared of soft tissue, using a perosteal elevator. The talonavicular and calcaneocuboid joints should be opened, so that all the available landmarks are clearly defined. Using an osteotome, the bar is then removed in its entirety as a rectangle, not as a wedge. Extensor digitorum brevis is allowed to fall back into place and the skin is sutured.

The foot is immobilized in below-knee non-weight-bearing plaster until the wound is healed. At 14 days, the cast is removed and the patient is encouraged to bear weight and use the foot normally.

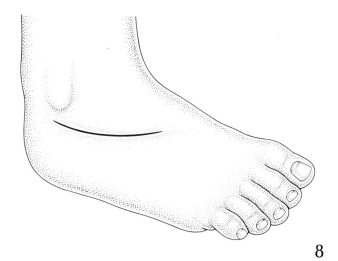

8

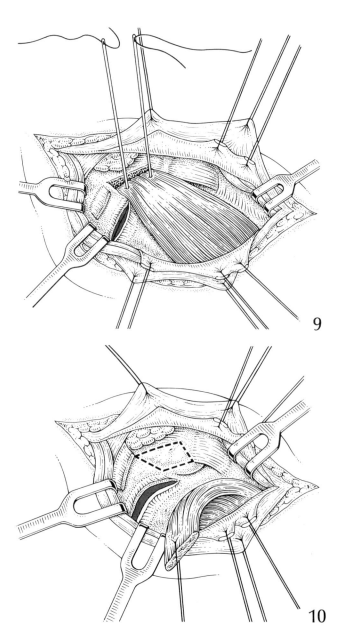

9

10

TENDON TRANSFER FOR RUPTURED TIBIALIS POSTERIOR TENDON

A grossly pronated foot may result from spontaneous rupture of the tibialis posterior tendon. In patients over 60 years of age, excellent correction of the deformity can be obtained by means of a medial displacement/rotation osteotomy of the calcaneum, as described for the idiopathic hypermobile flat foot. In the younger patient, the treatment of choice is a tendon transfer using the flexor digitorum longus as the motor power for inversion[5].

Technique

11 & 12

An incision is made on the medial side of the ankle, extending from the malleolus to the navicular. It is essential to confirm the diagnosis by opening the tendon sheath of tibialis posterior. The skin incision can then be extended proximally and distally. The abductor hallucis is reflected plantarward and the 'master knot' of Henry released, i.e. the site where flexor hallucis and flexor digitorum longus cross (with hallucis above the digitorum) and the origin of flexor hallucis brevis.

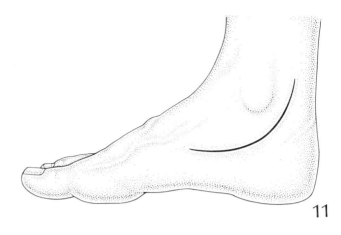

11

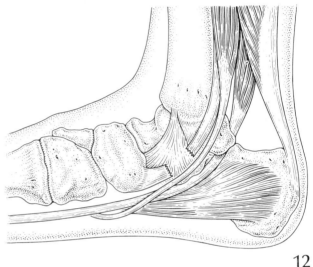

12

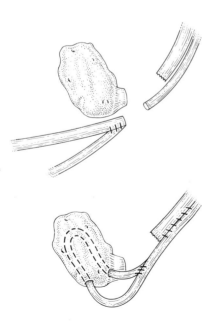

13

13

Flexor digitorum longus is divided at this point, and sutured distally to flexor hallucis longus. The proximal part of flexor digitorum longus is withdrawn from the site of division and rerouted through the sheath of tibialis posterior. It is attached to the navicular by passing it through a hole in the bone and tying the tendon to itself with the foot in equinus and inversion. The tendon should be sutured as tightly as possible. Side-to-side suture of flexor digitorum longus and the proximal part of the tendon of tibialis posterior should be attempted if possible. After wound closure, the foot is immobilized in a below-knee plaster in a position of equinovarus for 4 weeks and then placed in a plantigrade position in a walking cast for a further 4 weeks.

PES CAVUS

In the adult the indication for operative treatment is pain, while in the growing child the reason may be progressive deformity. The foot requires careful assessment to determine the main site of deformity which may be in the hind-, mid- or fore-foot, and these are sometimes combined.

If the heel is inverted and there is tightness of the plantar fascia, then a combination of a Steindler release and an osteotomy to remove a laterally based wedge from the calcaneum, as described by Dwyer[6], is the treatment of choice. With correctable clawing of the great toe and the lesser toes, a combination of Robert Jones' tendon transfer of extensor hallucis longus to the neck of the first metatarsal and Girdlestone's flexor to extensor tendon transfer will produce correction. When the hindfoot deformity is rigid, a triple arthrodesis is needed. On occasions, with mobile deformities, there is obvious tightness of the tendo Achillis which has to be lengthened to allow the foot to take up a plantigrade position. Very occasionally it may be thought necessary to carry out a mid-tarsal osteotomy, as described by Cole[7] and Japas[8] and, if so, then the alternative procedure of a tarsometa-tarsal truncated wedge, as described by Jahss[9], is preferable.

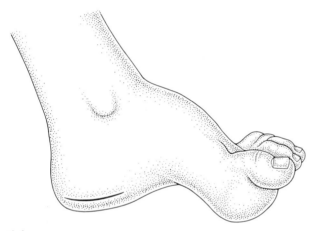

14

STEINDLER RELEASE OF PLANTAR FASCIA

14

This operation is usually combined with a laterally based Dwyer's osteotomy of the calcaneum. A longitudinal incision is made from the medial side of the posterior aspect of the heel to a point about 4 cm in front of the tubercle of the calcaneum.

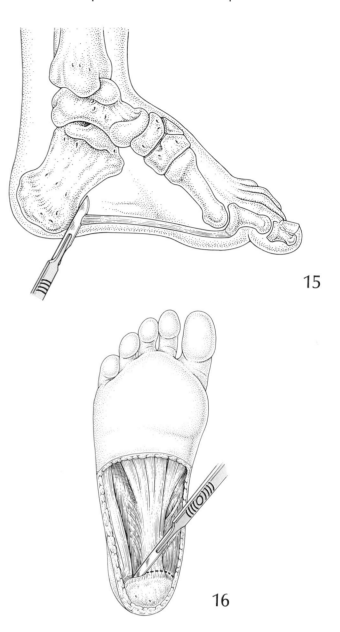

15

16

15 & 16

The upper surface of the plantar fascia is then dissected from the covering fat layer of the foot and freed across the width of the foot with a blunt instrument, such as artery forceps. The fascia is then incised at its insertion into the calcaneum. A sharp periosteal elevator is then inserted and a subperiosteal stripping of all structures is carried out. By keeping close to the medial tuberosity, the dissection is a safe distance from the vessels and nerves. The wound is then closed in layers.

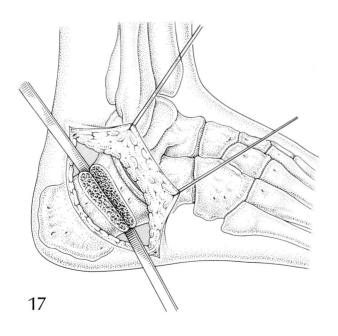

17

CALCANEAL OSTEOTOMY FOR PES CAVUS

17

The approach is the same as for the medial displacement/ rotation osteotomy used for the correction of the valgus hindfoot. The osteotomy is again carried out in a line parallel to the peroneal tendons extending from a point immediately anterior to the insertion of the tendo Achillis, and a sufficiently large wedge of bone is excised from the lateral aspect of the heel to correct the varus inclination. In order to close the wedge, an awl passed through the posterior section of the calcaneum provides leverage to produce good bony apposition, which can be made secure by the insertion of a staple.

TARSOMETATARSAL TRUNCATED WEDGE ARTHRODESIS[9]

18

Three longitudinal dorsal incisions are used. The medial incision is made with its centre over the tarsometatarsal joint of the first ray. The underlying joint is exposed. The distal osteotomy is done first, while the first metatarsal is still fixed in position. The proximal osteotomy of the medial cuneiform is then performed so that a small, dorsally truncated wedge is removed. It is safer to be conservative, as it is always possible to resect more bone if necessary.

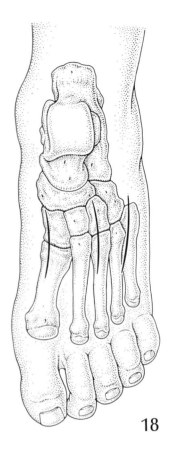

18

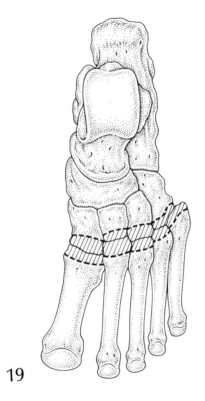

19

19 & 20

In a similar manner, further osteotomies of the second and third tarsometatarsal joints are made through a skin incision between the bases of the second and third metatarsals. It must be remembered that the base of the second metatarsal is more proximal than the adjacent metatarsals. The third incision is for osteotomies at the bases of the fourth and fifth metatarsal. The forefoot can then be dorsiflexed to close the wedges.

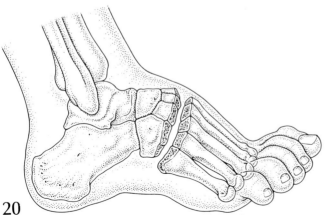

20

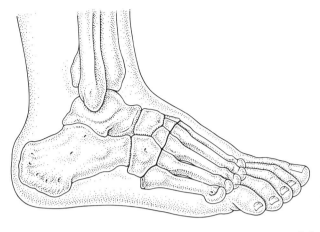

21 & 22

A finger is used to palpate the bone ends to check whether it is necessary to remove small segments of bone which block reduction. At the end of the operation, the forefoot should be at right angles to the tibia, and the metatarsal heads should all be level.

A padded plaster cast is applied, and the patient should not bear weight until the wound is healed. After 14 days the plaster cast is changed, and a walking plaster applied for a period of approximately 4 weeks. Provided union is sound, the plaster immobilization can be discontinued 6 weeks after the operation.

21

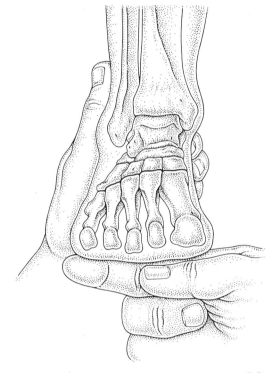

22

References

1. Rose GK. Pes planus. In: Jahss MH, ed. *Disorders of the foot.* Philadelphia: Saunders, 1982: 486–520.

2. Evans D. Calcaneo-valgus deformity. *J Bone Joint Surg [Br]* 1975; 57-B: 270–8.

3. Phillips GE. A review of elongation of os calcis for flat feet. *J Bone Joint Surg [Br]* 1983; 65-B: 15–8.

4. Mitchell GP, Gibson JMC. Excision of calcaneo-navicular bar for painful spasmodic flat foot. *J Bone Joint Surg [Br]* 1967; 49-B: 281–7.

5. Mann RA. Traumatic injuries to the soft tissues of the foot and ankle. In Mann RA, ed. *Surgery of the foot.* St Louis: C.V. Mosby Company, 1986; 476–80.

6. Dwyer FC. Osteotomy of the calcaneum for pes cavus. *J Bone Joint Surg [Br]* 1959; 41-B: 80–6.

7. Cole WH. The treatment of claw foot. *J Bone Joint Surg* 1940; 22: 895–908.

8. Japas LM. Surgical treatment of pes cavus by tarsal V-osteotomy. A preliminary report. *J Bone Joint Surg [Am]* 1968; 50-A: 927–44.

9. Jahss MH. Tarsometatarsal truncated wedge arthrodesis for pes cavus and equinovarus deformity of the fore part of the foot. *J Bone Joint Surg [Am]* 1980; 62-A: 713–22.

Operations for congenital talipes equinovarus

E. H. Bates FRCS, FRACS
Chairman, Section of Orthopaedics, Prince of Wales Children's Hospital, Sydney, Australia

Introduction

Roughly 50 per cent of club feet defy adequate correction by non-operative measures.

Timing

The timing of primary surgical intervention varies widely between 3 weeks and 12 months. Most surgeons prefer to manipulate and splint club feet for at least 3 months before abandoning non-operative treatment. Very early surgery carries greater risk of overcorrection and surgical trauma to a foot whose bones are largely cartilaginous.

Indications

The choice of primary soft tissue procedure is influenced by the child's age and by the type and extent of deformity.

Feet that are almost corrected by non-operative measures require less extensive surgery. A limited posterior release may be all that is required.

In general, however, feet requiring surgery should be subjected to those soft tissue releases required to correct subtalar rotation and to reduce the talonavicular joint.

Depending on the extent and site of major deformities, combinations of medial, posteromedial, plantar-medial and lateral releases may be required. In all cases, the object is to obtain full correction of each component of the deformity.

Operative position

With babies, the prone position provides excellent access for all soft tissue releases.

Operations

POSTERIOR SOFT TISSUE RELEASE

1

A transverse incision (a) just above the insertion of the Achilles tendon, or a longitudinal incision (b) just medial to the Achilles tendon, are equally effective.

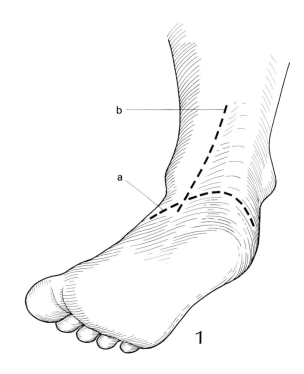

1

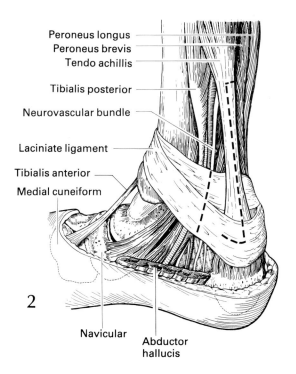

Peroneus longus
Peroneus brevis
Tendo achillis

Tibialis posterior

Neurovascular bundle

Laciniate ligament

Tibialis anterior
Medial cuneiform

2

Navicular   Abductor
hallucis

2

The Achilles tendon is elongated (Z-plasty) and the medial half of this tendon is detached from the calcaneum.

The neurovascular bundle is identified beneath the laciniate ligament between the Achilles tendon and the medial malleolus. Fine calcaneal branches may be sacrificed, but high division of the posterior tibial nerve is a common variation which should prompt careful dissection.

3

The deeper investing layer of fascia is divided in the midline and the flexor hallucis longus tendon is identified and traced downwards to the medial side of the subtalar joint. This tendon can be used to retract the neurovascular bundle medially.

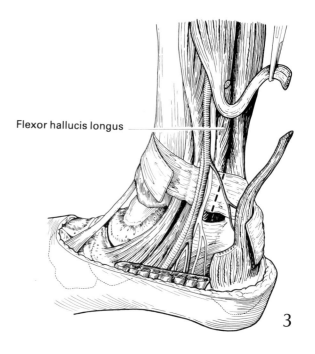

Flexor hallucis longus

3

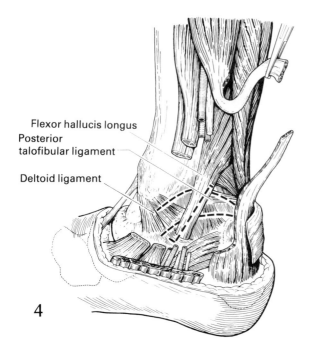

Flexor hallucis longus
Posterior
talofibular ligament

Deltoid ligament

4

Tibialis posterior and flexor digitorum longus tendons and the neurovascular bundle are resected in this diagram for clarity.

4

The ankle capsule is incised transversely and the arthrotomy extended medially to involve no more than the posterior quarter of the deltoid ligament. It is then extended laterally to the fibula, and the posterior talofibular ligament is divided.

The subtalar joint capsule is incised transversely and this arthrotomy extended medially and forwards to the flexor hallucis longus tendon, and then laterally deep to the peroneal tendon sheath.

The flexor hallucis longus tendon is elongated by dividing it obliquely over a length of 2–3 cm.

The tendons of tibialis posterior and flexor digitorum longus are exposed above and behind the medial malleolus, just in front of the neurovascular bundle. Z-lengthening of these tendons at their musculotendinous junction completes the posterior release operation.

MEDIAL SOFT TISSUE RELEASE

5

A horizontal curvilinear incision from the neck of the first metatarsal to a point just distal to the tip of the medial malleolus is made: (a) to leave a skin bridge between it and the longitudinal posterior incision, this bridge covering the neurovascular bundle; (b) to join up with the longitudinal posterior incision; or (c) to be extended to a full Cincinnatti-type exposure.

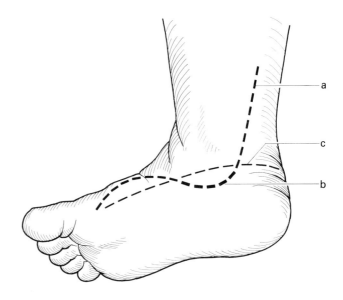

6

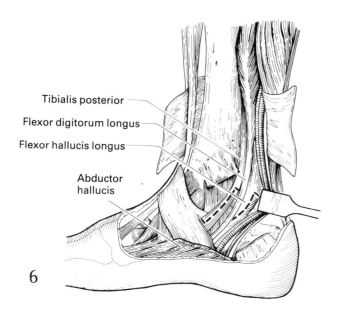

Tibialis posterior
Flexor digitorum longus
Flexor hallucis longus
Abductor hallucis

6

The neurovascular bundle is mobilized distally to ensure its protection during the medial subtalar arthrotomy. The abductor hallucis origin is detached from the flexor retinaculum. The insertion of the tibialis posterior tendon and the route of the flexor digitorum longus tendon, anterior to the neurovascular bundle, are exposed by dividing the thickened investing fascia. The tibialis posterior tendon is separated from all its insertions except that to the navicular and then it is Z-lengthened. With its division the talonavicular joint is exposed.

The flexor digitorum longus tendon is traced under the tarsus to expose Henry's knot and it is separated from the flexor hallucis longus tendon by sharp dissection.

7

The talonavicular joint is opened by medial capsulotomy and the arthrotomy extended dorsally to the lateral extent of the navicular and inferiorly to join the anterior part of the subtalar joint. The medial capsule of the subtalar joint is divided and the arthrotomy extended posteriorly, deep to the neurovascular bundle. This capsulotomy will then communicate with the posterior capsulotomy of the subtalar joint if a posterior release has been performed.

The capsule of the naviculocuneiform joint is incised medially, superiorly and inferiorly. In most cases the dissection to date will be adequate to permit easy reduction of the talonavicular joint.

Residual forefoot adduction may require a similar capsulotomy of the cuneiform–metatarsal joint. The tibialis anterior insertion should not be disturbed. In the event of persisting metatarsus varus, the tendon of abductor hallucis is identified near the neck of the first metatarsal and divided within the muscle fibres.

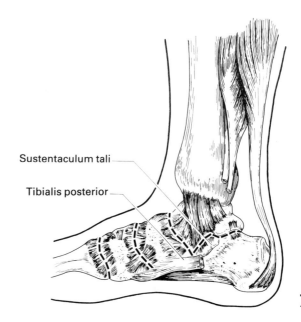

Sustentaculum tali
Tibialis posterior

7

PLANTAR SOFT TISSUE RELEASE

8

In feet with evidence of early cavus, especially repeat soft tissue operations, division of inferior structures may be required. If planned as an isolated procedure the incision in the illustration is preferred.

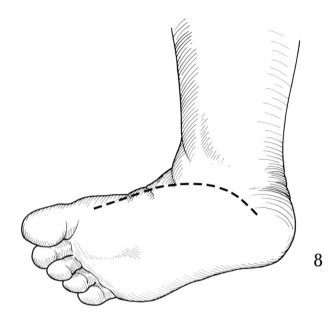

8

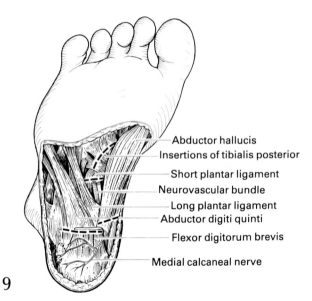

Abductor hallucis
Insertions of tibialis posterior
Short plantar ligament
Neurovascular bundle
Long plantar ligament
Abductor digiti quinti
Flexor digitorum brevis
Medial calcaneal nerve

9

9

The origin of the abductor hallucis is mobilized from the os calcis and flexor retinaculum, allowing the muscle to retract forwards with the neurovascular bundle. Care should be taken to avoid damage to the calcaneal branch of the posterior tibial nerve.

The proximal attachments of the plantar aponeurosis, flexor digitorum brevis and a variable portion of the abductor digiti quinti are divided (Steindler's operation).

The tendinous insertions of the posterior tibial tendon to the cuneiforms and metatarsals are divided. The inferior capsules of the talonavicular and naviculo-cuneiform joints are divided laterally under full vision, which involves division of the spring and short plantar ligaments.

LATERAL SOFT TISSUE RELEASE

Recent thought and writing suggests that derotation of the calcaneum beneath the talus is the prime object of club foot surgery. This subtalar mobilization involves posterior, medial and lateral releases.

10

The lateral release requires prolongation of the horizontal incision forward below the lateral malleolus toward the calcaneocuboid joint (a). If a longitudinal posterior incision has been used, then a separate lateral incision will be required (b).

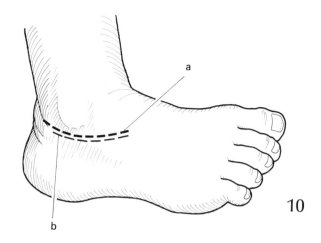

10

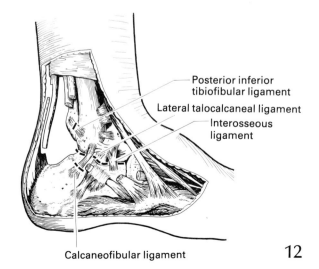

Peroneal tendon sheath

Peroneus tertius

11

Peroneus brevis
Peroneus longus
Inferior peroneal retinaculum

11

The peroneal tendons are mobilized to permit their retraction laterally; this is done by dividing part of their sheaths.

12

The subtalar capsulotomy is extended forwards to the sinus tarsi. The calcaneofibular ligament is divided. If the fibula remains posteriorly displaced it may be necessary to divide the posterior tibiofibular syndesmosis.

Posterior inferior tibiofibular ligament
Lateral talocalcaneal ligament
Interosseous ligament

Calcaneofibular ligament

12

Postoperative management

Maintenance of reduction and accommodation of swelling after soft tissue correction is best achieved using a Liverpool plaster. The foot should be reviewed (under general anaesthesia) at 2 weeks and if wound healing is complete, the definitive above-knee cast is applied for an initial period of 6 weeks.

Subsequently the plaster may be changed without anaesthesia and, if correction is adequate, a below-knee cast can be used for a further 6 weeks.

By this time the foot will fall readily into a corrected position and a Denis Browne's boot and bar splint are used to maintain this correction for most of the time until the child is standing or walking. It is the author's opinion that, for the walking child, persistence with this splint at night reduces the incidence of relapse if compliance is maintained and that it should be used until the age of 5 years.

SECONDARY CLUB FOOT SURGERY

Late presenting club foot and feet relapsing or inadequately corrected by primary surgery present some of the great challenges in club foot treatment. Innumerable 'secondary' procedures have been described. These include tendon transfers, tarsal osteotomies, bone resection and the final salvage procedure, triple arthrodesis.

TENDON TRANSFER

Despite their place in foot deformity of neuromuscular origin, the principles of tendon transfer do not support their use in idiopathic talipes equinovarus.

TARSAL OSTEOTOMIES

Osteotomies have been described for the calcaneum (Dwyer and Pandy), the talus (Hjelmstedt and J. Roberts) and the metatarsals (Green and Herndon).

BONE RESECTION

Dillwyn Evans' calcaneocuboid wedge resection and arthrodesis, performed as he described in conjunction with a medial soft tissue release, is probably the most reliable operation for secondary correction.

Wedge tarsectomy may be used in the older uncorrected foot to offset the need for triple arthrodesis.

Talectomy has also been used for secondary correction but is not recommended.

TRIPLE ARTHRODESIS

As a last resort, there are few feet that will not become plantigrade and functionally acceptable if a triple arthrodesis is performed.

Acknowledgement

I wish to thank my colleague, W. K. Chung, FRACS, for his assistance.

Further reading

Attenborough CG. Severe congenital talipes equino-varus. *J Bone Joint Surg [Br]* 1966; 48-B: 31–9.

Crawford AH, Marxen JL, Osterfeld DL. The Cincinatti incision: a comprehensive approach for surgical procedures of the foot and ankle in childhood. *J Bone Joint Surg [Am]* 1982; 64-A: 1355–8.

Evans D. The relapsed club foot. *J Bone Joint Surg [Br]* 1961; 43-B: 722–33.

Green AD, Lloyd-Roberts GC. The results of early posterior release in resistant club feet: a long term review. *J Bone Joint Surg [Br]* 1985; 67-B: 588–93.

McKay DW. New concept and approach to club foot treatment: principles and morbid anatomy. *J Paediatr Orthop* 1982; 2: 347–56.

Steindler A. Stripping of the os calcis. *J Orthop Surg* 1920; 2: 8–12.

Turco VJ. Surgical correction of the resistant club foot: one stage posteromedial release with internal fixation: a preliminary report. *J Bone Joint Surg [Am]* 1971; 53-A: 477–97.

Illustrations by Gillian Oliver after B. Hyams

The Robert Jones operation for clawing of hallux

B. Helal MChOrth, FRCS
Honorary Consultant Orthopaedic Surgeon, The Royal London Hospital and The Royal National Orthopaedic Hospital, London, and Enfield Group of Hospitals, UK

S. C. Chen FRCS
Consultant Orthopaedic Surgeon, Enfield Group of Hospitals, UK

Introduction

This operation is carried out for clawing of the big toe due to paralysis of the flexor hallucis brevis and weakness of dorsiflexion of the ankle. The extensor hallucis longus overacts and causes flexion at the interphalangeal joint and dorsiflexion of the big toe. If a callosity develops over the dorsum of the interphalangeal joint or under the metatarsal head correction is necessary.

Operation

Arthrodesis of interphalangeal joint

1a & b

A transverse incision is made across the interphalangeal joint of the big toe. The extensor hallucis longus tendon is identified and detached at its insertion.

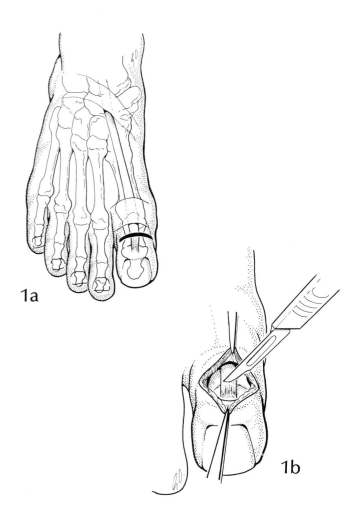

1a

1b

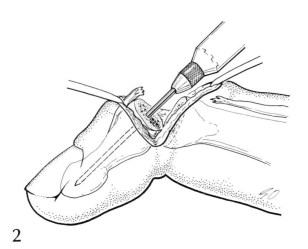

2

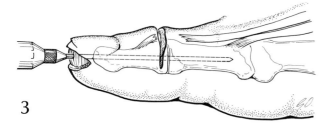

3

2 & 3

The interphalangeal joint is opened up and the articular cartilage removed. The distal phalanx is drilled in a retrograde manner and then the drill passed back again through the distal phalanx and the proximal phalanx drilled. The interphalangeal joint is arthrodesed using a screw.

Tendon transfer to metatarsal neck

4

A second incision is made along the dorsomedial side of the first metatarsal head and neck.

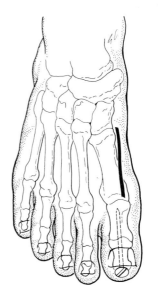

4

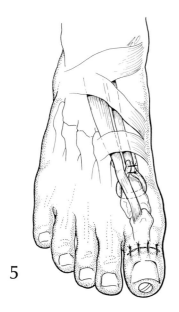

5

5

The neck of the first metatarsal is exposed. The surgeon drills transversely across the neck. The detached extensor hallucis longus tendon is pulled into the proximal wound and passed through the drill-hole in the neck of the first metatarsal. While an assistant pushes the head of the first metatarsal dorsally, with the tendon taut, it is sutured to itself using non-absorbable sutures.

Postoperative management

6

A plaster cast is applied from the tibial tuberosity to the big toe, with the big toe and the ankle in neutral position. The plaster is removed at 3 weeks and active exercises and weight-bearing started.

Reference

Jones R. The soldier's foot and the treatment of common deformities of the foot, Part II. Claw-foot. *Br Med J* 1916; 1: 749–53.

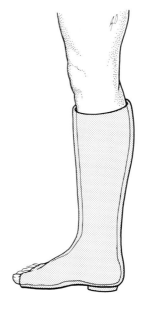

6

Illustrations by Gillian Oliver after B. Hyams

Flexor to extensor transfer for clawing of the lateral four toes (Girdlestone's operation)

B. Helal   MChOrth, FRCS
Honorary Consultant Orthopaedic Surgeon, The Royal London Hospital and The Royal National Orthopaedic Hospital, London, and Enfield Group of Hospitals, UK

S. C. Chen   FRCS
Consultant Orthopaedic Surgeon, Enfield Group of Hospitals, UK

Introduction

Claw toes, that is hyperextension of the metatarsophalangeal joint and flexion of the interphalangeal joints, are due either to overactivity of the toe extensors in the presence of normal toe flexors, caused by poliomyelitis or a peripheral neuropathy, or more commonly to loss of intrinsic foot muscle tone.

For the operation to be successful, the metatarsophalangeal and interphalangeal joints must be fully mobile.

Operation

Incisions

1

Dorsolateral incisions are made from the metatarsal neck to the distal interphalangeal joint of the lateral four toes. The surgeon starts on the second toe first and works laterally.

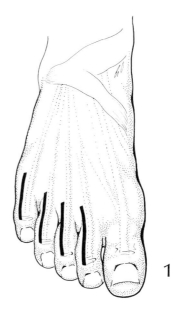

1

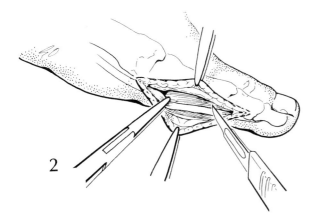

2

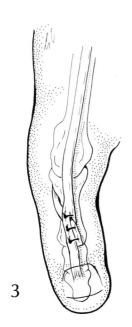

3

2

The lateral edge of the skin incision is retracted. The long and short flexor tendons are found and the long flexor tendon is held with artery forceps to prevent it from retreating proximally into the foot when it is divided at its insertion.

Tendon transfer[1]

3

The long flexor tendon is brought around the lateral side of the proximal phalanx well proximal and close to the bone so that the neurovascular structures are not compressed.

The extensor tendon is split and the long flexor tendon is passed through and sutured to it, proximal to the proximal interphalangeal joint and with the toe plantar-flexed at the metatarsophalangeal joint, using non-absorbable sutures.

Postoperative management

A padded crêpe bandage is applied to the foot. At the end of 2 weeks mobilizing exercises to the toes are started, and walking allowed. In older patients a below-knee plaster of Paris walking cast is necessary to hold the correction.

Reference

1. Taylor RG. The treatment of claw toes by multiple transfers of flexor into extensor tendons. *J Bone Joint Surg [Br]* 1951; 33-B: 539–42.

Illustrations by Gillian Oliver

Forefoot reconstruction

B. Helal MChOrth, FRCS
Honorary Consultant Orthopaedic Surgeon, The Royal London Hospital and The Royal National Orthopaedic Hospital, London, and Enfield Group of Hospitals, UK

S. C. Chen FRCS
Consultant Orthopaedic Surgeon, Enfield Group of Hospitals, UK

Introduction

In rheumatoid arthritis, the forefoot can be deformed by a combination of factors. There may be imbalance of muscle, as well as progressive damage to the metatarsophalangeal and interphalangeal joints of the toes, secondary to synovitis, synovial proliferation, effusion and bone erosion. These changes lead to clawing of the toes, i.e. hyperextension of the metatarsophalangeal joints and flexion of the interphalangeal joints. The metatarsophalangeal joints may be subluxated or dislocated, and the articular surfaces may be destroyed.

When the metatarsophalangeal joints only are affected and are at the subluxation stage, corrective procedures, such as the telescopic osteotomies of the second, third and fourth metatarsals can be carried out. When the metatarsophalangeal joints have dislocated but where the articular surfaces are still relatively normal, open reduction of the joints followed by telescopic osteotomies are feasible. When the articular surfaces are damaged, excision arthroplasties, such as the Fowler[1] or the Hoffmann[2] operations may be performed. The Fowler operation is technically more demanding, but it preserves more of the metatarsal bone. The Hoffmann operation is relatively easy to do, as the dislocated metatarsal heads present in the plantar wound, but more of the metatarsal bones are excised, although the proximal phalanges are not operated upon. In very severe cases, replacement of the metatarsophalangeal joints with a Silastic implant, like the Universal Small Joint Ball Spacer prosthesis (Corin Medical Ltd, Cirencester, UK) may be used.

TELESCOPIC OSTEOTOMIES OF THE SECOND, THIRD AND FOURTH METATARSALS

The objective of this operation is to redistribute the body weight from the prominent second, third and fourth metatarsal heads to all five. The principle of the technique is to perform an oblique osteotomy to the distal metatarsal shaft to allow the head and neck to rise to a more comfortable position. In addition, the oblique osteotomy allows the metatarsal shaft to shorten slightly.

Reduction of dislocated metatarsophalangeal joints

(If the joints are only subluxated, this stage is omitted.)

1a, b & c

Short incisions are made along the dorsum of the second, third and fourth metatarsophalangeal joints. The capsules are incised transversely, and the collateral ligaments released from the sides of the metatarsal heads. The extensor tendons are cut. The dislocated joints are reduced and held in place with Kirschner wires introduced obliquely across the joints in a downward and backward direction. It is important that the dislocations are reduced before proceeding to the telescopic osteotomies, as it would be difficult to reduce the dislocations after the osteotomies.

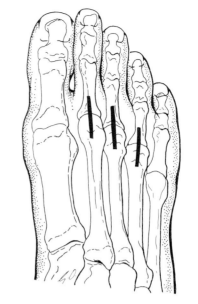

1a

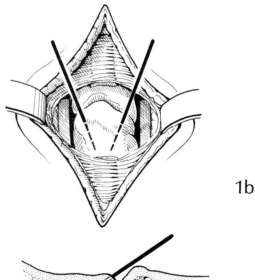

1b

1c

Incision for osteotomies

2

A 4 cm incision is made on the dorsum of the foot along the third metatarsal. The periosteum is incised along the shaft of the third metatarsal and stripped off the bone.

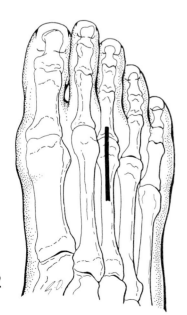

2

Siting the osteotomies

3

Retractors are placed on either side of the bone to protect the soft tissues. An oblique cut is made in the distal shaft of the metatarsal (not the neck), angled 45° downwards and forwards.

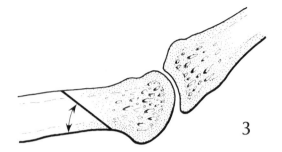

3

4

Through the same skin incision, the second metatarsal is exposed. The periosteum is incised along the shaft and stripped off. Trethowen ring–spike retractors are placed on either side of the bone and an oblique cut is made as described earlier.

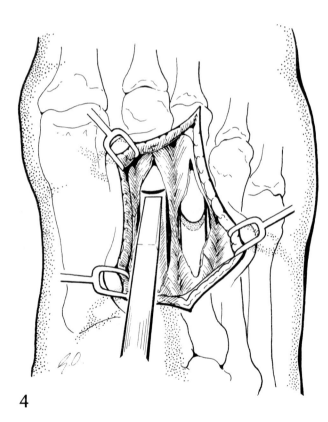

4

5a & b

Through the same skin incision, the fourth metatarsal is identified, and its periosteum stripped off. The spike retractors are placed on either side of the bone. At this stage the fifth metatarsal must not be mistaken for the fourth: this mistake is easily made as the bones are close together. By palpating the fifth metatarsal through the skin, a check may be made that the last bone exposed is indeed the fourth metatarsal.

Again, an oblique cut is made as described earlier. It is important to free the incarcerated metatarsal head from the underlying soft tissue by passing an osteotome between the bone and soft tissue.

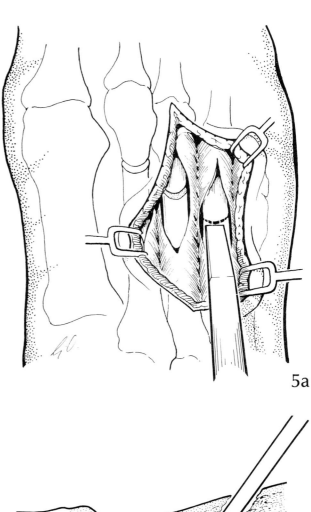

5a

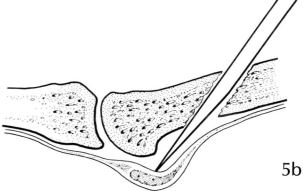

5b

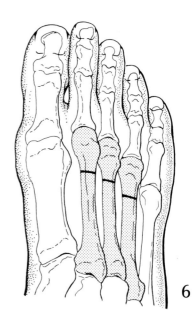

6

At the end of the procedure the three oblique osteotomies should describe a gentle curve which is convex distally. It is important that the soft tissues, especially the intrinsic muscles, are not damaged, or cross-union of the bones may occur.

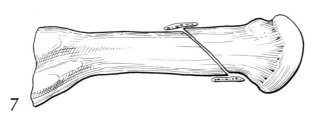

7

The sharp spikes of the distal cut ends of each metatarsal are nibbled away, and the bone chips deposited around the osteotomy sites to encourage bony union.

The skin wound is sutured, and a well padded bandage is applied to the foot and ankle.

Postoperative management

8

It is important that the middle three metatarsal heads are not raised too high, or undue pressure will fall on the first and fifth metatarsal heads, leading to painful callosities.

Early weight-bearing is desirable in the rheumatoid patient. Three days after the operation, the well-padded bandage is removed, and an adhesive dressing applied to the wound. The callosity under the middle three metatarsal heads helps elevation of the middle three metatarsal heads to the correct level. The patient is encouraged to walk, fully weight-bearing and wearing loose-fitting flat shoes for 3 months.

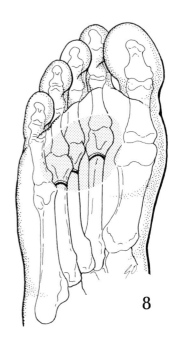

CORRECTION OF ASSOCIATED HALLUX VALGUS AND BUNIONETTE OF 5TH TOE

Once the metatarsal osteotomies have united, which usually takes about 3 months, the associated hallux valgus and bunionette, if present, are dealt with. It is important to stage these procedures to obtain optimum spread of weight when walking.

9a & b

A dorsomedial incision is made over the neck and distal shaft of the first metatarsal. An oblique osteotomy is made, directed laterally, posteriorly and inferiorly at 45°. The joint capsule is left untouched. The wound is sutured.

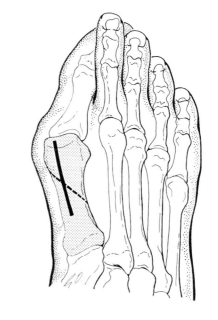

9a

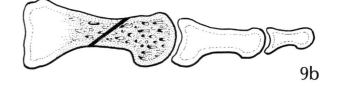

9b

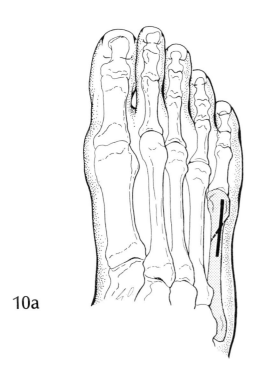

10a

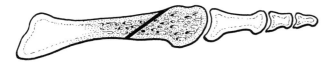

10b

10a & b

When a bunionette is present, it is ill-advised to excise the prominence, which is the metatarsal head, as there is not an exostosis as in hallux valgus.

A dorsolateral incision is made over the neck and distal shaft of the fifth metatarsal. An oblique osteotomy is made, directed medially, posteriorly and inferiorly at 45°. A below-knee walking plaster cast is applied with the big toe immobilized in valgus.

Postoperative management

The plaster cast is removed at the end of 8 weeks. Check radiographs are taken to make sure that bony union has taken place. Active toe exercises are started.

FOWLER OPERATION

11

A dorsomedial incision is made over the metatarsopha-langeal joint of the big toe. The joint is exposed. The proximal third of the proximal phalanx is excised. The dome of the metatarsal head is excised.

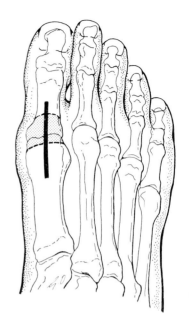

11

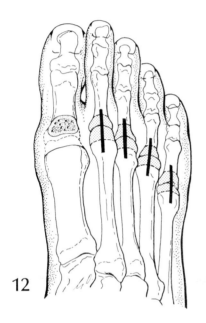

12

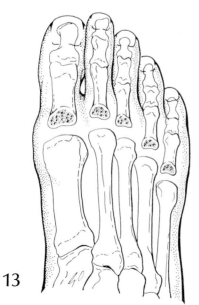

13

12 & 13

Longitudinal incisions are made over the metatarsopha-langeal joints of the second to fifth toes. The proximal third of the proximal phalanges and the metatarsal heads are excised, leaving the flare of the necks behind. The ends of the bones are rounded off by bone nibblers. At the end of the procedure, the ends of the metatarsals describe a gentle curve, convex distally. The level of the first metatarsal is checked to make sure that it is in line with the gentle curve described by the lateral four metatarsals. Only sufficient bone is removed to align it with the other metatarsals. Ideally, the sesamoid bones should still rest on bone. Any further adjustment of the lateral four metatarsals can also be made at this stage. The several wounds on the dorsum of the foot are now sutured.

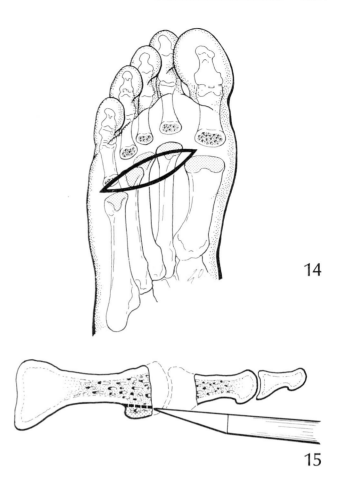

14 & 15

A transverse elliptical incision is made on the sole of the foot encompassing the callosities which are usually present. The undersurfaces of the second to fifth metatarsal heads are exposed by retracting the flexor tendons. The keel of each metatarsal beneath the neck is excised leaving a flat surface. The toes are brought down by suturing the elliptical skin wound with interrupted nylon sutures. A well-padded bandage is applied.

Postoperative management

The padded bandage is removed a week after surgery, and a lightly padded bandage is applied. The patient is encouraged to bear weight using a walking aid. At the end of 2 weeks, the dressings are taken down, and the skin sutures removed. Active plantarflexion exercises are started. The patient is advised to wear flat loose-fitting shoes.

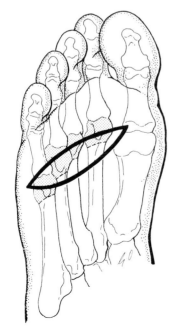

HOFFMANN OPERATION (Kates-Kessel technique[3])

16

A transverse elliptical incision is made on the sole of the foot, encompassing the callosities which are usually present. The flexor tendons are retracted, and the capsule of each joint is incised, exposing the dislocated metatarsal heads. These are excised at the level of the necks. The ends of the second to fifth metatarsals should describe a gentle curve, convex distally. (Kates and Kessel recommend removal of the first metatarsal head through the sole incision but this is technically more difficult and we recommend adherence to the Hoffmann technique.)

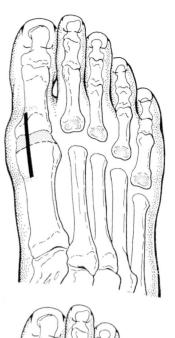

17

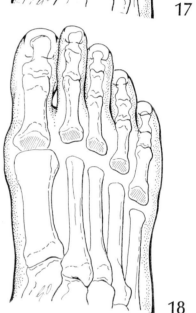

18

17 & 18

A dorsomedial incision is made over the metatarsophalangeal joint of the big toe. The first metatarsal head is excised in line with the other metatarsals. The skin incision is sutured, after repairing the joint capsule.

It is important to maintain the same relative lengths of the metatarsals to ensure a good result. Kates advised inspection by image intensifier at operation.

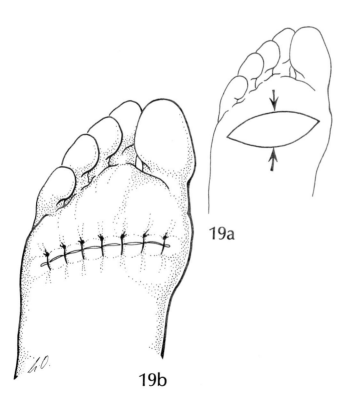

19a

19b

19a & b

The elliptical skin wound on the sole of the foot is now sutured with interrupted nylon stitches, bringing the toes down. A well-padded bandage is applied.

Postoperative management

A week after the operation, the well-padded bandage is taken down and the wounds inspected. A lightly padded bandage is applied, and the patient encouraged to walk using a walking aid. At the end of 2 weeks, the sutures are removed. The patient is advised to wear flat loose-fitting shoes.

PROSTHETIC REPLACEMENT OF THE METATARSOPHALANGEAL JOINTS

20

The Universal Small Joint Ball Spacer is a prosthesis made of silicone elastomer, and consists of a ball with truncated ends and two thin flexible stems, reinforced with Dacron ribbon (du Pont, UK). There are four sizes: No. 1 is 10 mm long and 15 mm wide, No. 2 is 9 × 13 mm, No. 3 is 8 × 11 mm and No. 4 is 7 × 9 mm.

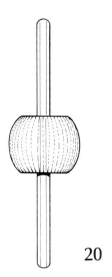

20

Prosthetic replacement in big toe

21

A straight dorsomedial incision is made across the metatarsophalangeal joint of the big toe. About 7.5 mm of the head is removed with a power saw, and the edges trimmed with a small bone nibbler. It is important not to remove too much of the head, otherwise the sesamoid bones will drop into the space created by the bone excision. Holes are made in the metatarsal and the proximal phalanx using a small Paton burr. It is important to site these holes in the centre of each bone and opposite each other. They should be along the longitudinal axes of the two bones.

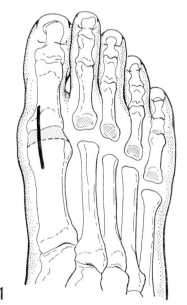

21

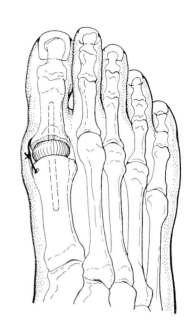

22a

22a & b

A drill hole is made in the medial side of the metatarsal stump. A suture of No. 1 PDS material (Ethicon, Edinburgh, UK) is placed in the capsule, either ventromedially or medially to correct any valgus with or without a rotational deformity. This suture is passed through the hole made in the medial side of the metatarsal. The correct size prosthesis (usually a No. 1) is inserted, making sure that it sits snugly in the space created. The big toe is moved up and down several times to make sure the prosthesis is well-seated.

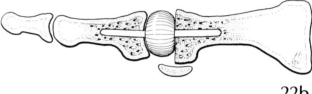

22b

22c

The capsule of the metatarsophalangeal joint of the big toe is attached to the metatarsal using the PDS suture already inserted in it. The capsules are sutured and the skin wounds closed.

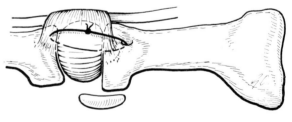

22c

Prosthetic replacement in lesser toes

23

Longitudinal incisions are made over the metatarsophalangeal joints of the lateral four toes. The metatarsal heads are excised so that they describe a gentle curve with the first metatarsal, convex distally. The proximal phalanges are brought down in line with the metatarsals. If necessary the collateral ligaments may have to be released from the sides of the metatarsals.

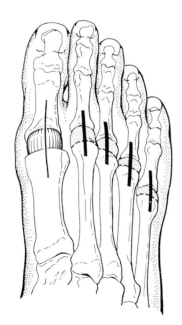

23

24

Holes are made in the metatarsals and proximal phalanges, in a similar fashion to the big toe. The correct size prostheses (usually No. 2 or 3) are inserted.

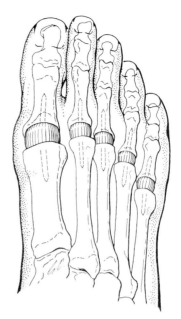

24

Closure

A transverse elliptical incision is made in the sole of the foot, encompassing the callosities which are usually present. The skin edges are sutured which results in the toes being brought down (*see Illustration 19a,b*). Well-padded bandages are applied.

Postoperative management

The bandages are removed a week after operation, and active and passive toe exercises are started. A lightly padded bandage is applied, and the patient is encouraged to walk. After a fortnight loose-fitting flat shoes are worn.

References

1. Fowler AW. A method of forefoot reconstruction: an operation for the relief of irreversible claw toes. *J Bone Joint Surg [Br]* 1959; 41-B: 507–13.

2. Hoffmann P. An operation for severe grades of contracted or clawed toes. *Am J Orthop Surg* 1912; 9: 441–9.

3. Kates A, Kessel L, Kay A. Arthroplasty of the forefoot. *J Bone Joint Surg [Br]* 1967; 49-B: 552–7.

Further reading

Chen SC, Ali MA. Metatarsal osteotomies: a comparison between the power saw and bone cutters. *J Bone Joint Surg [Br]* 1985; 67-B: 671.

Chen SC, Khan O. A comparative study of metatarsophalangeal osteotomies with and without open reduction of associated MTP joint dislocations. *J Bone Joint Surg [Br]* 1985; 67-B: 671.

Helal B. Metatarsal osteotomy for metatarsalgia. *J Bone Joint Surg [Br]* 1975; 57-B: 187.

Helal B. Surgery for adolescent hallux valgus. *Clin Orthop* 1981; 157: 50–63.

Helal B, Chen SC. Arthroplastik des Großzehengrundgelenks mit einer neuen Silastik – Endoprothese. *Orthopäde* 1982; 11: 200.

Helal B, Chen SC. Arthroplasty of the metatarso-phalangeal joint of the big toe using a new silicone elastomer prosthesis. *Med Chir Pied* 1986; 7: 95.

Helal B, Gupta SK, Gojaseni P. Surgery for adolescent hallux valgus. *Acta Orthop Scand* 1974; 45: 271–95.

Illustrations by Peter Cox after F. Price

Hallux valgus and hallux rigidus

H. Piggott FRCS
Consultant Orthopaedic Surgeon, United Birmingham Hospitals,
Royal Orthopaedic Hospital, Birmingham, and Warwickshire Orthopaedic Hospital, Coleshill, UK

HALLUX VALGUS

General considerations

The normal big toe is in slight valgus, determined by the shape of the metatarsal and proximal phalanx, but the articular surfaces of the metatarsophalangeal joint are everywhere in contact. Hallux valgus, by contrast, shows subluxation of the metatarsophalangeal joint, the phalanx being displaced laterally. A small intermediate group has the phalanx displaced to the lateral limit of the metatarsal head, leaving its medial border 'exposed'; this type sometimes progresses to subluxation. Although hallux valgus may develop in rheumatoid arthritis and some neurological disorders, in the great majority its cause is unknown and it starts insidiously in childhood and slowly progresses. There is a progressive buckling of the first skeletal ray, and later, presumably as a result of the altered mechanics, other forefoot changes appear, including depression of the second (and sometimes third and fourth) metatarsal head and dorsal subluxation or dislocation of the metatarsophalangeal joints, with hammer deformity of the proximal interphalangeal joints. Pes valgus is often present. Osteoarthritic changes may develop in the first metatarsophalangeal joint and a bunion forms over the medially projecting first metatarsal head, often with infective episodes.

Symptoms in this complex deformity are unpredictable and may be absent. The commonest complaints are: shoe pressure pain at the bunion, osteoarthritic symptoms in the first metatarsophalangeal joint, weight-bearing pain under the forefoot, shoe pressure on a hammer toe and a general foot ache on standing.

Choice of operation

With such a variable picture, selection of procedures must depend on overall assessment of symptoms, anatomical changes, way of life in relation to activity, shoe wear and personality. Some general guides are the following.

1. Physiological valgus is not a surgical problem; neither is a broad but otherwise normal forefoot.
2. In the early stages of deformity, when there is subluxation of the first metatarsophalangeal joint, but no secondary changes, treatment aims at permanent correction of the subluxation without damaging the joint.
3. In later stages when degenerative changes are present, surgery is determined by symptoms, and this may involve operation on the metatarsophalangeal joint or on other parts of the forefoot, or both.

This chapter considers only big toe operations.

Osteotomy

Osteotomy of the first metatarsal neck allows lateral displacement of the metatarsal head and slight shortening of the metatarsal shaft which slackens off the bowstrung long tendons so that the subluxation can be reduced without opening the joint. Division of the insertion of adductor hallucis and realignment of the tendon of extensor hallucis longus prevents recurrence of deformity. The operation is appropriate in the early stages before secondary changes have appeared.

Keller arthroplasty

The base of the proximal phalanx is excised to form a false joint and the medial prominence of the metatarsal head trimmed off. The false joint usually has enough mobility to allow a reasonable range of heel heights, but the big toe is short and push-off is weakened. This operation is suitable where symptoms arise from shoe pressure at the first metatarsal head or from degenerative changes in the first metatarsophalangeal joint, in a patient who does not need to walk long distances.

Arthrodesis

This gives a strong first ray, but the range of heel heights is limited and must be agreed preoperatively. It must *not* be done when the interphalangeal joint is stiff (unless excision arthroplasty of the latter is performed simultaneously). It is advised where symptoms arise from osteoarthritis of the joint, with or without metatarsal head pressure, in an active patient.

Exostectomy

Exostectomy has a limited place, where symptoms are restricted to shoe pressure discomfort. Postoperative recovery is more rapid than after arthroplasty or arthrodesis. It is not recommended for the younger patient with hallux valgus since it does nothing to prevent progression of the deformity.

INTERPHALANGEAL VALGUS

Valgus deformity is not uncommon at the interphalangeal joint of the big toe, and occasionally symptoms arise from shoe pressure on the prominent medial side of the joint. The deformity is due to the shape of the bones, not subluxation of the joint, and it can be corrected by osteotomy of the distal end of the proximal phalanx. Rarely, in late cases with degenerative osteoarthritis, arthrodesis is advisable.

HALLUX RIGIDUS

Hallux rigidus is a stiffening of the first metatarsophalangeal joint from arthritis, usually osteoarthritis, and may develop in quite young people. Transient episodes of pain and stiffness can occur and these should be treated conservatively, operation being reserved for persistent or frequently repeated symptoms.

The choice between arthrodesis, Keller arthroplasty and exostectomy depends on the same considerations as in hallux valgus, arthrodesis being for the vigorous who are content with a limited range of heel heights, arthroplasty for the less active and those who wish to wear high heels sometimes, while exostectomy is limited to the few whose symptoms are confined to shoe pressure on an exostosis, which in hallux rigidus is often dorsal, small and well localized.

Contraindications

1. Relative contraindications to all these procedures are severe diabetes, and arterial or venous insufficiency.
2. Stiffness of the metatarsophalangeal or the interphalangeal joint is a contraindication to arthrodesis of the other (though one of them may be arthrodesed and the other converted to a pseudarthrosis by excision of articular surfaces).
3. An infected bunion may delay surgery until it is controlled.

Preoperative

Position for operation

General anaesthesia is preferred. A pneumatic tourniquet is a great advantage but can be omitted on the rare occasions when there is circulatory doubt or any tendency to thrombosis. The patient is supine, and a slightly head-up position gives more comfortable access to the dorsum of the foot. Draping leaves the whole foot and ankle exposed; this is particularly important in assessing the position for arthrodesis. For most operations, the surgeon is more comfortable at the foot of the table facing the patient's head, but a right-handed operator may work conveniently on the left foot from that side of the table, an important point when bilateral procedures are performed simultaneously. A shelf clamped to the side of the foot of the table allows separation of the feet and further facilitates bilateral operation.

Operations

METATARSAL NECK OSTEOTOMY

Division of adductor hallucis

1

A straight dorsal incision is made from mid-phalanx to mid-metatarsal and the exposure deepened between the first and second metatarsal heads to expose the tendon of adductor hallucis at its insertion to the lateral sesamoid. This is facilitated by keeping close to the capsule of the first metatarsophalangeal joint while firm retraction is applied to the first and second metatarsals. The tendon is divided at its insertion.

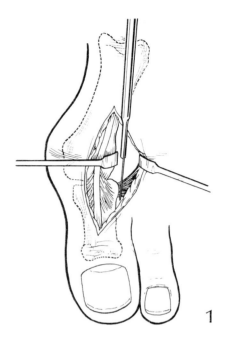

Line of osteotomy

2

The periosteum of the neck and distal shaft of the first metatarsal is approached by a longitudinal incision through the paratenon and extensor hood a few millimetres medial to the tendon of extensor hallucis longus, and the bone is then exposed subperiosteally. The neck is divided strictly transversely, immediately proximal to the joint capsule. It is essential to perform the osteotomy through this broad part of the bone to allow room for adequate lateral displacement of the head, which must be at least half its width. An oscillatory power saw is best but care must be taken to protect the extensor hallucis longus tendon. If power is not available, multiple small drill holes joined by cutting forceps are a good alternative.

Peg and socket

3a & b

The metatarsal head must be moved laterally by about half its diameter and the metatarsal shaft shortened about 8 mm to slacken off the long tendons, both flexor and extensor, which are bowstrung on the lateral side of the joint. Shortening in the long axis of the metatarsal would elevate the head slightly from the weight-bearing position and to avoid this (which would put excess strain on the lesser metatarsal heads), the head is displaced in a slightly plantar direction. To achieve this lateral and plantar displacement, the cortex of the proximal fragment is trimmed away to leave a stout projecting 8 mm lateroplantar peg. A socket is then made in the dorsomedial part of the cut surface of the head to fit the peg precisely. A small osteotome is used as a hand tool and the fit must be exact. The head is then displaced laterally and plantarwards, and peg and socket fitted and impacted. Finally, the now medially projecting distal part of the shelf is trimmed off smooth.

Fashioning and fitting the peg and socket must be precise and the immobilization is then very secure. The socket should be cut fractionally too small, 'lined up', and finally the peg trimmed to exactly the right size; a large peg should *not* be forced into a small socket – this will crush the cancellous bone of the head and result in a loose fit.

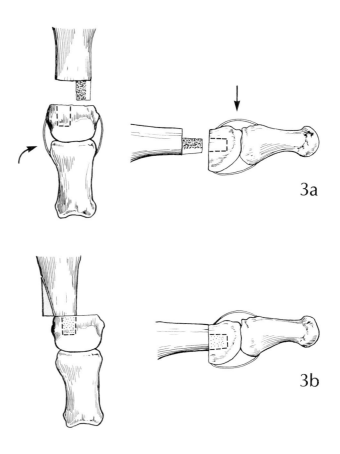

3a

3b

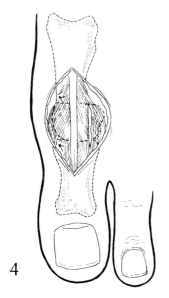

4

Realignment of extensor hallucis longus

4

The extensor hallucis longus tendon is now realigned centrally over the metatarsophalangeal joint. To do this the extensor hood is incised longitudinally on the lateral side of the tendon, and reefed medially. A plaster of Paris boot is applied with a cylindrical extension for the big toe, holding it in slight varus and flexion.

KELLER ARTHROPLASTY

Skin incision

5

The excision extends on the dorsum from the middle of the proximal phalanx to just proximal to the metatarsal head. The curve illustrated is a safeguard against contracture and is also concealed by the shoe. A bursa, if present, is excised at this stage, but if the overlying skin is adherent and thin, only its deep wall is removed.

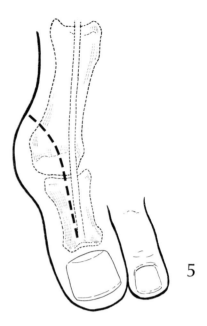

Capsular incision

6

The capsule is incised in the same line as the skin and detached with a scalpel from the sides of the base of the phalanx. Narrow spike retractors are inserted to protect the long tendons.

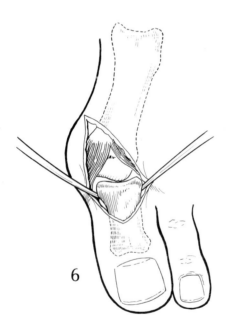

Dislocation of proximal phalanx

7

A sharp hook is inserted through the articular surface of the base of the phalanx and with help from the retractors serves to dislocate the joint with the phalanx in the strongly flexed position. A few touches of the knife on the plantar aspect release the phalanx from the capsule; by keeping very close to bone, the long flexor tendon is avoided.

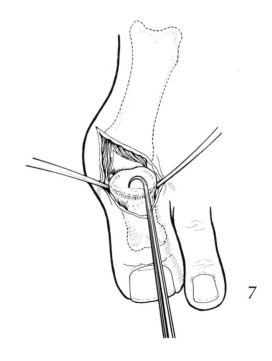

Excision of proximal phalanx

8

Approximately half the phalanx is excised. Sharp-pointed bone-cutting forceps may be used, taking small bites to avoid splintering; any rough edges are carefully smoothed off. The aim is a long fibrous joint to allow free mobility; hence adequate bony excision is essential, but removing more than half the phalanx is likely to give an obviously short toe and shoe pressure on the projecting second toe may result.

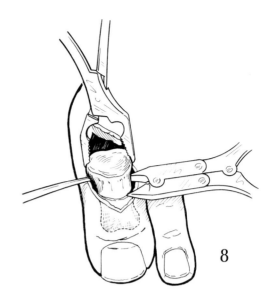

8

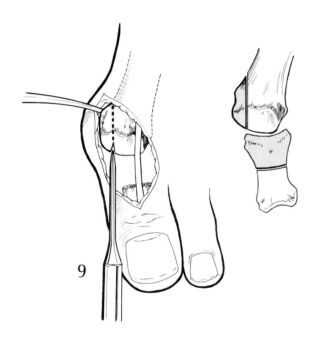

9

Excising exostosis

9

A narrow spike retractor under the metatarsal head holds the capsule clear and the 'exostosis' (really the non-articulating part of the metatarsal head) is removed with an osteotome, any resulting sharp edges being smoothed off with nibbling forceps. The line of osteotomy is determined by lining up the remains of the phalanx on the metatarsal head and removing enough of the latter to ensure there is no medial projection.

Elongating the extensor hallucis longus tendon or insertion of Kirschner wire

10a & b

If the big toe now lies comfortably straight, and with a gap of 4 mm or more at the pseudarthrosis, it remains only to suture the capsular incision and skin. However, sometimes the toe is found to flop into valgus, and sometimes the phalanx is held tightly against the metatarsal head by the tension of the longitudinal muscles. If the problem is valgus only, a Kirschner wire should be passed longitudinally across the pseudarthrosis. It is inserted in the cut proximal end of the phalanx and passed distally to emerge through the end of the toe, then pushed back into the first metatarsal shaft. Six millimetres are left projecting and bent plantarwards. If the pseudarthrosis is 'tight', in addition to inserting a Kirschner wire, the extensor hallucis longus tendon is lengthened by Z-plasty. The Kirschner wire is withdrawn 6 weeks later.

Wool and a firm crêpe bandage are applied with a spica configuration to hold the big toe in slight valgus.

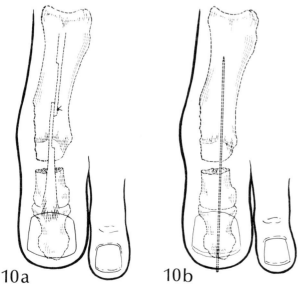

10a   10b

ARTHRODESIS

Incision

11

A dorsal longitudinal incision starts at the metatarsal neck and ends at the distal end of the proximal phalanx by curving plantarwards and medially. The capsule is opened in the line of incision, and the base of the proximal phalanx delivered as in the Keller procedure (*see Illustration 7*).

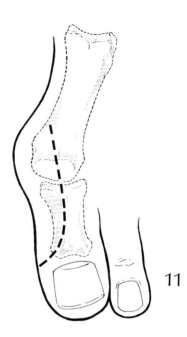

11

Excision of joint surfaces and alignment

12

Alignment of the phalanx is critical. Valgus should be such that the big toe lies alongside the second, nearly but not quite touching it. To determine the degree of dorsiflexion, the metatarsal is placed in the position it will take in shoes (the customary heel height having been agreed preoperatively), with the phalanx just clear of the ground.

Rotation must be avoided completely. The best way of ensuring a good fit is to remove both joint surfaces with an oscillating power saw, to leave flat cancellous surfaces fitting precisely in the desired alignment. The phalangeal surface is cut first, then the toe is lined up in the desired postoperative position and the plane of metatarsal section marked on the medial and dorsal surfaces of the head with a fine osteotome so that the two cut surfaces will be parallel. This needs much practice and a good eye, and there is no room for error. A good alternative is to remove articular cartilage and underlying cortical bone with nibbling forceps and small gouges, preserving the mutual curve of the articular surfaces, so that the phalanx may be aligned by ball and socket motion.

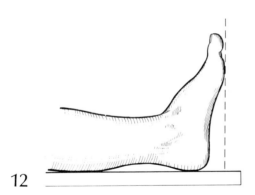

12

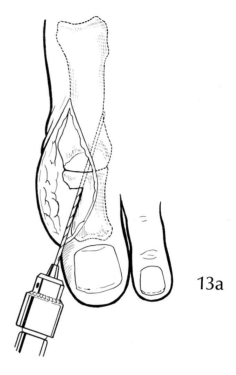

13a

Screw fixation

13a & b

A screw is inserted obliquely as shown. To allow accurate insertion of the drill and subsequent recessing of the screw head, a small notch is cut with nibbling forceps at the point of entry to the phalanx and the screw should engage the opposite cortex of the metatarsal shaft. The screw must be tightened only enough to prevent movement at the arthrodesis. Positioning of the joint and screw is critical and if the screw is incorrectly placed it is difficult to resite – second attempts usually pass along the original track. The cautious surgeon will therefore have in reserve a miniature Charnley compression apparatus.

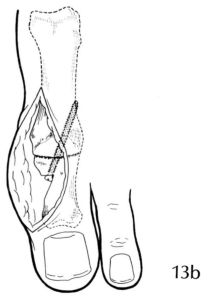

13b

EXOSTECTOMY

Line of osteotomy

14

The skin incision is as for the Keller procedure and similarly a bursa, if present, is excised. The capsule is incised in the same line but is detached from the medial side of the phalanx only enough to allow access for the osteotome. Plantarflexion and valgus deviation of the phalanx combined with a narrow spike retractor under the metatarsal head complete the exposure. The line of bone section should ensure that there is no projection beyond the line of the phalanx. Sharp edges are rounded off with nibbling forceps.

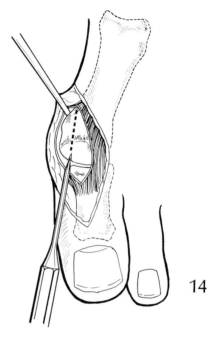

14

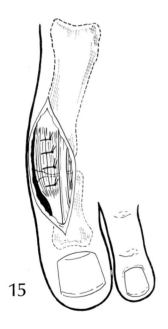

15

Capsular closure

15

The medial capsular flap is trimmed of any redundancy and then sutured back to effect a firm closure of the joint.

A small dorsal exostosis, most commonly seen in hallux rigidus, may be removed through a very limited curved or elliptical incision directly over it, skin and capsule being incised in the same line.

OSTEOTOMY OF NECK OF PROXIMAL PHALANX

16a & b

This is done only for interphalangeal valgus. A medial longitudinal incision extends from the base of the proximal to the middle of the distal phalanx; keeping to the 'mid-lateral' line of the toe will ensure that dissection is dorsal to the plantar digital nerve. The periosteum is incised and elevated from the distal part of the proximal phalangeal shaft, and a small wedge of bone, based medially, is excised with fine pointed bone-cutting forceps. The osteotomy is carried right through the lateral cortex, leaving only a bridge of periosteum – if the lateral cortex is left intact the wedge tends to spring open and correction is lost. It is then easy to close the wedge, and a strong catgut suture passed through small drill holes, as shown, will hold it closed. A fine Kirschner wire in a T-handle makes an excellent drill for this purpose. A padded malleable metal strip splint, curved to fit the toe, is adequate immobilization, but if there is any doubt about the stability of the suture, a Kirschner wire may be passed longitudinally from the tip of the toe across the osteotomy.

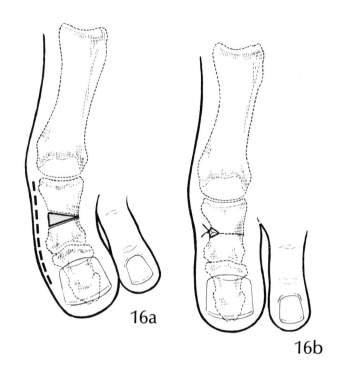

16a

16b

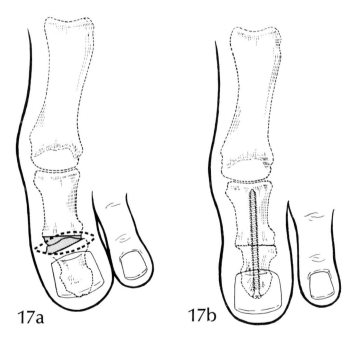

17a

17b

INTERPHALANGEAL ARTHRODESIS

17a & b

When osteoarthritic changes are present, with or without deformity, the interphalangeal joint may be arthrodesed, provided the metatarsophalangeal joint has full movement and is free of degenerative change. A dorsal transverse narrow elliptical incision is made, and the extensor tendon and dorsal joint capsule are incised transversely. The articular surfaces are trimmed off to expose cancellous bone and obtain a flush flat fit. Fixation may be secured by a longitudinal screw, or, if the distal phalanx is very small, by two longitudinal Kirschner wires.

Postoperative management

In all cases the foot is elevated in bed until pain and swelling have subsided, which is usually after 2–3 days. Pain may be quite severe and adequate analgesia is essential. Thereafter follows a progression from sitting out with feet elevated to crutch-walking in unilateral cases, or assisted walking in bilateral cases, to full weight-bearing and finally removal of dressings or plaster according to individual comfort and the mechanical needs of the different operations.

Metatarsal neck osteotomy and arthrodesis are immobilized immediately by a plaster of Paris boot or below-knee plaster cast with a cylindrical extension incorporating the big toe. Weight-bearing is permitted as soon as comfort permits, usually 4–5 days postoperatively, and the position is checked radiologically. Union is usually firm enough to permit removal of plaster 6 weeks after operation. If subcuticular sutures have been used, they may be left *in situ* until final removal of plaster.

At the conclusion of Keller arthroplasty or exostectomy, ample wool and a firm bandage are applied to hold the toe in slight varus and flexion. Patients are usually older than those selected for osteotomy or arthrodesis, skin quality may have been impaired by past inflammation, and after the Keller operation there is sometimes a tendency for the incision to sink a little into the gap created by the joint excision; for all these reasons interrupted skin sutures are preferred in these two operations and walking is prohibited, except for essential nursing needs, until healing is sound and sutures are removed, usually after about 2 weeks. For a Keller arthroplasty a thermoplastic splint is fitted to hold the big toe in slight overcorrection and is worn full-time for 6 weeks and at night for a further 6 weeks.

The interphalangeal operations, on the other hand, need only a malleable metal toe splint for 4 weeks, unless there is doubt about the security of fixation, in which case a plaster boot or below-knee plaster cast with a big toe spica extension is applied.

After all types of big toe operation, physiotherapy begins as soon as pain permits, usually about 24 hours postoperatively, and consists, as far as immobilization permits, of active exercises of intrinsic foot muscles, calf and dorsiflexors, and the antigravity exercises appropriate for any period of bed rest. The patient is taught these exercises *preoperatively*; he continues them through the whole period of immobilization and after that as long as any tendency to swelling remains, until full mobility is attained. Temporary elastic support of foot, ankle and leg may occasionally be necessary for swelling after removal of bandages or plaster boot.

Illustrations by Peter Cox

Dorsal nerve transfer for plantar digital neuroma (Morton's metatarsalgia)

W. N. Gilmour FRCS, FRACS
Emeritus Consultant Surgeon, Royal Perth Hospital and Princess Margaret Hospital for Children, Perth, Australia

Introduction

Morton, in his original description of pain occurring in the forefoot and radiating into the fourth toe, indicated this to be of neural origin.

Pathology

1 & 2

It has become clear that the pathology commences as an inflammation of the intermetatarsophalangeal bursa with secondary involvement of the plantar digital nerve – and also the vessel, creating an endarteritis. The nerve swelling is mostly due to oedema of the epineurium and surrounding tissue more than a true 'neuroma'. The space between the third and fourth toes is usually affected; that between the second and third less frequently. A transverse section shows the metatarsal heads with the bursa and its relationship to the plantar nerve and vessels.

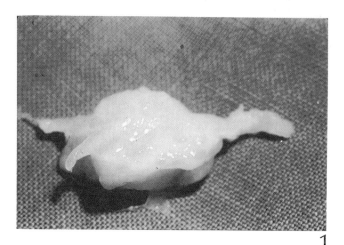

1

Mechanics

It is postulated that the reason for this difference is the movement which goes on between the third and fourth metatarsal heads. In the forefoot the first metatarsal and the paired fourth and fifth metatarsal heads are weight-bearing with the central second and third being elevated, making up the transverse arch.

The metatarsals function as three units. The gap between the first and second metatarsals avoids the necessity for a bursa; but maximum movement occurs between the third and the fourth heads, hence the bursa and its frequent enlargement.

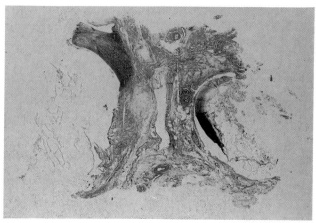

2

Preoperative

Diagnosis

The symptoms are of a pain which is burning and severe, radiating into the fourth or third toes and occurring at rest as well as when walking. At times it is described as knife-like.

The individual usually has a favourite pair of shoes and will be seen to remove the shoe at odd occasions.

The foot is usually architecturally normal. Some sensory loss may be determined and the 'neuroma' can be squeezed up between the metatarsal heads. Occasionally a dorsal lump will form or the toes will separate.

Principles of treatment

The bursitis and nerve involvement is reversible and may be assisted by (1) shoe selection, (2) metatarsal dome insole, and (3) infiltration with steroid. The conventional operation has been excision of the 'neuroma' through a plantar or dorsal incision. This results in the formation of a true end-neuroma which may repair distally into the weight-bearing area with the return of nerve symptoms. This may be dealt with by a second operation to dissect out the neuroma and implant it deeply in the muscles of the foot.

A more logical approach is to transfer the nerve from a plantar to a dorsal side.

Operation

The patient may select local or general anaesthesia. The operation is done in the supine position with the foot elevated.

Incision

3

A dorsal or a plantar incision may be chosen; it is remarkable how well the skin will heal without scar formation with a plantar incision.

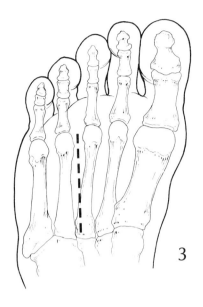

3

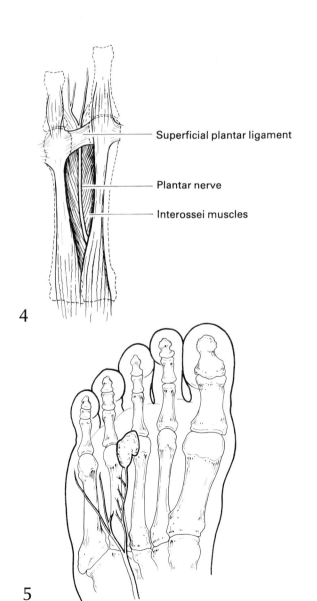

Superficial plantar ligament

Plantar nerve

Interossei muscles

4

Dissection

4 & 5

The nerve is found by dividing the superficial plantar ligament (which is a portion of the plantar fascia). The bursa is opened and the 'neuroma' dissected out from the surrounding tissue between the metatarsal heads. The distal dissection is taken well into the adjoining toes and along the proximal phalanx. The proximal dissection involves splitting the lumbrical. The nerve of the 3–4 space has a contribution from the medial plantar nerve and this is preserved. Small superficial twigs to the skin of the pad must be divided.

5

Nerve transposition

6

The bursa is opened and the space between the third and fourth metatarsals is opened by dividing the deep plantar ligament. The nerve can now be transposed onto the dorsum and above the metatarsophalangeal joint; it lies without tension if the proximal and distal dissection is adequate.

Postoperative management

The skin is closed and the foot bandaged to keep the metatarsal heads together.

Weight-bearing is allowed after 10 days, with the removal of the sutures. The foot is kept bound with adhesive strapping for 2 weeks.

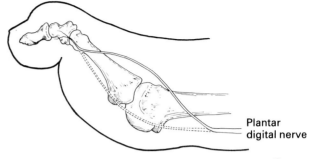

Plantar digital nerve

6

Illustrations by Peter Cox

Hammer and mallet toe

H. Piggott FRCS
Consultant Orthopaedic Surgeon, United Birmingham Hospitals,
Royal Orthopaedic Hospital, Birmingham, and Warwickshire Orthopaedic Hospital, Coleshill, UK

HAMMER TOE

Hammer toe is a flexion deformity of the proximal interphalangeal joint, most commonly affecting the second toe. Mobile at first, it later becomes fixed and may be associated with dorsal subluxation of the metatarsophalangeal joint. The distal interphalangeal joint may be normal or hyperextended; sometimes it is flexed. Hammer toe may occur in isolation or in association with hallux valgus; in the latter case, when deformity is extreme, the second toe may be so far dorsally displaced as to lie on top of the valgus big toe. Pain is caused by shoe pressure on the dorsum of the proximal interphalangeal joint, which develops a callosity and sometimes a small bursa.

Choice of operation

When the deformity and symptoms are limited to the proximal interphalangeal joint, it should be corrected by arthrodesis. *Mobile* dorsiflexion of the metatarsophalangeal joint can be treated simultaneously by subcutaneous extensor tenotomy and capsulotomy, but if this joint is subluxed, especially if irreducible, arthrodesis of the proximal interphalangeal joint is likely to result in an elevated 'anti-aircraft-gun toe' and excision of the proximal part of the proximal phalanx is preferred.

If the metatarsophalangeal joint is subluxed and the predominant symptom is weight-bearing pain under the metatarsal head, then reduction of the subluxation by metatarsal osteotomy (*see* p. 1264) is undertaken and the hammer toe corrected only if it still projects significantly when the metatarsal has been realigned.

Associated hallux valgus may need surgical correction at the same time as the second toe. Very occasionally, especially in the elderly, if the big toe abuts firmly on the third, if the intervening second toe, often hammered, is completely displaced dorsally and if symptoms are restricted to painful shoe pressure on that toe, surgery may be limited to amputating it.

MALLET TOE

This is a flexion deformity of the distal interphalangeal joint, most commonly affecting the second toe and usually occurring as an isolated deformity. Symptoms arise from pressure, either under the pulp from weight-bearing or on the dorsum from the shoe. Treatment is by arthrodesis of the distal interphalangeal joint.

Operations

SPIKE ARTHRODESIS

Incision

1

A dorsal ellipse of skin is excised over the apex of the deformity. The underlying extensor aponeurosis is similarly excised to open the joint.

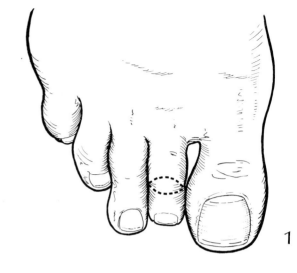

Division of collateral ligaments

2

The key to easy access is detachment of the collateral ligaments from the head of the proximal phalanx, cutting retrograde from within the joint, which is held strongly flexed.

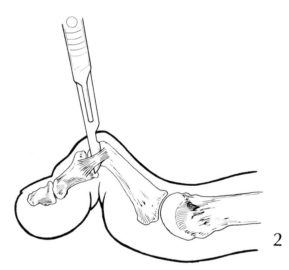

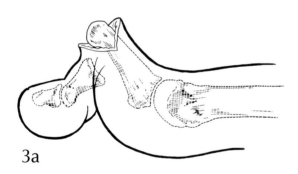

3a

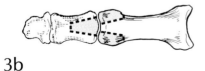

3b

Delivery, spike and socket

3a & b

The phalangeal head is then easily delivered and trimmed to make a stout spike. Small nibbling forceps are ideal and trimming starts most easily at the plantarolateral and plantaromedial aspects of the condyles; the dorsal cortex is left intact since strength of the spike depends on it. A matching conical hole is drilled in the proximal phalanx, starting with an awl and enlarging with burrs until a firm press-fit is obtained.

Suture and splintage

4

Two or three vertical mattress sutures close the incision, and a malleable padded metal toe splint or a plaster strip is applied.

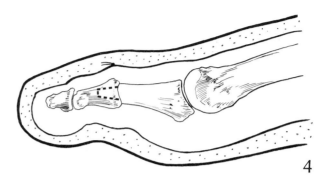

4

Kirschner wire method

5

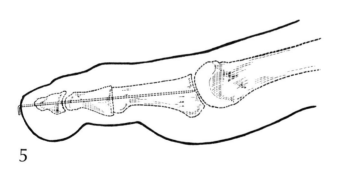

5

Spike arthrodesis shortens the toe a little, and if it is already short an alternative is to cut off the articular surfaces transversely and secure fixation with a longitudinal Kirschner wire passed from the joint distally, through both phalanges and the distal interphalangeal joint to emerge from the pulp, and then pushed retrograde into the proximal phalanx. It may be cut off subcutaneously or an 8 mm projection can be bent plantarwards, depending on the anticipated level of postoperative activity.

Mallet toe may similarly be corrected by spike arthrodesis of the distal interphalangeal joint, but the distal phalanx is not big enough for an adequate socket, and the Kirschner wire technique is more suitable. (When both interphalangeal joints are deformed, Kirschner wire arthrodesis of both may be performed simultaneously.)

PARTIAL EXCISION OF PROXIMAL PHALANX

6a, b & c

An S-incision is made to minimize risk of contracture. The extensor tendon is split longitudinally; and traction on the base of the phalanx with a strong towel clip, combined with a few touches of the scalpel to detach the capsule, allows easy delivery into the incision. The required amount of phalanx, usually about one-half, is removed with fine-pointed, bone-cutting forceps. If the toe tends to 'cock-up' the extensor expansion is divided transversely. Skin only is sutured and the toe is bandaged in slight plantarflexion.

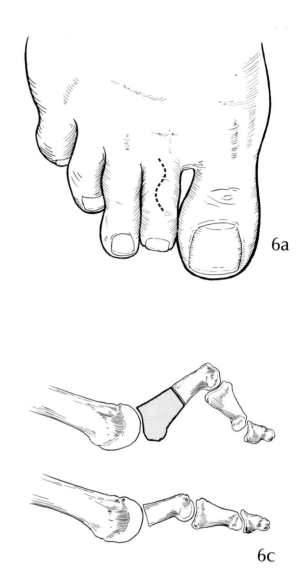

6a

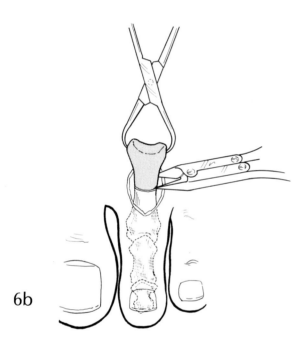

6b

6c

Postoperative management

The foot is elevated in bed until pain is minimal, usually 24–48 hours. Thereafter increasing walking is permitted, provided there is no pain or swelling. The position of a spike arthrodesis should be checked by X-ray at this stage. Sutures are removed after 12–14 days. Union of a spike is usually sound by 4 weeks and the splint may be removed then, but a 'flush-cut' Kirschner wire arthrodesis usually takes longer and the wire should remain *in situ* for 6–8 weeks. If the wire was cut off subcutaneously, local anaesthesia is required for its withdrawal, over the end of the wire if very superficial or as a digital block if it is more than 1–2 mm deep. Fine-pointed, short-nosed milliner's pliers facilitate withdrawal of the wire through a 4 mm stab incision which does not require suture.

Illustrations by Peter Cox after F. Price

Subluxation of the lesser metatarsophalangeal joints

H. Piggott FRCS
Consultant Orthopaedic Surgeon, United Birmingham Hospitals,
Royal Orthopaedic Hospital, Birmingham, and Warwickshire Orthopaedic Hospital, Coleshill, UK

Introduction

Some or all of the lesser metatarsophalangeal joints may become subluxed. This is most common in the second toe in association with hallux valgus, but also occurs in connection with hammer toe, while multiple subluxations may be a feature of rheumatoid arthritis or advanced pes cavus with clawing. The resulting pain on weight-bearing under the displaced metatarsal heads may demand surgical treatment and often has to be combined with correction of hallux valgus.

If only one or at the most two joints are subluxed surgery aims at correction of the displacement, but where all are affected there is little or no prospect of restoring normal anatomy, and forefoot arthroplasty by excision of all the metatarsophalangeal joints is preferred. Exceptionally, in the more active patient, and provided the interphalangeal joint of the great toe has a good range of movement, it may be preferable to combine excision arthroplasty of the second, third, fourth and fifth metatarsophalangeal joints with arthrodesis of the first.

Care must always be taken to distinguish the pressure symptoms of subluxation from intermittent claudication and Morton's metatarsalgia.

Operation is performed under general anaesthesia and with the use of a pneumatic tourniquet.

Operations

REDUCTION OF SINGLE METATARSOPHALANGEAL SUBLUXATION BY METATARSAL SHORTENING

The object is to shorten the metatarsal at the neck to allow the long toe tendons to slacken off, at the same time elevating the metatarsal head and reducing the subluxation so that the thick plantar capsule of the metatarsophalangeal joint is restored to its normal position under the head.

1a & b

Through a dorsal longitudinal S-incision, the metatarsal neck is exposed subperiosteally, divided transversely, trimmed down to a spike and impacted into a conical burr hole in the metatarsal head. The amount of shortening and elevation is determined by the extent of neck resection and should be just enough to bring the displaced metatarsal head into alignment with the others; usually it suffices to trim the neck and impact the spike without segmental resection.

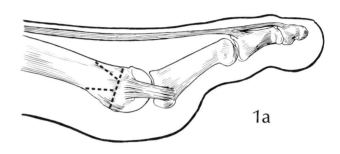

1a

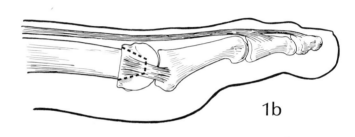

1b

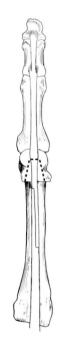

2a

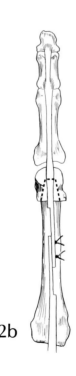

2b

2a & b

It is often necessary to elongate the extensor tendon. If the subluxation is passively reducible preoperatively the bone shortening may be all that is required, but more commonly it is found at completion of osteotomy that some degree of subluxation remains. If it can be reduced by simple flexion, Z-elongation of the extensor tendon is performed immediately proximal to the osteotomy.

3a & b

Often the subluxation is irreducible because of capsular contracture. In these cases the initial approach to the metatarsal neck is made by centering the extensor tendon Z-lengthening over the joint. The dorsal capsule is divided transversely and the collateral ligaments are severed from the metatarsal head by cutting retrogradely from inside the joint. The plantar capsule, if adherent, is separated from the undersurface of the head with a blunt curved elevator.

Suture of the extensor tendon with fine catgut and skin closure complete the operation.

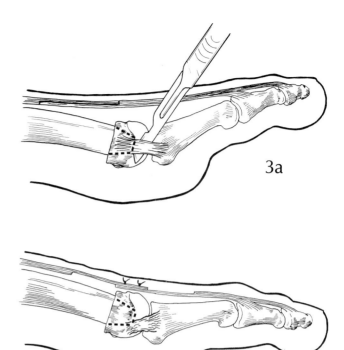

FOREFOOT ARTHROPLASTY

The incisions

4a & b

Three dorsal longitudinal incisions, each approximately 2 inches long, are made, one for the first joint and one for each pair of lesser joints. A separate elliptical incision is made in the sole 2–3 cm in width at its widest part, proximal to the weight-bearing skin.

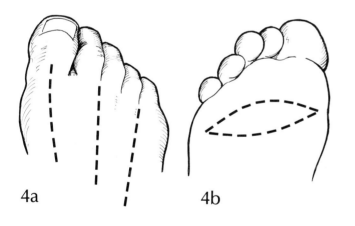

Bone excision

5a & b

The base of each proximal phalanx is exposed by incising the dorsal joint capsule, and, using a towel clip through the bone as a retractor, pulling it dorsally. It is freed from capsular attachments with a knife and the phalanx is divided near its middle with a small bone-cutting forceps. The base of the phalanx is discarded.

The metatarsal heads are trimmed to remove all palpable plantar prominences, leaving the five metatarsal heads as a whole forming a smooth curve convex distally.

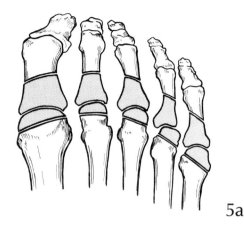

5a

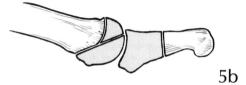

5b

Closure

6

Attention is now turned to the plantar elliptical incision, which is sited just proximal to the metatarsal heads. The whole ellipse of skin and underlying fat is discarded, and the incision closed. This has the effect of drawing the thick plantar capsules of the metatarsophalangeal joints, which have been displaced distally by the subluxation, back to their proper position under the refashioned metatarsal heads which are then properly cushioned against weight-bearing.

Finally, the dorsal incisions are closed.

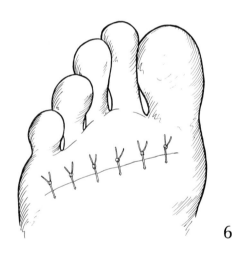

6

Postoperative management

This is similar for both operations described, but for single metatarsophalangeal reduction postoperative swelling is likely to be less and rehabilitation consequently faster than with forefoot arthroplasty. A well-padded plaster of Paris boot is applied, incorporating the toes in the straight position and moulded well upwards under the metatarsal heads. Considerable toe swelling may occur, so the plaster should be split and the foot well elevated. Unless other considerations prevail there should be no hurry to start weight-bearing, but usually about 2 weeks postoperatively swelling has subsided enough to allow removal of sutures and application of a close-fitting, well-moulded, plaster of Paris boot or wooden sandal in which walking may be started. This should be removed about 1 month postoperatively, and mobilizing exercises for the toes, foot and ankle are then begun.

Illustrations by Peter Cox after F. Price

Dorsally displaced fifth toe

H. Piggott FRCS
Consultant Orthopaedic Surgeon, United Birmingham Hospitals,
Royal Orthopaedic Hospital, Birmingham, and Warwickshire Orthopaedic Hospital, Coleshill, UK

Introduction

This is usually an isolated congenital anomaly, but care should be taken not to overlook clawing of all toes and early pes cavus, which require more extensive treatment. Symptoms arise from shoe pressure.

The Weedon–Butler operation described here is appropriate for most cases; but in an elderly patient with severe displacement, disarticulation through the metatarsophalangeal joint may be preferred. Lesser procedures involving skin only are not recommended since they do not correct the dorsal contracture of the deeper tissues.

Operation

(Weedon–Butler)

Incision

1a & b

An elliptical incision is made to surround the base of the toe, as for amputation, with proximal linear extensions at both ends; the plantar extension should incline slightly medially toward the centre of the sole. Dissection is deepened to expose the base of the phalanx and the joint capsule, care being taken to preserve the neurovascular bundles, which are most easily identified by blunt dissection with fine scissors.

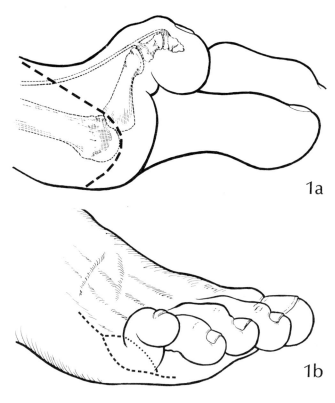

1a

1b

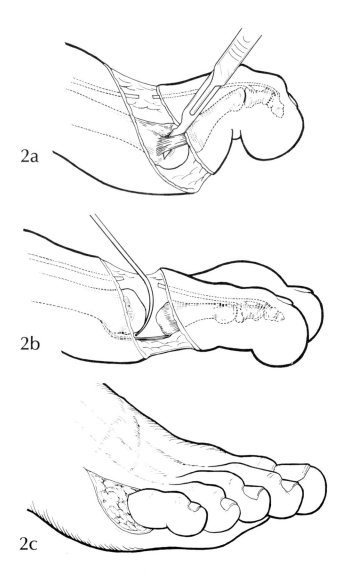

2a

2b

2c

Mobilization

2a, b & c

The extensor tendon and dorsal joint capsule are incised transversely and the collateral ligaments are detached from the metatarsal head by cutting them retrograde from within the joint. In some instances the whole lateral capsule may have to be released, and in severe cases the plantar capsule may be adherent to the undersurface of the metatarsal head from which it must be separated with a fine elevator. The toe will then lie in the corrected position in line with the other toes.

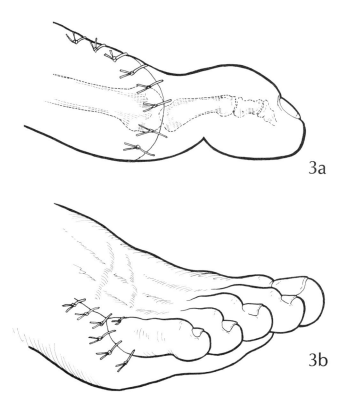

3a

3b

Closure

3a & b

The whole mobilized toe on its pedicle, consisting of neurovascular bundles, flexor tendons and plantar joint capsule, is now anchored in its corrected position by the plantar skin suture, the plantar linear extension of the incision being opened up in a V to receive the toe, while the dorsal end is closed behind it as a Y.

Postoperative management

The toe is carefully bandaged in the corrected position of slight plantar flexion. The circulation must be observed carefully and the bandages slackened if necessary. Elevation of the foot continues for 48–72 hours, when walking in an open-fronted shoe or sandal can begin. Sutures are removed after 14 days.

Illustrations by Peter Cox after F. Price

Ingrowing toe-nail

H. Piggott FRCS
Consultant Orthopaedic Surgeon, United Birmingham Hospitals,
Royal Orthopaedic Hospital, Birmingham, and Warwickshire Orthopaedic Hospital, Coleshill, UK

Introduction

The lateral or medial edge or both edges of the great toe-nail may be affected. The lesser toes are less commonly involved. While most cases occur in healthy individuals, the surgeon should look for neurological disease with sensory loss and for diabetes. An isolated episode may have been caused by careless nail-trimming and should be treated conservatively, but persistent or frequently repeated inflammation needs surgery. If only one edge of the nail is affected, excision of that edge and the underlying nail bed is sufficient, but involvement of both edges demands removal of the whole nail and germinal matrix to prevent regrowth. Neither operation should be performed in the presence of sepsis, which is most quickly cleared up by preliminary removal of the nail edge or whole nail, according to its extent.

For nail removal or wedge resection of matrix, a tubular tourniquet round the base of the toe suffices, but for total excision of nail and matrix a proximal pneumatic cuff is essential since a toe tourniquet prevents adequate skin mobilization.

Operations

WEDGE RESECTION

1a & b

The excision extends proximally to the base of the distal phalanx to ensure complete removal of germinal matrix within the wedge and deeply at the side to remove all epithelium and nail bed from the lateral gutter. Inadequate excision will be followed by regrowth of a troublesome nail spike.

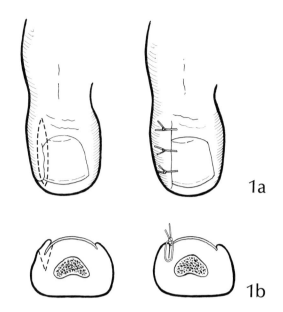

1a

1b

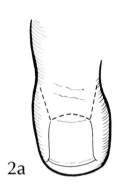

2a

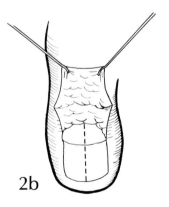

2b

THE ZADIK PROCEDURE

Exposure

2a & b

The lateral limbs of the incision extend proximally as far as the interphalangeal joint to allow complete exposure of germinal matrix and adequate mobility of the skin flap for advancement; the transverse limb is at the distal edge of the hangnail. The skin flap is elevated, with all the scanty subcutaneous fat, and turned proximally. The nail, if not previously removed, is split longitudinally with strong pointed scissors and avulsed.

Excision of germinal matrix

3

The whole germinal matrix must be excised or a stunted deformed nail fragment will regrow. The distal limit is indicated by the lunula, and to ensure complete removal proximally all the dense white matrix tissue must be dissected out to expose the underlying extensor tendon insertion. The nail bed distal to the lunula does not generate nail tissue and postoperatively will cover itself with ordinary cornified epithelium. The lateral recesses, if deep, may be excised at this stage as illustrated in wedge resection (*see above*).

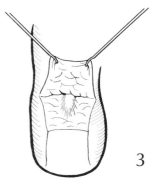

3

Closure

4

The skin flap, provided it has been adequately mobilized proximally, can be advanced to cover the small raw area corresponding to the lunula without tension. Fine atraumatic sutures are essential and insertion is easier if they are passed first through the skin flap, then brought out through the residual nail bed. A small longitudinal stab in the centre of the flap and a firm (but not too tight) dressing will prevent haematoma formation.

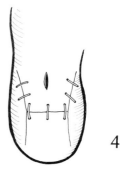

4

Postoperative management

After the Zadik procedure there is a risk of slow healing at the distal end and occasionally a little of the flap edge is lost. This can be minimized by elevation of the foot until pain-free, usually 48–72 hours, and avoiding weight-bearing until healing is complete, usually about 2 weeks. If this is impossible, a malleable splint or extended plaster of Paris boot should be fitted to prevent movement of the big toe.

Index

Abdomen,
  vascular injury to, 52
Abdominal tube pedicle skin flap, 8
Abscess,
  Brodie's, 61, 62–63
  paraspinal, 560
  subperiosteal, 55
Acetabuloplasty,
  Pemberton, 878
Acetabulum,
  dysplasia,
    innominate osteotomy for, 893
  fracture dislocation, 339
    reduction of, 344
    with stove-in hip, 321, 328
  Kocher–Langenbeck approach to, 342
  marginal fracture, 339
  posterior wall fracture, 343
  replacement of posterior rim, 339–345
    devices for, 360
    fixation, 345
    preoperative, 339
    postoperative management, 345
    special tools required, 341
Achilles tendon *See Tendo Achillis*
Acromioclavicular joint,
  chronic dislocation, 690
  injuries to, 686–691
    classification, 686
    indications for surgery, 687
    operations for, 687
    stabilization, 689
    Weaver–Dunn technique, 690
Amputation,
  See also under limb concerned
  antibiotics in, 399
  in children, 400
  complications, 400
  for Dupytren's contracture, 856, 863
  general principles, 397–401
  fingers, 193
  indications for, 397
  management of individual tissue, 399
  phantom limb pain in, 401
  preoperative, 398
  preparations for, 399
  rehabilitation, 401
  stump oedema, 401

Aneurysm,
  false, 50
Ankle,
  arthrodesis of, 1191–1197
    by anterior approach, 1192
    by lateral approach, 1193
    in haemophiliacs, 87
    tendon transfer in, 1198
  compression arthrodesis, 1195
  equinovarus deformity, 307
  equinus deformity in, 1172
    prevention of, 131
  fractures of, 284–294
    arthrodesis following, 1191
    in children, 365
    classification of, 284
    complications, 368
    exposure of fracture, 287, 292
    indications for lateral fixation, 286
    lateral complex, 287
    medial complex, 292
    non-union, 368
    partial growth arrest complicating, 368
    postoperative management, 294
    preoperative, 286
    reduction of, 288, 293
    type A injuries, 285, 293
    type B injuries, 285, 291, 293
    type C injuries, 286, 293
  pantalar arthrodesis, 1198
  surgical approach to, 58, 60
  trephine arthrodesis, 1197
Ankylosing spondylitis,
  hip in, 965
  hip replacement in, 945
Antibiotics,
  in amputation, 399
  in fractures from metastases, 385
  in osteomyelitis, 55, 56, 63, 64, 66
  in tendon injury, 17
Aorta,
  deceleration injury, 52
Arm,
  See also Forearm, etc.
  amputation through, 402–408
    above elbow, 407, 408
    below elbow, 403, 408
    disarticulation at elbow, 405, 408

Arm (*cont.*)
  amputation through (*cont.*)
    indications, 402
    postoperative management, 408
    preoperative, 402
    prosthetics for, 408
    skin flaps and cover, 405, 406
  compartment syndromes, 303
    Volkmann's ischaemic contracture
      following, 307
  decompression, 304
  fracture of long bones, 153–164
  ischaemia of muscles, 141
  traction systems, 141–144
Arteries,
  bypass injury, 41
  end-to-end anastomosis, 45, 46
  injuries,
    spasm following, 47
  ligation of, 40
  patching, 44
  reconstruction, 42
  repair of, 40
    patching, 44
    suturing, 43
    vein graft, 46
  suturing of, 43
Arteriovenous fistula, 51
Arthritis,
  septic, 54
Arthrography, 1057
Arthroscopy,
  See under joint concerned
Atherosclerosis,
  amputation for, 397
Atlantoaxial fractures and dislocations, 642
Atlantoaxial fusion, 476
Atlantoaxial instability, 472
Atlantoaxial joint,
  anatomy of, 454
Atlas,
  anatomy of, 454
  fracture of ring, 472
Avascular necrosis,
  following elbow fracture, 361
  following femoral neck fracture, 364
Avulsion flaps, 3

Axis,
    anatomy of, 454
Axontmesis, 295

Bankart operation, 681
Bateman's operation, 707
Bennett's fracture subluxation, 183
Berger's approach to forequarter
        amputation, 410
Biceps,
    rupture of, 709–712
        distal tendon, 711
        long head, 710
        postoperative management, 710, 712
    tenodesis, 703
Biceps tendon,
    redirection of, 751
Blood vessels,
    See also Arteries, Veins, etc.
    injury and repair, 39–53
    management in amputation, 400
Bone,
    cancer of, 1141
        biopsy in, 91
        diagnosis, 92
        management of, 1151
        metastases, 92, 96, 97, 394–396
        recurrence, 1151
        screening, 91
        staging, 92
    of children, 251
    healing and union, 101
    management in amputation, 400
    round cell tumours, 92, 96
Bone biopsy, 91–99
    aspiration, 94
    closed, 93
    complications, 97
    excisional, 93
    haemostasis, 97
    infection in, 98
    needles for, 94
    open, 93
    operation, 93, 94
    planning, 92
    postoperative management, 96
    trephine, 94
Bone grafting, 375–376
    for non-union, 371
    in fractures, 119
    obtaining bone for, 375
Bone infection,
    acute, 54–60
        draining in, 56
        pathology, 54
        postoperative management, 56
        principles of treatment, 55
        surgical treatment, 56
    chronic, 61–67
        two-stage procedure, 66
    microbiology of, 55
Bone metastases, 92, 96, 97, 394–396
    See also under Spine, Metastatic bone
            disease
    causing fractures, 384
        bone grafts for, 391
        cementing and compression fixation,
            386
        indications for operation, 384
        intramedullary nailing, 389
        operations for, 385

Bone metastases (cont.)
    causing fractures (cont.)
        plating for, 386
        plating with cement, 387
        realignment, 387
        stabilization, 391
    halo–body casts for, 487
Boutonnière deformity of finger, 819
    repair, 827
    secondary repair, 818
Bowstringing in tendon repair, 23
Boytchev procedure, 675
Brachial plexus,
    birth palsy, 705
    iatrogenic injury, 25, 452
    injuries to, 26
        nerve grafts for, 37
Brachioradialis,
    transfer to flexor digitorum
            profundus, 762
Bristow–Helfet procedure, 683
Brodie's abscess, 61, 62–63
Bryant's traction, 138
Buck's traction, 134
Bunnell criss-cross stitch, 812
Bunnell double right-angle stitch, 813
Bunnell withdrawal stitch, 814

Calcaneal osteotomy for pes cavus, 1217
Calcaneocavus deformity of foot, 1187
Calcaneonavicular synostosis, 1206
Calcaneonavicular bar,
    excision of, 1214
Calcaneum,
    beak fractures, 315
    correction of deformity, 316
    crush injuries, 315
    injuries to, 315
    medial displacement rotation
            osteotomy, 1213
    removal of, 318
    traction, 126
Capitellum,
    fracture of, 173–174
Carpal scaphoid,
    AO lag screw, 799
    fractures of, 794–804
        AO lag screw for, 799
        Herbert bone screw for, 801
        indications for operation, 795
        internal fixation of, 799
        Matte–Russe bone graft for, 796
        non-union, 795
        of proximal pole, 804
        operations, 796
Carpal tunnel decompression, 788, 789
Carpus,
    Lauenstein procedure, 773
Cauda equina, 533
    complicating reduction of
            spondylolisthesis, 558
Cerebral palsy, 512, 1152, 1169
    forearm paralysis in, 745
    hip adductors in, 926
    hip contracture in, 921
    hip extenders in, 936
    hip flexion deformity in, 931
    knee deformity in, 940, 981
    wrist and finger deformity in, 752

Cervical spine,
    anterior fusion, 463–470
        Bailey strut graft technique, 469
        Cloward dowel procedure, 466
        indications for, 463, 492
        operation, 464
        postoperative management, 470
        preoperative, 463
        Robinson block graft procedure, 468
    bilateral fracture dislocation, 630, 633
    fracture dislocations, 478, 630
        anterior stabilization, 637
        closed reduction, 630
        open posterior reduction, 635
        posterior fusion with plates or wires,
            640
        requiring fusion, 637
        spinal jacket for, 667
    Hodgson approach to, 561, 563
    infections, 561
    metastatic bone disease,
        anterior cord decompression, 575
        anterior stabilization, 577
        posterior decompression and
            stabilization, 579
    pathology of, 454
    posterior fusion, 471–481
        atlantoaxial, 476
        indications for, 492
        interspinous, 478
        occipitocervical, 472
        operations, 472
        postoperative management, 475, 477,
            479, 481
        preoperative, 471
    posterolateral fusion, 480
    problems,
        management of, 456
    Southwick and Robinson approach, 561–
            562
    transoral approach to, 453–462
        anterior, 456
        assessment of, 456
        operation, 457
        position of patient, 457
        preoperative, 455
        surgical exposure, 458
    unilateral dislocation, 631, 634
Charnley compression arthrodesis of
            ankle, 1195
Chemonucleosis for herniated
            intervertebral disc, 530–533
Children,
    amputation in, 400
    ankle fractures in, 365
    bones of, 351
    congenital dislocation of hip,
        operations for, 870–892
    fractures in,
        operative treatment, 351
    fracture of femoral neck in, 362
    high femoral osteotomy in, 900
    quadriceps contracture in, 1002
    recurrent dislocation of patella in,
            1103
    trigger finger and thumb in, 869
Chondromalacia patellae, 1032
    arthroscopic surgery for, 1030, 1039
    diagnostic arthroscopy for, 1036
Chondrosarcoma, 95
Christmas disease, 77
Claw toes, 1230

Club foot,
    bone resection, 1226
    lateral soft tissue release, 1225
    medial soft tissue release, 1223
    operations for, 1220–1231
        indications for, 1220
    plantar soft tissue release, 1224
    posterior soft tissue release, 1221
    postoperative management, 1226
    secondary surgery, 1226
    triple arthrodesis for, 1226
Colles' fracture, 163
    carpal tunnel compression following,
        788
Common peroneal nerve,
    care of, 299
    injury to, 25
Compartment syndromes, 49, 283, 295–308
    arm, 307
    evaluation and treatment, 298
    fasciotomy for, 295
        indications for, 296
    foot, 301
    forearm, 303
    hand, 305
    leg, 298, 307
    pain in, 295
    pathogenesis of, 295
    perifibular fasciotomy, 299
    thigh, 301
    tissue pressure, 296
        measurement, 297
    Volkmann's ischaemic contracture
        following, 307
Congenital anomalies,
    amputation for, 398
Costotransversectomy, 614
Cotrel–Dubousset instrumentation, 491
Coxa vara, 949
    after femoral neck fracture, 364
    congenital,
        correction of, 907
        high femoral osteotomy for, 900
Craniocervical junction,
    anatomy of, 454
    development of, 453
    movement of, 454
    radiography of, 455
    stabilization of, 460
Craniocleidodystostosis, 949
Cross-leg skin flaps, 10
Cruciate ligament,
    arthroscopy, 1014
Crush injuries,
    primary care of, 3
Cutaneous axial-pattern skin flap, 11

Darrach's procedure, 769
    postoperative management, 772
Degloving injuries, 4
Deltoid paralysis, 707
Denham pin, 125
de Quervain's disease, 787
Diabetes mellitus,
    amputations in, 397
    gangrene in, 444
Digital nerve,
    injury of, 25
Dillwyn Evans procedure,
    reversed, 1212

Dorsal nerve transfer,
    for plantar digital neuroma, 1255–1258
        operation, 1257
        postoperative management, 1258
        preoperative, 1256
Duchenne's muscular dystrophy, 512
Dunn device for stabilization of spine,
    665
Dupuytren's contracture, 855–864
    aetiology of, 855
    amputation for, 856
    clinical features of, 855
    dermofasciotomy, 856, 862
    extension, 864
    fasciotomy, 856, 863
    open-palm technique (McCash), 86
    operative principles, 857
        haemostasis, 862
        involving more than one ray, 860
        involving one ray, 857
    pathology of, 855
    postoperative management, 864
    preoperative, 856
    prognosis, 856
    recurrent, 862, 864
    selection of operation, 856
    Skoog technique, 860
    timing of surgery, 856
Dupuytren's diathesis, 855
Dural sac,
    care of, 528
Dynabrace Oxford Fixation System, 147

Elbow,
    amputation above, 407, 408
    amputation below, 403, 408
    arthroplasty, 729–735
        complications, 733
        indications and contraindications, 730
        infection following, 733
        insertion of prosthesis, 731
        loosening of prosthesis, 734
        postoperative management, 733
        results, 733
        skin problems following, 734
    biomechanics of joint, 730
    dislocation,
        following arthroplasty, 734
    fractures, 165–174
        in children, 354, 360
        complications of, 361
        diagnosis of, 165
        fixation, 165
        non-union, 361
        unstable, 360
    hemiarthroplasty, 729
    instability of, 76
    lateral condyle fracture in children, 354
    medial epicondyle fracture in children,
        356
    prosthesis for, 730, 731
    surgical approach to, 58, 59
    synovectomy,
        for rheumatic disease, 73
        indications and contraindications, 73
        postoperative management, 75, 76
        preoperative, 73
        technique, 74
        ulnar neuritis during, 75, 76

Elbow flexion,
    restoration by tendon replacement,
        736–744
        anterior transfer of triceps tendon,
            740
        Bunnell's modification, 739
        Steindler's flexorplasty, 737
        transfer of pectoralis major tendon,
            742
Epiphysiodesis, 1154
Epiphyses,
    fracture of, 352
    injuries to, 351
    premature union, 364
Equinus deformity, 989
Erb's palsy, 705–708
    Fairbank's operation,
        Sever's modification, 706
    postoperative management, 708
Extensor carpi radialis longus,
    transfer to flexor pollicis longus, 763
Extensor tendon repair, 21

Facial wounds, 4
Fairbank's operation,
    Sever's modification, 706
False aneurysms, 50
Fasciotomy,
    forearm, 304
    for trauma, 49
    hand, 305
    indications for, 296
    perifibular, 299
    postoperative management, 304
Femoral epiphysis,
    anatomy of, 910
    open replacement of, 914
    slipped,
        replacement of, 914
    upper, See Upper femoral epiphysis
Femoral osteotomy, 884
    for coxa vara, 888
Femur,
    avascular necrosis, 200
    biplane trochanteric osteotomy, 916
    condylar fracture, 394
    deformities, 992
    fractures of,
        bracing in, 110
        caused by metastases, 392
        in children, 136, 138
        skeletal traction for, 125, 134, 136
    fracture of neck,
        cervicotrochanteric, in children, 362
        complications, 364
        delay and non-union, 364
        hip replacement after, 950
        indication for operation, 362
        pertrochanteric, 362
        postoperative management, 364
        transcervical, 362
        transepiphyseal, 362
    geometric flexion osteotomy, 919
    high osteotomy, 900–908, 965
        postoperative management, 907, 908
    intracapsular fracture of neck, 199–208
        classification, 200
        closed reduction, 203
        fracture fixation, 205
        indications for internal fixation, 201

Femur (*cont.*)
  intracapsular fracture of neck (*cont.*)
    open reduction, 204
    operative technique, 202
    postoperative management, 208
    preoperative, 202
  lateral fracture in upper end, 139
  lengthening, 1154, 1159
    soft tissue release and corticotomy,
      1162
  lengthening osteotomy of, 382
  metastases in, 396
  plate removal from, 120
  preparation for knee arthroplasty, 1127
  replacement for tumour, 1142
    distal, 1145
    insertion of prosthesis, 1143, 1146
    postoperative management, 1144,
      1147
    proximal, 1142
  resection of lower end, 1133
    reversed wedge osteotomy, 905
  Robert Jones valgus osteotomy, 907
  rotation osteotomy, 901
    indications for, 901
    postoperative management, 903
    prevention of complications, 903
    with varus, 904
  shaft fracture, 1003
    availability of equipment for nailing, 240
    Küntscher's nailing technique,
      223–241
    Melbourne cross pinning technique,
      234, 240
    oblique spiral, 137
    postoperative management, 240
    preoperative, 223
    technical requirements, 224
    traction for, 137, 226
    transverse, 137
  shortening, 380, 906, 1154, 1157
  skeletal traction, 126
  subtrochanteric fracture, 216–222
    caused by metastases, 394
    classification, 217
    complications, 222
    indications for Zickel nail fixation, 216
    postoperative management, 222
    preoperative, 218
    Zickel nail fixation, 216, 218–221
  supracondylar fractures, 242–251
    bone grafting in, 250
    caused by metastases, 394
    classification, 243
    general considerations, 242
    indications for operation, 244
    internal traction, 242
    open, 244
    operation, 246
    pathological, 244, 250
    placement of lateral condylar window,
      247
    postoperative management, 251
    preoperative, 244
  trochanteric fractures, 209–215
    caused by metastases, 393
    classification, 209
    fixation, 210
    internal fixation, 210, 213
    operative details, 212
    postoperative management, 215
    preoperative, 211

Femur (*cont.*)
    T or Y bicondylar fractures, 244
    unicondylar fractures, 244
    wedge osteotomy, 908
Fibrin glue in nerve repair, 37
Fibula,
  compound fracture of, 14
Fibular osseocutaneous free skin grafts, 15
Fingers,
  amputation of, 193
  Boutonnière deformity, 819
    repair of, 827
    secondary repair, 818
  compartment syndrome, 305
  distal interphalangeal joint deformity,
    809
  extensor tendon injury, 809
  flexor digitorum profundus injury, 810
  flexor digitorum superficialis in, 811
  flexor tendons,
    blood supply, 828
  flexor tendon division, 828–835
    delay in primary repair, 832
    delayed repair, 832
    indications for operation, 830
    postoperative management, 834
    preoperative, 830
    technique of repair, 831
    tenolysis, 835
  flexor tendon injury, 827
    primary repair, 820, 828
    tendon graft operation, 820
  fractures,
    fixation, 178
    fixation by crossed K-wires, 177
    head of proximal phalanx, 181
    Kirschner wires in, 176–180
    Lister's intraosseous wiring, 180
    postoperative management, 179
    proximal phalanx shaft, 177
    shafts of metacarpals, 185
  gliding tendon implants, 839, 852
    pulley reconstruction, 843
  mallet deformity, 809, 827
  mallet fracture, 815
  metacarpals,
    fracture, 185
  paralysis of, 759
  proximal interphalangeal joint,
    deformity, 809
    dislocation of, 196
    fracture-subluxation, 184
  replantation of, 193
  rheumatoid disease,
    Swanson arthroplasty for, 68–72
  tendon injury,
    pulley reconstruction, 843
  tendon repairs, 18, 20
  tenography technique, 832
  transfer of extensor indicis to thumb,
    760
  trigger, 865–869
    in children, 869
    conservative treatment, 865
    operative details, 866
    postoperative management, 868
Fisk splint, 130
  suspension of, 133
Flat foot,
  See Pes planus
Flexor carpi ulnaris,
  transfer of, 746, 756

Flexor digitorum profundus,
  transfer of brachioradialis to, 762
Flexor pollicis longus,
  transfer of extensor carpi radialis longus
    to, 763
Flexor tendon repair, 21
Foot,
  amputations, 441
  arthrodesis of, 1199–1207
    Lambrinudi operation, 1201
    postoperative precautions, 1205
  calcaneocavus deformity of, 1187
  compartment syndromes in, 301
  correction of varus, 1199
  crush injury, 315, 320
  flat *See pes planus*
  fractures and dislocations, 309–320
    caused by metastases, 395
  Lambrinudi arthrodesis, 1191, 1201
  major disruptive lesions, 318
  pantalar arthrodesis, 1198
  reconstruction, 1232–1243
    correction of bunionette, 1237
    correction of hallux valgus, 1237
    Fowler operation, 1238
    Hoffmann operation, 1239
    osteotomies of metatarsals, 1233
    postoperative management, 1236,
      1240, 1242
    prosthetic replacement of joints and
      toe, 1241, 1242
  sole of,
    skin cover of wounds, 4
  stabilization of, 1199
  subluxation of lesser
    metatarsophalangeal joint,
      1263–1266
  surgical approach to, 58, 60, 310
  tendon transfer, 1215
  tendon transfer to heel, 1187
  transfer of tibialis posterior tendon to
    dorsum, 1184–1186
  triple arthrodesis, 1199
  valgus deformities, 1203
Foot drop, 307
Forearm,
  compound wound of, 15
  interosseous membrane of,
    release of, 750
  pronation deformity of, 746
  release of flexor muscles, 752
  supination deformity of, 750
  tendon reconstruction in, 745–764
    paralytic conditions, 753
    spastic conditions, 746
    triple transfer, 754
Forefoot,
  arthroplasty, 1265
  reconstruction, 1232–1343
    correction of hallux valgus, 1237
    Fowler operation, 1238
    Hoffmann operation, 1239
    osteotomies of metatarsals, 1233
    postoperative management, 1236,
      1240, 1242
    prosthetic replacement of joints and
      toe, 1241, 1242
Forequarter amputation, 409–413
  anterior approach (Berger), 410
  indications and contraindications, 409
  operation, 470
  posterior approach to (Littlewood), 413

Forequarter amputation (*cont.*)
  postoperative management, 413
  preoperative, 410
  prosthesis for, 413
Fowler operation, 1238
Fractures,
  See also under bone concerned
  bone grafting in, 119, 391
  bone healing and union, 101, 117, 370
  callus formation, 370
  caused by metastases, 384
    bone grafts for, 391
    cementing and compression fixation,
      386
    indications for operation, 384
    intramedullary nailing, 389
    operations, 385
    plating for, 386
    plating with cement, 387
    postoperative management, 395
    preoperative, 385
    prevention, 395
    realignment, 387
    stabilization, 391
  in children, 351
  complications of injury, 120
  compression, 103
  delayed union, mal- and non-union,
    122, 370, 371, 377–383
    atrophic, 370
    bone grafting for, 371
    causes of, 370
    hypertrophic, 370
  diagnosis, 104
    manipulation in, 105
  diaphyseal, 145
  external bridging callus, 101
  external skeletal fixation, 145–152
    applications, 146
    choice of frame, 145, 147, 149, 150
    indications for, 145
    postoperative management, 146, 148
    rehabilitation, 146
    removal of frame, 146
  external skeletal traction, 113
  failure of consolidation, 146
  healing, 117, 370
  history and mechanism of injury, 102
  implant removal, 120
  infection in, 122
  instability in, 145
  internal fixation, 114
  intramedullary nailing, 116
  Kirschner wires in, 115
  management,
    aims of, 100
    bracing, 110
    external skeletal fixation, 145–152
    general principles, 100–122
    grafting, 119
    internal fixation, 114
    in haemophilia, 89
    intramedullary nailing, 116
    methods of holding, 108
    plaster of Paris in, 109
    plate fixation, 117
    reduction, 107
    three-point fixation, 109
    traction *See Fractures, traction*
    wire fixation, 115
  medullary callus, 101

Fractures (*cont.*)
  of long bones,
    delayed union, mal- and non-union,
      369–383
  open, 120
  operative treatment,
    in children, 351–368
  pathological,
    *See also Fractures, caused by
      metastases*
    prevention of, 395
  plate fixation, 117
  primary callus response, 101
  radiology, 104
  rotational mal-union, 377
  screw fixation, 114
  self-stabilizing, 108
  skeletal traction, 111, 123, 125
    complications, 129
    sites of, 126
  skin traction, 111, 123, 124
  splints for, 129
  tendon injury and, 17
  traction, 123–144
    arm, 141
    Buck's, 134
    complications, 129
    Denham pin, 125
    duration of, 144
    external skeletal, 113
    fixed, 123
    Hamilton Russell, 135
    Kirschner wires in, 125
    leg, 134
    management of patient, 143
    ninety-ninety, 136
    Perkins', 134
    removal, 144
    skeletal, 111, 123, 124, 126, 129
    skin, 111, 124
    sliding, 123, 138
    Steinemann pin, 125
    Tulloch Brown, 135
    weights, 133
  union,
    following radiotherapy, 384
  wire fixation, 115
Fraser's approach to spine, 612

Galeazzi fracture, 160, 163
Gallé spinal fusion, 644
Gallows traction, 138
Ganglion,
  palmar, 791
  wrist, 790
Garré's sclerosing osteomyelitis, 62
Gastrocnemius,
  contracture, 1175
  distal division of, 1177
  proximal detachment of, 1175
  release, 989–992, 1169–1171
    indications and assessment, 1169
    operation, 1170
    postoperative management, 1171
    preoperative, 1169
Gastrocnemius tendon,
  exposure and division, 1171
Girdlestone's operation, 1230–1231
Girdlestone's pseudarthrosis of hip,
  965–969

Glenohumeral joint,
  arthroscopic appearance of, 694, 695,
    696
  dislocation of, 671
Goldthwaite–Roux operation, 1103
Grafts, skin, *See Skin grafts*
Grice–Green operation, 1203
  modification of, 1205
Growth plates,
  damage from traction, 129
  in epiphyseal fractures, 352
Gunshot injuries,
  primary care of, 3

Haemarthroses, 78, 80
Haemophilia,
  acquired, 77
  antifibrinolytic agents in, 79
  arthrodesis of hip in, 87
  arthrodesis of knee in, 83
  clinical signs, 78
  cysts and pseudotumours, 78, 89
  hip replacement in, 80
  management of fractures in, 89
  surgical procedures in, 77–90
    complications, 89
    postoperative management, 80
    preoperative, 78
    technique, 79
  synovectomy of knee in, 82
  types of, 77
Haemophilia A, 77
Haemophilia B, 77
Haemorrhage,
  control of,
    emergency, 39
    in haemophilia, 79
Hallux,
  clawing of, 1227–1229
Hallux rigidus, 1245–1254
  arthrodesis for, 1250
  exostectomy, 1252
  metatarsal neck osteotomy for, 1246
  osteotomy of neck of proximal phalanx,
    1253
  postoperative management, 1254
  preoperative, 1245
Hallux valgus, 444, 1244, 1245
  interphalangeal arthrodesis for, 1253
  Keller arthroplasty for, 1248
  osteotomy for, 1244
  postoperative management, 1254
Halo–body system, 486–490
  criteria for success, 490
  design of system, 488
  indications for, 487
  postapplication management, 490
  procedure, 489
  for transoral approach to cervical spine,
    460
Halofemoral traction, 482–485
  complications, 485
  application of halo, 483
  postoperative management, 485
Hamilton Russell traction, 135
Hammer toe, 1259, 1263
Hamstrings,
  transfer to quadriceps, 985–988
    complications, 988
    indications, 985
    postoperative management, 988

Hamstring,
  distal release, 981–984
    operation, 982
    postoperative management, 984
Hamstring,
  proximal release, 940–942
    operation, 941
    postoperative management, 942
Hand,
  acute injuries of, 188–198
    aetiology of, 188
    in children, 198
    operative treatment, 195
    postoperative management, 198
    primary treatment, 192
    skin closure, 197
    types of, 189
  blunt injury, 189
  compartment syndromes, 305
  extensor tendon reconstruction and
      repair, 827, 852
  flexor pollicis longus injury, 811
  flexor tendons,
    injury, 810
    in palm, 811, 827
    methods of repair, 820
    rheumatoid tenosynovitis of, 865
  flexor tendon reconstruction, 836, 839
    See also Hand, gliding tendon
        implants
  fractures and dislocations, 196
    See also specific bones, etc.
    caused by metastases, 392
    indications for operation, 176
    instruments for treatment, 176
    operative treatment, 175–187
  fracture-subluxation, 183
  gliding tendon implants, 836
    active programme, 853
    care of, 837
    complications, 848, 851
    contraindications, 838
    indications for, 838
    passive programme, 839
    postoperative management, 848, 851, 854
    preoperative, 839
    pulley reconstruction, 843
    replacement of implant, 849
    selection of tendon motor, 850
    special indications, 852
    stage I, 839
    tendon grafts, 849, 850
    testing pulley system, 847
  gunshot wounds, 191
    treatment, 195
  high-pressure injuries, 190, 191, 195
  infected wounds, 195
  injuries of,
    primary care, 4
  palmar ganglion, 791
  rheumatoid arthritis, 765
  roller injury, 190
  sharp injury, 190
  tendon graft attachment, 814
  tendon injuries, 808–827
    back of hand, 819, 827
    Bunnell criss-cross stitch, 812
    Bunnell double right-angle stitch, 813
    Bunnell withdrawal stitch, 814
    indications for operation, 809
    Kessler grasping stitch, 812
    operations for, 812

Hand (cont.)
  tendon injuries (cont.)
    in palm, 811, 825
    physiotherapy, 827
    postoperative management, 826
    problems, 808
    Pulvertaft interlacing method, 813
    sutures for, 812
    tenolysis, 851
    surgery of, 812
  tenolysis, 838
Harrington instrumentation, 550
  development of, 491
Harrington–Luque instrumentation, 518
Hartshill triangle, 661
Heel,
  tendon transfer to, 1187–1198
Hepatitis B, 78
Herbert bone screw, 801
Hindquarter amputation, 414–418
  indications and contraindications, 414
  operation, 415
  postoperative management, 418
  preoperative, 415
Hip,
  adductor release, 926–930
    indications and assessment, 926
    operation, 927
    partial neurectomy of obdurator
        nerve in, 929
    posterior adductor transfer, 929
    postoperative management, 930
  anterior approach to, 951
  anterolateral approach to, 951, 955
  arthritis of, 965
    arthrodesis for, 971
  arthrodesis of, 970–980
    bone graft, 978
    indications and contraindications, 971
    intra-articular, 971
    ischiofemoral, 975
    postoperative management, 974, 980
    preoperative, 971, 975
    special complications, 980
  arthrodesis,
    with iliofemoral graft, 971
  assessment of stability, 875
  congenital dislocation,
    arthrodesis for, 971
    assessment of stability, 875
    Chiari operation, 879
    closed adductor tenotomy, 872
    Colonna operation, 889
    femoral osteotomy, 884
    high femoral osteotomy for, 900, 901,
        904
    innominate osteotomy for, 893
    lateral shelf acetabuloplasty, 879, 882
    open reduction, 873
    operations for, 870–892
    Pemberton acetabuloplasty, 878
    replacement for, 947
    stability of, 875
  congenital dysplasia, 949
  degenerative conditions,
    replacement for, 948
  direct lateral approach to, 951, 957
  disarticulation of, 419–421
    operation for, 420
    postoperative management, 421
    preoperative, 419
    prosthetics, 421

Hip (cont.)
  dislocation after leg shortening, 1167
  flexion contracture, 921–925
    iliopsoas tenotomy, 923
    operations for, 922
    release of tight iliotibial tract, 922
    Soutter operation, 924
    posterior adductor transfer, 929
  flexor release,
    iliofemoral approach to, 931
    indications and assessment, 931
    operation, 932
    postoperative management, 935
    preoperative, 931
  Gibson approach, 952
  Girdlestone's pseudoarthrosis of,
      965–969
    Batchelor's modification, 968
    indications and contraindications, 965
    limitations, 965
    postoperative management, 969
  infratectal or juxtatectal transverse
      fractures, 328, 338
  lateral approach, 951
  Moore approach to, 952
  persistent fetal alignment of, 900
  posterior column fracture, 327
  replacement arthroplasty, 943–964
    anterolateral approach, 955
    anatomy of, 952
    direct lateral approach, 957
    for failed surgery, 950
    in haemophiliacs, 80
    indications, 943
    posterior approach, 952
    postoperative management, 962
    surgical approaches, 951
  septic arthritis, 948
  stove-in, 321–338
    acetabular fracture with, 328
    equipment for operation, 325
    extended iliofemoral approach, 336
    ilioinguinal approach, 330
    indications for operation, 323
    infratectal or juxtectal transverse
        fracture, 328, 338
    lateral approach, 336
    posterior approach, 326
    posterior column fracture, 327
    postoperative management, 338
    preoperative, 322
    replacement and fixation of fracture,
        334
    T-fractures, 329, 338
    surgical approach to, 58, 951
  T-fracture, 329, 338
  test of stability, 876
  tuberculosis of, 948
Hoffmann operation, 1239
Human immunodeficiency virus, 78
Humerus,
  See also Shoulder, etc.
  displaced fracture of greater tuberosity,
      155
  fractures of,
    bracing in, 110
    caused by metastases, 391
    compartment syndromes and, 303,
        307
    postoperative care, 155
    traction for, 112, 141, 142
    T–Y, 171

Humerus (*cont.*)
  fracture of neck,
    caused by metastases, 391
  fractures of shaft, 158
    closed intramedullary nailing, 160
    plating, 159
  metastases in, 396
  Neer hemiarthroplasty, 156
  proximal fractures, 153
    indications for operation, 153
    operation, 154
    two- and three-part, 158
  replacement of head, 716
  resection of head, 716
  supracondylar fracture, 307
    metastases causing, 392

Iliac bone for grafting, 66, 375
Iliac vein,
  injury to, 52
Iliopsoas tendon,
  anterolateral approach to, 933
  approach to, 937
  division, 934
  lengthening or recession, 936
    operation, 937
    postoperative management, 939
    preoperative, 936
Iliopsoas tenotomy, 923
Iliotibial tract,
  release of, 922
Infection,
  amputation and, 398, 400
Inferior radioulnar joint,
  capsulotomy of, 750
Infrapatellar fat pad,
  arthroscopy, 1013, 1033
Innominate osteotomy, 893–899
  indications and contraindications, 893
  operation, 894
  postoperative management, 899
  special requirements for, 893
Intercostobrachial nerve,
  damage to, 452
Interphalangeal valgus, 1245
Intervertebral disc,
  See also Lumbar disc, etc.
  degeneration, 463
  excision of, 508
  herniated, 530
  infection, 533
  resorption, 528
Ischaemia, 295
  amputation and, 398
  of limbs, 25
  signs of, 39

Jefferson fracture, 472
Jewett nail-plate, 215
Joints,
  bleeding into, 78
  contractures in amputations, 400
Joint infection,
  acute, 55
  aspiration of, 57
  chronic, 61–67
Jones operation, 1190

Kaneda device, 592
Kates–Kessel technique, 1239
Keller arthroplasty, 1248
Kessel prosthesis, 718
Kessler grasping stitch, 19, 812
Kienböck's disease of lunate, 791
Kirschner wires,
  in fractures, 115
  in traction, 125
Kleinert technique, 21
Klippel–Trenaunay syndrome, 1152
Knee,
  See also Patella
  acute osteochondral fracture, 1073
  amputation above, 398, 422
    indications and contraindications, 422
    operation, 423
    postoperative management, 426
    preoperative, 422
    prostheses, 426
  amputation below, 431
    anterior and posterior flaps, 435
    indications and contraindications, 431
    long posterior flap, 432
    postoperative management, 436
    preoperative, 431
    prosthetics, 436
  anatomy of, 1008
  anterior cavity,
    loose body removal, 1074
  anterior cruciate ligament,
    arthroscopy, 1014
    repair, 1085
  arthritis of,
    tibial osteotomy for, 1113–1118
  arthrodesis of,
    in haemophiliacs, 83
  arthroplasty of, 1119–1130
    complications, 1130
    correction of deformity, 1121
    extension gap, 1125
    flexion gap, 1123
    indications and contraindications,
      1119
    operation, 1120
    postoperative management, 1130
    preoperative, 1119
    preparation of femur, tibia and
      patella, 1127
  articular cartilage,
    arthroscopy, 1017
    surgical arthroscopy, 1027
  avascular necrosis of, 1073
  chronic anterior cruciate deficiency,
    1096
  clinical examination, 1079
  compression arthrodesis, 1131–1136
    complications, 1136
    indications and contraindications,
      1131
    operation, 1132
    postoperative management, 1136
    preoperative, 1131
  deformity, 940
  diagnostic arthroscopy of, 1007–1018
    anteromedial approach, 1016
    central approach, 1016
    indications for, 1009
    operation, 1011
    pathological findings, 1017
    posteromedial approach, 1017
    postoperative management, 1015

Knee (*cont.*)
  diagnostic arthroscopy of (*cont.*)
    preoperative, 1009
    preparation and position, 1010
  disarticulation at, 427, 430
    indications and contraindications, 427
    postoperative management, 430
    preoperative, 427
    prosthetics, 430
    using lateral flaps, 428
  excessive lateral pressure syndrome,
    1032
  fixed flexion deformity of, 86
  flexion contractures, 1061
  flexion deformity, 981
    correction, 984
  haemarthroses in, 82, 1112
  infrapatellar fat pad,
    diagnostic arthroscopy, 1033
  intercondylar notch
    arthroscopy, 1014
  lateral compartment,
    arthroscopy, 1015
  lateral gutter,
    arthroscopy, 1015
  ligament injury, 1079–1101
  limited flexion, 1003
  loose bodies in, 1073–1078
    arthroscopic removal, 1073
    diagnostic arthroscopy, 1035
    indications for removal, 1073
    in osteochondritis dissecans, 1077
    open removal, 1074
    posterior compartment, 1076
    suprapatellar pouch and anterior
      cavity, 1074
    symptoms and signs, 1073
  medial collateral ligament,
    repair of, 1080
  medial compartment,
    arthroscopy, 1013
  meniscus,
    diagnostic arthroscopy, 1033, 1034
    tears in, 1036
  open meniscectomy,
    indications, 1062
    medial, 1063
    preoperative, 1062
  osteoarthritis, 1036
    loose bodies in, 1073
  osteochondral fracture, 1073
    treatment of, 1078
  osteochondritis dissecans, 1073
    treatment, 1076
  pigmented villonodular synovitis, 1109
  posterior compartment,
    loose bodies in, 1031, 1076
  posterior cruciate ligament,
    repair of, 1083, 1093
  postoperative infection, 1061, 1112
  proximal hamstring release, 940
  rheumatoid arthritis, 1109
  suprapatellar pouch,
    loose body removal from, 1074
  surgical arthroscopy, 1019–1042
    See also Meniscectomy
    articular cartilage, 1027, 1039
    chondromalacia patellae, 1030, 1039
    division of synovial fold or shelf, 1025
    instruments, 1021
    lateral release, 1032
    removal of loose bodies, 1030, 1039

Knee (*cont.*)
  surgical arthroscopy (*cont.*)
    synovial tags, 1026, 1037, 1038
    synovium, 1023, 1037
    triangulation, 1–20
  synovectomy of, 1027, 1109–1112
    complications of, 1112
    operation, 1110
    postoperative management, 1112
    preoperative, 1109
  synovial biopsy, 1023, 1037
  synovial fold or shelf,
    division of, 1025
  synovial membrane,
    arthroscopy, 1017, 1033
  synovial osteochondromatosis, 1073
    treatment, 1078
  synovial tags,
    excision of, 1026, 1037, 1038
  tuberculosis, 1109
  valgus deformity, 1113, 1121
  varus deformity, 1121
Knee hinge, 130
Knock knee, 1113
Kocher–Langenbeck approach to
    acetabulum, 342
Küntscher's closed intramedullary nailing
    for femoral shaft fractures, 223–241
    availability of equipment, 240
    Melbourne cross pinning, 234, 240
    postoperative management, 240
    preoperative, 223
    technical requirements, 224
    traction, 226
Kyphosis,
  correction of, 662, 664

Lacerations, 2
Lambrinudi arthrodesis, 1191, 1201
Laminectomy,
  definition, 519
Lateral condyle,
  fracture of, 173
Latissimus dorsi,
  free flap from, 14
Lauenstein procedure, 773
Leg,
  amputation through, 422
    above knee, 422
    below knee, 431
    disarticulation at knee, 427
  avulsion flap, 3
  compartment syndromes in, 298
    perifibular fasciotomy for, 299
    postoperative management, 300
    Volkmann's ischaemic contracture
      following, 307
  diaphyseal lengthening, 1154
  epiphyseal lengthening, 1154
  insertion of Steinmann pin, 128
  lengthening, 1154, 1159–1167
    complications, 1167
    joint damage following, 1167
    muscle contractures, 1167
    pin-track infection, 1167
    soft tissue release and corticotomy,
      1162
    tibiofibular joint displacement after,
      1167

Leg (*cont.*)
  length inequality, 1152–1168
    aetiology of, 1152
    assessment of, 1152, 1153
    associated anomalies, 1153
    measurement, 1153
    monitoring patient, 1153
    preoperative, 1152
    procedures and indications, 1154
  massive replacement for tumours, 1137–
    1151
    See also specific bones
    assessment, 1138
    complications, 1151
    indications and contraindications,
      1137
    operation, 1142
    preoperative, 1138
    prosthetic failure, 1151
  prostheses for tumour surgery, 1138
  short,
    true and apparent, 1152
  shortening, 1154
    epiphysiodesis, 1154, 1155
    techniques, 1155
  traction systems, 134
  tumour surgery, 1137
    recurrences, 1151
Leprosy, 1184
Ligamentum patellae,
  rupture of, 995, 996, 998
Limb,
  ischaemia, 39, 49
  replacement, 53
  revascularization, 48
Lister's intraosseous wiring, 180
Littlewood's approach to forequarter
    amputation, 413
Ludloff approach to iliopsoas tendon, 936,
    937
Lumbar disc,
  central prolapse, 527
  extraforaminal prolapse, 528
  large subrhizal prolapse, 526
  prolapse, 519–529
    associated with special problems,
      528
    preoperative, 520
    indications for operation, 520
    operation, 523
    sequestered fragments, 527
    types of, 519
  small subrhizal prolapse, 526
Lumbar spine,
  approach to, 619
  fracture dislocation,
    closed reduction, 647
    open reduction and internal fixation,
      649
    spinal jacket for, 667
  infections, 568
  instability, 545
  metastatic bone disease,
    anterior decompression and
      stabilization, 587
    complications, 595
    posterior decompression and
      stabilization, 594
    posterior stabilization, 594
    supplementary instrumentation, 593
  paraspinal approach to, 622
posterior fusion, 539–544

Lunate,
  Keinbock's disease, 791
Luque instrumentation, 491
  for neuromuscular scoliosis, 512–518
    choice of procedure, 514
    exposure of spinous process, 515
    indications for, 512
    insertion of rods, 516
    postoperative management, 518
    preoperative, 513
    technique, 514

Magnuson–Stack procedure,
  modified, 683
Malleolus,
  fracture of, 286, 289, 291
    in children, 365
Mallet deformity of finger, 809
  repair of, 827
Mallet fracture of finger, 815
Mallet toe, 1259
Maquet operation, 1107
Matte–Russe bone graft of carpal
    scaphoid, 796
Medial cutaneous nerve,
  as donor nerve, 34
Medial malleolus,
  fractures, 365
Median nerve,
  compression, 788
  injuries, 25, 193, 789
  paralysis,
    combined with radial nerve paralysis,
      764
    combined with ulnar nerve paralysis,
      764
  repair by grafting, 32
  tendon reconstruction for palsy,
    759–763
Meniscectomy of knee, 1019, 1062–1072
  arthroscopic, 1040–1042, 1043–1055
    basic technique, 1044
  lateral, 1067
    postoperative management, 1069
  medial, 1063
    postoperative management, 1066
Meniscus,
  arthroscopic repair, 1056–1061
    complications, 1061
    contraindications, 1057
    indications, 1056
    inside-out technique, 1059
    investigations, 1057
    outside-in technique, 1060
    postoperative management, 1061
    technique, 1058
  bucket-handle tear, 1040, 1045
    excision, 1040, 1046
  diagnostic arthroscopy, 1033, 1034
  discoid lateral,
    arthroscopic surgery, 1054
    excision of, 1065
  excision of tag tears, 1041, 1048
  lateral,
    excision of posterior horn, 1070
    radial tears, 1042, 1052
    medial,
  medial,
    excision of retained posterior horn,
      1070
  parrot-beak tears, 1042, 1053

Meniscus (*cont.*)
  posterior horn cleavage tears, 1042, 1051
  posterior third bucket-handle tears,
    1041, 1042, 1049
  surface flap tear, 1055
  tears of,
    diagnostic arthroscopy, 1017, 1035
    torn cystic lateral, 1052
Mesh grafts, 3
Metacarpals,
  traction on, 127
Metacarpal head,
  resection of, 69
Metacarpal pin traction, 143
Metacarpophalangeal joint,
  Swanson arthroplasty, 68–72
    complications, 72
    dressings, 71
    in rheumatoid disease, 68–72
    insertion of implant, 70
    indications and contraindications, 68
    postoperative management, 72
    preoperative, 68
    technique, 69
Metaphyseal wedge osteotomy, 377
Metastatic bone disease, 92, 96, 97,
    384–396, 487, 571
Monteggia fracture, 160, 163, 169
  open reduction of radial head, 170
Morton's metatarsalgia,
  dorsal nerve transfer for, 1255–1258
Muscles,
  bleeding into, 78
  injury to, 48
  ischaemic, 48
  management in amputation, 399
Muscle autografts in nerve repair, 37
Muscle skin flaps, 13
Myelitis, 533
Myocutaneous skin flap, 13

Naughton Dunn's operation, 1199
Necrosis, 400
Neer hemi-arthroplasty, 156
Neer prosthesis, 719
Nerves,
  epineural repair, 37
  management in amputation, 400
  peripheral *See Peripheral nerves*
Nerve grafts,
  vascularized, 37
Nerve root anomalies, 528
Nerve transfer, 37
Neurapraxia, 25
  in compartment syndromes, 295
Neurolysis, 37
Ninety-ninety traction, 136

Obturator nerve,
  partial neurectomy, 929
Occipitoatlantal joints,
  anatomy of, 454
Odontoid,
  congenital anomalies, 476
  fractures, 486
    internal fixation, 642
Oedema of amputation stump, 401
Olecranon,
  fracture of, 167
  traction, 127, 142

Ollier's disease, 1152
Os calcis,
  osteomyelitis of, 66
Osteoarthrosis,
  hip replacement for, 944
Osteochondritis dissecans, 1073
  arthroscopic surgery of, 1027, 1031, 1038
    removal of fixation devices, 1028
    removal of fragments, 1027
  diagnostic arthroscopy, 1017
  treatment of, 1076
  with loose body, 1077
Osteoid osteoma, 91
Osteomyelitis,
  amputation for, 398
  chronic, 61
  chronic suppurative, 64
    postoperative management, 66
    preoperative, 64
    surgery of, 65
  diagnosis of, 55
  drainage in, 56
  Garré sclerosing, 62
  haematogenous, 64
  pathology of, 54
  presentation, 55
  principles of treatment, 55
  purulent, 61
  surgical treatment, 56
Osteoporosis, 595

Pain,
  from traction, 143
  in compartment syndromes, 295
Palmaris longus,
  transfer of, 758
Pantalar arthrodesis, 1198
Patella,
  See also Knee
  chondromalacia, 1032
    arthroscopic surgery, 1030, 1039
    diagnostic arthroscopy, 1036
  decompression and realignment, 1107
  fat pad,
    arthroscopy, 1013, 1033
  fractures of, 252–255, 955
    exposure of fracture, 253
    indications for operation, 252
    operative details, 253
    postoperative management, 255
    preoperative, 252
    rigid internal fixation, 254
  lateral subluxation, 1102
  Maquet operation, 1107
  preparation for knee arthroplasty, 1127
  recurrent dislocation of, 1102–1108
    in children, 1103
      Goldthwaite–Roux operation, 1103
    in teenagers and adults, 1106
  recurrent subluxation, 1032
  release and repositioning, 1103
  Trillat operation, 1108
Patellofemoral joint,
  arthroscopy of, 1013, 1033
  osteoarthritis, 1107
Pectoralis major tendon,
  transfer of, 742
Pelvic osteotomy, 879
  Chiari operation, 879
  Coventry screw and plate fixation, 887
  using four-hole plate, 886

Pelvis,
  cancer of, 414
  fractures of,
    external skeletal fixation, 150
Pemberton acetabuloplasty, 878
Peripheral nerves,
  epineural repair, 37
  grafting, 24, 32, 34
    donor nerve, 34
    indications for, 34
    partial repair, 36
    postoperative management, 36
    technique, 34
  iatrogenic injury, 25
  identification, 28
  injuries of, 25
    diagnosis, 25
    findings, 31
    vascular injuries and, 25
  primary repair of, 24
    postoperative management, 30
    primary sutures, 26
  repair of divisions, 24–38
    fibrin glue in, 37
    muscle autografts in, 37
    prognosis, 38
    rehabilitation in, 38
  secondary repair, 24, 30–33
    indications and contraindications, 30
    mobilization, 32
    postoperative management, 33
    resection and biopsy, 32
    technique, 31
Perkins' traction, 134
Perthes' disease,
  arthrosis following, 949
  high femoral osteotomy for, 900, 901
  innominate osteotomy for, 893
Pes cavus, 1216–1219
  calcaneal osteotomy for, 1217
  Steindler release of plantar fascia, 1216
  tarsometatarsal truncated wedge
    arthrodesis for, 1218
  wedge tarsectomy for, 1208
Pes planus, 1211–1215
  excision of calcaneonavicular bar, 1214
  preoperative, 1211
  reversed Dillwyn Evans procedure, 1212
Peyronie's disease, 855
Phalen's test, 788
Phantom limb, 401
Plantar digital neuroma,
  dorsal nerve transfer for, 1255–1258
Pneumothorax, 452
Poliomyelitis, 512, 936, 981, 1152, 1184
  hip deformity in, 931
Popliteal artery,
  damage to, 1061
Popliteal nerve injury, 1184
Posterior interosseous nerve,
  injury to, 25
Presacral nerve,
  care of, 556
Pressure garments, 86
Pridie technique, 87
Pronator teres,
  redirection of, 749
  transfer of, 758
Protrusio acetabuli,
  hip replacement for, 946
Proximal phalanx,
  fracture of shaft, 177

Pubic symphysis,
   exposure and fixation, 346–350
     apparatus required, 347
     indications for, 346
     operation, 348
     postoperative management, 350
     preoperative, 347
     reduction, 349
Pulvertaft interlacing method, 813
Putti–Platt operation, 675–679

Quadricepsplasty, 1003–1006
   complications of, 1006
   indications, 1003
   operation, 1004
   postoperative management, 1006
Quadriceps,
   contracture in infancy, 1002
   rupture of, 995–1002
     old lesions, 998
     recent lesions, 996
     transfer of hamstrings to, 985–988
Quadriceps tendon,
   lengthening and repair, 1001
   rupture of, 997, 1001

Radial nerve,
   care of, 790
   iatrogenic injury, 25
   paralysis,
     combined with median nerve
       paralysis, 764
     combined with ulnar nerve paralysis,
       764
     following synovectomy, 76
     tendon reconstruction, 753
Radial nerve repair palsy splint, 21
Radiotherapy,
   fracture union following, 384
Radius,
   deformities, 358
     of head, 358
   distal fractures, 163
     external skeletal fixation, 149
   excision of head, 166
   exposure of, 161
   fracture,
     caused by metastases, 392
     compartment syndromes and, 303
     postoperative management, 162, 164
     rigid plate fixation, 161
   fracture of head, 165–167
   fracture of neck in children, 358
   fracture of shaft, 160
   reduction of head, 170
   split head,
     reconstruction, 167
Respiratory distress syndrome, adult, 114
Reversed dynamic slings, 86
Rheumatoid arthritis, 765
   forefoot deformity, 1232
   hallux valgus, 1244
   halo–body cast in, 487
   hip replacement in, 944
   of hand and feet, 765
   of knee, 1109, 1119
   radio-ulnar joint involvement, 805
   Swanson arthroplasty for, 68–72
   synovectomy of elbow for, 73–76
   wrist arthroplasty for, 782

Robert Jones operation for clawing of
   hallux, 1227
Robert Jones valgus osteotomy, 907
Rotator cuff,
   repair, 697–704
     indications for, 697
     operation, 698
     postoperative management, 704
     principles of, 702
     surgical exposure of, 698

Salter–Harris classification, 352
Scaphoid,
   See Carpal scaphoid
Scoliosis,
   idiopathic, 482, 491–503
   indications for instrumentation, 491
   indications for posterior fusion, 491
   investigations, 492
   Luque instrumentation for, 512–518
     choice of procedure, 514
     exposure of spinous process, 515
     indications, 512
     insertion of rods, 516
     preoperative, 513
     technique, 514
   neuromuscular
     Luque instrumentation for, 518
   posterior procedures,
     bone grafting, 502
     excision of facet joints, 498
     exposure of laminae, 496
     insertion of Harrington hook, 497, 498
     insertion of Harrington rod, 501
     insertion of wires, 500
     operative details, 495
     planning fusion levels, 493
     postoperative management, 502
     preoperative, 492
     splitting spinous process tips, 495
     tightening of wires, 501
Semilunar cartilage
   See Meniscus
Septic arthritis, 54
Shoulder,
   See also Humerus, etc.
   arthrodesis of, 721–728
     alternative techniques, 726
     anterior operation, 721, 722, 728
     indications and contraindications, 721
     operation, 722
     posterior operation, 721, 727, 728
     postoperative management, 728
     preoperative, 721
   arthroplasty of, 713–720
     complications, 720
     excision, 713
     indications, 713
     loosening of prosthesis, 720
     Neer prosthesis, 719
     postoperative management, 720
     preoperative, 714
     total replacement, 713
     use of Kessel prosthesis, 718
     use of Stanmore prosthesis, 717, 718
   arthroscopy of, 692–696
     appearances of, 695–696
   dislocation following arthroplasty, 720
   distraction at joint, 721
   excision arthroplasty, 713
   hemiarthroplasty, 713

Shoulder (cont.)
   prosthesis for, 713
   recurrent anterior dislocation, 671–685
     aetiology, 671
     anterior apprehension test, 673
     approach to, 678
     Bankart operation, 681
     choice of operation, 675
     management of initial dislocation, 672
     modified Boytchev procedure, 684
     modified Bristow–Helfet procedure, 683
     modified Magnuson–Stack
       procedure, 683
     operations for, 676
     pathological, 675
     posterior stress test, 674
     postoperative management, 684
     preoperative, 673
     Putti–Platt operation, 675, 679
     structures to protect, 675
     sulcus sign, 674
     voluntary, 674
   resection of humeral head, 716
   surgical approach to, 58, 59
   tuberculosis, 721
Silfverskiöld operation, 1175
Silver's syndrome, 1152
Skeletal traction, 111, 123, 125
   complications of, 129
   sites of, 126
Skin,
   management in amputation, 399
Skin cover, 1–15
Skin flaps, 7–15
   abdominal tube pedicle, 8
   cross-leg, 10
   cutaneous axial-pattern, 11
   fasciocutaneous, 12
   free, 14
   local, 8
   muscle, 13
   principles of, 7
   regional, 8
Skin grafts,
   application of, 5
   delayed, 6
   mesh, 3, 6
   small split skin, 6
   split skin, 5
Skin loss, 5
Skoog technique, 860
Skull halo,
   preparation for, 625
   in spinal injuries, 624
Sliding traction, 123, 138
Soutter operation for hip contracture, 924
Spina bifida, 981, 1152
Spinal canal,
   opening, 524
Spinal fusion,
   vascular damage during, 53
Spinal stenosis,
   assessment, 534
   classification, 534
   lumbar disc prolapse with, 528
   posterior decompression for, 534–538
   posterior decompression,
     multiple level, 538
     postoperative management, 538
     preoperative, 534
     technique, 535
   presentation, 534

Spine,
  See also Cervical spine, Lumbar spine, etc.
  abscess, 560
  anterior approaches to, 598–615
    cervicothoracic area, 603
    Fraser's muscle splitting, 612
    retroperitoneal approach to L2–5, 610
    to C1–C2, 598
    to C3–T1, 600
    to T4–11, 605
    to thoracolumbar junction, 607
    to upper thoracic spine, 603
    transperitoneal midline approach to L4–S1, 613
  anterior decompression and fixation, for kyphosis, 662
  application of plaster of Paris jacket, 667
  approaches to, 597–623
    indications, 597
  cleft cleavage fractures, 652
  costotransversectomy, 614
  deformity, 482
    anterior instrumentation, 509
    anterior procedures, 504–511
    indications for operation, 504
    operations, 506
    postoperative management, 511
    preoperative, 505
  exposure of laminae, 496
  fractures and dislocations, 487
    Hartshill triangle, 661
    internal fixators, 655
    kyphotic deformities following, 662
    posterior fusion, 660
    postural reduction, 628
    spinal jacket for, 667
    spinal plates for, 659
    traction for, 125
    with locked facets, 647
  Fraser's muscle-splitting approach, 612
  fusion of Gallé type, 644
  infection, 487
    operations for, 559–570
  injuries, 624–669
    See also under Cervical spine, Lumbar spine etc
    application of halo and caliper, 624
    postural reduction plus maintenance, 628
    preparation for halo and calipers, 625
  instability, 463, 480, 487
  intertransverse fusion, 545–548
    postoperative management, 548
    with decompression, 548
    without decompression, 546
  intracranial fragments, 662
  metastatic bone disease of, 571–596
    aims of treatment, 571, 574
    anterior cord decompression, 575
    anterior decompression, 582, 587
    anterior stabilization, 577
    basic principles of treatment, 572
    complications of treatment, 595
    decompression in, 572
    failure of stabilization, 595
    indications for treatment, 571
    investigations, 574
    Kaneda device, 592
    laminar removal and replacement, 594
    posterior decompression and stabilization, 579

Spine (*cont.*)
  metastatic bone disease of (*cont.*)
    posterior spinal fusion in, 594
    posterior stabilization, 594
    postoperative treatment, 595
    preoperative, 574
    stabilization, 572, 573
    supplementary instrumentation, 593
    timing of surgery, 574
  paraspinal approach to lumbar spine, 622
  posterior approaches, 616–623
    to C1–7, 616
    to lumbar spine, 619
    to thoracic spine, 618
  rheumatoid arthritis of, 487
  thoracic,
    approaches to, 603, 618
  thoracolumbar junction,
    approach to, 607
  tongue-splitting approach to, 600
  transoral approach to, 598
  transperitoneal midline approach to, 613
  tuberculosis of, 559
  unstable fractures, 476
Splints, 129–133
  Fisk, 130
    suspension, 133
  preparation of, 131
  Thomas's, 129
    for femoral shaft fracture, 137
Spondylitis,
  pyogenic, 559
Spondylolisthesis,
  anatomical lesions, 551
  combined traction and fusion technique, 552
  disc prolapse and, 528
  gradual reduction, 554
  indications for surgery, 552
  intertransverse fusion for, 545–548
  measurements in, 551
  surgical reduction of, 549–558
    anterior lumbosacral fusion, 556
    bone grafting, 557
    complications, 558
    gradual, 554
    historical background, 550
    neurological examination, 555
    operations, 554
    postoperative management, 557
    preoperative, 552
    skull–femoral traction, 555
Stanmore prosthesis, 717
Steindler flexorplasty, 737
  Bunnell's modification, 739
Steindler release of plantar fascia, 1216
Steinmann pin,
  in fracture traction, 125
  insertion in leg, 128
Strayer operation, 1177
Subacromial space,
  approach to, 693, 698
  arthroscopic appearances of, 694
Subperiosteal abscess, 55
Subscapularis and interspinatus tendon transplantation, 703
Subtalar joint,
  approach to, 60
Sural nerve as donor nerve, 34, 35
Suturing wounds, 2

Swanson arthroplasty,
  of metacarpophalangeal joint, 68–72
    complications, 72
    dressings, 71
    indications and contraindications, 68
    insertion of implant, 70
    postoperative management, 72
    preoperative, 68
    technique, 69
Syme's amputation, 437–440
  alternatives to, 437
  indications and contraindications, 437
  postoperative management, 440
  preoperative, 437
  prosthetics, 440
  technique, 438
Synostosis,
  after elbow fracture, 361
Synovectomy, 1027
  of elbow, 73–76
  of knee in haemophilics, 82
Synovitis from tendon implants, 848

Talipes equinovarus,
  congenital, 1220
    indications for operation, 1220
    lateral soft tissue release, 1225
    medial soft tissue release, 1223
    operations for, 1220–1231
    plantar soft tissue release, 1224
    posterior soft tissue release, 1221
    postoperative management, 1226
    secondary surgery, 1226
Talocalcaneal synostosis, 1207
Talonavicular dislocation, 319
Talonavicular fracture-subluxation, 319
Talus,
  fracture dislocation, 312
  fracture of lateral process, 314
  fracture of neck, 311
  infection, 1191
  injuries to, 311
  inversion fracture, 313
  total dislocation of, 313
Tarsal osteotomies in club foot, 1226
Tarsectomy, 1208–1210
Tarsometatarsal disruption, 318
Tarsometatarsal truncated wedge arthrodesis, 1218
Tarsus,
  disruption of, 319
  fracture caused by metastases, 395
Tendo Achillis,
  acute rupture, 1179
    closed repair, 1180
    open repair, 1179
  incomplete tenotomy, 1172
  lengthening and repair, 1172–1183
  old rupture,
    repair of, 1182
  repair of, 1179
  Z-plasty, 1174
Tendons,
  care of during surgery, 21
  sheaths and pulleys, 18
Tendon injury,
  primary care, 17
Tendon repair, 16–23
  adhesions following, 23
  anchorage to bone, 20
  apical suture, 20

Tendon repair (*cont.*)
  associated injury, 17
  bowstringing, 23
  complications, 23
  contraindications, 17
  immobilization in, 22
  indications for, 17
  of unequal girth, 20
  preoperative, 17
  primary, 17
  protection after surgery, 21
  pulley reconstruction, 23
  replacement, 18
  suture materials, 19
  technique of, 19
  tension of, 22, 23
  timing of, 17
  transfer of, 18
Tendon transfer, 18
  to foot, 1184, 1187
Tenography technique, 832
Tenolysis, 835
Tetanus, 198
Thigh,
  cancer of, 414
  compartment syndromes, 301
Thomas arthrodesis of ankle, 1197
Thomas' splint, 129
  in femoral shaft fracture, 137
Thoracic outlet syndrome,
  anterior and posterior approach to, 452
  axillary approach to, 447–452
    choice of procedure, 448
    complications, 452
    indications and contraindications, 447
    postoperative management, 451
    preoperative, 448
    transaxillary first rib resection, 448
  recurrence, 452
Thoracic spine,
  costotransversectomy approach, 566
  fracture dislocations,
    closed reduction, 647
  infections of, 566
    operations for, 564
  metastatic bone disease,
    anterior decompression for, 582
    complications, 595
    posterior decompression and
      stabilization, 594
    posterior stabilization, 594
    stabilization, 587
Thoracolumbar spine,
  transpleural approach to, 564
Thorax,
  vascular injury of, 52
Thumb,
  Bennett's fracture-subluxation, 183
  flexor pollicis longus injury, 811
  transfer of extensor indicis to, 760
  trigger, 865–869
    in children, 869
    conservative treatment, 865
    operative details, 866
    postoperative management, 868
Tibia,
  anterolateral bone grafting, 371
  compound fractures of, 14
  diaphyseal fractures, 147
  fracture,
    bracing in, 110
    caused by metastases, 395

Tibia (*cont.*)
    external skeletal fixation, 147
    skeletal traction, 126
    traction for, 112, 134, 138
    traction weights, 133
  fractures of shaft, 268–283
    classification of open wounds, 269
    external fixation, 272, 275
    follow-up, 283
    internal fixation by intramedullary
      nailing, 278
    internal fixation by plating, 275
    non-operative management, 270
    operative treatment, 272
    postoperative management, 278, 283
    soft tissue injury in, 268
  lengthening, 1154, 1166
  medial condyle fracture, 258
  metaphyseal wedge osteotomy, 377
  metastases in, 396
  osteotomy,
    for arthritis of knee, 1113–1118
    operation, 1115
    postoperative management, 1118
  plateau fractures, 256–267
    approach to, 262
    associated fractures, 258
    bicondylar, 258, 266
    classification, 257
    cleavage, 257, 264
    depressed, 257, 258, 265
    laterally injured, 260
    medial condyle, 258
    medial injury, 261
    operative approach, 259
    postoperative management, 267
    preoperative, 259
    reconstruction and fixation, 264
    symptoms and signs, 259
  plate removal from, 120
  posterolateral bone grafting, 373
  preparation for knee arthroplasty,
    1127
  replacement for tumour, 1148–1150
  resection of upper end, 1133
  shortening, 1154
Tibialis posterior tendon,
  ruptures, 1215
  transfer of tendon to, 1215
  transfer to dorsum of foot, 1184–1186
Tibiofibular joint displacement,
  after leg lengthening, 1167
Tibiofibular syndesmosis, 290
Tillaux fracture, 290
Tissue pressure, 296
  measurement of, 297
Toes,
  amputation of, 444–446
  claw, 1230
  crush injuries, 320
  gangrene of, 397
  hammer, 1259, 1263
  mallet, 1259
  metatarsal shortening, 1264
  open fractures, 320
  ray resection, 444
  subungual haematoma, 320
Toe, big
  clawing of, 1227
  prosthetic replacement of, 1241
Toe, fifth
  dorsally placed, 1267–1269

Toe-nail
  ingrowing, 1270–1272
Transmetatarsal amputation, 441–443
Triceps disruption, 734
Triceps tendon,
  anterior transfer, 740
Trigger finger and thumb, 865–869
  in children, 869
  treatment, 865
  operative details, 866
  postoperative management, 868
  preoperative, 866
Trillat operation, 1108
Trochanteric osteosynthesis, 951
Trochanteric osteotomy, 963
Tauge's looped suture method, 19
Tuberculosis, 948
Tulloch Brown traction, 135
Tumours,
  amputation for, 398
  replacement surgery for leg, 1137–1151

Ulna,
  Darrach's procedure, 769
  excision of, 769
  exposure of, 162
  fracture, 169
    caused by metastases, 392
    compartment syndrome and, 303
    plating of, 162
    postoperative management, 162
  fracture of shaft, 160
  Lauenstein procedure, 773
Ulnar nerve,
  decompression of, 75
  injury to, 25, 734
  paralysis,
    combined with median nerve
      paralysis, 764
    combined with radial nerve paralysis,
      764
  repair by grafting, 32
  tendon reconstruction, 764
Ulnar neuritis, 75
Upper femoral epiphysis,
  anatomy of, 910
  slipped, 909–920
    acceptable deformity, 912, 913
    arthrodesis for, 971
    biplane trochanteric osteotomy for,
      916
    choice of treatment, 912
    geometric flexion osteotomy for, 919
    growth plate and, 912
    pinning *in situ*, 912
    technical errors, 913
    unacceptable deformity, 913, 919

Valgus deformity, 1113
Veins,
  injuries to, 48
Vein grafts,
  for arterial repair, 46
Vena cava laceration, 52
Venous insufficiency, 397
Volkmann's ischaemic contracture, 290,
  291
Volkmann's fracture, 290, 291
Volkmann's ischaemic contracture, 25, 37,
  141
  following compartment syndromes, 307

Walton manoeuvre, 631
Watson–Jones approach to hip, 951
Watson–Jones arthrodesis of ankle, 1192
Weaver–Dunn technique, 690
Weedon–Butler operation, 1268
Whoosh test, 43
Wounds,
    closure of, 1
    debridement, 2
    drainage, 2
    management of,
        in open fractures, 120
    mesh grafts, 3, 6
    nerve inury, 25
    primary care of, 48
    skin flaps for, 7–15
    skin grafts for, 5
    suturing, 2
    treatment of, 1
Wrist,
    arthrodesis of, 779, 791
        bone graft fixation, 792, 793

Wrist (cont.)
    arthrodesis of (cont.)
        indications for, 779
        internal fixation, 781
        limited, 782
        plate fixation, 793
        postoperative management, 782, 793
    arthroplasty, 782
        indications, 782
        postoperative management, 786
        procedure, 782
    Darrach's procedure, 769
    decompression procedures, 787
    de Quervain's disease, 787
    dorsal synovectomy, 766
    flexion deformity, 752
    flexor synovectomy, 777
    flexor tendon injury, 811, 827
    fractures caused by metastases, 392
    ganglion, 790
    Lauenstein procedure, 773
    limited arthrodesis, 782

    mobile radial deviation of, 805–807
    operations on, 766
    osteoarthritis of, 791
    panarthrodesis of, 791
    paralysis of, 759
    rheumatoid arthritis of, 765
    ruptured extensor tendons, 774, 776
    surgery of, 765–804
    tendon injury at, 826
    transfer of extensor indicis proprius, 775

Yount procedure, 922

Zadik procedure for ingrowing toe-nail,
    1271
Zickel nail fixation, 216–222
    complications, 222
    indications for, 216
    technique, 218